Study Guide and Procedure Checklist Manual for

Kinn's The Medical Assistant

An Applied Learning Approach

Fifteenth Edition

Brigitte Niedzwiecki, MSN, RN, RMA
Medical Assistant Program Director & Instructor
Chippewa Valley Technical College
Eau Claire, Wisconsin

Julie Pepper, BS, CMA (AAMA)
Medical Assistant Instructor
Chippewa Valley Technical College
Eau Claire, Wisconsin

ELSEVIER

ELSEVIER

3251 Riverport Lane
St. Louis, Missouri 63043

Study Guide and Procedure Checklist Manual for
Kinn's The Medical Assistant, Fifteenth Edition

ISBN: 978-0-323-87424-3

ISBN: 978-0-323-87424-3

Publishing Director: Kristin Wilhelm
Content Development Manager: Luke Held/Danielle Frazier
Senior Content Development Specialist: Sarah Vora
Publishing Services Manager: Julie Eddy
Senior Project Manager: Abigail Bradberry
Design Direction: Ryan Cook

Printed in India

Last digit is the print number: 9 8 7 6 5 4 3 2 1

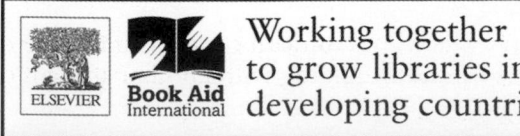

To the Student

This study guide was created to help you to achieve the objectives of each chapter in your text and establish a solid base of knowledge in medical assisting. Completing the exercises in each chapter in this guide will help reinforce the material studied in the textbook and learned in class.

STUDY HINTS FOR ALL STUDENTS

Ask Questions!

There are no stupid questions. If you do not know something or are not sure about it, you need to find out. Other people may be wondering the same thing but are too shy to ask. The answer could be a matter of life or death for your patient. That is certainly more important than feeling embarrassed about asking a question.

Chapter Objectives

At the beginning of each chapter in the textbook are learning objectives that you should have mastered by the time you have finished studying that chapter. Write these objectives in your notebook, leaving a blank space after each. Fill in the answers as you find them while reading the chapter. Review to make sure your answers are correct and complete. Use these answers when you study for tests. You should also do this for separate course objectives that your instructor has listed in your class syllabus.

Vocabulary

At the beginning of each chapter in the textbook are vocabulary terms that you will encounter as you read the chapter. These terms are in bold type the first time they appear in the chapter.

Summary of Learning Objectives

Use the Summary of Learning Objectives at the end of each chapter in the textbook to help you review for exams.

Reading Hints

As you read each chapter in the textbook, look at the subject headings to learn what each section is about. Read first for the general meaning and then reread parts you did not understand. It may help to read those parts aloud. Carefully read the information given in each table and study each figure and its legend.

Concepts

While studying, put difficult concepts into your own words to determine whether you understand them. Check this understanding with another student or the instructor. Write these concepts in your notebook.

Class Notes

When taking lecture notes in class, leave a large margin on the left side of each notebook page and write only on right-hand pages, leaving all left-hand pages blank. Look over your lecture notes soon after each class while your memory is fresh. Fill in missing words, complete sentences and ideas, and underline key phrases, definitions, and concepts. At the top of each page, write the topic of that page. In the left margin, write the key word for that part of your notes. On the opposite left-hand page, write a summary or outline that combines material from the textbook and the lecture. These can be your study notes for review.

Study Groups

Form a study group with other students so that you can help one another. Practice speaking and reading aloud. Ask questions about material you find unclear. Work together to find answers.

ADDITIONAL STUDY HINTS FOR ENGLISH AS A SECOND LANGUAGE (ESL) STUDENTS

Vocabulary

If you find a nontechnical word you do not know (e.g., drowsy), try to guess its meaning from the sentence (e.g., with electrolyte imbalance, the patient may feel fatigued and drowsy). If you are not sure of the meaning or if it seems particularly important, look it up in the dictionary.

Vocabulary Notebook

Keep a small alphabetized notebook or address book in your pocket or purse. Write down new nontechnical words you read or hear along with their meanings and pronunciations. Write each word under its initial letter so you can find it easily, as with a dictionary. For words you do not know or words that have a different meaning in medical assisting, write down how each word is used and how it is pronounced. Look up the meanings of these words in a dictionary or ask your instructor or first-language buddy (see the following section). Then write the different meanings or uses that you have found in your book, including the medical assisting meaning. Continue to add new words as you discover them.

First-Language Buddy

English as a second language (ESL) students should find a first-language buddy—another student who is a native speaker of English and who is willing to answer questions about word meanings, pronunciations, and culture. Maybe, in turn, your buddy would like to learn about your language and culture; this could be useful for their medical assisting career.

Contents

Competency Checklist

Student Name: _____

Admission Cohort: _____

Graduation Date: _____

CAAHEP Competency (2022)	Procedure	Date	Grade / Pass	Initial
I. Anatomy, Physiology, & Pharmacology				
I.P.1.a. Accurately measure and record: blood pressure	Procedure 20.9 Procedure 40.1			
I.P.1.b. Accurately measure and record: temperature	Procedure 20.1-20.6			
I.P.1.c. Accurately measure and record: pulse	Procedure 20.7, 20.8 Procedure 40.1			
I.P.1.d. Accurately measure and record: respirations	Procedure 20.8			
I.P.1.e. Accurately measure and record: height	Procedure 20.11			
I.P.1.f. Accurately measure and record: weight (adult and infant)	Procedure 20.11 Procedure 44.2			
I.P.1.g. Accurately measure and record: length (infant)	Procedure 44.2			
I.P.1.h. Accurately measure and record: head circumference (infant)	Procedure 44.1			
I.P.1.i. Accurately measure and record: oxygen saturation	Procedure 20.10			
I.P.2.a. Perform the following procedure: electrocardiography	Procedure 26.1			
I.P.2.b. Perform the following procedure: venipuncture	Procedures 48.1-48.3			
I.P.2.c. Perform the following procedure: capillary puncture	Procedure 48.4 Procedure 49.5-49.7 Procedure 50.5			
I.P.2.d. Perform the following procedure: pulmonary function testing	Procedure 41.1, 41.2			
I.P.3. Perform patient screening following established protocols	Procedure 31.1, 31.2, 31.5			
I.P.4.a. Verify the rules of medication administration: right patient	Procedure 30.1, 30.7-30.10 Procedure 31.3, 31.4, 31.6, 31.7 Procedure 41.3 Procedure 51.2, 51.3			

CAAHEP Competency (2022)	Procedure	Date	Grade / Pass	Initial
I.P.4.b. Verify the rules of medication administration: right medication	Procedure 30.1-30.10 Procedure 31.3, 31.4, 31.6, 31.7 Procedure 41.3 Procedure 51.1, 51.3			
I.P.4.c. Verify the rules of medication administration: right dose	Procedure 30.1-30.10 Procedure 31.3, 31.4, 31.6, 31.7 Procedure 41.3 Procedure 51.1, 51.3			
I.P.4.d. Verify the rules of medication administration: right route	Procedure 30.1-30.10 Procedure 31.3, 31.4, 31.6, 31.7 Procedure 41.3 Procedure 51.1, 51.3			
I.P.4.e. Verify the rules of medication administration: right time	Procedure 30.1-30.10 Procedure 31.3, 31.4, 31.6, 31.7 Procedure 41.3 Procedure 51.3			
I.P.4.f. Verify the rules of medication administration: right documentation	Procedure 30.1, 30.7-30.10 Procedure 31.3, 31.4, 31.6, 31.7 Procedure 41.3 Procedure 51.2, 51.3			
I.P.5. Select proper sites for administering parenteral medication	Procedure 30.7-30.10			
I.P.6. Administer oral medications	Procedure 30.1			
I.P.7. Administer parenteral (excluding IV) medications	Procedure 30.7-30.10			
I.P.8. Instruct and prepare a patient for a procedure or a treatment	Procedure 25.7, 25.8 Procedure 26.1, 26.2 Procedure 31.1-31.7 Procedure 36.4-36.9 Procedure 37.2, 37.3, 37.4 Procedure 40.1 Procedure 41.1-41.3 Procedure 42.2, 42.3 Procedure 43.1, 43.2			
I.P.9. Assist provider with a patient exam	Procedure 21.4-21.9, 21.11 Procedure 31.1, 31.2, 31.5 Procedure 37.1, 37.2 Procedures 43.1 Procedure 44.1, 44.2 Procedure 45.1			
I.P.10. Perform a quality control measure	Procedure 46.1 Procedure 47.4 Procedure 49.5-49.7 Procedure 50.4, 50.5, 50.7			
I.P.11.a. Collect specimens and perform: CLIA-waived hematology test	Procedure 49.1, 49.2, 49.4, 49.5			

CAAHEP Competency (2022)	Procedure	Date	Grade / Pass	Initial
I.P.11.b. Collect specimens and perform: CLIA-waived chemistry test	Procedure 49.6, 49.7			
I.P.11.c. Collect specimens and perform: CLIA-waived urinalysis	Procedures 47.1-47.3, 47.5, 47.7, 47.8			
I.P.11.d. Collect specimens and perform: CLIA-waived immunology test	Procedure 50.4			
I.P.11.e. Collect specimens and perform: CLIA-waived microbiology test	Procedure 50.2, 50.3 (collection only); 50.4			
I.P.12. Provide up-to-date documentation of provider/professional level CPR				
I.P.13.a. Perform first aid procedure for: bleeding	Procedure 27.5			
I.P.13.b. Perform first aid procedure for: diabetic coma or insulin shock	Procedure 27.1			
I.P.13.c. Perform first aid procedure for: stroke	Procedure 27.3			
I.P.13.d. Perform first aid procedure for: seizures	Procedure 27.3			
I.P.13.e. Perform first aid procedure for: environmental emergency	Procedure 27.1			
I.P.13.f. Perform first aid procedure for: syncope	Procedure 27.5			
II. Applied Mathematics				
II.P.1. Calculate proper dosages of medication for administration	Procedure 29.1 Procedure 30.1			
II.P.2. Record laboratory test results into the patient's record	Procedure 47.3, 47.5, 47.7, 47.8 Procedure 49.1, 49.2, 49.4-49.7 Procedure 50.4, 50.5, 50.7			
II.P.3. Document on a growth chart	Procedure 44.1, 44.2			
II.P.4. Apply mathematical computations to solve equations	Procedure 29.1			
II.P.5. Convert among measurement systems	Procedure 29.1			
III. Infection Control				
III.P.1. Participate in bloodborne pathogen training	Procedure 19.1			

CAAHEP Competency (2022)	Procedure	Date	Grade / Pass	Initial
III.P.2. Select appropriate barrier/ personal protective equipment (PPE)	Procedure 19.3 Procedure 30.7-30.10 Procedure 31.3, 31.4, 31.6, 31.7 Procedure 46.1 Procedure 47.2-47.8 Procedure 48.1-48.4 Procedure 49.1, 49.2, 49 4-49.7 Procedure 50.2-50.5, 50.7 Procedure 51.2, 51.4			
III.P.3. Perform handwashing	Procedure 19.2 Procedure 25.2			
III.P.4. Prepare items for autoclaving	Procedure 24.1			
III.P.5. Perform sterilization Procedure	Procedure 24.2			
III.P.6. Prepare a sterile field	Procedure 25.3-25.6			
III.P.7. Perform within a sterile field	Procedure 25.3-25.6			
III.P.8. Perform wound care	Procedure 25.6, 25.7			
III.P.9. Perform dressing change	Procedure 25.7			
III.P.10.a. Demonstrate proper disposal of biohazardous material: sharps	Procedure 25.6, 25.8 Procedure 30.2-30.10 Procedure 48.1-48.4 Procedure 49.1, 49.2, 49.4-49.7 Procedure 50.5 Procedure 51.2, 51.4			
III.P.10.b. Demonstrate proper disposal of biohazardous material: regulated wastes	Procedure 25.6-25.8 Procedure 48.1-48.4 Procedure 49.1, 49.2, 49.4-49.7 Procedures 50.2-50.5, 50.7			
IV. Nutrition				
IV.P.1. Instruct a patient regarding a dietary change related to patient's special dietary needs	Procedure 23.1			
V. Concepts of Effective Communication				
V.P.1. Respond to nonverbal communication	Procedure 2.1-2.4 Procedure 21.2			
V.P.2. Correctly use and pronounce medical terminology in healthcare interactions	Procedure 21.1			
V.P.3.a. Coach patients regarding: office policies	Procedure 9.3			

CAAHEP Competency (2022)	Procedure	Date	Grade / Pass	Initial
V.P.3.b. Coach patients regarding: medical encounters	Procedure 22.1 Procedure 34.1, 34.2 Procedure 36.1-36.9 Procedure 39.1 Procedure 42.1 Procedure 43.2 Procedure 50.1, 50.6, 50.8			
V.P.4. Demonstrate professional telephone techniques	Procedure 8.1			
V.P.5. Document telephone messages accurately	Procedure 8.2			
V.P.6. Using technology, compose clear and correct correspondence	Procedure 7.1-7.5			
V.P.7. Use a list of community resources to facilitate referrals	Procedure 22.2			
V.P.8. Participate in a telehealth interaction with a patient	Procedure 21.3			
VI. Administrative Functions				
VI.P.1. Manage appointment schedule using established priorities	Procedure 9.1, 9.2, 9.4			
VI.P.2. Schedule a patient procedure	Procedure 9.5			
VI.P.3. Input patient data using an electronic system	Procedure 10.1, 10.2			
VI.P.4. Perform an inventory of supplies	Procedure 11.3			
VII. Basic Practice Finances				
VII.P.1.a. Perform accounts receivable Procedure to patient accounts including posting: charges	Procedure 16.1			
VII.P.1.b. Perform accounts receivable Procedure to patient accounts including posting: payments	Procedure 16.1, 16.3			
VII.P.1.c. Perform accounts receivable Procedure to patient accounts including posting: adjustments	Procedure 16.3			
VII.P.2. Input accurate billing information in an electronic system	Procedure 9.2 Procedure 16.1, 16.3			
VII.P.3. Inform a patient of financial obligations for services rendered	Procedure 15.6 Procedure 16.2			
VIII. Third-Party Reimbursement				
VIII.P.1. Interpret information on an insurance card	Procedure 12.1			
VIII.P.2. Verify eligibility for services	Procedure 15.1, 15.6			

CAAHEP Competency (2022)	Procedure	Date	Grade / Pass	Initial
VIII.P.3. Obtain precertification or preauthorization including documentation	Procedure 15.1			
VIII.P.4. Complete an insurance claim form	Procedure 15.2, 15.3			
VIII.P.5. Assist a patient in understanding an Explanation of Benefits (EOB)	Procedure 15.5			
IX. Procedural and Diagnostic Coding				
IX.P.1. Perform procedural coding	Procedure 14.1, 14.2			
IX.P.2. Perform diagnostic coding	Procedure 13.1			
IX.P.3. Utilize medical necessity guidelines	Procedure 15.4			
X. Legal Implications				
X.P.1. Locate a state's legal scope of practice for medical assistants	Procedure 3.2			
X.P.2.a. Apply HIPAA rules in regard to: privacy	Procedure 4.1 Procedure 8.1			
X.P.2.b. Apply HIPAA rules in regard to: release of information	Procedure 4.2			
X.P.3. Document patient care accurately in the medical record	Procedure 8.1, 8.2 Procedure 21.1, 21.3 Procedure 22.1, 22.2 Procedure 25.6- 25.8 Procedure 26.1, 26.2 Procedure 27.1-27.6 Procedure 30.1, 30.7-30.10 Procedure 31.3, 31.4, 31.6, 31.7 Procedure 34.1, 34.2 Procedure 36.1-36.9 Procedure 37.1. 37.3, 37.4 Procedure 39.1 Procedure 40.1 Procedure 41.1-41.4 Procedure 42.1-42.3 Procedure 43.2 Procedure 44.1, 44.2 Procedure 48.1-48.4 Procedure 49.1, 49.2, 49.4-49.7 Procedure 50.1-50.3, 50.6, 50.8 Procedure 51.2, 51.4			
X.P.4. Complete compliance reporting based on public health statutes	Procedure 4.3			

CAAHEP Competency (2022)	Procedure	Date	Grade / Pass	Initial
X.P.5. Report an illegal activity following the protocol established by the healthcare setting	Procedure 4.4			
X.P.6. Complete an incident report related to an error in patient care	Procedure 4.5			
XI. Ethical Considerations				
XI.P.1. Demonstrate professional response(s) to ethical issues	Procedure 5.1, 5.2			
XII. Protective Practices				
XII.P.1. Comply with safety practices	Procedure 46.1, 46.3 Procedures 47.1-47.8 Procedure 49.1, 49.2, 49.4-49.7 Procedure 50.2-50.5			
XII.P.2.a. Demonstrate proper use of: eyewash equipment	Procedure 46.2			
XII.P.2.b. Demonstrate proper use of: fire extinguishers	Procedure 11.6			
XII.P.3. Use proper body mechanics	Procedure 11.3 Procedure 21.10			
XII.P.4. Evaluate an environment to identify unsafe conditions	Procedure 11.4 Procedure 46.3			
Affective Competencies				
A.1. Demonstrate critical thinking skills	Procedure 8.1 Procedure 9.2, 9.5 Procedure 15.5, 15.7 Procedure 26.1 Procedure 27.2 Procedure 34.1 Procedure 48.1-48.3			
A.2. Reassure patients	Procedure 47.9			
A.3. Demonstrate empathy for patients' concerns	Procedure 2.1-2.4 Procedure 4.1 Procedure 9.2 Procedure 15.5, 15.6, 15.7 Procedure 16.2 Procedure 21.1 Procedure 23.1 Procedure 26.1 Procedure 45.1 Procedure 48.5			

CAAHEP Competency (2022)	Procedure	Date	Grade / Pass	Initial
A.4. Demonstrate active listening	Procedure 2.1-2.4 Procedure 4.1 Procedure 21.1 Procedure 22.1 Procedure 47.9 Procedure 48.5			
A.5. Respect diversity	Procedure 2.1-2.4 Procedure 43.2			
A.6. Recognize personal boundaries	Procedure 2.1-2.4 Procedure 21.1			
A.7. Demonstrate tactfulness	Procedure 14.3 Procedure 15.5, 15.6, 15.7 Procedure 16.2			
A.8. Demonstrate self-awareness	Procedure 11.5			

The Professional Medical Assistant and the Healthcare Team

chapter

1

CAAHEP Competencies	Assessments
XI.C.4 Identify professional behaviors of a medical assistant	Skills and Concepts – B. 1
V.C.10 Identify the role of the medical assistant as a patient navigator	Workplace Application – 2
X.C.1. Identify scope of practice and standards of care for medical assistants	Skills and Concepts – C. 1, 2
X.C.2. Understand the provider role in terms of standard of care	Skills and Concepts – C. 1, 2
V.C.9. Identify the principles of self-boundaries	Skills and Concepts – K. 2
ABHES Competencies	**Assessments**
1. General Orientation	Skills and Concepts – A. 1, 2
a. Describe the current employment outlook for the medical assistant	
b. Compare and contrast the allied health professions and understand their relation to medical assisting	Skills and Concepts – H. 1-19
c. Describe and comprehend medical assistant credentialing requirements, the process to obtain the credential and the importance of credentialing	Skills and Concepts – D. 1
d. List the general responsibilities and skills of the medical assistant	Skills and Concepts – A. 3
5. Human Relations	Skills and Concepts – J. 2
f. Demonstrate an understanding of the core competencies for Interprofessional Collaborative Practice; i.e., values/ethics, roles/responsibilities, interprofessional communication, teamwork	
g. Partner with health care teams to attain optimal patient health outcomes	Skills and Concepts – K. 1
h. Display effective interpersonal skills with patients and health care team members	Skills and Concepts – K. 1
i. Demonstrate cultural awareness	Skills and Concepts – B. 1

ABHES Competencies	Assessments
8. Clinical Procedures i. Identify community resources and Complementary and Alternative Medicine practices (CAM)	Skills and Concepts – G. 3

VOCABULARY REVIEW

Using the word pool on the right, find the correct word to match the definition. Write the word on the line after the definition.

Group A

1. Adhering to ethical standards or right conduct standards _____

2. The way an individual perceives and processes information to learn new material _____

3. To learn or memorize beyond the point of proficiency or immediate recall _____

4. The process of sorting patients to determine medical need and the priority of care _____

5. A person who identifies patients' needs and barriers, then assists by coordinating care and identifying community and healthcare resources to meet the needs _____

6. How an individual internalizes new information and makes it their own _____

7. A learning device (e.g., an image, a rhyme, or a figure of speech) that a person uses to help them remember information _____

8. Meticulous, careful _____

9. How an individual looks at information and sees it as real _____

10. The process of thinking about new information to create new ways of learning _____

11. Harmful _____

12. Conduct expected of a reasonably prudent person acting under similar circumstances; it falls below the standards of behavior established by law for the protection of others against unreasonable risk of harm _____

Word Pool
- patient navigator
- detrimental
- integrity
- conscientious
- triage
- negligence
- perceiving
- processing
- learning style
- reflection
- overlearn
- mnemonic

Group B

1. A group of diverse medical and healthcare systems, practices, and products that are not generally considered part of conventional medicine; some are used in combination with conventional medicine and others are used instead of conventional medicine

   _____

2. Emotional or mental condition with respect to cheerfulness or confidence _____

3. A system of medical practice that treats disease by the use of remedies such as medications and surgery to produce effects different from those caused by the disease under treatment

   _____

4. Dependable; able to be trusted _____

5. The process by which something becomes harmful or unusable through contact with something unclean

   _____

6. The ability to determine what needs to be done and take action on your own _____

7. A form of healing that considers the whole person (i.e., body, mind, spirit, and emotions) in individual treatment plans

   _____

8. A concept of care that involves health professionals and volunteers who provide medical, psychological, and spiritual support to terminally ill patients and their loved ones

   _____

9. Behavior toward others; outward manner

   _____

10. The constant practice of considering all aspects of a situation when deciding what to believe or what to do

    _____

11. An important point or group of statistical values that, when evaluated, indicates the quality of care provided in a healthcare facility _____

Word Pool
- critical thinking
- contamination
- allopathic
- holistic
- complementary and alternative medicine (CAM)
- hospice
- indicators
- demeanor
- initiative
- reliable
- morale

ABBREVIATIONS

Write out what each of the following abbreviations stands for.

1. CAAHEP _____

2. CAM _____

3. EHR _____

4. ECG _____

5. CLIA _____

6. OSHA _____

7. IV _____

8. AAMA _____

9. CEU _____

10. AMT _____

11. NHA _____

12. MD _____

13. DO _____

14. OMT _____

15. DC _____

16. NP _____

17. RN _____

18. PA _____

19. IDS _____

20. ED _____

21. PCMH _____

22. AHRQ _____

23. HHS _____

24. IT _____

SKILLS AND CONCEPTS

Answer the following questions. Write your answer on the line or in the space provided.

A. Responsibilities of the Medical Assistant

1. According the U.S. Bureau of Labor Statistics, employment opportunities for medical assistants is expected to grow _____ through _____.

2. List factors for the expected growth in job opportunities for medical assistants. _____

    _____

    _____

    _____

    _____

    _____

3. List five clinical and five administrative skills that are part of the job description for an entry-level medical assistant.

Clinical skills include: _____

_____

_____

_____

_____

_____

Administrative skills include: _____

_____

_____

_____

_____

_____

B. Characteristics of Professional Medical Assistants

1. What methods can the medical assistant use to treat others with courtesy and respect? _____

_____

_____

_____

_____

_____

C. Scope of Practice and Standards of Care for Medical Assistants

1. What is the difference between scope of practice and standards of care? _____

_____

_____

_____

_____

_____

_____

2. Describe the difference between standard of care for a provider and a medical assistant._____

_____

_____

_____

_____

_____

3. Identify five practices that are beyond the scope of practice of medical assistants._____

_____

_____

_____

_____

_____

D. Professional Medical Assisting Organizations, Credentials, and Continuing Education

1. What are some of the differences between the AAMA and AMT? What credentials can be granted by each?

_____

_____

_____

_____

_____

_____

2. Is the NHA involved in medical assistant program curriculum development or accreditation? What service does this company provide?

_____

_____

_____

_____

_____

_____

E. How to Succeed as a Medical Assistant Student

1. Choose three study skills from your reading and describe how you think they will help you learn.

    _____

    _____

    _____

    _____

    _____

2. What test-taking strategies might help you improve your scores?_____

    _____

    _____

    _____

3. Describe what it means to be a critical thinker. _____

    _____

    _____

    _____

    _____

    _____

F. The History of Medicine

1. Describe how the profession of medical assisting began. Why are medical assistants defined as *multi-skilled* healthcare workers?

    _____

    _____

    _____

    _____

    _____

G. Medical Professionals

1. _____ physicians, or DOs, complete requirements similar to those for MDs to graduate and practice medicine.

2. _____ provide direct patient care services under the supervision of licensed physicians and are trained to diagnose and treat patients as directed by the physician.

3. Identify five complementary and alternative medicine therapies. _____

_____

_____

_____

_____

4. Explain the role of the hospitalist. _____

_____

_____

_____

_____

H. Allied Health Professionals

Match the following descriptions with the appropriate healthcare occupation.

1. _____ Provides services such as injury prevention, assessment, and rehabilitation
2. _____ Is qualified to implement exercise programs designed to reverse or minimize debilitation and enhance the functional capacity of medically stable patients
3. _____ Practices medicine under the direction and responsible supervision of a medical doctor or doctor of osteopathy
4. _____ Performs diagnostic examinations and therapeutic interventions of the heart or blood vessels, both invasive and noninvasive
5. _____ Assists licensed pharmacists by performing duties that do not require the expertise of a pharmacist
6. _____ Assists in developing and implementing the anesthesia care plan
7. _____ Helps improve patient mobility, relieve pain, and prevent or limit permanent physical disabilities
8. _____ Helps patients use their leisure in ways that enhance health, functional abilities, independence, and quality of life
9. _____ Identifies patients who have hearing, balance, and related ear problems
10. _____ Integrates and applies the principles from the science of food, nutrition, biochemistry, food management, and behavior to achieve and maintain health
11. _____ Evaluates, treats, and manages patients of all ages with respiratory illnesses and other cardiopulmonary disorders

a. audiologist
b. diagnostic cardiovascular technologist
c. therapeutic recreation specialist
d. physical therapist
e. pharmacy technician
f. dietetic technician
g. anesthesiology assistant
h. blood bank technology specialist
i. diagnostic medical sonographer
j. kinesiotherapist
k. occupational therapist
l. orthoptist
m. physician assistant
n. surgical technologist
o. respiratory therapist
p. athletic trainer
q. medical technologist
r. emergency medical technician
s. nuclear medicine technologist

12. _____ Evaluates disorders of vision, eye movement, and eye alignment

13. _____ Performs routine and standardized tests in blood center and transfusion services

14. _____ Uses equipment that produces sound waves, resulting in images of internal structures

15. _____ Uses the nuclear properties of radioactive and stable nuclides to make diagnostic evaluations of the anatomic or physiologic conditions of the body

16. _____ Helps prepare patients for surgery and maintain the sterile field in the surgical suite, making sure all members of the surgical team follow sterile technique

17. _____ Assists in helping patients compensate for loss of function

18. _____ Performs diagnostic testing on blood, body fluids, and other types of specimens to assist the provider in arriving at a diagnosis

19. _____ Provides medical care to patients who have suffered an injury or illness outside the hospital setting

I. Types of Healthcare Facilities

1. Hospitals are classified according to the type of care and services they provide to patients. Describe the three different levels of hospitalized care.

   a. _____

   _____

   _____

   _____

   b. _____

   _____

   _____

   _____

   c. _____

   _____

   _____

   _____

J. The Healthcare Team

1. Define a patient-centered medical home (PCMH) and its five core functions and attributes. _____

   _____

   _____

   _____

   _____

   _____

   _____

   _____

2. Define *teamwork* in your own words. _____

   _____

   _____

   _____

   _____

K. Professionalism as a Team Member

1. Summarize three obstructions to professionalism.

   a. _____

   _____

   _____

   _____

   b. _____

   _____

   _____

   _____

   c. _____

   _____

   _____

   _____

2. Identify the principles of self-boundaries. How do they relate to the field of medical assisting? _____

_____

_____

_____

_____

_____

_____

_____

3. Describe four time-management techniques medical assistants can use in the healthcare environment to meet the demands of a busy practice.

a. _____

b. _____

c. _____

d. _____

CERTIFICATION PREPARATION
Circle the correct answer.

1. The first national organization formed for medical assistants was
   a. CAAHEP.
   b. ABHES.
   c. AMT.
   d. AAMA.

2. Which healthcare professional is trained to practice medicine under the supervision of a physician?
   a. Medical technologist
   b. Paramedic
   c. Medical assistant
   d. Physician assistant

3. The allied health specialist who performs ultrasound diagnostic procedures under the supervision of a physician is called a(n)
   a. cytotechnologist.
   b. diagnostic medical sonographer.
   c. electroneurodiagnostic technologist.
   d. perfusionist.

4. A method of prioritizing patients so that the most urgent cases receive care first is called
   a. case management.
   b. accreditation.
   c. triage.
   d. quality control.

5. The health professional who provides basic patient care services, including diagnosing illnesses and prescribing medications, is a
   a. nurse practitioner.
   b. nurse anesthetist.
   c. licensed practical nurse.
   d. vocational nurse.

6. One factor is absolutely true about all practicing medical assistants—they are not independent practitioners. Whether certified or not, regardless of length of training or experience, every medical assistant must practice under the direct supervision of a physician or other licensed practitioner (e.g., nurse practitioner or physician assistant).
   a. Both statements are true.
   b. Both statements are false.
   c. The first statement is true; the second is false.
   d. The first statement is false; the second is true.

7. Which mind maps would display the cause and effect of events?
   a. Spider map
   b. Fishbone map
   c. Chain-of-events map
   d. Cycle map

8. Which is *not* part of critical thinking?
   a. Sorting out conflicting information
   b. Weighing your knowledge about the information
   c. Deciding on a reasonable belief or action
   d. Incorporating personal beliefs

9. Deciding which tasks are most important is called
   a. modification.
   b. teaching.
   c. prioritizing.
   d. procrastinating.

10. Which statement about professionalism is true?
   a. It must be practiced at all times in the workplace.
   b. It can lead to wage increases and promotions.
   c. Unacceptable behavior is detrimental to the medical assistant's career.
   d. All of the above are true.

WORKPLACE APPLICATIONS

1. You are employed by a primary care physician who is investigating the possibility of forming a PCMH with other practitioners and allied health professionals in the community. Refer to the Department of Health and Human Services PCMH Resource Center at http://pcmh.ahrq.gov/. Research the meaning of PCMH and review the research that supports the PCMH model of care. What did you learn? Share this information with your class.

2. What does it mean to operate as a patient navigator? Why are medical assistants who are skilled in both administrative and clinical areas ideally suited to help patients navigate complex healthcare systems? How could you help the patient described below?

   Mrs. Kate Glasgow is an 82-year-old patient in the family practice where you work. Mrs. Glasgow recently suffered a mild cerebrovascular accident (CVA) and her son is trying to help coordinate her care. Mrs. Glasgow does not understand when or how to take her new medications, she is concerned about whether her health insurance will cover the cost of frequent clinic appointments and assistive devices, she doesn't understand how to prepare for magnetic resonance imaging (MRI) the provider ordered, and she dislikes having to comply with getting blood drawn every week.

3. Martin Smith is a patient who always disrupts the clinic. He constantly complains about everything from the moment he enters until the moment he leaves. Karen is at the desk when he arrives to check out and pay his bill. When she tells him that he has a previous balance from a claim that his insurance did not pay, he argues that Karen filed the claim incorrectly. Karen is not in charge of filing insurance claims and did not handle any part of the claim in question. How can she be courteous to this patient?

INTERNET ACTIVITIES

1. Choose one of the early medical pioneers discussed in this chapter and research the person using the internet. After conducting the research, create a poster presentation, a PowerPoint presentation, or write a paper and present the results of your research to the class.

2. Research professionalism requirements for other health professions. Talk about the ways that those requirements are similar to or different from those of a medical assistant. Compare professionalism in the healthcare industry to that in other professions such as law enforcement or education. Talk about why medical professionalism is so critical.

Therapeutic Communication

chapter

2

CAAHEP Competencies	Assessment
V.C.1. Identify types of verbal and nonverbal communication	Skills and Concepts – C. 1, 3-11; D. 1, 4; Certification Preparation – 1, 2
V.C.2. Identify communication barriers	Skills and Concepts – F. 1 a-h; Certification Preparation – 3
V.C.3. Identify techniques for overcoming communication barriers	Skills and Concepts – F. 2-9; Certification Preparation – 4
V.C.4. Identify the steps in the sender-receiver process	Skills and Concepts – D. 2-3
V.C.5. Identify challenges in communication with different age groups	Skills and Concepts – F. 10-12, 21-28
V.C.9. Identify the principles of self-boundaries	Skills and Concepts – H. 1
V.C.11. Identify coping mechanisms	Skills and Concepts – I. 12-20; Certification Preparation – 5; Internet Activities – 4
V.C.13.a. Understand the basic concepts of the following theories: Maslow	Skills and Concepts – I. 1-9 a-h; Certification Preparation – 8-9; Internet Activities – 3
V.C.13.b. Understand the basic concepts of the following theories: Erikson	Skills and Concepts – F. 13-29; Certification Preparation – 6
V.C.13.c. Understand the basic concepts of the following theories: Kübler-Ross	Skills and Concepts – F. 30-35; Certification Preparation – 7
V.C.14. Identify issues associated with diversity as it relates to patient care	Skills and Concepts – B. 1-9
X.C.10.c. Identify: Americans with Disabilities Act Amendments Act (ADAAA)	Skills and Concepts – J. 1
V.P.1. Respond to nonverbal communication	Procedures 2.1, 2.2, 2.3, 2.4
A.3. Demonstrate empathy for patients' concerns	Procedures 2.1, 2.2, 2.3, 2.4
A.4. Demonstrate active listening	Procedures 2.1, 2.2, 2.3, 2.4
A.5. Respect diversity	Procedures 2.1, 2.2, 2.3, 2.4
A.6 Recognize personal boundaries	Procedure 2.5

ABHES Competencies	Assessment
5. Human Relations a. Respond appropriately to patients with abnormal behavior patterns	Skills and Concepts – F. 3, H. 4-5
b. Provide support for terminally ill patients 1) Use empathy when communicating with terminally ill patients	Skills and Concepts – F. 9
2) Identify common stages that terminally ill patients experience	Skills and Concepts – F. 10 a-e
d. Adapt care to address the developmental stages of life	Skills and Concepts – F. 6, 7, 8 a-i; Certification Preparation – 6
e. Analyze the effect of hereditary and environmental influences on behavior	Skills and Concepts – I. 1-3
h. Display effective interpersonal skills with patients and healthcare team members	Procedures 2.1, 2.2, 2.3, 2.4, 2.5
i . Demonstrate cultural awareness	Internet Activities – 1-2; Procedures 2.2, 2.3
7. Administrative Procedures g. Display professionalism through written and verbal communications	Procedures 2.1, 2.2, 2.4
8. Clinical Procedures j. Make adaptations for patients with special needs (psychological or physical limitations)	Review of Concepts – F. 2b-c, e, g, 6
k. Make adaptations to care for patients across their lifespan	Review of Concepts – F. 7, 8a-h

VOCABULARY REVIEW

Using the word pool on the right, find the correct word to match the definition. Write the word on the line after the definition.

1. The ability to understand another's perspective, experiences, or motivations _____

2. The act of sticking to something _____

3. A type of communication that occurs through body language and expressive behaviors rather than with verbal or written words

   _____

4. The inherent worth or state of being worthy of respect

   _____

5. Having a deep awareness of the suffering of another and the wish to ease it _____

6. The differences and similarities in identity, perspective, and points of view among people _____

7. Having a composed and self-assured manner

   _____

Word Pool
- adherence
- communication
- compassion
- coping mechanisms
- defense mechanisms
- dignity
- diversity
- empathy
- nonverbal communication
- hierarchy
- poised
- rapport
- respect
- stress
- therapeutic communication

8. A relationship of harmony and accord between the patient and the healthcare professional _____

9. To show consideration or appreciation for another person _____

10. A condition that causes physical and/or emotional tension _____

11. Exchange of information, feelings, and thoughts between two or more people using spoken words or other methods _____

12. A process of communicating with patients and family members in healthcare _____

13. Things arranged in order or rank _____

14. Unconscious mental processes that protect people from anxiety, loss, conflict, or shame _____

15. Behavioral and psychological strategies used to deal with or minimize stressful events _____

ABBREVIATIONS
Write out what each of the following abbreviations stands for.

1. ADA _____

2. ADAAA _____

SKILLS AND CONCEPTS
Answer the following questions.

A. Introduction and First Impressions and High-Quality Patient Care

1. _____ is a process of communicating with patients and family members in healthcare.

2. What factors are involved in creating a first impression?
   a. Physical appearance or dress
   b. Attitude and compassion
   c. Therapeutic communication skills
   d. All of the above

B. Respecting Diverse Populations

Match the description with the correct type of diversity. Answers can be used more than once.

1. _____ Includes the general customs, norms, values, and beliefs held by a group of people.

2. _____ Can make it more difficult for people to access healthcare and receive quality healthcare.

3. _____ Relates to a common ancestry, culture, religion, traditions, nationality, and language shared by a group of people.

4. _____ Pertains to the country where the person was born and holds citizenship.

5. _____ Can impact patient care if healthcare professionals assume patients will conform to the mainstream values and the patient's health beliefs are not considered.

6. _____ A person's lifestyle choice may influence the care they receive.

7. _____ Pertains to immigrants to the United States who lack insurance for healthcare.

8. _____ Relates to a group of people who have the same physical characteristics.

9. _____ All the ways a person is different from others (e.g., lifestyle, religion, tastes, and preferences).

a. nationality
b. race
c. culture
d. ethnicity
e. social factors
f. culture and ethnicity

Select the correct answer.

10. To show respect, a healthcare professional should
    a. smile and make eye contact if appropriate when first meeting a person.
    b. be courteous, sincere, polite, and welcoming.
    c. use a calm tone of voice and proper grammar without slang.
    d. all of the above

C. Nonverbal Communication

1. We communicate _____ through nonverbal behaviors (our body language and expressive behaviors) than through our words.

2. What is involved with nonverbal communication?
    a. Nonverbal behaviors
    b. Nonverbal communication delivery factors
    c. Cultural differences and spatial distance
    d. All of the above

3. Which is considered a negative, closed nonverbal behavior?
    a. Being at the level of the other person and angled toward them
    b. Arms crossed in front of the body or hands behind the person's back
    c. Poised and shoulders relaxed
    d. Light touch on the person's hand

4. Which is considered a positive, open nonverbal behavior?
    a. Professional appearance
    b. Fidgeting and looking at the clock
    c. Lowered eyebrows or one raised eyebrow
    d. Avoiding eye contact

Match the nonverbal delivery factor with the definition.

5. _____ Describes the emotion in the voice.
6. _____ Refers to the speed at which the speaker talks.
7. _____ Pertains to how the word is said.
8. _____ Refers to the loudness of the speaker's voice.
9. _____ Includes the highness and lowness of the voice.
10. _____ Describes the melodic pattern or the pitch variation.
11. _____ Relates to the quality of the voice.

a. rate
b. clarity
c. volume
d. pitch
e. tone
f. intonation
g. pronunciation

Select the correct answer or fill the answer in on the line.

12. Which of the following is *not* a professional expectation when speaking with patients?
    a. Use a moderate rate and volume.
    b. Speak in a clear voice.
    c. Vary your pitch.
    d. Use medical terminology and generational terms.

13. How can a medical assistant respect a person from another cultural group that is unfamiliar?
    a. Follow the other person's lead in terms of nonverbal behaviors and personal space.
    b. Use gestures cautiously.
    c. Refrain from touching a child's head.
    d. All of the above

14. When medical assistants talk with patients, they should be _____ away from the patients, which is considered the _____ space.

15. When medical assistants perform procedures on patients, they are _____ away from patients, which is considered the _____ space.

16. A person will move _____ if they want to increase the space between themselves and other people.

D. Verbal Communication

1. Two types of verbal communication include _____ and _____.

2. Describe the steps in the communication cycle (or sender-receiver process)._____

_____

_____

3. We decode messages based on _____ and _____.

4. Which of the following is a type of written communication?
    a. Texts and written phone messages
    b. Letters and emails
    c. Informational flyers
    d. All of the above

Match style of oral communication with the correct description. Answers can be used more than once.

5. _____ When working with this type of communicator, a person should avoid being controlled and respectfully maintain their position.

6. _____ This type of communicator tries to dominate others and may glare, frown, and purposefully invade others' personal space.

7. _____ This type of communicator clearly states their needs and wants.

8. _____ This type of communicator avoid expressing feelings or opinions, fails to assert themselves, and allows others to infringe on their rights.

9. _____ This type of communicator uses a medium pitch, speed, and volume of voice and positive, open nonverbal behaviors.

10. _____ When working with this type of communicator, a person may need to use humor and try to have a positive discussion.

11. _____ This type of communicator is cunning, tries to control others, and maybe demeaning or condescending.

12. _____ This type of communicator denies problems and may speak in a sugary-sweet voice, look innocent, and pretend to be warm and friendly.

13. _____ When working with this type of communicator, a person should remain calm and attempt to see the other person's point of view.

14. _____ This type of communicator speaks in a soft voice, fidgets, and belittles their contribution.

15. _____ A healthcare professional needs to be this type of communicator.

16. _____ When working with this type of communicator, a person should use a firm approach and be assertive.

a. passive communicator
b. aggressive communicator
c. passive-aggressive communicator
d. manipulative communicator
e. assertive communicator

E. Therapeutic Communication

1. What is the advantage of using therapeutic communication in a healthcare setting?
    a. It is an interactive relationship that conveys acceptance and respect without judgment or blame.
    b. It encourages healthcare professionals to build rapport with patients, which is helpful in building the relationship.
    c. When that bond develops and grows, patients are more comfortable expressing their feelings, ideas, and concerns.
    d. All of the above

2. Which is correct regarding active listening and passively hearing what a speaker is saying?
   a. With active listening, we fully concentrate on what is being said and how it is being said.
   b. The speaker can easily see the person is actively listening.
   c. With passive hearing, we hear what the patient is saying, but we are distracted by our own thoughts.
   d. All of the above

3. What is a nonverbal behavior that *cannot* be used during active listening?
   a. Eye contact and nodding your head
   b. Body position and facial expression
   c. Looking at the clock and yawning
   d. All of the above

4. Which is *not* correct regarding closed questions or statements?
   a. Asks for general information or states the topic to be discussed
   b. Closed questions limit the patient's answer to one or two words
   c. Used to confirm specific facts
   d. Answers to closed questions may include yes and no

5. Which is *not* correct regarding open questions or statements?
   a. Used as a communication tool to begin a conversation with a patient
   b. Used to introduce a new section of questions
   c. A poor method to use when wanting additional details from the patient about their problem
   d. Used when a person introduces a new topic

6. _____ allows the listener to get additional information.

7. _____ or _____ means to reword or rephrase a statement to check the meaning and interpretation.

8. _____ allows the listener to recap and review what was said.

9. _____ allows time to gather thoughts and answer questions.

10. _____ means to put words to the person's emotional reaction, which acknowledges the person's feelings.

F. Barriers to Effective Communication

1. For each description below, identify the type of barrier to communication.

   a. Noise, lack of privacy, temperature _____

   b. Fear and anxiety related to being judged by the healthcare professional or the inability to explain personal feelings _____

   c. Unable to read or write _____

   d. Hunger, pain, anger, tiredness _____

   e. Unable to see written communication _____

   f. Unable to hear verbal communication _____

   g. Functioning at a lower age level _____

   h. English is not the patient's primary language _____

Match the communication barrier with the correct way the medical assistant can help overcome the barrier.

2. _____ Help make the patient comfortable. Provide food and drink if available. Administer pain medications as ordered.

3. _____ Use audio recordings, screen magnifiers, large-print materials, and screen reader software.

4. _____ Provide privacy for patients. Talk with patients in a quiet room with the door closed. Make sure the room temperature is comfortable.

5. _____ Use print materials and written instructions. Use videos with captions. Have text telephones (TTYs) available. Use a sign language interpreter.

6. _____ Use "functioning age" -appropriate language and materials. Provide information also to the guardian/caregiver.

7. _____ Use interpreters and translated materials. Limit medical terminology and define medical terms that must be used. Use culturally appropriate materials and visuals (pictures, graphs, and models).

8. _____ Use pictures and models. Draw pictures and use simple language.

9. _____ Provide a warm, caring environment. Make sure your body language reflects an open and caring manner. Gain the person's trust. Keep voice at normal level.

a. hearing impairment
b. non-English–speaking
c. illiteracy
d. internal distractions
e. environmental distractions
f. visual impairment
g. emotional distraction
h. intellectual disability

Match the challenges in communication with the correct development stage.

10. _____ Does not comprehend cause and effect or the impact in the future

11. _____ Unable to process medical information

12. _____ Understands concrete examples versus hypothetical situations

a. sensory motor
b. preoperational
c. concrete operations

Match the goal of the stage with the correct psychosocial developmental stages.

13. _____ Encouraged to try new activities. Must assume responsibilities and learn new skills. Will make child feel purposeful and increase self-esteem.

14. _____ To know who you are as a person and how you fit into the world around you. Creates a meaningful self-image.

15. _____ Must develop trust, with the ability to mistrust should the need arise.

16. _____ Must seek to finish tasks. Recognition for accomplishments is important.

a. trust versus mistrust
b. autonomy versus shame and doubt
c. initiative versus guilt
d. industry versus inferiority
e. identity versus role confusion
f. intimacy versus isolation
g. generativity versus stagnation
h. ego integrity versus despair

17. _____ Must explore and manipulate things in their "world" to develop autonomy and self-esteem.

18. _____ Develops friendships; takes on commitments.

19. _____ Reflects on one's life and comes to terms with it, instead of regretting the past.

20. _____ Achieves a balance between the concern for the next generation (having a family) and being self-absorbed.

Match the communication tip with the correct psychosocial developmental stages.

21. _____ Use short simple sentences. Encourage questions. Use imitation, play, and role playing.

22. _____ Communicate with dignity and respect. Limit slang and "generational" terms. Use simpler language. Speak clearly. Allow time to respond.

23. _____ Identify motivating factors and use them as needed during communication. Realize person may be juggling a lot of obligations.

24. _____ Use calm and soothing voice, hold child securely. Loud voices and noises can startle a child.

25. _____ Use engaging simple tools to communicate information (videos, gaming software, pamphlets). Encourage discussion and questions.

26. _____ Provide privacy and independence. Encourage responsible decision making. Encourage discussion and questions.

27. _____ Identify motivating factors and use them as needed during communication. Realize person may be juggling a lot of obligations.

28. _____ Use simple language. Allow child to touch and explore objects. Allow child to play and make choices.

a. trust versus mistrust
b. autonomy versus shame and doubt
c. initiative versus guilt
d. industry versus inferiority
e. identity versus role confusion
f. intimacy versus isolation
g. generativity versus stagnation
h. ego integrity versus despair

Answer the following questions.

29. Discuss how Erikson's theory of psychosocial developmental relates to communicating with patients.

_____

_____

_____

30. Discuss how Kübler-Ross's theory relates to communicating with patients. _____

_____

_____

_____

Match the description with the correct stage of Kübler-Ross's theory.

31. _____ Person feels sad, fearful, and uncertain. May not participate in normal activities. Distances self from others.

32. _____ Refuses to accept the fact (e.g., diagnosis or prognosis). Defense mechanism that allows the person to ignore what is happening.

33. _____ Has come to terms with situation.

34. _____ Can be directed at self or others.

35. _____ Attempts to bargain with the higher power the person believes in (e.g., God).

a. denial
b. anger
c. bargaining
d. depression
e. acceptance

G. Communicating in the Workplace

1. When speaking with providers, what guideline should the medical assistant follow?
   a. Speak confidently, clearly, and concisely.
   b. Start with the patient's name and age if appropriate.
   c. Discuss the situation in an organized manner.
   d. All of the above

2. When speaking with providers, what guideline should the medical assistant follow?
   a. If the situation relates to a series of events, start with what occurred first, then second, and so on.
   b. Write down any information the provider gives.
   c. Read information written down back to the provider to ensure accuracy.
   d. All of the above

H. Personal and Professional Boundaries with Communication

1. What is a principle of self-boundaries (personal boundaries)?
   a. They are also called personal boundaries.
   b. They are the limits people use to protect themselves.
   c. Include mental, emotional, physical, and social factors.
   d. All of the above

2. The relationship between the patient and the medical assistant must be professional. What should the medical assistant do to keep this relationship professional?
   a. Share personal issues, struggles, life stories, or other personal intimate information.
   b. Befriend the patient on social media.
   c. Refrain from contacting the patient outside of the work environment.
   d. All of the above

I. Understanding Behavior

1. What is correct regarding Maslow's Hierarchy of Needs theory?
   a. This is a motivational theory that depicts eight levels of needs.
   b. Each level must be satisfied before we can move up to the next level.
   c. The needs include "Deficiency" needs and "Growth" needs.
   d. All of the above

Match the description with the correct needs from Maslow's Hierarchy of Needs theory. Answers can be used more than once.

2. _____ These needs are considered coping behaviors.

3. _____ Needs must be fulfilled to cope with life and survival.

4. _____ Top four levels of needs.

5. _____ We are all motivated to meet these unmet needs.

6. _____ These needs relate to making ourselves a better person.

7. _____ Fulfillment of these needs leads to long-lasting happiness.

8. _____ Fulfillment of these needs leads to instant short-term gratification.

a. "growth" needs
b. "deficiency" needs

9. For the following descriptions, identify the level of need according to Maslow's theory.

   a. Includes air, food, drink, shelter, and warmth _____

   b. Includes friendship and intimacy _____

   c. Includes protection form the elements and security _____

   d. Includes knowledge, curiosity, and understanding _____

   e. The appreciation of and search for beauty and balance _____

   f. Includes self-esteem and achievement _____

   g. The need to realize one's potential _____

   h. Which needs are met by helping others achieve their very best? _____

10. _____ are unconscious mental processes that protect people from anxiety, loss, conflict, or shame.

11. Identify the defense mechanism based on the following descriptions.

    a. Completely rejects the information. _____

    b. The person comes up with various explanations to justify their response. _____

    c. Transfers the emotion toward one person to another person or thing. _____

    d. Simply forgets something that is bad or hurtful. _____

Match the description or coping mechanism with the correct type of coping mechanism. Answers can be used more than once.

12. _____ Reduce the feelings associated with stress for a short time.

13. _____ Improve our functioning level and reduce stress level

14. _____ Hostility and aggression

15. _____ Eat healthy, well-balanced meals

16. _____ Drug and alcohol use

17. _____ Gambling

18. _____ Social withdrawal and isolation

19. _____ Talk and share with others

20. _____ Exercise, drink water, and get plenty of sleep

a. adaptive (healthy) coping mechanisms
b. maladaptive (unhealthy) coping mechanisms

J. Closing Comments

1. Discuss the impact of the Americans with Disabilities Act Amendments Act (ADAAA) in relationship to communication barriers in healthcare.

   _____

   _____

   _____

   _____

   _____

2. Discuss three ways that healthcare providers can meet their federal obligation for accommodating patients with communication disabilities.

   _____

   _____

   _____

CERTIFICATION PREPARATION

Circle the correct answer.

1. What is a type of nonverbal communication?
   a. Body language
   b. Oral communication
   c. Email
   d. Letter

2. What is a type of verbal communication?
   a. Written message
   b. Oral communication
   c. Email
   d. All of the above

3. Hunger, pain, anger, and tiredness are considered which type of barrier to communication?
   a. Environmental distractions
   b. Internal distractions
   c. External distractions
   d. Hearing impairment

4. What is a way to overcome environmental distractions?
   a. Help make the patient comfortable.
   b. Use audio recordings and large-print materials.
   c. Provide privacy for patients.
   d. Use pictures and models.

5. What is a maladaptive coping mechanism?
   a. Passive-aggressive behavior
   b. Drug and alcohol use
   c. Denial
   d. All of the above

6. Erikson's theory places a 4-year-old child in which developmental stage?
   a. Trust versus mistrust
   b. Autonomy versus shame and doubt
   c. Initiative versus guilt
   d. Industry versus inferiority

7. According to Kübler-Ross, when a person feels sadness, fear, and uncertainty, they are in which stage of grief?
   a. Denial
   b. Anger
   c. Bargaining
   d. Depression

8. Which level of Maslow's Hierarchy of Needs includes protection from the elements, security, and stability?
   a. Physiologic needs
   b. Safety needs
   c. Love and belongingness needs
   d. Esteem needs

9. Which level of Maslow's Hierarchy of Needs includes knowledge, curiosity, understanding, and exploration?
   a. Cognitive needs
   b. Aesthetic needs
   c. Self-actualization needs
   d. Transcendence needs

10. A person is using which defense mechanism when they revert to an old, immature behavior to express their feelings?
    a. Denial
    b. Repression
    c. Regression
    d. Displacement

WORKPLACE APPLICATIONS

1. When Christi was doing her orientation, she observed Sally rooming patients. With the patient seated in the room, Sally stood near the patient collecting the patient's information. She smiled occasionally as she talked with the patient. Christi noticed Sally had poor posture and yawned several times during the patient interview. At times, Sally used appropriate light touch with the patient and used small hand gestures. Describe the positive nonverbal behaviors that Christi observed.

   _____

   _____

   _____

   _____

2. Using #1 above, list the negative and closed nonverbal behaviors that Christi observed. For each type of negative behavior, indicate the correct positive and open behavior that should have been used.

_____

_____

_____

3. Christi is following Samantha during orientation as they work with a Hmong provider. Most of the patients are Hmong. Describe specific cultural differences with nonverbal behaviors that would apply to the Hmong community.

_____

_____

_____

INTERNET ACTIVITIES

1. Using online resources, research a specific culture different than your own. Create a poster presentation, a PowerPoint presentation, or write a paper summarizing your research. Include the following points in your project:
    a. Description of the culture (e.g., origin, typical family structure)
    b. Culture, beliefs, religion, and ethnic customs that influence healthcare discussions, treatments, and care
    c. Beliefs that impact verbal and nonverbal communication
2. Using online resources, research four cultures different than your own. Focus your research on cultural beliefs that impact communication in the healthcare environment. Create a poster presentation, a PowerPoint presentation, or write a paper summarizing your research. Include tips for a medical assistant to remember when working with a patient from each of the cultures.
3. Research Maslow's Hierarchy of Needs. Create a poster presentation, a PowerPoint presentation, or write a paper summarizing the theory and describe its importance to medical assistants. Cite two appropriate references used.
4. Research adaptive (healthy) and maladaptive (nonadaptive, unhealthy) coping mechanisms. Create a list of eight adaptive and eight maladaptive coping mechanisms. Discuss the importance of using adaptive coping mechanisms. Cite two appropriate references used.

Procedure 2.1   Use Feedback Techniques and Demonstrate Respect for Individual Diversity: Gender and Appearance

Name _____ Date _____ Score _____

Tasks: Use feedback techniques (e.g., reflection, restatement, and clarification) to obtain patient information. Respond to nonverbal communication. Communicate respectfully with patients with individual diversity related to gender and appearance. Demonstrate empathy, active listening, and nonverbal communication.

Background: When working with a transgender patient, ask the patient privately which pronouns the person prefers. Make sure to add this information into the patient's health record for future reference.

Scenario: You are rooming Crystal Green. You can see that she has expertly applied her makeup, has long red fingernails, long blonde hair, and is wearing three-inch heels. You are surprised to see that her birth sex is male. This is the first time you have roomed a transgender patient. You are uncomfortable in this situation because you have strong personal beliefs that birth sex should be maintained throughout a person's life.

Directions: Using the scenario, role-play with a peer the rooming process (obtain the patient's chief complaint [main reason for the visit], allergies, pregnancy history, and current medications). The partner (patient) should make up any information required.

Equipment and Supplies:
- Patient health record
- History form (optional) (Work Product 2.1)
- Pen

Standard: Complete the procedure and all critical steps in _____ minutes with a minimum score of 85% within two attempts (*or as indicated by the instructor*).

Scoring: Divide the points earned by the total possible points. Failure to perform a critical step, indicated by an asterisk (*), results in grade no higher than an 84% (*or as indicated by the instructor*).

Time: Began_____ Ended_____ Total minutes: _____

Steps	Possible Points	Attempt 1	Attempt 2
1. Greet the patient. Identify yourself. Verify the patient's identity with full name and date of birth. Explain the procedure in a manner that is understood by the patient. Answer any questions the patient may have on the procedure.	10		
2. Demonstrate respect for the patient. Be sincere, courteous, polite, and welcoming. Maintain the patient's dignity. Demonstrate professional, nonjudgmental verbal and nonverbal communication. Ask appropriate questions as information is obtained. (*Refer to the Affective Behaviors Checklist – **Respect** and the Grading Rubric*)	15*		
3. Using appropriate closed and open-ended questions and statements, obtain the patient's chief complaint (main reason for the visit) and history of present illness, allergies, pregnancy history, medical history, and current medications. Document the information in the health record or on the history form.	10		

4.	Use feedback techniques, including reflection, restatement, and clarification as information is obtained.	**10***		
5.	Respond to the patient's nonverbal communication by using feedback techniques (e.g., reflection). If the patient's nonverbal communication is interpreted differently than the patient's oral statements, clarify the information with the patient.	**10***		
6.	Use active listening skills. Remain neutral and refrain from interrupting. Allow for periods of silence. Smile and nod your head to show interest. Use appropriate eye contact. Focus on the patient and avoid distractions (e.g., looking at the clock, fidgeting). (*Refer to the Affective Behaviors Checklist – **Active Listening** and the Grading Rubric*)	**15***		
7.	Use professional, positive nonverbal communication behaviors. Use a clear voice, with a moderate rate and volume. Use a varying pitch and an accepting or a neutral tone. Use words the patient can understand. Correctly pronounce the words. Be at the same eye level as the patient's. Smile and have a poised posture. Use light touch on the hand if appropriate. Maintain proper eye contact if culturally appropriate. (*Refer to the Affective Behaviors Checklist – **Nonverbal Communication** and the Grading Rubric*)	**15***		
8.	Demonstrate empathy by listening to the patient and learning about their experiences and concerns. Use therapeutic communication techniques and positive nonverbal behaviors. Show your support and respect. (*Refer to the Affective Behaviors Checklist – **Empathy** and the Grading Rubric*)	**15***		
	Total Score	**100**		

Affective Behavior	**Affective Behaviors Checklist** **Directions:** *Check behaviors observed during the role-play.*					
Respect	**Negative, Unprofessional Behaviors**	**Attempt**		**Positive, Professional Behaviors**	**Attempt**	
		1	**2**		**1**	**2**
	Rude, unkind, fake/false attitude, disrespectful, impolite, unwelcoming			Courteous, sincere, polite, welcoming		
	Unconcerned with person's dignity; brief, abrupt			Maintained person's dignity; took time with person		
	Unprofessional verbal communication; inappropriate questions			Professional verbal communication		
	Negative nonverbal behaviors, poor eye contact			Positive nonverbal behaviors, proper eye contact		
	Other:			Other:		

Active Listening	Biased, offensive			Remained neutral		
	Interrupted			Refrained from interrupting		
	Did not allow for silence or pauses			Allowed for periods of silence		
	Negative nonverbal behaviors (rolled eyes, yawned, frowned, avoided eye contact)			Positive nonverbal behaviors (smiled, nodded head, appropriate eye contact)		
	Distracted (looked at watch, phone)			Focused on patient, avoided distractions		
	Other:			Other:		
Nonverbal Communication	Muffled voice; rate too fast or slow; too loud or too soft; unaccepting tone			Clear voice with moderate rate and volume; varying pitch; accepting or neutral tone		
	Incorrectly pronounced words; used words the person did not understand (e.g., medical terminology, generational phrases)			Correctly pronounced words; used words person can understand		
	Stood while patient was sitting; slouching, lack of poised posture			Was at the same position of the patient; had a poised posture		
	Frowned, lack of proper eye contact, inappropriate touch			Smiled, maintained proper eye contact, used light touch on hand when appropriate		
	Other:			Other:		
Empathy	Did not listen to patient's responses			Listened to patient; learned about patient		
	Lack of respect and support demonstrated			Showed respect and support		
	Lack of therapeutic communication techniques used			Used therapeutic communication techniques		
	Negative nonverbal behaviors (e.g., positioning, frowning, poor eye contact)			Positive nonverbal behaviors (e.g., at the same level as patient, smiled, good eye contact)		
	Other:			Other:		

Grading Rubric for the Affective Behaviors Checklist **Directions:** *Based on checklist results, identify the points received for the procedure checklist. Indicate how the behaviors demonstrated met the expectations.*		**Points for Procedure Checklist**	**Attempt 1**	**Attempt 2**
Does not meet Expectation	• Response lacked respect, active listening, professional nonverbal communication, and/or empathy. • Student demonstrated more than 2 negative, unprofessional behaviors during the interaction.	0		
Needs Improvement	• Response lacked respect, active listening, professional nonverbal communication, and/or empathy. • Student demonstrated 1 or 2 negative, unprofessional behaviors during the interaction.	0		
Meets Expectation	• Response was respectful and empathetic. Demonstrated active listening, professional nonverbal communication. No negative, unprofessional behaviors observed. • More practice is needed for behavior to appear natural and for student to appear comfortable and at ease.	15		
Occasionally Exceeds Expectation	• Response was respectful and empathetic. Demonstrated active listening, professional nonverbal communication. No negative, unprofessional behaviors observed. • At times student appeared comfortable and at ease; but more practice is needed for behavior to become natural and consistent with a professional medical assistant.	15		
Always Exceeds Expectation	• Response was respectful and empathetic. Demonstrated active listening, professional nonverbal communication. No negative, unprofessional behaviors observed. • Student's behaviors appeared natural and comfortable. Behaviors are consistent with a professional medical assistant.	15		

Comments

CAAHEP Competencies	Step(s)
V.P.1. Respond to nonverbal communication	5
A.3. Demonstrate empathy for patients' concerns	8
A.4. Demonstrate active listening	6
A.5. Respect diversity	2
ABHES Competencies	**Step(s)**
5. Human Relations h. Display effective interpersonal skills with patients and healthcare team members	Entire role-play
7. Administrative Procedures g. Display professionalism through written and verbal communications	Entire role-play

Work Product 2.1   History Form for Established Patient

Name _____   **Date** _____   **Score** _____

(To be used with Procedure 2.1)

MEDICAL HISTORY FORM	DATE		MRN:
NAME	DOB	AGE	
CHIEF COMPLAINT			
HX OF PRESENT ILLNESS			
ALLERGIES	CURRENT MEDICATIONS		
FEMALES: PREGNANT YES NO LMP: _____ Do you feel safe in your home? YES NO	UPDATED TO MEDICAL HISTORY SINCE LAST VISIT **NICOTINE / TOBACCO** USE: YES NO PRODUCT: AMOUNT DAILY: NUMBER OF YEARS OF USE: :_____		

Procedure 2.2   Use Feedback Techniques and Demonstrate Respect for Individual Diversity: Race

Name _____   Date _____   Score _____

Tasks: Use feedback techniques (e.g., reflection, restatement, and clarification) to obtain patient information. Respond to nonverbal communication. Communicate respectfully with patients with individual diversity related to race. Demonstrate empathy, active listening, and nonverbal communication.

Background: When working with an interpreter, allow time for the person to translate the information to the patient. Also, focus on the patient and do not look at the interpreter when speaking to the patient.

Scenario: You are rooming Maria Hernandez. She is always late for her appointments, and today she was 20 minutes late. She also does not speak English and you need to use a Spanish interpreter for the visit. You are uncomfortable in this situation because you have not worked with an interpreter before. You are also feeling rushed because she was late for her appointment.

Directions: Role-play the scenario with two peers. One peer is the patient, and the other peer is the translator. While acting as the translator, the information can be repeated in English. You need to obtain a brief medical history on this patient (e.g., chief complaint, allergies, and current medications). The peer (patient) should make up any information required.

Equipment and Supplies:
- Patient health record
- History form (optional) (Work Product 2.2)
- Pen

Standard: Complete the procedure and all critical steps in _____ minutes with a minimum score of 85% within two attempts (*or as indicated by the instructor*).

Scoring: Divide the points earned by the total possible points. Failure to perform a critical step, indicated by an asterisk (*), results in grade no higher than an 84% (*or as indicated by the instructor*).

Time: Began_____ Ended_____ Total minutes: _____

Steps	Possible Points	Attempt 1	Attempt 2
1. Greet the patient. Identify yourself. Verify the patient's identity with full name and date of birth. Explain the procedure in a manner that is understood by the patient. Answer any questions the patient may have on the procedure.	10		
2. Demonstrate respect for the patient. Focus on the patient, not on the interpreter. Pause to give the interpreter and patient time to answer. Be sincere, courteous, polite, and welcoming. Maintain the patient's dignity. Demonstrate professional, nonjudgmental verbal and nonverbal communication. Ask appropriate questions as information is obtained. (*Refer to the Affective Behaviors Checklist – **Respect** and the Grading Rubric*)	15*		
3. Using appropriate closed and open-ended questions and statements, obtain the patient's chief complaint (main reason for the visit) and history of present illness, allergies, pregnancy history, medical history, and current medications. Document the information in the health record or on the history form.	10		

4.	Use feedback techniques including reflection, restatements, and clarification as information is obtained.	10*		
5.	Respond to the patient's nonverbal communication by using feedback techniques (e.g., reflection). If the patient's nonverbal communication is interpreted differently than the patient's oral statements, clarify the information with the patient.	10*		
6.	Use active listening skills. Remain neutral and refrain from interrupting. Allow for periods of silence. Smile and nod your head to show interest. Use appropriate eye contact. Focus on the patient and avoid distractions (e.g., looking at the clock, fidgeting). *(Refer to the Affective Behaviors Checklist – **Active Listening** and the Grading Rubric)*	15*		
7.	Use professional, positive nonverbal communication behaviors. Use a clear voice, with a moderate rate and volume. Use a varying pitch and an accepting or a neutral tone. Use words the patient can understand. Correctly pronounce the words. Be at the same position as the patient. Smile and have a poised posture. Use light touch on the hand if appropriate. Maintain proper eye contact if culturally appropriate. *(Refer to the Affective Behaviors Checklist – **Nonverbal Communication** and the Grading Rubric)*	15*		
8.	Demonstrate empathy by listening to the patient and learning about their experiences and concerns. Use therapeutic communication techniques and positive nonverbal behaviors. Show your support and respect. *(Refer to the Affective Behaviors Checklist – **Empathy** and the Grading Rubric)*	15*		
	Total Score	100		

Affective Behavior	Affective Behaviors Checklist **Directions:** *Check behaviors observed during the role-play.*					
Respect	**Negative, Unprofessional Behaviors**	**Attempt**		**Positive, Professional Behaviors**	**Attempt**	
		1	2		1	2
	Rude, unkind, fake/false attitude, disrespectful, impolite, unwelcoming			Courteous, sincere, polite, welcoming		
	Unconcerned with person's dignity; brief, abrupt			Maintained person's dignity; took time with person		
	Focused on the interpreter; rushed the conversation; did not give the patient and interpreter time to talk			Focused on the patient; gave adequate time for the patient and interpreter to respond		
	Unprofessional verbal communication; inappropriate questions			Professional verbal communication		
	Negative nonverbal behaviors, poor eye contact			Positive nonverbal behaviors, proper eye contact		
	Other:			Other:		

Active Listening	Biased, offensive			Remained neutral		
	Interrupted			Refrained from interrupting		
	Did not allow for silence or pauses			Allowed for periods of silence		
	Negative nonverbal behaviors (rolled eyes, yawned, frowned, avoided eye contact)			Positive nonverbal behaviors, smiled, nodded head, appropriate eye contact		
	Distracted (looked at watch, phone)			Focused on patient, avoided distractions		
	Other:			Other:		
Nonverbal Communication	Muffled voice; too fast or slow of rate; too loud or too soft; unaccepting tone			Clear voice with moderate rate and volume; varying pitch; accepting or neutral tone		
	Incorrectly pronounced words; used words the person did not understand (e.g., medical terminology, generational phrases)			Correctly pronounced words; used words person can understand		
	Stood while patient was sitting; slouching, lack of poised posture			Was at the same position as the patient; had a poised posture		
	Frowned, lack of proper eye contact, inappropriate touch			Smiled, maintained proper eye contact, used light touch on hand when appropriate		
	Other:			Other:		
Empathy	Did not listen to patient's responses			Listened to patient; learned about patient		
	Lack of respect and support demonstrated			Showed respect and support		
	Lack of therapeutic communication techniques used			Used therapeutic communication techniques		
	Negative nonverbal behaviors (e.g., positioning, frowning, poor eye contact)			Positive nonverbal behaviors (e.g., at the same level as patient, smiled, good eye contact)		
	Other:			Other:		

Grading Rubric for the Affective Behaviors Checklist **Directions:** *Based on checklist results, identify the points received for the procedure checklist. Indicate how the behaviors demonstrated met the expectations.*	**Points for Procedure Checklist**	**Attempt 1**	**Attempt 2**
Does not meet Expectation • Response lacked respect, active listening, professional nonverbal communication, and/or empathy. • Student demonstrated more than 2 negative, unprofessional behaviors during the interaction.	0		
Needs Improvement • Response lacked respect, active listening, professional nonverbal communication, and/or empathy. • Student demonstrated 1 or 2 negative, unprofessional behaviors during the interaction.	0		
Meets Expectation • Response was respectful and empathetic. Demonstrated active listening, professional nonverbal communication. No negative, unprofessional behaviors observed. • More practice is needed for behavior to appear natural and for student to appear comfortable and at ease.	15		
Occasionally Exceeds Expectation • Response was respectful and empathetic. Demonstrated active listening, professional nonverbal communication. No negative, unprofessional behaviors observed. • At times student appeared comfortable and at ease; but more practice is needed for behavior to become natural and consistent with a professional medical assistant.	15		
Always Exceeds Expectation • Response was respectful and empathetic. Demonstrated active listening, professional nonverbal communication. No negative, unprofessional behaviors observed. • Student's behaviors appeared natural and comfortable. Behaviors are consistent with a professional medical assistant.	15		

Comments

CAAHEP Competencies	**Step(s)**
V.P.1. Respond to nonverbal communication	5
A.3. Demonstrate empathy for patients' concerns	8
A.4. Demonstrate active listening	6
A.5. Respect diversity	2
ABHES Competencies	**Step(s)**
5. Human Relations h. Display effective interpersonal skills with patients and healthcare team members	Entire role-play
i. Demonstrate cultural awareness.	Entire role-play
7. Administrative Procedures g. Display professionalism through written and verbal communications	Entire role-play

Work Product 2.2 History Form for Established Patient

Name _____ Date _____ Score _____

(To be used with Procedure 2.2)

MEDICAL HISTORY FORM	DATE		MRN:	
NAME	DOB	AGE		
CHIEF COMPLAINT				
HX OF PRESENT ILLNESS				
ALLERGIES	CURRENT MEDICATIONS			
FEMALES: PREGNANT YES NO LMP: _____ Do you feel safe in your home? YES NO	UPDATED TO MEDICAL HISTORY SINCE LAST VISIT **NICOTINE / TOBACCO** USE: YES NO PRODUCT: AMOUNT DAILY: NUMBER OF YEARS OF USE: :_____			

Procedure 2.3 Demonstrate Respect for Individual Diversity: Religion and Appearance

Name _____ Date _____ Score _____

Tasks: Respond to nonverbal communication. Communicate respectfully with patients with individual diversity related to religion and appearance. Demonstrate empathy, active listening, and nonverbal communication.

Background: The Sikh religion was founded in northern India. Sikhs believe in one god, the equality of males and females, justice, and community service. Turbans and kachera are worn at all times for religious reasons. Turbans or scarves cover the uncut hair. If the turban or scarf needs to be removed, an alternative head covering should be provided. A turban or scarf should be treated with respect. Placing it on the floor or near shoes would be a sign of disrespect. Kachera are undershorts/undergarments, and at least one leg is to remain in the kachera at all times.

Scenario: You are preparing a patient for an examination. The patient is Sikh. The provider always wants the patient to completely undress, wear a gown, and be seated on the exam table before she comes into the room. You are uncomfortable in this situation because you have never worked with a patient who is Sikh.

Directions: Role-play the scenario with a peer. Instruct the peer (patient) how to prepare for the examination.

Equipment and Supplies:
- Gown and drape sheet (optional)
- Exam table (optional)

Standard: Complete the procedure and all critical steps in _____ minutes with a minimum score of 85% within two attempts (*or as indicated by the instructor*).

Scoring: Divide the points earned by the total possible points. Failure to perform a critical step, indicated by an asterisk (*), results in grade no higher than an 84% (*or as indicated by the instructor*).

Time: Began_____ Ended_____ Total minutes: _____

Steps	Possible Points	Attempt 1	Attempt 2
1. Greet the patient. Identify yourself. Verify the patient's identity with full name and date of birth. Explain the procedure (undressing) in a manner that is understood by the patient. Answer any questions the patient may have on the procedure.	20		
2. Demonstrate respect for the patient. Be sincere, courteous, polite, and welcoming. Maintain the patient's dignity. Demonstrate professional, nonjudgmental verbal and nonverbal communication. *(Refer to the Affective Behaviors Checklist – **Respect** and the Grading Rubric)*	15*		
3. Respond to the patient's nonverbal communication by using feedback techniques (e.g., reflection). If the patient's nonverbal communication is interpreted differently than the patient's oral statements, clarify the information with the patient.	20*		

4. Use active listening skills. Remain neutral and refrain from interrupting. Smile and nod your head to show interest. Use appropriate eye contact. Focus on the patient and avoid distractions (e.g., looking at the clock, fidgeting). *(Refer to the Affective Behaviors Checklist – Active Listening and the Grading Rubric)*	**15***			
5. Use professional, positive nonverbal communication behaviors. Use a clear voice, with a moderate rate and volume. Use a varying pitch and an accepting or a neutral tone. Use words the patient can understand. Correctly pronounce the words. Be at the same eye level as the patient's. Smile and have a poised posture. Use light touch on the hand if appropriate. Maintain proper eye contact if culturally appropriate. *(Refer to the Affective Behaviors Checklist – Nonverbal Communication and the Grading Rubric)*	**15***			
6. Demonstrate empathy by listening to the patient and learning about their experiences and concerns. Use therapeutic communication techniques and positive nonverbal behaviors. Show your support and respect. *(Refer to the Affective Behaviors Checklist – Empathy and the Grading Rubric)*	**15***			
Total Score	**100**			

Affective Behavior	Affective Behaviors Checklist **Directions**: *Check behaviors observed during the role-play.*					
	Negative, Unprofessional Behaviors	**Attempt**		**Positive, Professional Behaviors**	**Attempt**	
Respect		**1**	**2**		**1**	**2**
	Rude, unkind, fake/false attitude, disrespectful, impolite, unwelcoming			Courteous, sincere, polite, welcoming		
	Unconcerned with person's dignity; brief, abrupt			Maintained person's dignity; took time with person		
	Unprofessional verbal communication; inappropriate questions			Professional verbal communication		
	Negative nonverbal behaviors, poor eye contact			Positive nonverbal behaviors, proper eye contact		
	Other:			Other:		
Active Listening	Biased, offensive			Remained neutral		
	Interrupted			Refrained from interrupting		
	Did not allow for silence or pauses			Allowed for periods of silence		
	Negative nonverbal behaviors (rolled eyes, yawned, frowned, avoided eye contact)			Positive nonverbal behaviors, smiled, nodded head, appropriate eye contact		
	Distracted (looked at watch, phone)			Focused on patient, avoided distractions		
	Other:			Other:		

Nonverbal Communication	Muffled voice; too fast or slow of rate; too loud or too soft; unaccepting tone			Clear voice with moderate rate and volume; varying pitch; accepting or neutral tone		
	Incorrectly pronounced words; used words the person did not understand (e.g., medical terminology, generational phrases)			Correctly pronounced words; used words person can understand		
	Stood while patient was sitting; slouching, lack of poised posture			Was at the same position of the patient; had a poised posture		
	Frowned. Lack of proper eye contact. Inappropriate touch.			Smiled. Maintained proper eye contact. Used light touch on hand when appropriate.		
	Other:			Other:		
Empathy	Did not listen to patient's responses			Listened to patient; learned about patient		
	Lack of respect and support demonstrated			Showed respect and support		
	Lack of therapeutic communication techniques used			Used therapeutic communication techniques		
	Negative nonverbal behaviors (e.g., positioning, frowning, poor eye contact)			Positive nonverbal behaviors (e.g., at the same level as patient, smiled, good eye contact)		
	Other:			Other:		

Grading Rubric for the Affective Behaviors Checklist **Directions**: *Based on checklist results, identify the points received for the procedure checklist. Indicate how the behaviors demonstrated met the expectations.*	**Points for Procedure Checklist**	**Attempt 1**	**Attempt 2**
Does not meet Expectation	• Response lacked respect, active listening, professional nonverbal communication, and/or empathy. • Student demonstrated more than 2 negative, unprofessional behaviors during the interaction.	0		
Needs Improvement	• Response lacked respect, active listening, professional nonverbal communication, and/or empathy. • Student demonstrated 1 or 2 negative, unprofessional behaviors during the interaction.	0		
Meets Expectation	• Response was respectful and empathetic. Demonstrated active listening, professional nonverbal communication. No negative, unprofessional behaviors observed. • More practice is needed for behavior to appear natural and for student to appear comfortable and at ease.	15		

Occasionally Exceeds Expectation	• Response was respectful and empathetic. Demonstrated active listening, professional nonverbal communication. No negative, unprofessional behaviors observed. • At times student appeared comfortable and at ease; but more practice is needed for behavior to become natural and consistent with a professional medical assistant.	15		
Always Exceeds Expectation	• Response was respectful and empathetic. Demonstrated active listening, professional nonverbal communication. No negative, unprofessional behaviors observed. • Student's behaviors appeared natural and comfortable. Behaviors are consistent with a professional medical assistant.	15		

Comments

CAAHEP Competencies	Step(s)
V.P.1. Respond to nonverbal communication	3
A.3. Demonstrate empathy for patients' concerns	6
A.4. Demonstrate active listening	4
A.5. Respect diversity	2
ABHES Competencies	**Step(s)**
5. Human Relations h. Display effective interpersonal skills with patients and healthcare team members	Entire role-play

Procedure 2.4   Use Feedback Techniques and Demonstrate Respect for Individual Diversity: Age, Economic Status, and Appearance

Name _____ Date _____ Score _____

Tasks: Use feedback techniques (e.g., reflection, restatement, and clarification) to obtain patient information. Respond to nonverbal communication. Communicate respectfully with patients with individual diversity related to age, economic status, and appearance. Demonstrate empathy, active listening, and nonverbal communication.

Scenario: You are rooming Mr. Abraham Black (79 years old), who has recently been diagnosed with dementia. He likes to talk about things that happened long before you were born, and you are not interested in those events. He also has a hard time hearing your questions, and you frequently repeat questions. Mr. Black has poor personal hygiene. His clothes are dirty and torn. He has an unpleasant body odor. Mr. Black tells you he cannot afford to eat if he buys his medications. He does not believe in government programs and refuses to take "handouts." You have worked with Mr. Black in the past and have heard this all before, numerous times. You would prefer to work with the younger generation and with patients who have better hygiene.

Directions: Using the scenario, role-play the rooming process with a peer (patient). Obtain the patient's chief complaint, allergies, and current medications. The patient should make up any information required.

Equipment and Supplies:
• Patient health record
• History form (optional) (Work Product 2.3)
• Pen

Standard: Complete the procedure and all critical steps in _____ minutes with a minimum score of 85% within two attempts (*or as indicated by the instructor*).

Scoring: Divide the points earned by the total possible points. Failure to perform a critical step, indicated by an asterisk (*), results in grade no higher than an 84% (*or as indicated by the instructor*).

Time: Began_____ Ended_____ Total minutes: _____

Steps	Possible Points	Attempt 1	Attempt 2
1. Greet the patient. Identify yourself. Verify the patient's identity with full name and date of birth. Explain the procedure in a manner that is understood by the patient. Answer any questions the patient may have on the procedure.	10		
2. Demonstrate respect for the patient. Be sincere, courteous, polite, and welcoming. Maintain the patient's dignity. Demonstrate professional, nonjudgmental verbal and nonverbal communication. Ask appropriate questions as information is obtained. *(Refer to the Affective Behaviors Checklist – **Respect** and the Grading Rubric)*	15*		
3. Using appropriate closed and open-ended questions and statements, obtain the patient's chief complaint (main reason for the visit) and history of present illness, allergies, pregnancy history, medical history, and current medications. Document the information in the health record or on the history form.	10		

4.	Use feedback techniques including reflection, restatement, and clarification as information is obtained.	**10***		
5.	Respond to the patient's nonverbal communication by using feedback techniques (e.g., reflection). If the patient's nonverbal communication is interpreted differently than the patient's oral statements, clarify the information with the patient.	**10***		
6.	Use active listening skills. Remain neutral and refrain from interrupting. Allow for periods of silence. Smile and nod your head to show interest. Use appropriate eye contact. Focus on the patient and avoid distractions (e.g., looking at the clock, fidgeting). *(Refer to the Affective Behaviors Checklist – **Active Listening** and the Grading Rubric)*	**15***		
7.	Use professional, positive nonverbal communication behaviors. (Use a clear voice, with a moderate rate and volume. Use a varying pitch and an accepting or neutral tone. Use words the patient can understand. Correctly pronounce the words. Be at the same eye level as the patient's. Smile and have a poised posture. Use light touch on the hand if appropriate. Maintain proper eye contact if culturally appropriate. *(Refer to the Affective Behaviors Checklist – **Nonverbal Communication** and the Grading Rubric)*	**15***		
8.	Demonstrate empathy by listening to the patient and learning about their experiences and concerns. Use therapeutic communication techniques and positive nonverbal behaviors. Show your support and respect. *(Refer to the Affective Behaviors Checklist – **Empathy** and the Grading Rubric)*	**15***		
	Total Score	**100**		

Affective Behavior	Affective Behaviors Checklist **Directions:** *Check behaviors observed during the role-play.*					
Respect	**Negative, Unprofessional Behaviors**	**Attempt**		**Positive, Professional Behaviors**	**Attempt**	
		1	**2**		**1**	**2**
	Rude, unkind, fake/false attitude, disrespectful, impolite, unwelcoming			Courteous, sincere, polite, welcoming		
	Unconcerned with person's dignity; brief, abrupt			Maintained person's dignity; took time with person		
	Unprofessional verbal communication; inappropriate questions			Professional verbal communication		
	Negative nonverbal behaviors, poor eye contact			Positive nonverbal behaviors, proper eye contact		
	Other:			Other:		

Active Listening	Biased, offensive			Remained neutral		
	Interrupted			Refrained from interrupting		
	Did not allow for silence or pauses			Allowed for periods of silence		
	Negative nonverbal behaviors (rolled eyes, yawned, frowned, avoided eye contact)			Positive nonverbal behaviors (smiled, nodded head, appropriate eye contact)		
	Distracted (looked at watch, phone)			Focused on patient, avoided distractions		
	Other:			Other:		
Nonverbal Communication	Muffled voice; too fast or slow of rate; too loud or too soft; unaccepting tone			Clear voice with moderate rate and volume; varying pitch; accepting or neutral tone		
	Incorrectly pronounced words; used words the person did not understand (e.g., medical terminology, generational phrases)			Correctly pronounced words; used words person can understand		
	Stood while patient was sitting; slouching, lack of poised posture			Was at the same position of the patient; had a poised posture		
	Frowned. Lack of proper eye contact. Inappropriate touch.			Smiled. Maintained proper eye contact. Used light touch on hand when appropriate.		
	Other:			Other:		
Empathy	Did not listen to patient's responses			Listened to patient; learned about patient		
	Lack of respect and support demonstrated			Showed respect and support		
	Lack of therapeutic communication techniques used			Used therapeutic communication techniques		
	Negative nonverbal behaviors (e.g., positioning, frowning, poor eye contact)			Positive nonverbal behaviors (e.g., at the same level as patient, smiled, good eye contact)		
	Other:			Other:		

Grading Rubric for the Affective Behaviors Checklist **Directions:** *Based on checklist results, identify the points received for the procedure checklist. Indicate how the behaviors demonstrated met the expectations.*		**Points for Procedure Checklist**	**Attempt 1**	**Attempt 2**
Does not meet Expectation	• Response lacked respect, active listening, professional nonverbal communication, and/or empathy. • Student demonstrated more than 2 negative, unprofessional behaviors during the interaction.	0		
Needs Improvement	• Response lacked respect, active listening, professional nonverbal communication, and/or empathy. • Student demonstrated 1 or 2 negative, unprofessional behaviors during the interaction.	0		
Meets Expectation	• Response was respectful and empathetic. Demonstrated active listening, professional nonverbal communication. No negative, unprofessional behaviors observed. • More practice is needed for behavior to appear natural and for student to appear comfortable and at ease.	15		
Occasionally Exceeds Expectation	• Response was respectful and empathetic. Demonstrated active listening, professional nonverbal communication. No negative, unprofessional behaviors observed. • At times student appeared comfortable and at ease; but more practice is needed for behavior to become natural and consistent with a professional medical assistant.	15		
Always Exceeds Expectation	• Response was respectful and empathetic. Demonstrated active listening, professional nonverbal communication. No negative, unprofessional behaviors observed. • Student's behaviors appeared natural and comfortable. Behaviors are consistent with a professional medical assistant.	15		

Comments

CAAHEP Competencies	**Step(s)**
V.P.1. Respond to nonverbal communication	5
A.3. Demonstrate empathy for patients' concerns	8
A.4. Demonstrate: active listening	6
A.5. Respect diversity	2
ABHES Competencies	**Step(s)**
5. Human Relations h. Display effective interpersonal skills with patients and healthcare team members	Entire role-play
7. Administrative Procedures g. Display professionalism through written and verbal communications	Entire role-play

Work Product 2.3 History Form for Established Patient

Name _____ **Date** _____ **Score** _____

(To be used with Procedure 2.4)

MEDICAL HISTORY FORM	DATE		MRN:
NAME	DOB	AGE	
CHIEF COMPLAINT			
HX OF PRESENT ILLNESS			
ALLERGIES	CURRENT MEDICATIONS		
FEMALES: PREGNANT YES NO LMP: _____ Do you feel safe in your home? YES NO	UPDATED TO MEDICAL HISTORY SINCE LAST VISIT **NICOTINE / TOBACCO** USE: YES NO PRODUCT: AMOUNT DAILY: NUMBER OF YEARS OF USE: :_____		

Procedure 2.5 Demonstrate Appropriate Self-Boundaries

Name _____ Date _____ Score _____

Task: Use respectful and tactful communication while demonstrating the principles of self-boundaries.

Background: For the medical assistant to have a professional therapeutic relationship with a patient, the medical assistant must guard against crossing self-boundaries, which are also called *professional boundaries*. The relationship between the medical assistant and the patient needs to be professional. It cannot be a dual relationship, where the medical assistant also becomes a friend to the patient. This means the medical assistant cannot share personal intimate information, contact the patient outside of the work environment, befriend the patient on social media, or engage in a flirty or romantic relationship with the patient.

Scenario #1: You are rooming Morgan, who frequently sees the provider you work for. You have gotten to know Morgan over the time you have worked for the provider. Today, Morgan asks you for your personal phone number and social media information.

Scenario #2: You are rooming Sam, whom you have gotten to know well over the time you have worked for your provider. Sam is outgoing, enjoys talking, and has many of the same interests as you do. You have just split up with your significant other and have been feeling a bit down. Sam asks you if you would be available for coffee sometime.

Directions: Role-play the scenarios with a peer. Your peer will play the patient in the scenario and you are the medical assistant.

Standard: Complete the role-play in _____ minutes with a minimum score of 100% within two attempts (*or as indicated by the instructor*).

Scoring: Divide the points earned by the total possible points. Met competency: 100% (10 points). Not met competency: 0% (0 points).

Time: Began_____ Ended_____ Total minutes: _____

Affective Behavior	Affective Behaviors Checklist Directions: *Check behaviors observed during the role-play.*					
Respect	**Negative, Unprofessional Behaviors**	**Attempt**		**Positive, Professional Behaviors**	**Attempt**	
		1	**2**		**1**	**2**
	Rude, unkind, disrespectful, and/or impolite			Courteous and polite		
	Unconcerned with person's dignity			Maintained person's dignity		
	Poor eye contact			Proper eye contact		
	Negative nonverbal behaviors			Positive nonverbal behaviors		
	Other:			Other:		

Tactful	Improper and/or inappropriate.			Proper and appropriate.		
	Spoke and/or acted in a manner that was offensive to others.			Spoke and acted without offending others.		
	Failed to address the self-boundaries/professional boundary issue or followed through on what the patient wanted.			Addressed the self-boundaries/professional boundary issue in a clear and diplomatic way.		
	Failed to show awareness of the patient's personal space; was too close to the patient during the interaction.			Showed awareness of the patient's personal space and maintained a comfortable distance.		
	Lacked courtesy; demonstrated unprofessional behaviors (verbal or nonverbal) during a difficult situation.			Showed courtesy and professionalism in a difficult situation.		
	Other:			Other:		

Grading Rubric for the Affective Behaviors Checklist **Directions:** *Based on checklist results, identify the points received for the procedure checklist. Indicate how the behaviors demonstrated met the expectations.*		**Point Value**	**Attempt 1**	**Attempt 2**
Does Not Meet Expectation	• Response was disrespectful and/or not tactful. • Student demonstrated more than two negative, unprofessional behaviors during the interaction.	0		
Needs Improvement	• Response was disrespectful and/or not tactful. • Student demonstrated one or two negative, unprofessional behaviors during the interaction.	0		
Meets Expectation	• Response was respectful and tactful; no negative, unprofessional behaviors observed. • More practice is needed for behavior to appear natural and for student to appear comfortable and at ease.	10		
Occasionally Exceeds Expectation	• Response was respectful and tactful; no negative, unprofessional behaviors observed. • At times student appeared comfortable and at ease; but more practice is needed for behavior to become natural and consistent with a professional medical assistant.	10		
Always Exceeds Expectation	• Response was respectful and tactful; no negative, unprofessional behaviors observed. • Student's behaviors appeared natural and comfortable. Behaviors are consistent with a professional medical assistant.	10		

Comments

CAAHEP Competencies	Step(s)
A.6 Recognize personal boundaries	Entire role-play
ABHES Competencies	**Step(s)**
5. Human Relations h. Display effective interpersonal skills with patients and healthcare team members	Entire role-play

Legal Principles

CAAHEP Competencies	Assessment
X.C.1. Identify scope of practice and standards of care for medical assistants.	Skills and Concepts – K. 16-17
X.C.2. Identify the provider role in terms of standard of care.	Skills and Concepts – C. 18
X.C.4. Identify the standards outlined in The Patient Care Partnership	Skills and Concepts – J. 2-4
X.C.5. Identify licensure and certification as they apply to healthcare providers	Skills and Concepts – K. 1-7
X.C.6. Identify criminal and civil law as they apply to the practicing medical assistant	Skills and Concepts – B. 9
X.C.7.a. Define: negligence	Skills and Concepts – C. 8
X.C.7.b. Define: malpractice	Skills and Concepts – C. 11
X.C.7.c. Define: statute of limitations	Skills and Concepts – D. 4; Certification Preparation – 2
X.C.8. Identify the purpose of medical malpractice insurance.	Skills and Concepts – F. 1
X.C.13.a. Define the following medical legal terms: informed consent	Skills and Concepts – I. 1
X.C.13.b. Define the following medical legal terms: implied consent	Skills and Concepts – I. 5; Certification Preparation – 10
X.C.13.c. Define the following medical legal terms: expressed consent	Skills and Concepts – I. 2; Certification Preparation – 10
X.C.13.d. Define the following medical legal terms: patient incompetence	Skills and Concepts – G. 12
X.C.13.e. Define the following medical legal terms: emancipated minor	Skills and Concepts – G. 14
X.C.13.f. Define the following medical legal terms: mature minor	Skills and Concepts – I. 3; Certification Preparation – 8
X.C.13.g. Define the following medical legal terms: subpoena duces tecum	Skills and Concepts – E. 16; Certification Preparation – 6

CAAHEP Competencies	Assessment
X.C.13.h. Define the following medical legal terms: respondeat superior	Skills and Concepts - H. 4; Certification Preparation – 9
X.C.13.i. Define the following medical legal terms: res ipsa loquitur	Skills and Concepts – E. 5
X.C.13.j. Define the following medical legal terms: locum tenens	Skills and Concepts – K. 13; Certification Preparation – 7
X.C.13.k. Define the following medical legal terms: defendant-plaintiff	Skills and Concepts - B. 2, 3
X.C.13.l. Define the following medical legal terms: deposition	Skills and Concepts – E. 13
X.C.13.m. Define the following medical legal terms: arbitration-mediation	Skills and Concepts – E. 6, 8; Certification Preparation – 1
X.P.1. Locate a state's legal scope of practice for medical assistants	Procedure 3.2

ABHES Competencies	Assessment
4. Medical Law and Ethics c. Follow established policies when initiating or terminating medical treatment	Skills and Concepts – H. 1-2e
4.d. Distinguish between employer and personal liability coverage	Skills and Concepts – F. 2-6
4.f. Comply with federal, state, and local health laws and regulations 1) Define the scope of practice for the medical assistant within the state where employed	Procedure 3.2
4.f.2) Describe what procedures can and cannot be delegated to the medical assistant and by whom within various employment settings	Skills and Concepts – K. 18a-f

VOCABULARY REVIEW

Using the word pool on the right, find the correct word to match the definition. Write the word on the line after the definition.

Group A

1. Prone to lawsuits _____

2. A bill that has passed becomes this; also found in the name of a specific law _____

3. A rule of conduct or action prescribed or formally recognized as enforceable by a controlling authority _____

4. Used more to refer to the contents of the actual law _____

5. A piece of legislation passed by a municipality or local government _____

6. A prior court decision that serves as a model for similar legal cases in the future _____

Word Pool
- act
- case law
- common law
- constitutional law
- law
- litigious
- ordinance
- precedent
- statute
- statutory law

7. Derived from legal precedents and common law
   _____

8. Derived from the federal and state constitutions, which give power to federal and state governments _____

9. Unwritten laws that come from judicial decisions based on societal traditions and customs _____

10. Refers to the laws enacted by state and federal legislatures
    _____

Group B

1. Legally responsible or obligated _____

2. A strategy used by the defendant to avoid liability in a lawsuit
   _____

3. Lack of actions _____

4. Statutes that define actions or omissions (lack of actions) that threaten and / or harm public safety and welfare
   _____

5. Actions or omissions that are prohibited by criminal laws (and the government) _____

6. Protect and define private rights _____

7. A civil wrongdoing that causes harm to a person or property, excludes breach of contract _____

8. The individual or entity who committed the tort, either intentionally or as a result of negligence _____

9. Laws related to procedures, regulations, and rules of governmental administrative agencies _____

10. A monetary settlement the defendant pays the plaintiff in a civil case for loss or injury _____

Word Pool
- civil laws
- crimes
- criminal law
- damages
- defense
- liable
- omissions
- regulatory and administrative law
- tort
- tortfeasor

Group C

1. A court order by which an individual or institution is required to perform or refrain from performing a certain act
   _____

2. A settlement for a specific dollar amount that directly relates to medical bills _____

3. A court judgment that defines the legal rights of the parties involved _____

4. The process of settling disputes outside of litigation
   _____

5. A legal obligation _____

6. The person or company purchasing the insurance policy
   _____

Word Pool
- alternative dispute resolution
- declaratory judgment
- injunction
- insured
- insurer
- legally binding
- nominal damages
- premium
- special damages
- third party

7. Very small settlement because the plaintiff's injury was slight

   _____

8. The payment the insured pays to the insurance company

   _____

9. Another name for the insurance company

   _____

10. When the insurer pays the plaintiff, the plaintiff is known as
    the _____

Group D

1. One party voluntarily agrees with another party's proposition or
   plan _____

2. An agreement between two parties _____

3. Person voluntarily gives up license _____

4. License is terminated and the person can no longer practice in that
   occupation in the state _____

5. Person's license is monitored for a specific period of time

   _____

6. Person cannot practice in that occupation for a specific period of
   time _____

7. Person is sent a warning or letter of concern

   _____

Word Pool
- contract
- consent
- license revoked
- license surrendered
- license suspended
- probation
- reprimand

ABBREVIATIONS
Write out what each of the following abbreviations stands for.

1. DOB _____

2. VIS _____

3. CMA _____

4. LPN _____

5. NP _____

6. CNM _____

7. RN _____

8. PA _____

9. MD _____

10. DO _____

11. OWI _____

12. OUI _____

13. ADR _____

14. CDC _____

15. CAAHEP _____

SKILLS AND CONCEPTS

Answer the following questions. Write your answer on the line or in the space provided.

A. Sources of Law

1. A(n) _____ is a rule of conduct or action prescribed or formally recognized as enforceable by a controlling authority.

2. The _____ is the supreme law of the United States.

3. The _____ branch includes the Supreme Court and interprets laws according to the U.S. Constitution.

4. The _____ branch includes Congress and makes new laws.

5. The president administers the _____ branch and issues executive orders, appoints judges, and makes treaties with other nations.

6. Case law was derived from legal _____ and _____.

B. Criminal and Civil Law

1. _____ law determines the rights and obligations of the people and _____ laws must be followed when investigating and prosecuting unlawful acts.

2. _____ is an individual or party who brings the suit to court.

3. _____ is an individual or business against whom a lawsuit is filed

4. In criminal law, the wrongdoing is called a(n) _____ and in civil law it can be called a(n) _____ or a(n) _____.

5. A(n) _____, a serious criminal offense, is punishable by a substantial fine and _____ time _____ 1 year.

6. A(n) _____, a lesser criminal offense, is punishable by a substantial fine and possible _____ time _____ 1 year.

7. Contract issues, divorce, child custody, product liability, and accidents are common types of disputes handled in the _____ court system.

8. If the matter is brought to court, in the _____ court system, most of the time there is a trial by jury; whereas with the _____ court system, cases are decided by the judge and many times there is no jury.

9. Describe criminal and civil law as they apply to the practicing medical assistant. Your answer should also provide an example of a criminal and civil matter that relates to medical assistants. (Provide examples other than those in the textbook.)

_____

_____

_____

_____

_____

C. Tort Law

1. With _____ torts, the plaintiff must prove the defendant had specific intent to perform the action that caused the injury and _____ or _____ torts result when a person's conduct falls below the standard of behavior expected of a reasonable person in the same situation.

Define the following terms by matching the definition with the term.

2. _____ Disclosing private facts without the consent of the individual or intrusion into a person's personal life

3. _____ The intentional restraint of another individual without consent or reason

4. _____ Deceiving or lying to a person or party for monetary gain

5. _____ Intentionally saying something or writing something false about another person that causes harm

6. _____ Written defamation

7. _____ Spoken defamation

8. _____ Failure to act as a reasonably prudent person would under similar circumstances; such conduct falls below the standards of behavior established by law for the protection of others against unreasonable risk of harm

9. _____ Uses reasonable behavior as an objective test to measure another's actions or lack of actions

10. _____ Refers to the level and type of care an ordinary, prudent healthcare professional, having the same training and experience in a similar practice, would have provided under a similar situation.

11. _____ A type of negligence in which a licensed professional fails to provide the standard of care, causing harm to a person

12. _____ Failure to act when one had a legal duty to act

13. _____ Performance of an unlawful, wrongful act

14. _____ Improper performance of a lawful act that causes damage or injury

15. _____ Range of responsibilities and practice guidelines that determine the boundaries within which a healthcare worker practices

a. fraud
b. defamation
c. false imprisonment
d. slander
e. scope of practice
f. invasion of privacy
g. unintentional torts
h. malfeasance
i. nonfeasance
j. misfeasance
k. reasonable person standard
l. malpractice
m. standard of care
n. libel

Answer the following questions.

16. Explain the "reasonable person" standard and how it can determine negligent acts._____

_____

_____

17. How does medical malpractice differ from negligence?_____

_____

_____

18. Discuss the provider's role in terms of standard of care. _____

_____

_____

_____

D. Defenses to Liability

1. Which of the following is a type of defense?
   a. Technical
   b. Denial
   c. Affirmative
   d. All of the above

2. Which is a requirement for Good Samaritan Law protection?
   a. A person must provide treatment in a true emergency.
   b. Care must be provided outside of a place with necessary medical equipment.
   c. The provider cannot bill the patient for the care provided.
   d. All of the above

Define the following terms by matching the definition with the term.

3. _____ Latin for "a thing decided;" once a case has been decided by the court, it cannot be litigated again

4. _____ The length of time legal action can be taken after an event has occurred

5. _____ Used when none of the facts are true

6. _____ The defendant can show evidence that the plaintiff knew about the risks involved and consented to proceed with the activity

7. _____ The defendant admits to wrongdoing, but their attorney introduces facts that support the defendant's conduct

8. _____ The plaintiff's action or lack of action caused the injury to a certain percent

a. assumption of risk
b. affirmative defense
c. comparative negligence
d. denial defense
e. *res judicata*
f. statute of limitations

E. Resolving a Civil Lawsuit

Define the following terms by matching the definition with the term.

1. _____ The healthcare professional has a legal obligation to the patient.

2. _____ The breach of duty of care directly causes the patient's injury.

3. _____ A monetary settlement the defendant pays the plaintiff in a civil case for loss or injury. Also, one of the 4 Ds of negligence, meaning the patient suffers a legally recognized injury.

4. _____ The healthcare professional breaches (violates) the duty of care to the patient.

5. _____ A Latin term meaning "the thing speaks for itself." A legal concept under which the plaintiff's burden to prove malpractice is minimal since the jury can clearly understand the details of the injury.

6. _____ The process in which conflicting parties in a dispute submit their differences to a court-appointed person, who submits a legally binding decision.

7. _____ Monetary payment to the plaintiff for losses suffered.

8. _____ The process of facilitating conflicting parties to make an agreement, settlement, or compromise.

9. _____ A person who observed the situation and testifies in court about the facts of the case.

10. _____ Large payments made to the plaintiff by the defendant as ordered by the court and meant to punish the defendant.

11. _____ Monetary payments to the plaintiff for emotional pain and anguish.

12. _____ A person who is educated and knowledgeable in the area of concern and provides their opinion in court.

13. _____ A sworn testimony made before a court-appointed officer; it is used in the discovery process and may be used in the trial.

14. _____ Written or oral questions that must be answered under oath.

15. _____ A court order requiring a person to appear in court at a specific time to testify in a legal case.

16. _____ A legal document commanding a person to bring a piece of evidence (e.g., the plaintiff's health record) to court.

a. dereliction
b. arbitration
c. expert witness
d. fact witness
e. damages
f. *res ipsa loquitur*
g. direct cause
h. duty of care
i. mediation
j. punitive damages
k. compensatory damages
l. general damages
m. interrogatory
n. *subpoena duces tecum*
o. subpoena
p. deposition

F. Professional Liability Insurance

1. Describe the purpose of medical malpractice insurance. _____

_____

_____

_____

_____

Match the description with the insurance-related term.

2. _____ A type of liability coverage used by professionals to protect themselves against liability suits incurred because of errors and omissions while performing their professional services

3. _____ A type of liability coverage that protects against claims related to harm other than bodily injury

4. _____ A type of liability coverage purchased by companies. It protects businesses from lawsuits for property loss and bodily injury from nonemployees

5. _____ An insurance policy that covers claims made during the policy year

6. _____ An insurance policy that covers claims for wrongful acts that occurred during the policy year

a. general liability insurance
b. occurrence policy
c. personal injury insurance
d. professional liability insurance
e. claims-made policy

G. Contracts
Match the description with the element required for a legally binding contract.

1. _____ The second party agrees to the offer.
2. _____ A person entering a contract must have legal capacity.
3. _____ The consideration must be legal.
4. _____ Made by one party.
5. _____ Each party exchanges something of value.

a. offer
b. consideration
c. competency and capacity
d. legal subject matter
e. acceptance

Select the correct answer.

6. What is a condition related to competency and capacity that would invalidate a contract?
   a. Underage (minor)
   b. Incompetence
   c. Intoxicated or under the influence of drugs
   d. All of the above

7. Which of the following activities can an emancipated minor *not* do?
   a. Be a party in a contract and sue
   b. Vote and buy alcohol
   c. Keep earned income and apply for public benefits
   d. Make all of their own healthcare decisions

Define the following terms by matching the definition with the term.

8. _____ A common law concept that requires specific types of contracts must be in writing to avoid fraud and to be binding.

9. _____ The parties have agreed to the terms of the contract through their actions and behaviors.

10. _____ One who has not reached adulthood.

11. _____ The parties have specifically stated the terms of the contract in writing, orally, or both.

12. _____ A patient who lacks the ability to manage personal affairs due to mental deficiency; an appointed guardian or conservator manages the patient's affairs.

13. _____ Occurs when the terms of the contract are not fulfilled by one party without a legitimate legal reason.

14. _____ A minor who has been granted emancipation by the court; the minor can assume the rights and responsibilities of adulthood.

a. breach of contract
b. implied contract
c. expressed contract
d. patient incompetence
e. emancipated minor
f. statute of frauds
g. minor

H. Provider-Patient Relationship

1. Which is a reason providers terminate the provider-patient relationship?
   a. Retirement or moving
   b. Patient isn't paying for the services provided
   c. Due to patient's behavior or if the patient isn't following the provider's treatment plan
   d. All of the above

2. Complete the description of the termination process for the provider-patient relationship. Write the word or phrase on the line.

   a. _____ must notify the patient in writing of the withdrawal of care.

   b. A(n) _____ must be indicated for the termination and there must be an adequate period of coverage to allow the patient to find another provider.

   c. The termination letter should be sent as a(n) _____ with return receipt requested.

   d. A(n) _____ and the return receipt need to be placed or scanned into the patient's health record.

   e. _____ should be notified of the termination date so no appointments are made after that date.

3. Providers can be charged with _____ if they do not follow the proper termination procedure.

4. _____ is a common law doctrine that means "let the master answer" and means that the employer/provider is liable for actions that the employee did or did not do within the scope of employment.

5. How can a medical assistant protect the provider from charges of patient abandonment? _____

_____

_____

I. Consents

Define the following terms by matching the definition with the term.

1. _____ A legal process that ensures the patient or guardian understands the treatment and gives consent for the treatment

2. _____ Consent that is given either by the spoken or written word

3. _____ A person under the age of adulthood who demonstrates the maturity to make a personal healthcare decision and can give informed consent for treatment

4. _____ One party voluntarily agrees with another party's proposition or plan

5. _____ Consent that is inferred based on signs, actions, or conduct of the patient rather than oral communication

a. informed consent
b. implied consent
c. expressed consent
d. consent
e. mature minor

Select the correct answer.

6. The elements that must be present for informed consent include that the patient or guardian
   a. is competent to understand and decide and voluntarily decides to agree to or refuse the treatment.
   b. understands the diagnosis, reason for treatment, proposed treatment, and the risks of the treatment.
   c. understands the alternative treatments available, the risks of the treatments, and the risks if treatment is delayed or not done.
   d. signs a treatment consent form.
   e. All of the above

7. Who can give informed consent?
   a. Adults with sound mind
   b. Married minors and minor parents
   c. Emancipated minors and mature minors
   d. All of the above

8. Who *cannot* give informed consent?
   a. Patients under the influence of alcohol or drugs
   b. A minor
   c. A patient who is mentally incompetent
   d. A patient who speaks little to no English and no interpreter service was provided
   e. All of the above

9. What is the medical assistant's role with informed consent?
   a. Prepare the informed consent form.
   b. Educate the patient on the procedure.
   c. Educate the patient on alternative procedures.
   d. All of the above

J. Patient's Rights and Responsibilities

1. The Affordable Care Act's Patient's Bill of Rights focuses on rights related to _____.

2. The _____ document helps patients understand the expectations for patients and the patients' rights and responsibilities.

3. The Patient Care Partnership document replaces the _____, though it covers the same topics.

4. Which topic(s) is/are included in the Patient's Bill of Rights and the Patient Care Partnership document?
    a. The patient's rights related to medical care, respectful treatment, privacy and confidentiality, identity, explanation of care, informed consent, research projects, and safe environment
    b. The patient's rights to be informed of the facility's conduct rules and regulations
    c. The patient's responsibilities (e.g., providing information, respect and consideration, compliance with medical care, medical records, responsibilities based on the clinic's rules and regulations, and reporting of patient complaints)
    d. All of the above

5. A patient refuses an injection of medication ordered by the provider. Describe the steps that need to be followed by the medical assistant.

_____

_____

_____

_____

K. Practice Requirements

Match the licensure and certification for the following healthcare professionals. Answers may be used more than once.

1. _____ Doctor of medicine (MD)
2. _____ Physician assistant (PA)
3. _____ Doctor of osteopathy (DO)
4. _____ Nurse practitioner (NP)
5. _____ Registered nurse (RN)
6. _____ Medical assistant (MA)
7. _____ Licensed practical nurse (LPN)

   a. Must pass a licensure exam to practice.
   b. National certification exam is optional.
   c. Obtains the certification after passing the national exam. Must obtain a state license to practice.
   d. Must pass all three parts of the U.S. Medical Licensing Exam and obtain a state license to practice.

Define the following terms by matching the definition with the term.

8. _____ The state's laws and regulations that govern the practice of medicine

9. _____ A voluntary process indicating that a person has met predetermined criteria

10. _____ A state board grants a license to a person who is currently licensed in another state that has the same or stricter standards

11. _____ A state has a written agreement with another state to recognize licenses issued by that state without additional review of the person's credentials

12. _____ People working in a specific occupation have their name entered into an official registry

   a. reciprocity
   b. Medical Practice Act
   c. endorsement
   d. *locum tenens*
   e. telemedicine
   f. certification
   g. registration
   h. licensure

13. _____ Latin for "to substitute for;" the term refers to physicians or advanced-practice professionals who temporarily contract to provide healthcare services when a facility has a vacancy, vacation, or a leave of absence.

14. _____ A mandatory process established by state law that ensures a person has met the legal standards for practicing an occupation in that state.

15. _____ The use of telecommunication technology to provide healthcare services to patients at a distance; it is usually used in rural communities.

Answer the following questions.

16. Describe the scope of practice for medical assistants. _____

_____

_____

_____

17. Describe the standard of care for medical assistants. _____

_____

_____

_____

18. For the following activities, identify if the medical assistant could be delegated (assigned) by the provider to do the activity. Write "yes" on the line if the medical assistant could be delegated the activity. Write "no" on the line if the medical assistant could not do the activity.

    a. Prepare the informed consent paperwork. _____

    b. Discuss the procedure with the patient for the informed consent. _____

    c. Prepare waived laboratory testing. _____

    d. Answer phone calls. _____

    e. Prescribe medications for the patient's condition. _____

    f. Diagnose the patient's condition. _____

L. Accreditation

1. _____ is a recognition granted by a specific organization to educational, healthcare, or managed care organizations that have demonstrated compliance with standards.

Match the organization with its role.

2. _____ Accredits ambulatory care facilities, hospitals, behavioral healthcare facilities, home healthcare agencies, and laboratory services

3. _____ Accredits medical laboratories

4. _____ Accredits health plans

    a. National Committee for Quality Assurance

    b. The Joint Commission

    c. College of American Pathologists Laboratory Accreditation Program

CERTIFICATION PREPARATION

Circle the correct answer.

1. Which is a type of alternative dispute resolution where the final decision is legally binding?
   a. Dereliction
   b. Mediation
   c. Arbitration
   d. Summary judgment

2. Which varies by state and indicates the length of time legal action can be taken after an event has occurred?
   a. *Res judicata*
   b. *Res ipsa loquitur*
   c. Release of tortfeasor
   d. Statute of limitations

3. Which is a negligent act classification that means the person failed to act when he or she had a legal duty to act?
   a. Misfeasance
   b. Nonfeasance
   c. Malpractice
   d. Malfeasance

4. Which type of defense involves the defendant admitting wrongdoing and the defense attorney introduces facts that support the defendant's conduct?
   a. Denial defense
   b. Comparative defense
   c. Technical defense
   d. Affirmative defense

5. Which is not one of the "Ds" of negligence?
   a. Duty of care
   b. Dereliction
   c. Deposition
   d. Damages

6. Which is a legal document ordering a person to bring the plaintiff's health record to court?
   a. Subpoena
   b. *Subpoena duces tecum*
   c. *Res ipsa loquitur*
   d. Statute of limitations

7. Which is a physician or advanced-practice professional temporarily contracted to provide healthcare services when a facility has a vacancy, vacation, or a leave of absence?
   a. Telemedicine
   b. Injunction
   c. *Respondeat superior*
   d. *Locum tenens*

8. A person younger than the age of adulthood who demonstrates the maturity to make a personal healthcare decision and can give informed consent for treatment is called a(n)
   a. mature minor.
   b. emancipated minor.
   c. incompetence.
   d. *respondeat superior.*

9. Which means "let the master answer;" thus, the employer/provider is legally responsible for the wrongful actions or lack of actions of the employees if done within the scope of employment?
   a. Tortfeasor
   b. *Res ipsa loquitur*
   c. *Respondeat superior*
   d. *Res judicata*

10. _____ consent is inferred based on signs or conduct of the patient, whereas _____ consent is given either by the spoken or written word.
    a. Implied; informed
    b. Informed; expressed
    c. Implied; expressed
    d. Expressed; informed

WORKPLACE APPLICATIONS

1. Cara has just graduated from a medical assistant program and decides to take out a professional liability insurance policy. She wants a policy that she can stop paying at retirement and will still be covered for past situations. Describe what type of policy she should purchase.

   _____

   _____

   _____

   _____

2. Dr. Smith and Dr. Brown are family practice providers who trained at the same college. Dr. Smith practices in Los Angeles, CA and Dr. Brown practices in Bayfield, WI (a city of fewer than 600 people). Would the standard of care be the same for these two family practice providers? Explain your answer.

   _____

   _____

   _____

3. Jane is a medical assistant who works with Dr. Walden. She identifies herself as "Dr. Walden's nurse" to patients. Discuss how this might impact the standard of care.

   _____

   _____

4. Ken Thomas was notified by a medical supplier that the mesh that was used for his hernia surgery was faulty. They paid Ken a monetary compensation after Ken signed a release to give up the right to sue the company in the future. Five years later, Ken had to go through surgery to remove the mesh. Ken wanted to sue the company for his pain and suffering. What technical defense would be used to prevent the lawsuit? Discuss this technical defense.

   _____

   _____

   _____

5. Bella, a new CMA, is working with a patient who is undergoing minor surgery. The provider explained the procedure and stepped out of the room. She needs to get the informed consent form signed. When she asks the patient if she has any questions before signing, the patient states she does. How should Bella handle this situation?

   _____

   _____

   _____

INTERNET ACTIVITIES

1. Using the internet, find a local healthcare facility that has their Patient's Bill of Rights posted online. Create a poster presentation or a PowerPoint presentation summarizing the areas addressed in the facility's Patient's Bill of Rights.

2. Using online resources, research how an MD and/or DO can renew their license in your state. Write a brief summary of what is required to renew a medical doctor's license in your state. Cite the website(s) used.

3. Credentialed medical assistants need to maintain their credentials through continuing education. Using online resources, identify two sites that offer continuing education for medical assistants. Briefly summarize your findings and cite the websites used.

Procedure 3.1   Apply the Patient's Bill of Rights

Name _____ Date _____ Score _____

Tasks: Apply the Patient's Bill of Rights in scenarios related to choice of treatment, consent for treatment, and refusal of treatment. Demonstrate sensitivity to the patients' rights.

Scenario 1 (Choice of treatment): Julia Berkley (DOB 07/05/19XX) saw Dr. Angela Perez during her entire pregnancy. Julia is experiencing some complications. Dr. Perez explained the choices Julia had for delivery. She stated that with the complications, a cesarean delivery (C-section) may be the best option. Because you are working with Dr. Perez, you prepare the consent form for the C-section. You go into the exam room to have Julia sign the consent form. As you discuss the form, Julia tells you that she is fearful of a C-section and wants a vaginal delivery.

Scenario 2 (Consent for treatment): Ken Thomas (DOB 10/25/19XX) sees Jean Burke, NP, before leaving on a week-long trip out of the country. He is leaving in 3 days and wants a hepatitis A vaccine injection. The area he is traveling to has a high risk for hepatitis A. Jean Burke orders immunoglobulin for Ken, which will provide immediate protection against hepatitis A. You prepare the injection and enter the exam room. As you are telling Ken about the side effects of the medication, he asks, "What is immunoglobulin?" You reply that it is a sterile medication made of antibodies from blood. Ken states that he is a Jehovah's Witness and cannot receive blood products.

Scenario 3 (Refusal of treatment): Aaron Jackson (DOB 10/17/20XX) is brought in by his mother for his well-child checkup. His records indicate that he is due for his first varicella vaccine injection. You bring the Varicella (Chickenpox) Vaccine VIS (vaccine information statement) and the vaccine authorization form to the exam room. As you start to discuss the vaccine, Aaron's mother, Patricia, interrupts you and tells you she is not interested in having Aaron get his chickenpox vaccination.

Equipment and Supplies:
- Patient health records
- Patient's Bill of Rights (Figure 3.3)
- General procedure consent form (Figure 3.4)
- Varicella (Chickenpox) VIS (available at *https://www.cdc.gov*)
- Vaccine authorization form (Figure 3.5)

Standard: Complete the procedure and all critical steps in _____ minutes with a minimum score of 85% within two attempts (*or as indicated by the instructor*).

Scoring: Divide the points earned by the total possible points. Failure to perform a critical step, indicated by an asterisk (*), results in grade no higher than an 84% (*or as indicated by the instructor*).

Time: Began_____ Ended_____ Total minutes: _____

Steps:	Point Value	Attempt 1	Attempt 2
1. Review the Patient's Bill of Rights. Apply the Patient's Bill of Rights as you role-play each of the three scenarios.	10*		
2. Using Scenario 1, role-play the situation with a peer. You are the medical assistant. Demonstrate how a medical assistant should handle the situation. Apply the Patient's Bill of Rights to the situation by remembering the rights of the patient. a. Show sensitivity to the patient by being respective and professional. Be open and accepting in your verbal and nonverbal body language. (*Refer to the Checklist for Affective Behaviors.*)	10*		
b. Ask the patient if she has any questions about the procedures. Let the provider know if the patient has questions.	10		
c. Ask the patient what she would like to do. Based on her answer, follow up as necessary.	10*		
d. Using the health record, document the patient's decision and the name of the provider notified.	5		
3. Using Scenario 2, role-play the situation with a peer. You are the medical assistant. Demonstrate how a medical assistant should handle the situation. Apply the Patient's Bill of Rights to the situation by remembering the rights of the patient. a. Show sensitivity to the patient regarding his right to refuse. Be respectful and professional. Be open and accepting in your verbal and nonverbal body language. Be accepting of his beliefs and his refusal. (*Refer to the Checklist for Affective Behaviors.*)	10*		
b. When the patient refuses the medication, be respectful in your body language and words. Notify the provider.	10*		
c. Using the health record, document the patient's decision and the name of the provider notified.	5		
4. Using Scenario 3, role-play the situation with a peer. You are the medical assistant. Demonstrate how a medical assistant should handle the situation. Apply the Patient's Bill of Rights to the situation by remembering the rights of the patient. a. Show sensitivity to the mother of the patient by being respectful and professional. Be open and accepting in your verbal and nonverbal body language. (*Refer to the Checklist for Affective Behaviors.*)	10*		
b. Ask the mother if she has any questions about the vaccine. Let the provider know if the mother has questions.	5		
c. Ask the mother what she would like to do. Based on her answer, follow up as necessary.	10*		
d. Using the health record, document the mother's decision and the name of the provider notified.	5		
Total Points	100		

Checklist for Affective Behaviors

Affective Behavior	Directions: *Check behaviors observed during the role-play.*				
Sensitivity	**Negative, Unprofessional Behaviors**	**Attempt** 1	2	**Positive, Professional Behaviors**	**Attempt** 1	2
	Poor eye contact			Proper eye contact		
	Distracted; not focused on the other person			Focuses full attention on the other person		
	Judgmental attitude; not accepting attitude			Nonjudgmental, accepting attitude		
	Fails to clarify what the person verbally or nonverbally communicated			Uses summarizing or paraphrasing to clarify what the person verbally or nonverbally communicated		
	Fails to acknowledge what the person communicated			Acknowledges what the person communicated		
	Rude, discourteous			Pleasant and courteous		
	Disregards the person's dignity and rights			Maintains the person's dignity and rights		
	Other:			Other:		

Grading for Affective Behaviors		Point Value	Attempt 1	Attempt 2
Does not meet Expectation	• Response lacked sensitivity. • Student demonstrated more than 2 negative, unprofessional behaviors during the interaction.	0		
Needs Improvement	• Response lacked sensitivity. • Student demonstrated 1 or 2 negative, unprofessional behaviors during the interaction.	0		
Meets Expectation	• Response was sensitive; no negative, unprofessional behaviors observed. • More practice is needed for behavior to appear natural and for student to appear comfortable and at ease.	10		
Occasionally Exceeds Expectation	• Response was sensitive; no negative, unprofessional behaviors observed. • At times student appeared comfortable and at ease; but more practice is needed for behavior to become natural and consistent with a professional medical assistant.	10		
Always Exceeds Expectation	• Response was sensitive; no negative, unprofessional behaviors observed. • Student's behaviors appeared natural and comfortable. Behaviors are consistent with a professional medical assistant.	10		

Documentation – Scenario 1

Documentation – Scenario 2

Documentation – Scenario 3

Comments

Procedure 3.2   Locate the Medical Assistant's Legal Scope of Practice

Name _____ Date _____ Score _____

Tasks: Search online to locate the legal scope of practice for a medical assistant practicing in your state. Summarize the scope of practice.

Equipment and Supplies:
- Computer and printer with word processing software and internet access

Standard: Complete the procedure and all critical steps with a minimum score of 85% within two attempts (*or as indicated by the instructor*).

Scoring: Divide the points earned by the total possible points. Failure to perform a critical step, indicated by an asterisk (*), results in grade no higher than an 84% (*or as indicated by the instructor*).

Steps:	Point Value	Attempt 1	Attempt 2
1. Using the internet, search for the medical assistant's scope of practice in your state. Read the scope of practice for your state.	20		
2. Using the word processing software, create a short paper summarizing the medical assistant's scope of practice. Address the following points: a. Can medical assistants give injections? If so, what type of injections? b. Can medical assistants give oral, topical, and/or inhaled medications? c. Can medical assistants calculate drug dosages? d. What is the medical assistant's role with prescriptions? e. Describe additional duties that a medical assistant can legally do in your state. f. Include the website address(es) you used for this paper. *Note:* If your instructor does not provide you with different guidelines for the paper, follow these. Create at least a one-page paper, using double line spacing, a 10- or 12-point font, and 1-inch margins.	70		
3. After completing the paper, proofread the paper. Use correct spelling, punctuation, sentence structure, and capitalization. Make any changes required. Based on your instructor's directions, submit the paper to the instructor.	10		
Total Points	100		

Comments

CAAHEP Competencies	Step(s)
X.P.1. Locate a state's legal scope of practice for medical assistants	Entire procedure
ABHES Competencies	**Step(s)**
4. Medical Law and Ethics f. Comply with federal, state, and local health laws and regulations as they relate to healthcare settings. 1) Define the scope of practice for the medical assistant within the state where employed	Entire procedure

Healthcare Laws

chapter

4

CAAHEP Competencies	Assessments
X.C.3. Identify components of the Health Information Portability & Accountability Act (HIPAA)	Skills and Concepts – B. 1-8, C. 1-8, D. 1-5; Certification Preparation – 4-7; Workplace Application – 1a-d, 2-3
X.C.7.d. Define: Good Samaritan Act(s)	Skills and Concepts – H. 4; Certification Preparation – 1
X.C.7.e. Define: Uniform Anatomical Gift Act	Skills and Concepts – H. 8; Certification Preparation – 2
X.C.7.h. Define: Patient Self Determination Act (PSDA)	Skills and Concepts – H. 6; Certification Preparation – 1
X.C.7.i. Define: risk management	Skills and Concepts – M. 4
X.C.9. Identify legal and illegal applicant interview questions	Skills and Concepts – K. 4-5; Certification Preparation – 9
X.C.10.a. Identify: Health Information Technology for Economic and Clinical Health (HITECH) Act	Skills and Concepts – E. 1-2
X.C.10.b. Identify: Genetic Information Nondiscrimination Act of 2008 (GINA)	Skills and Concepts–E. 3, K. 2
X.C.10.c. Identify: Americans with Disabilities Act Amendments Act (ADAAA)	Skills and Concepts – L. 3; Certification Preparation – 10
X.C.11.a. Identify the process in compliance reporting: unsafe activities	Skills and Concepts – K. 6
X.C.11.b. Identify the process in compliance reporting: errors in patient care	Skills and Concepts – M. 5
X.C.11.c. Identify the process in compliance reporting: conflicts of interest	Skills and Concepts – J. 9
X.C.11.d. Identify the process in compliance reporting: incident reports	Skills and Concepts – M. 1-3
X.C.12.a. Identify compliance with public health statutes related to: communicable diseases	Skills and Concepts – I. 1-4
X.C.12.b. Identify compliance with public health statutes related to: abuse, neglect, and exploitation	Skills and Concepts – I. 6-10, 12 ; Workplace Application – 4
X.C.12.c. Identify compliance with public health statutes related to: wounds of violence	Skills and Concepts – I. 5
X.P.2.a. Apply HIPAA rules in regard to: privacy	Procedure 4.1

CAAHEP Competencies	Assessments
X.P.2.b. Apply HIPAA rules in regard to: release of information	Procedure 4.2
X.P.4. Perform compliance reporting based on public health statutes	Procedure 4.3
X.P.5. Report an illegal activity following the protocol established by the healthcare setting	Procedure 4.4
X.P.6. Complete an incident report related to an error in patient care	Procedure 4.5
A.3. Demonstrate empathy for patients' concerns.	Procedure 4.1
A.4. Demonstrate active listening.	Procedure 4.1
ABHES Competencies	**Assessments**
4. Medical Law and Ethics b. Institute federal and state guidelines when: 1) Releasing medical records or information	Procedures 4.1, 4.2
4.b.2) Entering orders in and utilizing electronic health records	Procedure 4.3
4.e. Perform risk management procedures	Procedure 4.5
4.f. Comply with federal, state, and local health laws and regulations as they relate to healthcare settings	Procedures 4.1 through 4.4
4.h. Demonstrate compliance with HIPAA guidelines, the ADA Amendments Act, and the Health Information Technology for Economic and Clinical Health (HITECH) Act	Procedures 4.1, 4.2

VOCABULARY REVIEW

Using the word pool on the right, find the correct word to match the definition. Write the word on the line after the definition.

Group A

1. Step-by-step directions _____

2. The electronic exchange of information between two agencies to accomplish financial or administrative healthcare activities _____

3. An organization that accepts the claim data from the provider, reformats the data to meet the specifications outlined by the insurance plan, and submits the claim _____

4. A system designed to use characters (i.e., numbers and letters) to represent something like a medical procedure or a disease _____

5. Written principles that provide goals for the employees and the facility _____

Word Pool
- claims clearinghouse
- coding system
- confidentiality
- electronic health record
- electronic transaction
- invasion of privacy
- policies
- precedence
- privacy
- procedures

6. Being free from unwanted intrusion _____

7. The top priority _____

8. A legally protected right of patients _____

9. The disclosing of private facts without the consent of the individual _____

10. Conforms to nationally recognized standards and contains health-related information about a specific patient; it can be created, managed, and consulted by authorized clinicians and staff from more than one healthcare organization

_____

Group B

1. Individually identifiable health information stored or transmitted by covered entities or business associates

_____

2. Protected health information that has had all of the direct patient identifiers removed _____

3. Reasons that the health information can be released

_____

4. Healthcare providers, health (insurance) plans, and claims clearinghouses that transmit protected health information electronically _____

5. A form that must be completed by the patient before information can be shared with another person; also called an *authorization to disclose* form _____

6. To remove all direct patient identifiers from the PHI information

_____

7. A form that must be completed by the patient before the patient records can be transferred _____

8. A person or business that provides a service to a covered entity that involves access to PHI _____

9. Safeguards that include a security officer who is responsible for creating and carrying out security policies and procedures

_____

10. Safeguards that include facility, workstation, and device security

_____

Word Pool
- administrative safeguards
- business associate
- covered entities
- de-identify
- disclosure authorization
- limited data set
- permission
- physical safeguards
- protected health information
- record release form

Group C

1. Disclosure of protected health information, without a reason or permission, which compromises the security or privacy of the information _____

2. Leaving a place; exit route _____

3. Diseases spread from person to person by either direct contact or indirect contact _____

4. An action that purposely harms another person _____

5. Written instructions about healthcare decisions in case a person is unable to make them _____

6. Failure to provide proper attention or care to another person _____

7. The act of using another person for one's own advantage _____

8. Communication that cannot be disclosed without authorization of the person involved; includes provider-patient and lawyer-client communications _____

9. People between the ages of 18 and 64 who have a mental or physical impairment that prevents them from doing normal activities or protecting themselves _____

10. Getting back at others for something they did to you _____

Word Pool
- abuse
- advance directives
- breach
- communicable diseases
- dependent adults
- egress
- retaliation
- exploitation
- neglect
- privileged communication

Group D

1. Any financial interest, personal or professional activity, or obligation that impacts a person's objectivity when performing the job _____

2. Punishment inflicted on someone as vengeance for a wrong or criminal act; the act of taking revenge _____

3. A deceitful action that causes another to give up something of value _____

4. The employer can end employment at any time for any reason _____

5. Legal reason for firing an employee _____

6. Employer did not have just cause for firing the employee _____

7. Unfair treatment of another person based on the person's age, gender (sex), ethnicity, sexual orientation, disability, marital status, or other selective factors _____

8. Continued, unwanted, and annoying actions done to another person _____

9. A person (usually an employee) who reports a violation of the law within the organization; the person reports the information to the public or to a person in authority _____

Word Pool
- conflict of interest
- discrimination
- employment-at-will
- fraud
- harassment
- just cause
- retribution
- whistleblower
- wrongful termination

ABBREVIATIONS

Write out what each of the following abbreviations stands for.

1. HIPAA _____

2. EHR _____

3. HHS _____

4. OCR _____

5. CPT _____

6. ICD _____

7. NPI _____

8. HPI _____

9. EIN _____

10. PHI _____

11. ePHI _____

12. FDA _____

13. DEA _____

14. PPSA _____

15. CMS _____

16. CLIA _____

17. OSH Act _____

18. OSHA _____

19. OPIM _____

20. PPE _____

21. CAPTA _____

22. VAERS _____

23. CDC _____

24. VICP _____

25. UDDA _____

26. UAGA _____

27. NOTA _____

28. OPTN _____

SKILLS AND CONCEPTS
Answer the following questions.

A. Privacy and Confidentiality

1. If your state's confidentiality laws are stricter than the federal laws, the state laws need to be followed. This is known as _____.

2. Healthcare professionals have the duty *not* to disclose what type of information unless authorized by the patient?
   a. medical
   b. financial
   c. insurance
   d. all of the above

B. Health Insurance Portability and Accountability Act
Match the following components to the correct HIPAA standard. Answers can be used more than once.

1. _____ Relates to unique identifiers including the National Provider Identifier, Health Plan Identifier, and the Employer Identification Number.

2. _____ Relates to standard transactions for electronic exchange of administrative healthcare information.

3. _____ Relates to the Security Rule.

4. _____ Relates to code sets including CPT and ICD.

5. _____ Relates to the Privacy Rule.

   a. Standard 1
   b. Standard 2
   c. Standard 3
   d. Standard 4

Select the correct answer.

6. Which of the following is *not* a covered entity?
   a. Healthcare provider
   b. Nursing home
   c. Pharmacy
   d. Legal firm representing the healthcare facility

7. Which of the following is *not* a business associate?
   a. Insurance company
   b. Accounting firm used by the healthcare facility
   c. Accreditation agency used by the healthcare facility
   d. Claims processing agency used by the healthcare facility

8. Which of the following is *not* a direct patient identifier?
   a. Patient's name
   b. Social Security number
   c. Contact information
   d. Patient's healthcare provider's name

C. Privacy Rule

1. The main purpose of the _____ is to define and limit the situations in which a patient's information can be used or disclosed.

2. Patients have the right to
   a. examine their health information.
   b. obtain a copy of their health records.
   c. request corrections to be made if information is incorrect.
   d. All of the above

3. Which of the following statements is correct?
   a. Covered entities must comply with the Privacy Rule.
   b. PHI can be given to business associates only after the written agreement regarding the safekeeping of PHI is signed.
   c. Only PHI required for the business associate's job can be given.
   d. All of the above

4. Which of the following do *not* require written authorization from the patient to release the PHI?
   a. Treatment, payment, and healthcare operations
   b. Uses and disclosures with opportunity to agree or object
   c. Incidental use and disclosure
   d. All of the above

5. When patients are being treated for emotional or mental conditions, the _____ allows providers to use professional judgment to determine if the records should be released to the patients.

6. The only permission that requires written authorization from patients is disclosing the PHI to a(n) _____.

7. Which of the following parts of a health record must be held to a higher level of confidentiality?
   a. Psychotherapy notes
   b. Substance abuse information
   c. Human immunodeficiency virus information
   d. All of the above

8. The federal statute called _____ restricts the release and use of patient records that include substance use diagnoses and services.

D. Security Rule

1. The _____ covers patient records that are created, used, received, and maintained by the covered entities.

Match the description to the safeguard. Answers can be used more than once.

2. _____ Audits to track activities of users
3. _____ Workstation and device security
4. _____ Potential risks to the ePHI are identified
5. _____ Encryption of data on mobile devices

a. physical safeguard
b. administrative safeguard
c. technical safeguard

E. Other Privacy Laws

1. The _____ contains provisions that increased the enforcement of the privacy and security of electronic transmission and health information.

2. How did the HITECH Act modify HIPAA?
   a. Prohibited the sale of PHI without the patient's authorization.
   b. Made business associates directly liable for compliance with HIPAA.
   c. Created a tiered violation category with related violation penalties and breach notification requirements.
   d. All of the above

3. The _____ modified HIPAA by clarifying that genetic information is health information and prohibited the use and disclosure of genetic information by covered health plans.

F. Drug Laws

1. The _____ enforces the Food, Drug, and Cosmetic Act.

2. The _____ is responsible for the safety, effectiveness, security, and quality of drugs, cosmetics, and food.

3. The FDA is responsible for which of the following areas?
   a. Medications
   b. Vaccines and blood components
   c. Medical devices and dietary supplements
   d. All of the above

4. The _____ enforces the Controlled Substances Act.

5. The _____ oversees the manufacturing, importation, possession, use, and distribution of controlled _____ _____.

6. Drugs on Schedule _____ have the highest potential for abuse and those on Schedule _____ have the lowest potential for abuse.

7. Each provider prescribing scheduled medications needs to have a unique _____ that needs to be renewed every _____.

G. Workplace Safety Laws

1. Occupational Safety and Health Act of 1970 is enforced by the _____.

2. _____ sets workplace standards and conducts inspections to ensure employee safety.

3. The goal of the _____ was to reduce the risk of healthcare workers' exposure to bloodborne diseases and this act required OSHA to update its Bloodborne Pathogens Standard.

4. The impact of the Needle Safety and Prevention Act includes
   a. healthcare workers must use safer medical devices.
   b. the Exposure Control Plan must include a sharps injury log documenting all instances of injuries from sharps.
   c. used sharps must be put in sharps disposal containers and PPE must be worn when there is a risk of blood or body fluid exposure.
   d. all of the above

H. Additional Healthcare Laws and Regulations

1. The _____ is commonly known as the Affordable Care Act.

2. Which of the following is *not* a goal of the Affordable Care Act?
   a. Provide Americans with affordable health insurance.
   b. Provide confidentiality standards in the healthcare insurance industry.
   c. Attempt to reform the healthcare system and reduce healthcare spending.
   d. All of the above

3. _____ establishes quality standards and regulates laboratory testing.

4. _____ are state laws that provide legal protection for those assisting an injured person during an emergency.

5. Which of the following relates to Good Samaritan laws?
   a. The injured person does not pay for the care given.
   b. The injured person needs to agree to the help if possible.
   c. The person assisting the injured person must exercise the same standard of care of their profession within the limits of the emergency.
   d. All of the above

6. _____ requires most healthcare institutions to inform patients of their right to make decisions and the facility's policies respecting advance directives.

7. _____ served as a guide for state lawmakers to create their own laws that define death.

8. The purpose of the _____ was to make organ donation easier for people.

9. _____ established the Organ Procurement and Transplant Network (OPTN) and also established a national registry for organ matching.

I. Compliance Reporting

For each of the following, match how a provider complies with the public health statutes when a communicable disease is diagnosed.

1. _____ If the disease is an urgent public health concern, what must be done?

2. _____ If the disease is a less urgent communicable disease, what must be done?

3. _____ How are HIV and AIDS reported by the provider?

a. May be reported electronically by mail or fax within 3 days.
b. The provider may need to mail the paperwork to increase confidentiality.
c. Reporting must be done immediately, usually by phone or fax.

Select the correct answer for the following questions.

4. Which of the following is *incorrect* regarding reporting communicable diseases?
   a. The state's public health department must be notified.
   b. The notification process is called *disease reporting*.
   c. Only the provider can report the new reportable disease case.
   d. The reporting process can vary by each state.

5. Which of the following is correct regarding compliance with wounds of violence reporting?
    a. State statutes vary from state to state regarding wounds of violence reporting.
    b. Reportable cases include wounds caused by gunshots and stabbing.
    c. Reportable cases include specific types of burns and nonaccidental wounds caused by a knife, an axe, or a sharp-pointed instrument.
    d. All of the above

6. Which of the following is *incorrect* regarding compliance reporting child abuse, neglect, and exploitation?
    a. Only some states require child maltreatment to be reported.
    b. In most states, healthcare providers need to report any child maltreatment.
    c. Most state statutes do not consider abuse and neglect information as privileged communication.
    d. The Child Welfare Information Gateway website can be used as a resource for state reporting information.

For each of the following, match the type of child maltreatment.

7. _____ Failure to provide adequate nutrition, clothing, shelter, and hygiene.

8. _____ Failure to provide needed care for injury, impairment, or illness.

9. _____ Fractures or burns that are unexplained or do not match the explanation given.

10. _____ Failure to enroll child in school or to home-school child.

a. physical abuse
b. sexual abuse
c. medical neglect
d. educational neglect
e. physical neglect

Select the correct answer or fill in the blank for the following questions.

11. The purpose of the _____ was to maintain the rights and dignity of the older person.

12. Which of the following do all states have?
    a. Adult or elder protective services statutes that provide reporting and investigating procedures for elder abuse in the state.
    b. Statutes that establish a Long-Term Care Ombudsman Program that advocates for the safety and rights of long-term care facility residents.
    c. General criminal statutes on fraud, sexual assault, battery, and other abuses that can relate to elder abuse.
    d. All of the above

13. The _____ will dictate who are mandated reporters, when to report, and how to report the situation.

14. _____ is a national surveillance program that monitors vaccine safety by collecting information on unusual vaccine side effects.

15. The _____ provides compensation for children injured by childhood vaccines.

J. Compliance Programs

1. A(n) _____ or corporate compliance is a program within a business that detects and prevents violations of state and federal laws.

2. _____ occurs when someone sells or uses another person's personal information for financial gain.

3. _____ relates to any financial interest, personal or professional activity, or obligation that affects a person's objectivity when performing the job.

4. The _____ prohibits intentionally receiving or giving anything of value to get referrals or generate federal healthcare program business.

5. The _____ prohibits a person from submitting false or fraudulent Medicare or Medicaid claims for payment.

6. The _____ prohibits a healthcare provider from referring a Medicare patient for services to a facility in which the provider or the provider's immediate family has a financial relationship.

7. The _____ prohibits intentionally defrauding any healthcare benefit program.

8. Describe the process in compliance reporting for violations or illegal activities related to fraud.

   _____

   _____

   _____

9. Describe the process in compliance reporting for a conflict of interest. _____ _____

   _____

   _____

   _____

K. Employment Concerns

1. The _____ prohibits employment discrimination based on color, race, gender, religion, or national origin.

2. The _____ prohibits employment discrimination based on the person's genetic information.

3. Describe how a medical assistant should handle violations noticed in the workplace. _____

   _____

   _____

4. Which of the following questions would be considered illegal to ask during an interview?
   a. "Are you eligible to work in this state?"
   b. "Are you pregnant?"
   c. "What medications are you taking?"
   d. b and c

5. Which of the following questions would be considered legal to ask during an interview?
   a. "Can you work on Sundays?"
   b. "How old are you?"
   c. "Have you ever been arrested?"
   d. "What diseases or conditions do you have?"

6. Describe how a medical assistant should handle unsafe activities or practices in the workplace.

_____

_____

_____

L. Laws Protecting Patients Against Discrimination

1. The _____ prohibits discrimination against individuals with disabilities in everyday activities, including getting healthcare.

2. The _____ prohibits discrimination against individuals with disabilities in services that receive federal financial assistance and requires that healthcare agencies make their services accessible to people with disabilities.

3. The _____ expanded the meaning and interpretation of the definition of disability and ensures that individuals with disabilities and certain conditions, such as cancer and diabetes, receive protection under the law.

M. Incident Reports and Risk Management

1. Which of the following is correct regarding incident reports?
   a. An incident report is an internal document that needs to be completed whenever an unexpected event occurs.
   b. The purpose is to gather information about the situation in case of a future lawsuit.
   c. The purpose is to communicate issues for risk-management procedures.
   d. All of the above

2. Which of the following is _incorrect_?
   a. An incident report should be completed for patient complaints, medication errors, and medical device malfunction.
   b. List the facts and your conclusions when completing an incident report.
   c. Do not mention the incident report in the patient's health record.
   d. Complete the incident report by the end of the day when the situation occurred.

3. Usually, the incident report is given to the _____ to review before it is sent to the risk-management team.

4. _____ involves techniques used to reduce or eliminate accidental loss to the healthcare facility and involves identifying, assessing, and controlling risks.

5. The wrong medication was given to the patient. Describe the process in compliance reporting for errors in patient care.

_____

_____

_____

CERTIFICATION PREPARATION

Circle the correct answer.

1. Which state law provides legal protection for those assisting an injured person during an emergency?
   a. Uniform Anatomical Gift Act
   b. Good Samaritan Act
   c. Patient Self-Determination Act
   d. Genetic Information Nondiscrimination Act

2. Which act makes organ donation easier?
   a. Uniform Determination of Death Act
   b. National Organ Transplant Act
   c. Uniform Anatomical Gift Act
   d. Patient Self-Determination Act

3. Which act requires most healthcare institutions to inform patients of their rights to make decisions and the facility's policies about advance directives?
   a. Uniform Determination of Death Act
   b. National Organ Transplant Act
   c. Uniform Anatomical Gift Act
   d. Patient Self-Determination Act

4. Which HIPAA standard requires healthcare facilities, insurance companies, and others to protect patient information that is electronically stored and transmitted?
   a. Standard 1 related to transactions and code sets
   b. Standard 2 related to the Privacy Rule
   c. Standard 3 related to the Security Rule
   d. Standard 4 related to unique identifiers

5. Individually identifiable health information stored or transmitted by covered entities or business associates is the definition of which term?
   a. Permission
   b. PHI
   c. Covered entities
   d. Limited data set

6. Under HIPAA, healthcare providers, health (insurance) plans, and claims clearinghouses must transmit PHI electronically. What are these entities called under HIPAA?
   a. Covered entities
   b. PHI
   c. Business associates
   d. Permission

7. Under HIPAA, which is a reason for releasing or disclosing patient information?
   a. De-identify
   b. Business associates
   c. PHI
   d. Permission

8. Which psychotherapy notes are held at a higher level of confidentiality?
   a. Prescriptions for medications treating mental health disorders
   b. Results of the clinical tests related to mental health disorders
   c. Types and frequency of treatments ordered for mental health disorders
   d. What the patient said during the session and the provider's analysis of the statements and the situation

9. Which question is illegal during an interview?
   a. "Are you eligible to work in this state?"
   b. "Can you perform the essential job functions of a medical assistant with or without reasonable accommodation?"
   c. "When did you move to the United States?"
   d. "Can you work on weekends?"

10. Which act expanded the meaning and interpretation of the definition of disability and included people with cancer, diabetes, attention-deficit/hyperactivity disorder, learning disabilities, and epilepsy?
    a. ADA
    b. OSHA
    c. ADAAA
    d. Stark Law

WORKPLACE APPLICATIONS

1. The billing department supervisor at Walden-Martin Family Medical Clinic wants to hire ACE Coders to assist with the billing processes. Answer the following questions using this scenario.

    a. Who is the covered entity? _____

    b. Who is the business associate? _____

    c. What must be in done before the business associate obtains patient information? _____

    _____

    d. Can the business associates have unlimited access to all patient information? Explain why or why not.

    _____

    _____

2. Mrs. Smith asked Bella to call and talk with her daughter, Rosie. Mrs. Smith wanted Bella to tell Rosie the results of her blood test. Mrs. Smith stated that Rosie was a nurse and would understand the information. Can Bella give Mrs. Smith's information to Rosie? If not, what could be done so Rosie could get the information?

    _____

    _____

3. Mr. Green had before-and-after pictures taken as he was going through bariatric surgery and weight loss. He requests that these pictures be given to his new provider. What is the typical process to transfer pictures to another agency?

    _____

    _____

4. Mr. Thomas is a 39-year-old dependent adult. During the rooming process, the medical assistant suspects that Mr. Thomas is a victim of neglect. What should the medical assistant do?

    _____

    _____

INTERNET ACTIVITIES

1. Using the internet, research your state's disease reporting public health statutes. Create a poster presentation, PowerPoint presentation, or paper summarizing the reporting process for each category of diseases (e.g., urgent public health concern, less urgent, and HIV and AIDS). List three diseases for the urgent and less urgent categories.

2. Using the internet, review the Child Welfare Information Gateway website (www.childwelfare.gov) for content related to your state. You can also use government websites from your state. Create a poster presentation, PowerPoint presentation, or paper summarizing child protection in your state. Focus on related statutes, the reporting process, and who mandatory reporters are.

3. Using the internet, research prevention of elder abuse, neglect, and exploitation. Focus on resources in your state. Briefly summarize your findings and cite the websites used.

Procedure 4.1   Protecting a Patient's Privacy

Name _____ Date _____ Score _____

Tasks: Apply HIPAA rules and protect a patient's privacy. Demonstrate active listening skills and empathy to a patient.

Scenario: Ken Thomas (date of birth [DOB] 10/25/19XX) saw Jean Burke, nurse practitioner (NP), this past week. He was diagnosed with acute leukemia after several tests. You work with Ms. Burke, and you were involved with arranging Ken's tests. Today, Ken's adult child, Alex Thomas, calls you. Alex wants to know what is going on with Ken. You look at Ken's health record and see that Alex is not on the disclosure authorization form. Per the facility's policy, for information to be given to a patient's family, a disclosure authorization form must be completed.

Later Ken calls and asks why you did not update Alex on his condition. He sounds upset while he is talking with you.

Directions: Role-play the scenario with a peer. You are the medical assistant in the scenario. Your peer will play Alex and then Ken.

Equipment and Supplies:
- Patient's health record
- Disclosure authorization form (electronic or paper) (See Figure 4.2)

Standard: Complete the procedure and all critical steps in _____ minutes with a minimum score of 85% within two attempts (*or as indicated by the instructor*).

Scoring: Divide the points earned by the total possible points. Failure to perform a critical step, indicated by an asterisk (*), results in grade no higher than an 84% (*or as indicated by the instructor*).

Time: Began_____ Ended_____ Total minutes: _____

Steps:	Point Value	Attempt 1	Attempt 2
1. You realized that Alex is not on the disclosure authorization form. Inform Alex that his name is not on a disclosure authorization form. Discuss the purpose of the disclosure authorization form. Be professional and respectful as you apply HIPAA rules to the situation. *(Refer to the Affective Behaviors Checklist – **Respect** and the Grading Rubric)*	20*		
2. Explain to Alex how you would be able to give him information. Encourage Alex to talk with his father about the situation.	15		
Scenario update: Your peer will now play the part of Ken, the patient. 3. When Ken calls, be professional and empathetic as you listen to his complaints. Inform Ken that you understand his frustration. Be respectful to his feelings and his rights. Explain why you could not give information to Alex. *(Refer to the Affective Behaviors Checklist – **Empathy** and the Grading Rubric)*	20*		

4.	Demonstrate active listening skills when interacting with Ken. Remain neutral and refrain from interrupting. Keep your voice even and do not raise the volume. Focus on the patient and avoid distractions. *(Refer to the Affective Behaviors Checklist – **Active Listening** and the Grading Rubric)*	**20***		
5.	Discuss with Ken how you could prepare the disclosure authorization form. Make plans for how Ken would sign the form.	**10**		
6.	Document the phone call with Alex and Ken. Describe the facts and the plan to complete the disclosure authorization form.	**15**		
	Total Points	**100**		

Affective Behavior	**Affective Behaviors Checklist** **Directions:** *Check behaviors observed during the role-play.*					
Respect	**Negative, Unprofessional Behaviors**	**Attempt**		**Positive, Professional Behaviors**	**Attempt**	
		1	**2**		**1**	**2**
	Rude, unkind, fake/false attitude, disrespectful, impolite, unwelcoming			Courteous, sincere, polite, welcoming		
	Unconcerned with person's dignity; brief, abrupt			Maintained person's dignity; took time with person		
	Unprofessional verbal communication; inappropriate questions			Professional verbal communication		
	Negative nonverbal behaviors, poor eye contact			Positive nonverbal behaviors, proper eye contact		
	Other:			Other:		
Active Listening	Biased, offensive; raised volume of voice			Remained neutral, kept voice even and did not raise volume		
	Interrupted			Refrained from interrupting		
	Did not allow for silence or pauses			Allowed for periods of silence		
	Distracted			Focused on patient, avoided distractions		
	Other:			Other:		
Empathy	Did not listen to patient's responses			Listened to patient		
	Lack of respect and support demonstrated			Showed respect and support		
	Lack of therapeutic communication techniques used			Used therapeutic communication techniques		
	Other:			Other:		

Grading Rubric for the Affective Behaviors Checklist **Directions:** *Based on checklist results, identify the points received for the procedure checklist. Indicate how the behaviors demonstrated met the expectations.*		**Points for Procedure Checklist**	**Attempt 1**	**Attempt 2**
Does not meet Expectation	• Response lacked respect, active listening, and/or empathy. • Student demonstrated more than 2 negative, unprofessional behaviors during the interaction.	0		
Needs Improvement	• Response lacked respect, active listening, and/or empathy. • Student demonstrated 1 or 2 negative, unprofessional behaviors during the interaction.	0		
Meets Expectation	• Response was respectful and empathetic. Demonstrated active listening. No negative, unprofessional behaviors observed. • More practice is needed for behavior to appear natural and for student to appear comfortable and at ease.	20		
Occasionally Exceeds Expectation	• Response was respectful and empathetic. Demonstrated active listening. No negative, unprofessional behaviors observed. • At times student appeared comfortable and at ease; but more practice is needed for behavior to become natural and consistent with a professional medical assistant.	20		
Always Exceeds Expectation	• Response was respectful and empathetic. Demonstrated active listening. No negative, unprofessional behaviors observed. • Student's behaviors appeared natural and comfortable. Behaviors are consistent with a professional medical assistant.	20		

Documentation

Comments

CAAHEP Competencies	Step(s)
X.P.2.a. Apply HIPAA rules in regard to: privacy	1-3, 5
A.3. Demonstrate empathy for patients' concerns.	3
A.4. Demonstrate active listening.	4
ABHES Competencies	**Step(s)**
4. Medical Law and Ethics b. Institute federal and state guidelines when: 1) Releasing medical records or information	Entire procedure
4.f. Comply with federal, state, and local health laws and regulations as they relate to healthcare settings	1-3, 6
4.h. Demonstrate compliance with HIPAA guidelines, the ADA Amendments Act, and the Health Information Technology for Economic and Clinical Health (HITECH) Act	1-3, 6

Procedure 4.2 Completing a Release of Record Form for a Release of Information

Name _____ Date _____ Score _____

Tasks: Apply HIPAA rules and complete a release of record form for a release of information.

Scenario: Aaron Jackson was seen at Walden Hospital for a high fever. You need to help Aaron's mother complete a records release form so his record from the emergency department visit can be sent to the clinic. She needs to request all records from the visit on the first of this month. The clinic information is on the form. The release will expire in 1 month.

AARON'S INFORMATION	WALDEN HOSPITAL'S INFORMATION
Date of birth: 10/17/20XX Social Security number: 164-72-4618 Address: 555 McArthur Avenue Anytown, AL 12345-1234 Phone: (123) 814-7844 Mother: Patricia Jackson	Address: Walden Hospital 123 Healing Way Anywhere, AL 12345-1234 Phone: (123) 814-4563 Fax: (123) 814-6544

Directions: You will complete the medical record release form. You will role-play the scenario with you as the medical assistant and a peer as the mother.

Equipment and Supplies:
- Records release form (electronic or paper) (See Work Product 4.1)
- Patient's health record

Standard: Complete the procedure and all critical steps in _____ minutes with a minimum score of 85% within two attempts (*or as indicated by the instructor*).

Scoring: Divide the points earned by the total possible points. Failure to perform a critical step, indicated by an asterisk (*), results in grade no higher than an 84% (*or as indicated by the instructor*).

Time: Began_____ Ended_____ Total minutes: _____

Steps:	Point Value	Attempt 1	Attempt 2
1. Using the medical record release form, complete the patient information (Work Product 4.1). Add the patient's name, DOB, and social security number (SSN). Include the current address and phone number that is found in the patient's health record. If an electronic form is used, select the correct patient and the fields will auto-populate.	10*		
2. Complete the parts of the form that specify who authorizes the release and who is to release the information.	15*		
3. Check the box(es) of the information that needs to be released. If required, write in what other records need to be released.	15*		
4. Add the date of the visit. Add the name and contact information for the facility where the records need to be sent.	15*		
5. Indicate how the released information will be used.	15		

6.	Indicate when the authorization should expire. Proofread the form for accuracy. If using an electronic form, save the form to the patient's record. Print the form so the mother can sign.	**10**		
7.	During a role-play with the patient's mother, explain what the provider is requesting. Ensure she can understand and read English. Have the mother read the form.	**10**		
8.	Ask the mother if she has any questions. Answer any questions and then explain where she needs to sign if she agrees with the documentation.	**10**		
	Total Points	**100**		

Comments

CAAHEP Competencies	**Step(s)**
X.P.2.b. Apply HIPAA rules in regard to: release of information	Entire procedure
ABHES Competencies	**Step(s)**
4. Medical Law and Ethics b. Institute federal and state guidelines when: 1) Releasing medical records or information	Entire procedure
4. f. Comply with federal, state, and local health laws and regulations as they relate to healthcare settings	Entire procedure
4.h. Demonstrate compliance with HIPAA guidelines, the ADA Amendments Act, and the Health Information Technology for Economic and Clinical Health (HITECH) Act	Entire procedure

Work Product 4.1   Records Release Form

Name _____ Date _____ Score _____

WALDEN-MARTIN
FAMILY MEDICAL CLINIC
1234 ANYSTREET | ANYTOWN, ANYSTATE 12345
PHONE 123-123-1234 | FAX 123-123-5678

Medical Records Release

Patient Name: _____ **Date of Birth:** _____

SSN: _____ **Phone:** _____

Address:

I, _____ authorize _____

to disclose/release the following information (check all applicable):

☐ All Records   ☐ Abstract/Summary

☐ Laboratory/pathology records   ☐ Pharmacy/prescription records

☐ X-ray/radiology records   ☐ Other

☐ Billing records

Note: If these records contain any information from previous providers or information about HIV/AIDS status, cancer diagnosis, drug alcohol abuse, or sexually transmitted disease, you are hereby authorizing disclosure of this information. A copy of this signed authorization must be given to the individual.

These records are for services provided on the following date(s):_____

Please send the records listed above to (use additional sheets if necessary):

Name: _____ **Phone:** _____

Address: **Fax:** _____

The information may be used/disclosed for each of the following purposes:

☐ At patient's request   ☐ For employment purposes

☐ For patient's health care   ☐ Other

☐ For payment/insurance

This authorization shall expire no later than: _____ **or upon the following event** _____ **, and may not be valid for greater than one year from the date of signature for medical records.**

I understand that after the custodian of records discloses my health information, it may no longer be protected by federal privacy laws. I understand that this authorization is voluntary and I may refuse to sign this authorization which will not affect my ability to obtain treatment; receive payment; or eligibility for benefits unless allowed by law. By signing below I represent and warrant that I have authority to sign this document and authorize the use or disclosure of protected health information and that there are no claims or orders that would prohibit, limit, or otherwise restrict my ability to authorize the use or disclosure of this protected health information.

_____   _____

Patient signature   **Date**
(or patient's personal representative)

_____   _____

Printed name of patient representative   **Representative's authority to sign for patient**
                                                            (i.e. parent, guardian, power of attorney, executor)

Procedure 4.3   Perform Disease Reporting

Name _____   Date _____   Score _____

Tasks: Research the state's disease reporting public health statutes and complete the disease reporting paperwork based on public health statutes. Document the activity in the patient's health record.

Scenario: Jean Burke, NP, received the test results for Ken Thomas. He tested positive for gonorrhea. She wants you to file the report with the public health department. Here is the information from his health record and the clinic. For any missing information, follow the instructor's directions (or if no directions are provided for this exercise, make up the information).

Patient Information	Provider and Lab Information	Health Record Information
Ken Thomas 398 Larkin Avenue Anytown, AL 12345-1234 Anycounty Email: k.thomas@anytown.mail Phone: (123) 784-1118 DOB: 10/25/19XX Race: Multiple races Ethnicity: Unknown Marital status: Single, living with Sandy Brown, who was not treated	**Provider:** Jean Burke, N.P. Walden-Martin Family Medical Clinic 1234 Anystreet Anytown, AL 12345-1234 Phone: (123) 123-1234 Fax: (123) 123-5678 **Lab:** Walden-Martin Family Medical Clinic Lab	**Diagnosis:** Gonorrhea **Symptoms:** Started 5 days ago, greenish discharge from penis, burning with urination **Test:** Urine specimen was collected yesterday; gonorrhea nucleic acid amplification test NAAT test done yesterday, results are positive **Treatment:** Patient treated today with ceftriaxone 250 mg intramuscular (IM) single dose and azithromycin 1 g orally single dose

Equipment and Supplies:
- Computer with internet access and printer
- Patient's health record (see table with information)
- Black pen

Standard: Complete the procedure and all critical steps in _____ minutes with a minimum score of 85% within two attempts (*or as indicated by the instructor*).

Scoring: Divide the points earned by the total possible points. Failure to perform a critical step, indicated by an asterisk (*), results in grade no higher than an 84% (*or as indicated by the instructor*).

Time: Began_____ Ended_____ Total minutes: _____

Steps:	Point Value	Attempt 1	Attempt 2
1. Using the internet, search for the disease reporting procedure in your state's public health department or similar facility. Read the procedure.	10		
2. Identify which form is required based on the patient's diagnosis. Print the form.	10		

3.	Use a black pen to complete the form. Neatly complete the patient's demographic information section using the information from the health record.	25		
4.	Complete the diagnosis, symptoms, testing, and treatment information.	25		
5.	Complete the rest of the form. Review the form for accuracy. Make any changes required before submitting the form to the instructor.	20		
6.	Document in the patient's health record that the disease reporting paperwork was completed and submitted.	10		
	Total Points	**100**		

Documentation

Comments

CAAHEP Competencies	Step(s)
X.P.4. Perform compliance reporting based on public health statutes	Entire procedure
ABHES Competencies	**Step(s)**
4. Medical Law and Ethics f. Comply with federal, state, and local health laws and regulations as they relate to healthcare settings	Entire procedure
4.b.2) Entering orders in and utilizing electronic health records	6

Procedure 4.4   Report Illegal Activity

Name _____ Date _____ Score _____

Task: Report an illegal activity in the healthcare setting following proper protocol.

Scenario: You witness a coworker, Sally Brown, taking medical samples from the supply cabinet. You see her sticking them into her purse. She sees you and states, "This was the same medication I had to pay $200 for the last time I was sick. I don't see why we need to pay for medications when we have samples that we give free to patients. We should be able to use them also." You know the facility's professional policy prohibits taking medical samples from the sample cabinet for personal reasons.

Facility's Compliance Reporting Protocol:

Walden-Martin Family Medical Clinic's Compliance Program has a phone number and email address for employees to report suspected violations, suspected illegal activity, fraud, abuse, theft, and workplace safety concerns. Concerns can be left on the voicemail or emailed without fear of retribution or retaliation. Please include as many details as possible, including dates, names, and the situation.

Any employee who seeks retribution or retaliation against another employee for reporting an offense needs to be aware of criminal penalties for such actions.

Equipment and Supplies:
- Computer with email and internet access or phone
- Instructor's email address or voicemail phone number
- Pen and paper
- Facility's compliance reporting protocol (See box)

Standard: Complete the procedure and all critical steps with a minimum score of 85% within two attempts (*or as indicated by the instructor*).

Scoring: Divide the points earned by the total possible points. Failure to perform a critical step, indicated by an asterisk (*), results in grade no higher than an 84% (*or as indicated by the instructor*).

Steps:	Point Value	Attempt 1	Attempt 2
1. Read the facility's corporate compliance reporting protocol.	10		
2. Using the paper and pen, write down the facts of what you witnessed.	10		
3. Using the paper and pen, compose the message you want to email or leave on the voicemail for the compliance office.	30		
4. Proofread the message and make any changes required. Make sure to include the date, names of people involved, and the details of the situation.	20		
5. Using your email or phone, send a message to the corporate compliance office. Use the email address or phone number provided by your instructor.	30		
Total Points	**100**		

Comments

CAAHEP Competencies	Step(s)
X.P.5. Report an illegal activity following the protocol established by the healthcare setting	Entire procedure
ABHES Competencies	**Step(s)**
4. Medical Law and Ethics f. Comply with federal, state, and local health laws and regulations as they relate to healthcare settings	Entire procedure

Procedure 4.5   Complete Incident Report

Name _____ Date _____ Score _____

Task: Complete an incident report form for a medication error.

Scenario: Johnny Parker (DOB 06/15/20XX) sees Jean Burke, NP, for a well-child visit. Johnny is off-schedule with his hepatitis B vaccine series, and today he is to get his last hepatitis B booster. You (a medical assistant) prepare the medication and give the injection in his right deltoid muscle. Later in the day, you realize that hepatitis B has been out of stock for 1 week. You must have given a hepatitis A booster to Johnny. You realize that you failed to read the label three times during preparation of the medication. You report the mistake to Jean Burke, NP, and your supervisor. Your supervisor calls Lisa Parker, Johnny's mother. They will come back next week for the hepatitis B vaccine. You need to complete the incident report.

Equipment and Supplies:
- Incident report form (Work Product 4.2) and black pen or computer with internet access and SimChart for the Medical Office (SCMO)

Standard: Complete the procedure and all critical steps in _____ minutes with a minimum score of 85% within two attempts (*or as indicated by the instructor*).

Scoring: Divide the points earned by the total possible points. Failure to perform a critical step, indicated by an asterisk (*), results in grade no higher than an 84% (*or as indicated by the instructor*).

Time: Began_____ Ended_____ Total minutes: _____

Steps:	Point Value	Attempt 1	Attempt 2
1. **SCMO method:** Access SCMO and enter the Simulation Playground. If a popup window appears, select "Return to previous session with saved patient information" and click Start. On the Calendar screen, click on the Form Repository icon. Click on Office Forms on the left Info Panel and select Incident Report. **For both methods:** Accurately complete the information from the date down to the reason for the patient's visit.	20		
2. **For both methods:** Specify the incident description, immediate action and outcome, and contributing factors, and fill in the prevention boxes. Provide as much detail as possible. Be honest and concise with your facts.	20		
3. **For both methods:** Complete the reported by, position, and contact phone number sections. Your information should be in these fields. (For this exercise, make up a contact phone number.)	20		
4. **For both methods:** Complete the other persons involved, position, and contact phone number sections. Jean Burke's information should be in these fields. (Make up her contact phone number.)	20		
5. **For both methods:** Review the form for accuracy. Make any changes required before submitting the form to the instructor. (**For the SCMO method**: Save or print the form based on your instructor's directions.)	20		
Total Points	100		

Comments

CAAHEP Competencies	Step(s)
X.P.6. Complete an incident report related to an error in patient care	Entire procedure
ABHES Competencies	**Step(s)**
4. Medical Law and Ethics e. Perform risk management procedures	Entire procedure

Work Product 4.2   Incident Report Form

Name _____ Date _____ Score _____

WALDEN-MARTIN
FAMILY MEDICAL CLINIC
1234 ANYSTREET | ANYTOWN, ANYSTATE 12345
PHONE 123-123-1234 | FAX 123-123-5678

Incident Report

Date: _____   Time: _____

Incident Type: ☐ Staff   ☐ Patient   ☐ Visitor   ☐ Equipment/Property

Witness: ☐ Staff   ☐ Patient   ☐ Visitor

Department: _____   Exact Location: _____

Medical Team: _____

Patient Reason for Visit: _____   Medication Incident: ☐ Yes   ☐ No

Incident Description: [   ]   Immediate Actions and Outcome: [   ]

Contributing Factors: [   ]   Prevention: [   ]

Next of kin / guardian notified / patient?   ☐ Yes   ☐ No   ☐ N/A   Medical staff notified?   ☐ Yes   ☐ No   ☐ N/A

Reported By: _____   Position: _____

Contact Phone Number: _____

Other Persons Involved: _____   Position: _____

Contact Phone Number: _____

Medical Report (Document patient's assessment and list investigations and treatments):

_____

Provider: _____   Designation: _____

Provider Signature: _____   Date/Time: _____

Healthcare Ethics

CAAHEP Competencies	Assessment
V.C.13.c. Identify the basic concepts of the following theories: Kübler-Ross	Skills and Concepts – I. 1-8; Certification Preparation – 6
X.C.7.e. Define: Uniform Anatomical Gift Act	Skills and Concepts – M. 1; Certification Preparation – 10
X.C.7.f. Define: living will/advanced directives	Vocabulary Review – D. 3, 5; Skills and Concepts – J. 2-3; Certification Preparation – 7
X.C.7.g. Define: medical durable power of attorney	Vocabulary Review – D. 4; Skills and Concepts – J. 5
X.C.7.h. Define: Patient Self Determination Act (PSDA)	Skills and Concepts – J. 1
XI.C.1.a. Define: ethics	Vocabulary Review – D. 1; Certification Preparation – 1
XI.C.1.b. Define: morals	Vocabulary Review – D. 2; Certification Preparation – 2
XI.C.2. Identify personal and professional ethics	Vocabulary Review – A. 1, 5; Skills and Concepts – A. 1-2; B. 1-2, 4; Certification Preparation – 3
XI.C.3. Identify potential effects of personal morals on professional performance	Skills and Concepts – A. 3
XI.P.1. Demonstrate professional response(s) to ethical issues	Procedures 5.1, 5.2
ABHES Competencies	Assessment
4. Medical Law and Ethics g. Display compliance with the Code of Ethics of the profession	Skills and Concepts – B. 4; Procedures 5.1, 5.2

VOCABULARY REVIEW

Using the word pool on the right, find the correct word to match the definition. Write the word on the line after the definition.

Group A

1. Codes of conduct stated by an employer or professional association _____

2. Basic units of heredity _____

3. Rod-shaped structures found in the cell's nucleus; they contain genetic information _____

4. A set of rules about good and bad behavior _____

5. An individual's code of conduct _____

6. The freedom to determine one's own actions and decisions _____

7. People who study the ethical effect of biomedical advances _____

8. To treat patients fairly and give them care that is due and appropriate _____

9. The moral obligation to act for the good or benefit of others _____

10. To do no harm _____

Word Pool
- autonomy
- beneficence
- bioethicists
- chromosomes
- code of ethics
- genes
- justice
- nonmaleficence
- personal ethics
- professional ethics

Group B

1. The inability to get pregnant after 1 year of unprotected intercourse _____

2. Nonreproductive cells; they do not include sperm and egg cells _____

3. Cells can make copies of themselves _____

4. Sperm and egg cells _____

5. Cells can develop into specialized cells _____

6. The process of creating a genetically identical biological entity _____

7. The entire genetic makeup of an organism _____

8. A branch of medicine involved with using patients' genomic information as part of their clinical care _____

9. A branch of pharmacology that studies the genetic factors that influence a person's response to a medication _____

10. The manipulation of genetic material in cells to change hereditary traits or produce a specific result _____

Word Pool
- cloning
- differentiate
- genetic engineering
- genome
- genomic medicine
- germline cells
- infertility
- pharmacogenomics
- self-renew
- somatic cells

Group C

1. A competent adult can appoint a person to make healthcare decisions in the event they are unable to do so
_____

2. Withholding a life-saving treatment (e.g., feeding tube) and letting the person die _____

3. A branch of knowledge, learning, or instruction; for instance, medicine, nursing, social work, and physical therapy
_____

4. Incorporating the most current and valid research results into the practice of healthcare, thus providing the best patient care
_____

5. Latin for "father of the country," a doctrine that gives the courts the power to make decisions for people who cannot make their own decisions _____

6. Involves removing egg cells from a female's ovaries, fertilizing them with sperm outside of the body, and then implanting the fertilized egg in the uterus _____

7. To help relieve the symptoms of a serious illness
_____

8. A type of palliative care for people who have about 6 months or less to live _____

9. Bringing to an end _____

10. The act of killing a person who is suffering from an incurable disease _____

11. To preserve by freezing at low temperatures
_____

12. A physician who has graduated from medical school and is finishing specialized clinical training _____

13. An immature ovum _____

14. A person who acts on behalf of another person or takes the place of another person _____

15. A group composed of members from a variety of disciplines that analyzes ethical issues _____

16. Any procedure where nonhuman cells, tissues, or organs are implanted or infused into a person _____

Word Pool

- cessation
- cryopreservation
- discipline
- ethics committees
- euthanasia
- evidence-based practices
- healthcare proxy
- hospice
- in vitro fertilization
- oocyte
- palliative
- *parens patriae*
- passive euthanasia
- resident
- surrogate
- xenotransplantation

Group D

Fill in the blank with the word or phrase that is defined.

1. _____ are rules of conduct that differentiate between acceptable and unacceptable behavior.

2. _____ are internal principles that distinguish between right and wrong.

3. _____ are written instructions about healthcare decisions should a person be unable to make them.

4. _____ is similar to a living will but includes all healthcare decisions.

5. _____ provides instructions about life-sustaining medical treatment to be administered or withheld when the patient has a terminal condition.

ABBREVIATIONS

Write out what each of the following abbreviations stands for.

1. AMA _____

2. CEJA _____

3. AAMA _____

4. GMOs _____

5. FDA _____

6. ART _____

7. IUI _____

8. STI _____

9. PSDA _____

10. DNR _____

11. CPR _____

12. POLST _____

13. UDDA _____

14. UAGA _____

15. NOTA _____

16. OPTN _____

SKILLS AND CONCEPTS

Answer the following questions.

A. Personal Ethics

1. _____ includes an individual's honesty, fairness, commitment, integrity, and accountability; it also includes doing what one considers to be correct.

2. Our _____ affect how we conduct ourselves or, in other words, our personal ethics.

3. Which of the following statements is correct regarding personal morals and professional performance?
   a. Personal morals affect professional performance.
   b. Personal morals that align with professional characteristics will positively affect one's professional performance.
   c. Personal morals can negatively affect professional performance.
   d. All of the above

B. Professional Ethics

1. _____ are codes of conduct stated by an employer or a professional association.

2. Which of the following statements is *incorrect* regarding professional ethics?
   a. The employee handbook may indicate how employees need to conduct themselves in the workplace.
   b. Codes of ethics are published by professional associations.
   c. Professional ethics can be violated without consequences.
   d. A code of ethics exists for medical assistants.

3. Which of the following statements is correct?
   a. The care a medical assistant provides must reflect respect for that patient.
   b. The medical assistant is legally and ethically obligated to keep patient information confidential.
   c. The medical assistant must uphold the standards of the profession.
   d. All of the above

4. Which of the following points is *not* included in the Medical Assistant Code of Ethics?
   a. Render service with full respect for the dignity of humanity.
   b. Respect confidential information obtained through employment unless legally authorized or required by responsible performance of duty to divulge such information.
   c. Uphold the honor and high principles of the profession and accept its disciplines.
   d. Endeavor to be more effective and aspire to render greater service.

C. Separation Plan

1. How can a medical assistant approach a situation if it involves their biases? _____
   _____
   _____

2. When looking for employment, why is it important to consider one's biases before applying for certain jobs?
   _____
   _____

D. Principles of Healthcare Ethics

Match the ethical principle with the description. Answers may be used more than once.

1. _____ Healthcare professionals promote health in patients and assist patients to recover from illness.

2. _____ Healthcare professionals are obligated not to inflict intentional harm on patients.

3. _____ The medical assistant ensures the environment is both physically and psychologically safe for others and that safety hazards are reported and corrected.

4. _____ The medical assistant promotes health and prevention of diseases.

a. autonomy
b. nonmaleficence
c. beneficence
d. justice

5. _____ The medical assistant must protect patients' privacy.

6. _____ Professional behaviors of the medical assistant include providing equal respect and courtesy to all people.

7. _____ Healthcare professionals must respect and honor the patient's decision.

E. Ethical Issues Related to Genetics

1. Which of the following is an important advance in genomic medicine?
   a. Pharmacogenetics
   b. Stem cell transplants
   c. Genetic testing
   d. All of the above

2. Which of the following is *not* a type of genetic testing?
   a. Newborn screening
   b. Prenatal testing
   c. Bariatric testing
   d. Carrier testing

3. Which of the following is correct regarding stem cells?
   a. Embryonic stem cells are derived from bone marrow, brain, skin, and heart tissue.
   b. Embryonic stem cells are derived from umbilical cord blood.
   c. Adult stem cells are thought to cause fewer rejection issues with transplants if a person's own stem cells are used.
   d. All of the above

4. _____ is currently an experimental technique that uses genes to prevent or treat diseases.

5. _____, or genome editing, is a specific gene therapy that can remove, add, or alter sections of the gene.

F. Reproductive Ethical Issues
Match the term with the correct description.

1. _____ Specially prepared sperm is placed into a woman's uterus using a long, narrow tube

2. _____ A woman carries and gives birth for another couple

3. _____ Egg freezing or egg banking

4. _____ The deliberate termination of a pregnancy

5. _____ Occurs when the egg is from a surrogate and the sperm is from the father

6. _____ Occurs when the sperm and egg come from the intended parents or are donated, and the surrogate is not related to the baby

a. surrogacy
b. cryopreservation of oocytes
c. gestational surrogacy
d. traditional surrogacy
e. intrauterine insemination
f. elective abortion

G. Childhood Ethical Issues
Match the term with the correct description.

1. _____ No contact between the adoptive parents and the birth parents

2. _____ Used for children or adults who are incompetent and when parents refuse healthcare for a child

3. _____ Allows a person to give up an unwanted infant anonymously

4. _____ Adoptive parents meet and may stay in contact with the birth parents

a. closed adoption
b. open adoption
c. *parens patriae*
d. Safe Haven infant protection laws

H. Research Trials and Ethical Issues
Match the description with the correct answer. Answers may be used more than once.

1. _____ Addressed the importance of human research, the obligations of the physicians involved, the importance of informed consent, and the protection of the participants

2. _____ Human experiments require voluntary consent, the results must be for the good of society, and the experiments must be based on prior knowledge and should avoid all unnecessary physical and mental suffering

3. _____ Researched the natural history of syphilis on African American men

4. _____ Outlined what was legal when conducting human experiments

5. _____ Identified basic ethical principles and guidelines regarding human subject research

a. Nuremberg Code
b. Belmont Report
c. Declaration of Helsinki
d. Tuskegee Study

I. End-of-Life Issues
Match the description and emotions with the correct state of grief and dying. Answers may be used more than once.

1. _____ Tom blames the drug company for his cancer.

2. _____ Tia feels sad, fearful, and uncertain as her mother is dying.

3. _____ Dan experienced disbelief and numbness when he heard the prognosis.

4. _____ Sally makes a deal with God so she can live for another 6 months.

5. _____ John, diagnosed with incurable cancer, distances himself from his friends.

6. _____ Sam's mother is dying of cancer. He has come to terms with the situation.

7. _____ Alice refuses to accept the breast cancer diagnosis.

a. denial
b. anger
c. bargaining
d. depression
e. acceptance

Select the correct answer.

8. Which of the following is correct regarding the stages of grief and dying as defined by Dr. Elisabeth Kübler-Ross?
    a. The grieving stages include denial, anger, bargaining, depression, and acceptance.
    b. Some people may not experience all of the grieving stages.
    c. People may move through the stages differently, and some may switch back and forth among the stages.
    d. All of the above

J. Patient Self-Determination Act

1. The Patient Self-Determination Act requires
    a. healthcare institutions to provide patients with a written document of their rights to make decisions and the facility's policies respecting advance directives.
    b. that patients are asked if they have advance directives at the time of admission.
    c. documentation of the patient's advance directive status in the health record.
    d. all of the above

2. _____ are written instructions about healthcare decisions should a person be unable to make them.

3. A(n) _____ provides instructions about life-sustaining medical treatment to be administered or withheld when the patient has a terminal condition.

4. With a(n) _____, a competent adult can appoint a person to make healthcare decisions in the event they are unable to do so.

5. The _____ is similar to a living will but includes all healthcare decisions, names a healthcare proxy, and can include healthcare wishes.

6. _____ the person refuses cardiopulmonary resuscitation if they stop breathing or have no pulse.

K. Ethical Issues Related to Dying

1. The Uniform Determination of Death Act
    a. served as a guide for federal lawmakers.
    b. provided a definition of death.
    c. declared death if reversible cessation of circulatory and respiratory functions occurs.
    d. declared death if reversible cessation of all function of the brain occurs.

2. If providers have questions regarding life-sustaining treatments, they should
    a. support the decision of the patient or surrogate.
    b. review the patient's advance directive.
    c. seek advice from an ethics committee.
    d. all of the above

Match the types of euthanasia with the description.

3. _____ The patient consents to the euthanasia action.

4. _____ Another person kills the patient.

5. _____ Killing the person using an injection.

6. _____ The patient does not consent to the action.

7. _____ Withholding a lifesaving treatment and letting the person die.

8. _____ The patient kills him- or herself.

9. _____ The patient kills him- or herself with the assistance of another person.

a. active euthanasia
b. passive euthanasia
c. voluntary euthanasia
d. involuntary euthanasia
e. self-administered euthanasia
f. other-administered euthanasia
g. assisted euthanasia

L. Organ Donation and Ethical Issues

1. Which of the following organs and tissues can be donated?
   a. Intestines, pancreas, and lung
   b. Tendons, bone marrow, and corneas
   c. Kidney, liver, and heart
   d. All of the above

2. With _____, the donor specifically names the person to receive the donation.

3. In _____, a pair of organs is involved and the transplant candidates do not match the donor they know, but match the other donor; thus, the organs are swapped or traded.

4. With _____, the organ donor does not know the person nor is related to the person.

M. Organ Donation Laws

1. The Uniform Anatomical Gift Act
   a. makes it easier for people to donate organs.
   b. was enacted by states and differences exist among states.
   c. provides uniformity in organ and tissue donations across the nation.
   d. all of the above

2. The National Organ Transplant Act
   a. established the Organ Procurement and Transplant Network.
   b. established a national registry for organ matching.
   c. was passed by Congress in 1984.
   d. all of the above

CERTIFICATION PREPARATION

Circle the correct answer.

1. Which term means "rules of conduct that differentiate between acceptable and unacceptable behavior"?
   a. Ethics
   b. Justice
   c. Morals
   d. Code of ethics

2. Which term means "internal principles that distinguish between right and wrong"?
   a. Ethics
   b. Morals
   c. Justice
   d. Nonmaleficence

3. _____ are codes of conduct stated by an employer or professional association.
   a. Personal ethics
   b. Morals
   c. Professional ethics
   d. Code of ethics

4. Which term means "to do no harm"?
   a. Autonomy
   b. Justice
   c. Nonmaleficence
   d. Beneficence

5. What is the process of creating a genetically identical biological entity?
   a. Genetic engineering
   b. Cloning
   c. Genetic testing
   d. Pharmacogenetics

6. Which Kübler-Ross stage of grief and dying involves the person refusing to accept the fact?
   a. Anger
   b. Depression
   c. Bargaining
   d. Denial

7. Which advance directive provides instructions about life-sustaining medical treatment to be administered or withheld when the patient has a terminal condition?
   a. Medical durable power of attorney
   b. Healthcare proxy
   c. Living will
   d. Organ donation

8. Which advance directive allows a competent adult to appoint a person (called a proxy or agent) to make healthcare decisions in the event the patient is unable to do so?
   a. Medical durable power of attorney
   b. Healthcare proxy
   c. Living will
   d. Organ donation

9. Which is the type of euthanasia where the patient consents to the action?
   a. Active
   b. Passive
   c. Voluntary
   d. Involuntary

10. Which act provides uniformity in organ and tissue donations across the nation?
    a. Patient Self-Determination Act
    b. Uniform Anatomical Gift Act
    c. Uniform Determination of Death Act
    d. National Organ Transplant Act

WORKPLACE APPLICATIONS

1. Mrs. Johnson called Walden-Martin Family Medical Clinic and Daniela answered the phone. Mrs. Johnson requested an appointment. She stated that she has experienced sleep changes, difficulty concentrating, sadness, and appetite changes since her husband died. Based on what you have read in this chapter, what might be occurring with Mrs. Johnson?

    _____

    _____

2. Jean is graduating from a medical assistant program. During her practicum, she heard about the dangers of narcotic medications. She does not believe that patients should receive narcotic medications. Jean is an advocate of alternative medications and feels there are reasonable alternatives to narcotic medications. How should Jean approach finding a job, given her bias?

    _____

    _____

3. Jan, a certified medical assistant, was discussing advance directives with a patient. The patient asked Jan to explain the importance of advance directives. How would you explain the importance of advance directives?

    _____

    _____

    _____

INTERNET ACTIVITIES

1. Using the internet, research your state's advance directive forms. Create a poster presentation, PowerPoint presentation, or paper summarizing the topic areas on the advance directive forms. Cite your resource(s).

2. Using the internet, research your state's Safe Haven laws for children. If your state does not have these laws, select a state that does. Create a poster presentation, PowerPoint presentation, or paper summarizing the Safe Haven laws. Focus on related statutes, maximum age of the child, and locations where the child can be brought. Cite your resource(s).

3. Using the internet, research an ethical issue. Create a poster presentation, PowerPoint presentation, or paper summarizing your findings. In your project, summarize the ethical issue and provide the advocates' and opponents' views of the issue.

Procedure 5.1   Developing an Ethics Separation Plan

Name _____   Date _____   Score _____

Task: To develop a plan for separation of personal and professional ethics.

Scenario: You are working at WMFM Clinic. Your provider sees many children, including teens. New state laws allow confidential healthcare for minors. The agency has now adopted policies and procedures to allow providers to see teens 16 years or older without parental consent. The teens can be seen for sexually transmitted infections (STIs) and reproductive issues (including birth control). All health records related to these visits are confidential, meaning parents cannot be told about their child's visit.

Your personal belief is that parents should always be allowed to know what is occurring with their children. They are responsible for the child until age 18, and they pay the bills. You also believe that children under 18 are too young to be in an intimate relationship, which should be reserved for adults who are committed to each other. You do not believe in birth control.

Equipment and Supplies:
- Paper and pen
- Medical Assisting Code of Ethics (see box in the textbook)

Standard: Complete the procedure and all critical steps with a minimum score of 85% within two attempts (*or as indicated by the instructor*).

Scoring: Divide the points earned by the total possible points. Failure to perform a critical step, indicated by an asterisk (*), results in grade no higher than an 84% (*or as indicated by the instructor*).

Steps/Criteria:	Point Value	Attempt 1	Attempt 2
1. Read the code of ethics for medical assistants. Write down key themes or phrases.	15		
2. Using the scenario, write down the professional ethics involved in the situation.	15		
3. Using the scenario, write down the personal ethics involved in the situation.	15		
4. Compare the lists. Identify the personal ethics that conflict with the code of ethics and the professional ethics of the agency.	15		
5. For each area of conflict, create a plan for how you will separate your personal and professional ethics. Remember, as a professional, you need to follow the professional ethics of the agency and the profession. Address how you will handle the situation and what your options would be if you were in the situation.	20*		
6. Describe how the personal ethics and morals in this scenario would impact patient care. • Describe how a medical assistant's personal ethics and morals could impact how that person provides care. • Describe how patient care may be altered or not up to the standard of care required. • Describe how a medical assistant could respond in a professional manner and maintain the standard of care and personal integrity.	20*		
Total Points	**100**		

Comments

CAAHEP Competencies	Step(s)
XI.P.1. Demonstrate professional response(s) to ethical issues	5
ABHES Competencies	**Step(s)**
4. Medical Law and Ethics g. Display compliance with the Code of Ethics of the profession	5

Procedure 5.2 Demonstrate Appropriate Response to Ethical Issues

Name _____ Date _____ Score _____

Tasks: Identify ethical issues and demonstrate professional responses. Recognize the impact of personal ethics and morals on the delivery of healthcare.

Scenario 1: You are working at WMFM Clinic. You are responsible for collecting payments from patients. Mr. Smythe, who is visually impaired, paid for his visit in cash. He gives you $500 for a $402 bill. You make change and give him a receipt. At the end of the day, you notice that you have $60 more than what you should have, and some of the bills were mixed up in the cashbox. You realize you gave Mr. Smythe the incorrect amount of money.

Scenario 2: You are setting up a laceration repair tray for Dr. Martin to use. As you are preparing the sterile equipment, one of the instruments becomes contaminated. You know Dr. Martin urgently needs the tray. You do nothing about the contamination, which you realize can cause an infection. You finish setting up the tray.

Equipment and Supplies:
- Paper and pen

Standard: Complete the procedure and all critical steps in _____ minutes with a minimum score of 85% within two attempts (*or as indicated by the instructor*).

Scoring: Divide the points earned by the total possible points. Failure to perform a critical step, indicated by an asterisk (*), results in grade no higher than an 84% (*or as indicated by the instructor*).

Time: Began_____ Ended_____ Total minutes: _____

Steps:	Point Value	Attempt 1	Attempt 2
1. Read both scenarios. Identify and write down the ethical issues involved.	20		
2. With a peer, role-play scenario 1. Demonstrate a professional and appropriate ethical response to this situation. a. Explain the situation to the supervisor. b. Describe how you felt the error occurred and who received the incorrect change. c. Explain how you would like to handle the situation and correct the error.	30		
3. With a peer, role-play scenario 2. During the role-play, demonstrate a professional and appropriate ethical response to this situation.	30		
4. In a written response, discuss the potential implication for the patient's health related to not reporting or correcting the error in scenario 2.	20		
Total Points	100		

- Ethical issue(s) identified in scenario 1:_____

_____

_____

_____

- Ethical issue(s) identified in scenario 2:_____

  _____

  _____

  _____

- Discuss the potential implication for the patient's health related to not reporting or correcting the error.

  _____

  _____

  _____

  _____

  _____

  _____

  _____

  _____

  _____

Comments

CAAHEP Competencies	Step(s)
XI.P.1. Demonstrate professional response(s) to ethical issues	1-3
ABHES Competencies	**Step(s)**
4. Medical Law and Ethics g. Display compliance with the Code of Ethics of the profession	Entire procedure

Technology

CAAHEP Competencies	Assessment
V.C.15. Identify the medical assistant's role in telehealth	Skills and Concepts – I. 19
VI.C.5. Identify the importance of data back-up	Skills and Concepts – J. 6-7
VI.C.6. Identify the components of an Electronic Medical Record, Electronic Health Record, and Practice Management System	Skills and Concepts – I. 10-17; Certification Preparation – 4-5
XII.C.7.b. Identify principles of: ergonomics	Skills and Concepts – H. 1-8

ABHES Competencies	Assessment
7. Administrative Procedure h. Perform basic computer skills	Procedure 6.2
8. Clinical Procedures a. Practice standard precautions and perform disinfection/sterilization techniques	Procedure 6.1

VOCABULARY REVIEW

Using the word pool on the right, find the correct word to match the definition. Write the word on the line after the definition.

Group A

1. Any peripheral hardware that allows the user to provide data to the computer _____

2. A set of electronic instructions to operate and perform different computer tasks _____

3. A pen-shaped device with a variety of tips that is used on touchscreens to write, draw, or enter commands

   _____

4. An electronic record that conforms to nationally recognized standards and contains health-related information about a specific patient; can be created, managed, and consulted by authorized clinicians and staff from more than one healthcare organization

   _____

Word Pool
- electronic health record (EHR)
- hardware
- input device
- optical character recognition
- output device
- patient portal
- secondary storage devices
- software
- stylus
- telemedicine

5. Computer hardware that displays the processed data from the computer (e.g., monitors and printers) _____

6. The remote diagnosis and treatment of patients using technology _____

7. A secure online website that gives patients 24-hour access to personal health information using a username and password _____

8. Scanners convert images to digital text through this process _____

9. Media (e.g., jump drive, flash drive, hard drive) capable of permanently storing data until they are replaced or deleted by the user

    _____

10. Physical equipment of the computer system required for communication and data processing functions

    _____

Group B

1. A computer application that allows the user to enter demographic information, schedule appointments, maintain lists of insurance payers, perform billing tasks, and generate reports

    _____

2. A system that links personal computers and peripheral devices to share information and resources _____

3. Peripheral computer hardware that connects to the router to provide internet access to the network or computer

    _____

4. A personal computer that doesn't contain a hard drive and allows the user only limited functions including access to software, the network, or the internet _____

5. Files are copied onto many servers in various locations

    _____

6. Computer hardware and software that perform data analysis, storage, and archiving; also called a *database server*

    _____

7. A private computer network that can only be accessed by authorized people _____

8. A collection of data or program records stored as a unit with a specific name _____

9. Used to allow multiple devices to be on the same network to send and receive information _____

10. A communication system for connecting several computers so information can be shared _____

Word Pool
- computer network
- data server
- downtime
- dumb terminal
- electronic medical record (EMR)
- ethernet
- file
- intranet
- modem
- practice management software (PMS)
- protected health information
- redundancy
- router

11. An electronic record of health-related information about an individual that can be created, gathered, managed, and accessed by authorized clinicians and staff members within a single healthcare organization; also called *EMR*

    _____

12. The interval of time during which something, such as hardware or software, is not functioning _____

13. Individually identifiable health information stored or transmitted by covered entities or business associates. Includes verbal, paper, or electronic information _____

ABBREVIATIONS

Write out what each of the following abbreviations stands for.

1. EHR_____

2. PC _____

3. ADF_____

4. NPP _____

5. LCD_____

6. CPU_____

7. ROM _____

8. RAM _____

9. HDD _____

10. USB _____

11. RW_____

12. TB _____

13. LAN _____

14. WAN_____

15. ISP _____

16. DSL _____

SKILLS AND CONCEPTS

Answer the following questions. Write your answer on the line or in the space provided.

A. Computers

Match the type of computer to the description.

1. _____ Large tower computers that are used by large organizations to store large quantities of information

2. _____ Smaller computers that have their own central processing unit (CPU)

3. _____ Expensive, very large computers that have incredibly fast processing speeds

4. _____ Large multiprocessing machines that support about 200 users at a time

5. _____ Computers that can be carried, such as laptops, netbooks, tablets, and smartphones

a. mobile computer
b. personal computer
c. minicomputer
d. mainframe computer
e. supercomputer

Fill in the blank.

6. A server can also be a(n) _____.

7. The personal computer is a(n) _____, or the primary computer equipment and all other forms of physical equipment used with the PC are called _____.

B. Input Devices

1. Which is *not* an input device?
   a. Printer and monitor
   b. Keyboard and mouse
   c. Touchscreen and signature pad
   d. Webcam and microphone

Fill in the blank.

2. For a radiofrequency connection to work, a(n) _____ must be plugged into the Universal Serial Bus (USB) drive on the device.

3. _____ uses shortwave radio frequencies to interconnect wireless electronic devices.

4. A touchscreen allows a person to interact with the computer by touching the display screen with a finger or _____.

5. A(n) _____ or smart pen is a battery-operated device that looks like and functions like a regular pen but can also digitally capture handwriting or drawing.

6. The remote diagnosis and treatment of patients using technology is called _____, a form of telehealth.

7. Scanners convert images to digital text through a process called _____.

C. Output Devices

1. Which of the following is an output device?
   a. Monitor
   b. Speakers
   c. Printer
   d. All of the above

Fill in the blank.

2. Images are created on monitors using _____; the _____ the number, the sharper the image.

3. A laser printer uses a(n) _____, _____, and _____ to produce images on paper.

D. Internal Computer Components
Fill in the blank.

1. The _____ is the "brain" of the computer and it sits on the _____.

2. The hard drive, _____ of the computer, contains the operating system and the re-lated system fields.

Match the primary memory with the correct description.

3. _____ Main working memory; lost if power is turned off

4. _____ Provides temporary use of information; contains data and instructions for opened programs

5. _____ Contains memory that has hardwire instructions. Not lost if power is cut, since a small long-life battery supports it

6. _____ Used for loading and running programs

7. _____ Allows programs to operate more quickly and efficiently

8. _____ Used to boot a computer or start the system diagnostic checks

a. read-only memory (ROM)
b. cache memory
c. random access memory (RAM)

E. Secondary Storage Devices and Cloud Storage

1. A(n) _____ is usually considered a character, such as a number, letter, or symbol.

2. Put these data storage capacities in order from smallest to largest: MB, GB, TB, KB_____

   _____

3. _____, also called file sharing or online storage; allows computer files to be stored using the internet and a third-party service.

4. The advantage of having the healthcare facility's computer environment on the cloud is
    a. the user can access the healthcare facility's computer environment from any location with web access and through a wired or wireless connection.
    b. Access can occur at any time of the day.
    c. All of the above

F. Network and Internet Access Devices

1. The intranet allows the employers to _____ with each other and share _____.

2. Only _____ can access the intranet or network in a healthcare facility.

3. A(n) _____ must be used to allow multiple devices to be on the same network.

4. For a healthcare facility's computer network to access the internet, they need to subscribe to a(n) _____ and to have its router connected to a(n) _____.

G. Maintaining Computer Hardware

1. What is a way to prevent computer problems?
    a. Hardware should be located on a stable, even surface, away from heat sources.
    b. Ventilation slots should be clear, allowing air to flow into the device to cool the components.
    c. Cables and electric cords should be securely plugged in.
    d. Liquids and food should be kept away from the hardware.
    e. All of the above

2. How should the hardware's casing be cleaned?
    a. Use a damp lint-free cloth to wipe the hardware's casing to remove the grime and dirt.
    b. Wipe clean all vents and air holes.
    c. All of the above

3. What is an infection control practice for technological devices in the ambulatory care facility?
    a. Disinfect keyboards daily.
    b. Healthcare professionals should sanitize hands before and after using keyboards.
    c. Gloves should not be worn during computer use.
    d. Touchscreen computer monitors and signature pads should be cleaned and disinfected daily per the manufacturer's guidelines.
    e. All of the above

H. Computer Workstation Ergonomics

1. _____ is the field of study that involves reducing strain and injuries by improving workstation design.

2. The _____ should help support the upper body and the backrest lumbar support area should be fitted to the small of the back

3. The _____ should support the forearms with the shoulders in a relaxed position.

4. The torso and neck should be _____ and _____.

5. The feet need to be _____ on the floor or a footrest.

6. The monitor should be directly in front of the person with the _____ of the monitor at or just below eye level.

7. The work surface and mouse should be at _____ for typing.

8. The wrist should be supported by a foam _____.

I. Software Used in Ambulatory Care

1. _____ is a collection of programs that operate and control the computer.

2. The _____ loads on the computer and operates in the background while application software is used.

3. _____ allows the user or other applications to perform specific tasks.

Match the description with the correct application software. Answers can be used more than once.

4. _____ Microsoft Access and EHR software
5. _____ Microsoft Excel and Google Sheets
6. _____ Microsoft Word and Google Docs
7. _____ PMS
8. _____ Corel WordPerfect

a. word processing software
b. spreadsheet software
c. database software

Select the correct answer.

9. What task is done with PMS?
   a. Scheduling appointments
   b. Patient registration
   c. Billing and coding medical charges
   d. Managing finances
   e. All of the above

10. Which of the following is a component of PMS?
    a. Claim denial management and electronic claim submission
    b. Financial and management reporting
    c. Scheduler and insurance eligibility verification
    d. Medical coding or encoder
    e. All of the above

Match the description with the correct PMS features.

11. _____ Used to detect errors on insurance claims before they are electronically submitted

12. _____ Used to verify patients' insurance benefits quickly

13. _____ Used to create customized business reports to show the amount of revenue the provider brought into the business

14. _____ Used to select diagnostic and procedural codes during the billing process

15. _____ Used to manage the provider's schedule and to schedule patient appointments

a. claim denial management and electronic claim submission
b. financial and management reporting
c. scheduler
d. medical coding or encoder
e. insurance eligibility verification

Select the correct answer or fill in the blank.

16. The _____ is a digital version of the paper medical record and contains limited information usually related to medical treatment for one healthcare facility.

17. What is a component of the EHR?
    a. Patient's past medical history and family history
    b. Visit information
    c. Laboratory and diagnostic imaging reports
    d. Hospital documents and consultation reports
    e. All of the above

18. A(n) _____ is a secure website that allows a patient 24-hour access to their health information

19. What is the medical assistant's role in virtual visits (telehealth)?
    a. Scheduling the visit for the patient
    b. Providing patients directions on how to access the software
    c. Explain the virtual visit process to the patient
    d. Update the patient's information during the visit
    e. All of the above

J. Computer Network Privacy and Security

1. The _____ include administrative policies, procedures, and actions to manage the security measures to protect electronic health information.

2. _____ involves identifying potential computer network breach threats and the likelihood that they will occur.

3. _____ include the physical measures, policies, and procedures used to protect the computer network and related buildings and equipment from hazards and unauthorized access.

4. _____ include technology, policies, and procedures that protect the ePHI and access to it.

5. _____ is software used to encode or change the information into nonreadable or encrypted data and the reader will need to enter a password for decryption to occur and to make the text readable again.

6. _____ is a process in which the network files are copied using an external hard drive, a server, or an online backup system.

7. What is the importance of data backup?
   a. It protects the data from a disaster in the medical facility.
   b. The data backup file can be used if the facility's data is compromised by errors, natural causes, or human causes.
   c. All of the above

8. _____ are devices that attach to the monitor that allow visualization of the screen contents only if the user is directly in front of the screen; also called monitor filters or privacy screens.

9. A(n) _____ is a record of computer activity used to monitor users' actions within software, including additions, deletions, and viewing of electronic records.

10. _____ means that each employee with network access must log in using a unique password.

11. A(n) _____ is a program or hardware device that acts as a barrier or filter between the network and the internet.

K. Recognizing and Preventing Phishing Attacks

1. _____ is defined as a generic cyberattack toward many individuals or organizations with the intent to steal confidential data or install malware on the users' devices.

2. _____ is defined as a customized cyberattack toward an individual or organization with the intent to steal confidential data or install malware on the user's device.

3. _____ is to assume or mimic the identity of another user to gain access to a computer system.

4. _____ is malicious software that can infiltrate the computer system and any network.

5. How can a person protect against phishing attacks?
   a. Use virus protection software.
   b. Do not respond to any text or email that asks for your username or password.
   c. Do not click on anything in unsolicited email or text messages.
   d. Be careful of the information shared online and on social media.
   e. All of the above

L. Continual Technologic Advances in Healthcare
Match the description with the correct term.

1. _____ The use of electronic software to communicate with pharmacies and send prescribing information

2. _____ Something designed to be used at or near where the patient is seen

3. _____ A method used to gather patient data outside of the traditional healthcare environment by using technologic devices

a. remote patient monitoring
b. point-of-care
c. e-prescribing

CERTIFICATION PREPARATION

Circle the correct answer.

1. What is one kilobyte equivalent to?
   a. 1024 bytes
   b. 1024 MB
   c. 1024 GB
   d. 1024 TB

2. Which software protects computers against viruses?
   a. Database software
   b. Presentation software
   c. Anti-malware software
   d. Spreadsheet software

3. What is a physical safeguard that is used over monitors to prevent others from seeing the information?
   a. Firewalls
   b. Screen savers
   c. Authentication
   d. Privacy filters

4. Which is a type of software that allows the user to enter demographic information, schedule appointments, maintain lists of insurance payers, perform billing tasks, and generate reports?
   a. EHR
   b. EMR
   c. PMS
   d. Microsoft Word and Excel

5. What is an electronic version of a patient's paper record?
   a. EHR
   b. EMR
   c. PMS
   d. a and b

6. What are records of computer activity used to monitor users' actions within software, including additions, deletions, and viewing of electronic records?
   a. Automatic log-off
   b. Authentication
   c. Firewalls
   d. Audit trails

7. What is malicious software designed to damage or disrupt a system (e.g., a virus)?
   a. Decryption
   b. Ethernet
   c. Hacker
   d. Malware

8. What means potential threats to the computer system security are identified, the likelihood of such occurrence is determined, and additional safeguards are implemented?
   a. Firewalls
   b. Security risk analysis
   c. Authentication
   d. Privacy filters

9. What makes a strong password?
   a. Using a person's name
   b. Consisting of eight or more characters
   c. A random combination of upper- and lowercase letters, numbers, and symbols
   d. b and c

10. Which is the computer memory used for loading and running programs?
    a. ROM
    b. RAM
    c. Cache
    d. Hard drive

WORKPLACE APPLICATIONS

1. As part of her role, Christiana is learning about security measures to keep the network secure and confidential. Identify the security measures described.

   a. Records of computer activity used to monitor users' actions within software, including additions, deletions, and viewing of electronic records.

    b.   A program or hardware device that acts as a barrier or filter between the network and the internet.

    _____

    c.   After a period of inactivity, the workstation logs off. _____

    _____

    d.   Potential threats of network breaches are identified and action plans are instituted to prevent the breaches.

    _____

    e.   Used to encode or change the information into nonreadable or encrypted data. _____

    _____

2.   Christiana is evaluating the scanners in the reception area and the health information management department, which handles scanning documents into EHRs. Discuss types of scanners that might be used in both of these areas.

    _____

    _____

    _____

3.   Christiana would like to have a computer with internet access available for patients to use in the reception area. What are things that she will need to consider?

    _____

    _____

INTERNET ACTIVITIES

1.   Review the content of one of the patient education websites listed in the chapter. Create a poster presentation, a PowerPoint presentation, or write a paper summarizing your research.

2.   Select a disease. Find two reputable patient education websites that provide information on the disease, diagnostic tests, and treatments. One of your websites must be different than those listed in the chapter. Create a poster presentation, a PowerPoint presentation, or write a paper summarizing your research and include the websites used.

3.   You need to purchase a printer for your department. Research a business-sized laser printer and an inkjet printer. Create a poster presentation, a PowerPoint presentation, or write a paper summarizing your research and include the websites used. Include the following points for each printer:
    a.   Name and model number of the printer
    b.   Cost of the printer
    c.   Cost of a new printer cartridge
    d.   Speed of the printer
    e.   Additional features of the printer that would be useful in a business setting

Procedure 6.1   Prepare a Workstation

Name _____   **Date** _____   **Score** _____

Tasks: Perform infection control procedures and create an ergonomically friendly workstation.

Equipment and Supplies:
- Nonabrasive disinfectant (hospital grade) wipes or specially made wipes for computer hardware or as indicated by the keyboard manufacturer
- Gloves (if required for using wipes)
- User guide for keyboard or facility's infection control procedure for computer hardware
- Desktop computer with adjustable monitor
- Office chair with an adjustable seat, armrest, and backrest
- Footrest (if needed)
- Foam wrist rest
- Document holder (optional)
- Hand sanitizer (optional)

Standard: Complete the procedure and all critical steps in _____ minutes with a minimum score of 85% within two attempts (*or as indicated by the instructor*).

Scoring: Divide the points earned by the total possible points. Failure to perform a critical step, indicated by an asterisk (*), results in grade no higher than an 84% (*or as indicated by the instructor*).

Time: Began_____ Ended_____ Total minutes: _____

Steps:	Point Value	Attempt 1	Attempt 2
1. While sitting in the chair, adjust the backrest so it supports the upper body and the lumbar support area fits to the small of the back. Adjust the seat pan height so the feet are flat on the floor or footrest. Adjust the armrest to support the forearms with the shoulders in a relaxed position.	20		
2. Adjust the monitor so it is directly in front of the person and the top of the monitor is at or just below the eye level. If using a document holder, position it so it is at the same distance and height as the monitor.	20		
3. Place the keyboard at a height and an angle to allow the wrists to be in a neutral position. Position the mouse so it is at elbow level for typing. Support the wrists with a foam wrist rest.	20		
4. While sitting with your torso and neck vertically and in line, identify if everything is positioned correctly and comfortably. Make any adjustments as needed.	10		
5. Using the keyboard user guide or the facilities' infection control procedure for computer hardware, determine the product to use to disinfect the keyboard. Don gloves if needed. Using a disinfectant wipe, clean the surface using friction for 5 seconds in each area. Discard gloves if worn.	20*		
6. Wash hands or use hand sanitizer before using the keyboard.	10*		
Total Points	100		

Comments

ABHES Competencies	Step(s)
8. Clinical Procedures a. Practice standard precautions and perform disinfection/ sterilization techniques	5

Procedure 6.2   Identify a Reliable Patient Education Website

Name _____   Date _____   Score _____

Tasks: Research a disease or condition and evaluate a patient education website.

Equipment and Supplies:
- Computer with internet access, word processing software, and printer

Standard: Complete the procedure and all critical steps in _____ minutes with a minimum score of 85% within two attempts (*or as indicated by the instructor*).

Scoring: Divide the points earned by the total possible points. Failure to perform a critical step, indicated by an asterisk (*), results in grade no higher than an 84% (*or as indicated by the instructor*).

Time: Began_____ Ended_____ Total minutes: _____

Steps:	Point Value	Attempt 1	Attempt 2
1. Select a disease or condition. Using the internet, find a website with information about the disease or condition. Do not use a website listed in this chapter.	10*		
2. Identify the mission or purpose of the website, who supports or runs the website, and whether there is advertising present on the page. If advertising is present, is the advertising mixed in with the content or text?	20		
3. Determine if the information is current or less than 3 years old.	10		
4. Identify the author(s) and the person's background. Does a panel of healthcare experts review the content?	20		
5. Identify if a person needs to enter personal information to view pages of the website. If so, what does the website's host do with the personal information?	20		
6. Compose a one-page paper on your findings. Use double line spacing and a 12-point font size. Include the website you used. Discuss if the website is reliable and if the content is updated. Proofread and spell-check your document prior to printing it.	20		
Total Points	**100**		

Comments

ABHES Competencies	Step(s)
7. Administrative Procedure h. Perform basic computer skills	Entire procedure

Written Communication

CAAHEP Competencies	Assessment
V.C.7. Identify different types of electronic technology used in professional communication	Skills and Concepts – E. 1; H. 1
V.P.6. Using technology, compose clear and correct correspondence	Procedures 7.1, 7.2, 7.3, 7.4, 7.5

ABHES Competencies	Assessment
7. Administrative Procedures g. Display professionalism through written and verbal communications	Procedures 7.1, 7.2, 7.3, 7.4, 7.5, 7.6
h. Perform basic computer skills	Procedures 7.1, 7.2, 7.3, 7.4, 7.5

VOCABULARY REVIEW

Using the word pool on the right, find the correct word to match the definition. Write the word on the line after the definition.

Group A

1. Types of communication _____

2. A word or group of words that describes a noun or pronoun

   _____

3. A word or group of words that answers *how, where, when*, or *to what extent*, thus further describing a verb, adjective, or adverbs

   _____

4. Often begin with words such as *although, since, when, because,* and *if*; needs a subject and verb to be a complete sentence

   _____

5. A word that indicates a relationship or location between a noun or pronoun and the rest of the sentence _____

6. A group of words without a subject or verb

   _____

Word Pool
- adjective
- adverb
- copy notation
- dependent clauses
- media
- phrase
- practice management software
- preposition
- reference notation
- template

7. Notes the initials of the person who composed the letter in uppercase followed by the initials of the person who keyed (typed) the letter in lowercase _____

8. Used to notify the letter's recipient who else received a copy of the letter _____

9. A type of software that allows the user to enter demographic information, schedule appointments, maintain lists of insurance payers, perform billing tasks, and generate reports

   _____

10. A document or file that has a preset format

    _____

Group B

1. A person who has written documentation that he or she can accept a shipment for another individual _____

2. An electronic record that conforms to nationally recognized standards and contains health-related information about a specific patient _____

3. The most common layout for a printed page; the height of the paper is greater than its width _____

4. Documents sent to a patient explaining that the provider is ending the physician-patient relationship and the patient needs to see another provider _____

5. The measurement around something; when referring to mail, it is the measurement around the middle of the package that is being shipped _____

6. A region or geographic area used for shipping

   _____

7. A term describing employees for whom an employer has obtained a fidelity bond from an insurance company that will cover losses from any dishonest acts (e.g., embezzlement, theft) committed by those employees _____

Word Pool
- authorized agent
- bonded
- electronic health record
- girth
- portrait orientation
- termination letters
- zone

SKILLS AND CONCEPTS
Answer the following questions either by filling in the blank or selecting the correct answer.

A. Parts of Speech

1. A(n) _____ is a word or phrase for a person, place, thing, or idea.

2. A(n) _____ is a word or a phrase that shows action or a state of being.

3. A(n) _____ is a phrase without a main clause and is a major error in writing.

4. A(n) _____ is a word or group of words that describes a noun or pronoun; may come before or after the noun or pronoun it describes.

5. A(n) _____ is a word or group of words that answers *how, where, when,* or *to what extent,* thus further describing a verb, adjective, or other adverbs.

6. A(n) _____ is a word that indicates a relationship or location between a noun or pronoun and the rest of the sentence.

B. Common Communication Errors

1. _____ are words that sound alike.

2. Which of the following statements contains a noun and pronoun mismatch?
   a. The providers see patients in the exam room.
   b. The receptionists asks patients for their updated insurance cards.
   c. The medical assistants room patients and obtain their vital signs.
   d. All of the above

3. Which statement is grammatically *incorrect*?
   a. Sally works as a receptionist at the dental clinic.
   b. The affect of the bad weather, patients arrived late.
   c. "Your good at your job," stated the patient.
   d. b and c

4. Which statement is grammatically correct?
   a. Tom went to room the patient.
   b. Jess was late, too.
   c. Two patients were left in the reception area.
   d. All of the above
   e. a and c

5. Which statement is grammatically *incorrect*?
   a. There were three exam rooms opened.
   b. Their provider was running late after doing hospital rounds.
   c. They're out to lunch.
   d. Their are two providers off today.

C. Punctuation
Fill in the blank.

1. Use a(n) _____ for a sentence that makes a statement.

2. Use a(n) _____ after a direct question.

3. Use a(n) _____ for sentences that express strong emotion.

4. A(n) _____ is a common punctuation mark used in professional letters and documentation.

5. A(n) _____ is used to introduce a series of items either in the sentence or a bulleted list.

6. _____ are used to set off direct quotes.

7. A(n) _____ is used to show ownership.

Match the error in the statement with the correct answers. Answers can be used more than once.

8. _____ Zac the receptionist greeted the patients when they arrived.

9. _____ My retirement is set for March 30 2027.

10. _____ Marie and I arrived early at the medical office

11. _____ Yes I will need your new insurance card.

12. _____ Thank you Katie for all your hard work.

a. missing a comma
b. missing two commas
c. missing a period

D. Capitalizations and Number

1. Which is a situation where capitalization is needed?
   a. The first letter of the first word in a sentence or question
   b. The pronoun "I"
   c. The first letter of proper nouns
   d. All of the above

2. Spell out all numbers at the _____ of a sentence.

E. Written Correspondence

1. How does the medical assistant use electronic technology in professional communication?
   a. They may communicate with vendors or supply companies.
   b. They may also need to send written communication to patients and other providers.
   c. They will compose letters and emails.
   d. All of the above

2. Professional letters use _____ paper or letterhead paper.

3. The letter typically has _____ margins on all four sides, although shorter letters may use larger margins.

4. The entire letter should be written using _____ line spacing.

5. What information is found in the sender's address?
   a. Facility's name, street address, or post office box
   b. City, state, and ZIP code
   c. May also include phone numbers, website address, and an email address
   d. All of the above

6. What is the correct format for the date in a professional letter?
   a. January 6, 2027
   b. January 6th 2027
   c. 01/06/2027
   d. January 6 2027

7. What punctuation mark is used after the greeting in a professional letter?
   a. Period
   b. Colon
   c. Semicolon
   d. Comma

8. How is the reference notation keyed if Kayla Smith typed the letter for Dr. James Martin?
   a. KS/JM
   b. JM/ks
   c. JM:ks
   d. JM:KS
   e. b and c

9. _____ is used to notify the letter's recipient who else received a copy of the letter.

10. _____ is used if the sender does not want the recipient to know a copy was sent to another person.

11. What should be on a continuation page?
    a. Recipient's name
    b. Page number
    c. Date
    d. All of the above

F. Business Letter Formats

1. Professional letters use "_____" punctuation, meaning all parts of the letter use punctuation marks.

2. Informal letters sometimes use "open" punctuation, which means the only punctuation used is found in the _____ of the letter.

3. With a full block letter format, all lines start flush with the _____ margin.

4. The semi-block format _____ the paragraphs in the body of the letter.

G. Memoranda

1. Letters and memos use _____ orientation.

2. Which of the following headings is *not* used in a memorandum?
   a. To
   b. Sender
   c. Date
   d. Subject

3. The headings are _____ justified with a blank line between each header.

4. The headings in a memorandum are
   a. keyed in bold font.
   b. keyed in capital letters.
   c. followed by a colon.
   d. all of the above

H. Professional Emails

1. Why do medical assistants need to know how to compose a professional email?
   a. Professional emails are used to communicate with providers and other staff members.
   b. Professional emails are now used more often to communicate with patients.
   c. All of the above

2. What is *not* an appropriate greeting for a professional email?
   a. "Good morning, Mr. Jones,"
   b. "Dear Mr. Jones,"
   c. "Hey Mr. Jones,"

3. You are sending an email to Mr. Black and Dr. Martin asked that you blind-copy him on the email. To do this, you would add Dr. Martin's name to _____ address line.

4. Refrain from using all _____ letters, since the reader may feel you are shouting at them.

5. When sending an email to several people, separate each email address by a(n) _____.

6. Add an email address to the _____ line if another person needs to receive a courtesy copy of the email.

7. How do you end a professional email?
   a. "Kind regards"
   b. "Thank you"
   c. "Sincerely"
   d. All of the above

I. Faxed Communications

1. When sending a fax regarding a patient, which federal law does *not* apply?
   a. HIPAA
   b. HITECH
   c. Confidentiality Act
   d. a and c

2. What information is included on a typical fax face sheet?
   a. Sender's name and phone number
   b. Receiver's name, company, fax number, and phone number
   c. Number of pages, date, and subject
   d. All of the above

3. When sending a fax, the medical assistant should
   a. include the fax cover sheet in the page count.
   b. fax the cover sheet last.
   c. All of the above

J. Preparing Mail

1. Business letters should be enclosed in standard _____ envelopes, which measure _____.

2. An automated mail processing machine reads the address on an envelope
   a. top line (the person's name) first.
   b. second address line (the street address) first.
   c. bottom line (i.e., city, state, and ZIP code) first.

3. When addressing mail, the medical assistant should
   a. use a simple black font of at least 10-point size.
   b. use all uppercase letters and no punctuation marks.
   c. left-justify the address.
   d. use only approved abbreviations.
   e. all of the above

4. When addressing mail, what should *not* be done?
   a. Use the # sign.
   b. Put one space between the city and state and two spaces between the state and ZIP code.
   c. Use the ZIP+4 code.
   d. Include an attention line below the last line of the delivery address.

K. Outgoing and Incoming Mail

1. Which factor affects the postage rate of mail?
   a. Weight and size of the item
   b. Urgency for arrival
   c. Delivery zone
   d. Services required
   e. All of the above

2. A(n) _____ shows the date when the item was mailed and additional information on when the delivery occurred and the recipient's signature.

3. Termination letters are sent by _____.

4. _____ is an optional mail service that protects against loss or damage and the cost is based on the declared value of the item.

5. _____ is an optional mail service that requires the addressee or authorized agent to verify identity when signing for the delivery.

6. _____ is an optional mail service that requires the recipient to pay for the merchandise and shipping when the package is received.

CERTIFICATION PREPARATION
Circle the correct answer.

1. Which is a word or group of words that describes a noun or pronoun?
   a. Adverb
   b. Adjective
   c. Verb
   d. Noun

2. Which needs to be capitalized?
   a. The first letter of the first word in a sentence or question
   b. The first letter of proper nouns
   c. The pronoun "I"
   d. All of the above

3. When should a comma be used?
   a. Before a coordinator (and, but, yet, nor, for, or, so) that links two main clauses
   b. To separate items in a list of three or more things
   c. After certain words (e.g., yes, no) at the start of a sentence
   d. All of the above

4. What punctuation is used at the end of the salutation in a professional letter?
   a. Colon
   b. Semicolon
   c. Comma
   d. Period

5. What includes the initials of the person who composed the letter?
   a. Enclosure notation
   b. Reference notation
   c. Copy notation
   d. Attachment notation

6. Which type of business letter format has the sender's and inside addresses and paragraphs left-justified and the date, closing, and signature block starts at the center point?
   a. Semi-block
   b. Memo
   c. Modified block
   d. Full block

7. Which is the most common mail service used for envelopes weighing up to 13 ounces, and provides delivery in 3 days or less?
   a. Priority Mail
   b. Priority Mail Express
   c. First-Class Mail
   d. Media Mail

8. Which optional mail service is used to protect expensive items, a mailing receipt is provided, and upon request, an electronic verification of delivery or delivery attempt can be sent?
   a. Registered Mail
   b. Standard Insurance
   c. Certified Mail
   d. Return Receipt

9. Dr. James Smith composed a letter and Cathy Black keyed the letter. What is the correct format for the notation in the letter?
   a. cb:JS
   b. JS:cb
   c. CB:js
   d. js:CB

10. Which is *not* a header in a memo?
    a. TO
    b. FROM
    c. DEPARTMENT
    d. SUBJECT

Workplace Applications

1. Christiana is composing the following letters. Indicate the name that should appear in the signature block.

   a. A letter from her to the office supply company. _____

   b. A letter to Mrs. White from Dr. James Martin. _____

   c. A referral letter about a patient from Dr. James Martin to Dr. Robert Black. _____

   _____

2. When Christiana Zwellen is composing a letter for Dr. James Martin, indicate two ways she can create the reference notation.

   _____

   _____

3. Christiana needs to fold a letter for a #10 envelope. Describe how this is done. _____

_____

_____

_____

INTERNET ACTIVITIES

1. Research professional email etiquette. Describe five ways you can improve your written communication with patients and professionals.

_____

_____

_____

2. Research the two-letter postal abbreviations for the states. Write each address provided as it should appear on an envelope. Use only approved U.S. Postal Service standard street abbreviations and the two-letter postal abbreviation for states.

   a. Walden-Martin Family Medical Clinic, 1234 Any Street, Anytown, Alabama 14453 _____

   _____

   _____

   b. John Smith, 383 E. Center, Anytown, Nebraska 13333-2232 _____

   _____

   _____

   c. Sally Black, 39291 S. Parkway, Anytown, Wisconsin 54334-6443_____

   _____

   _____

   d. Jeff Jones, 454 Boulevard, Anytown, Minnesota 49932-1234_____

   _____

   _____

   e. Sam House, 599 State Highway, Anytown, Illinois 69532-1651 _____

   _____

   _____

3. Use the ZIP code look-up tool on www.usps.com to find the ZIP codes for the following cities. Write the ZIP code on the line to the right of the city.

   a. Chicken, AK _____

   b. Rabbit Hash, KY _____

   c. Oatmeal, TX _____

   d. Turkey, TX _____

   e. Popcorn, IN _____

   f. Toast, NC _____

   g. Corn, OK _____

   h. Cucumber, WV _____

   i. Chili, WI _____

   j. Cream, WI _____

Procedure 7.1   Compose a Professional Business Letter Using the Full Block Letter Format

Name _____ Date _____ Score _____

Tasks: Compose a professional letter using technology. Use the full block letter format and closed punctuation. Address the envelope and fold the letter.

Scenario: Jean Burke, NP (nurse practitioner), has requested that you compose a letter to the parent (Lisa Parker) of Johnny Parker (date of birth [DOB]: 06/15/20XX) to let her know that Johnny's throat culture from last Wednesday was negative. If he is not improving or if she has any questions, she should call the office. Lisa Parker's address is 91 Poplar Street, Anytown, AL 12345-1234. You are working at Walden-Martin Family Medical Clinic. The healthcare facility's address is 1234 Anystreet, Anytown, AL 12345. The phone number is 123-123-1234 and the fax number is 123-123-5678.

Equipment and Supplies:
- Patient's health record
- Computer with word processing software and printer
- Paper
- #10 envelope

Standard: Complete the procedure and all critical steps with a minimum score of 85% within two attempts *(or as indicated by the instructor).*

Scoring: Divide the points earned by the total possible points. Failure to perform a critical step, indicated by an asterisk (*), results in grade no higher than an 84% *(or as indicated by the instructor).*

Steps:	Point Value	Attempt 1	Attempt 2
1. Obtain the intended recipient's contact information and determine the message you want to convey. Using the computer and word processing software, compose the letter using the full block letter format. Use 1-inch margins on all four sides, portrait orientation, and single line spacing throughout the letter. Use an easy-to-read font (e.g., Times New Roman or Calibri) in a 10- or 12-point size.	5		
2. Create a letterhead in the header of the document. Include the clinic's name, street address or post office box, city, state, and ZIP code.	10		
3. Key (type) the date starting at the left margin. Have one blank line between the date line and the last line of the letterhead.	10		
4. Key the inside address starting at the left margin and use the correct spelling and punctuation. Leave one to nine blank lines between the date and the inside address to center the body of the letter on the page.	10*		
5. Key the salutation starting at the left margin and use the correct spelling and punctuation. Leave one blank line between the inside address and the salutation.	10		
6. Use your critical thinking skills to compose a concise, accurate message. Type the message in the body of the letter starting at the left margin. Leave one blank line between the salutation and the first line of the body and then between each paragraph of the body. The message should be clear, concise, and professional. Use proper grammar, punctuation, capitalization, and sentence structure.	10		
7. Key a proper closing starting at the left margin and use correct spelling and punctuation. Leave one blank line between the last line of the body and the closing.	10		

8.	Key the signature block starting at the left margin and use the correct spelling and punctuation. Leave four blank lines between the closing and the signature block. If you are preparing the letter for a provider, you must include a reference notation.	**10**		
9.	Spell-check and proofread the document. Check for the proper tone, grammar, punctuation, capitalization, and sentence structure. Check for proper spacing between the parts of the letter. Make any final corrections. Print the document.	**5**		
10.	Address the envelope, using either the computer and word processing software or a pen and following the correct format.	**10**		
11.	When using a #10 envelope, fold the letter by pulling up the bottom end until it reaches just below the inside address or two-thirds of the way up the letter. Crease at the fold. Then, fold the top of the letter down so that it is flush with the bottom fold and crease the paper.	**5**		
12.	File a copy of the letter in the paper medical record or upload an electronic copy of the letter to the electronic health record (EHR).	**5**		
	Total Points	**100**		

Comments

CAAHEP Competencies	Step(s)
V.P.6. Using technology, compose clear and correct correspondence	Entire procedure
ABHES Competencies	**Step(s)**
7. Administrative Procedures g. Display professionalism through written and verbal communications	Entire procedure
7.h. Perform basic computer skills	Entire procedure

Procedure 7.2   Compose a Professional Business Letter Using the Modified Block Letter Format

Name _____ **Date** _____ **Score** _____

Tasks: Compose a professional letter using technology. Use the modified block letter format (with the center point option). Address the envelope (if needed) and fold the letter.

Scenario: Julie Walden, MD, has requested that you compose a letter to Carl C. Bowden (DOB: 04/05/19XX) to let him know that his hepatitis C laboratory test was negative. If he has any questions, he should call the office. His address is 19 Beale Street, Anytown, AL 12345-1234. You are working at Walden-Martin Family Medical Clinic. The healthcare facility's address is 1234 Anystreet, Anytown, AL 12345. The phone number is 123-123-1234 and the fax number is 123-123-5678.

Equipment and Supplies:
- Patient's health record
- Computer with word processing software and printer
- Paper
- #10 envelope or window business envelope

Standard: Complete the procedure and all critical steps with a minimum score of 85% within two attempts *(or as indicated by the instructor).*

Scoring: Divide the points earned by the total possible points. Failure to perform a critical step, indicated by an asterisk (*), results in grade no higher than an 84% *(or as indicated by the instructor).*

Steps:	Point Value	Attempt 1	Attempt 2
1. Obtain the intended recipient's contact information and determine the message you want to convey. Using the computer and word processing software, compose the letter using the modified block letter format. Use 1-inch margins on all four sides, portrait orientation, and single line spacing throughout the letter. Use an easy-to-read font (e.g., Times New Roman or Calibri) in a 10- or 12-point size.	5		
2. Create a letterhead in the header of the document. Include the clinic's name, street address or post office box, city, state, and ZIP code.	10		
3. Key (type) the date starting at the center point of the line, which is usually about 3.25 inches from the margin. Have one blank line between the date line and the last line of the letterhead.	10		
4. Key the inside address starting at the left margin and use the correct spelling and punctuation. Leave one to nine blank lines between the date and the inside address to center the body of the letter on the page. If using a window business envelope, adjust the address position to fit the window.	10*		
5. Key the salutation starting at the left margin and use the correct spelling and punctuation. Leave one blank line between the inside address and the salutation.	10		

6.	Use your critical thinking skills to compose a concise, accurate message. Type the message in the body of the letter starting at the left margin. Leave one blank line between the salutation and the first line of the body and then between each paragraph of the body. The message should be clear, concise, and professional. Use proper grammar, punctuation, capitalization, and sentence structure.	**10**		
7.	Key a proper closing. Start the closing at the center point of the line. (The first letter of the closing should align vertically with the first letter of the date.) Use correct spelling and punctuation. Leave one blank line between the last line of the body and the closing.	**10**		
8.	Key the signature block. Start the signature block at the center point of the line. (The first letter of the signature block should align vertically with the first letter of the date and closing.) Use the correct spelling and punctuation. Leave four blank lines between the closing and the signature block. If you are preparing the letter for a provider, you must include a reference notation.	**10**		
9.	Spell-check and proofread the document. Check for the proper tone, grammar, punctuation, capitalization, and sentence structure. Check for proper spacing between the parts of the letter. Make any final corrections. Print the document. If needed, address the envelope, using either the computer and word processing software or a pen and following the correct format.	**10**		
10.	When using a #10 envelope, fold the letter by pulling up the bottom end until it reaches just below the inside address or two-thirds of the way up the letter. Crease at the fold. Then, fold the top of the letter down so that it is flush with the bottom fold and crease the paper. For window business envelopes, have the letter's print side facing up and place the envelope over the top third of the letter. Fold the bottom edge of the paper up to the bottom edge of the envelope and crease at the fold. Then, remove the envelope and flip the letter over and fold the top of the letter down to the prior crease line and crease at the fold. Place the letter in the envelope so that the recipient's address shows through the window.	**10**		
11.	File a copy of the letter in the paper medical record or upload an electronic copy of the letter to the electronic health record (EHR).	**5**		
	Total Points	**100**		

Comments

CAAHEP Competencies	Step(s)
V.P.6. Using technology, compose clear and correct correspondence	Entire procedure
ABHES Competencies	**Step(s)**
7. Administrative Procedures g. Display professionalism through written and verbal communications	Entire procedure
7.h. Perform basic computer skills	Entire procedure

Procedure 7.3   Compose a Professional Business Letter Using the Semi-Block Letter Format

Name _____   Date _____   Score _____

Tasks: Compose a professional letter using technology. Use the semi-block letter format (with the center point option). Address the envelope and fold the letter.

Scenario: Julie Walden, MD, has requested that you compose a letter to Amma Patel (DOB: 01/14/19XX) to let her know that her thyroid test was normal, but her vitamin D level was low. Dr. Walden would like Amma to take 15 mcg of vitamin D each morning. She can purchase this over the counter. She needs to have her vitamin D rechecked in 6 months. She can call to schedule a blood test closer to that time. If she has any questions, she should call the office. Her address is 1346 Charity Lane, Anytown, AL 12345-1234. You are working at Walden-Martin Family Medical Clinic. The healthcare facility's address is 1234 Anystreet, Anytown, AL 12345. The phone number is 123-123-1234 and the fax number is 123-123-5678.

Equipment and Supplies:
- Patient's health record
- Computer with word processing software and printer
- Paper
- #10 envelope or #6¾ envelope

Standard: Complete the procedure and all critical steps with a minimum score of 85% within two attempts *(or as indicated by the instructor).*

Scoring: Divide the points earned by the total possible points. Failure to perform a critical step, indicated by an asterisk (*), results in grade no higher than an 84% *(or as indicated by the instructor).*

Steps:	Point Value	Attempt 1	Attempt 2
1. Obtain the intended recipient's contact information and determine the message you want to convey. Using the computer and word processing software, compose the letter using the semi-block letter format. Use 1-inch margins on all four sides, portrait orientation, and single line spacing throughout the letter. Use an easy-to-read font (e.g., Times New Roman or Calibri) in a 10- or 12-point size.	5		
2. Create a letterhead in the header of the document. Include the clinic's name, street address or post office box, city, state, and ZIP code.	10		
3. Key (type) the date starting at the center point of the line, which is usually about 3.25 inches from the margin. Have one blank line between the date line and the last line of the letterhead.	10		
4. Key the inside address starting at the left margin and use the correct spelling and punctuation. Leave one to nine blank lines between the date and the inside address to center the body of the letter on the page.	10*		
5. Key the salutation starting at the left margin and use the correct spelling and punctuation. Leave one blank line between the inside address and the salutation.	10		

6. Use your critical thinking skills to compose a concise, accurate message. Type the message in the body of the letter starting at the left margin. Leave one blank line between the salutation and the first line of the body and then between each paragraph of the body. Each paragraph should be indented five spaces. The message should be clear, concise, and professional. Use proper grammar, punctuation, capitalization, and sentence structure.	10			
7. Key a proper closing. Start the closing at the center point of the line. (The first letter of the closing should align vertically with the first letter of the date.) Use correct spelling and punctuation. Leave one blank line between the last line of the body and the closing.	10			
8. Key the signature block. Start the signature block at the center point of the line. (The first letter of the signature block should align vertically with the first letter of the date and closing.) Use the correct spelling and punctuation. Leave four blank lines between the closing and the signature block. If you are preparing the letter for a provider, you must include a reference notation.	10			
9. Spell-check and proofread the document. Check for the proper tone, grammar, punctuation, capitalization, and sentence structure. Check for proper spacing between the parts of the letter. Make any final corrections. Print the document.	5			
10. Address the envelope, using either the computer and word processing software or a pen and following the correct format.	10			
11. When using a #10 envelope, fold the letter by pulling up the bottom end until it reaches just below the inside address or two-thirds of the way up the letter. Crease at the fold. Then, fold the top of the letter down so that it is flush with the bottom fold and crease the paper. When using a #6{3/4} envelope, pull the bottom edge of the letter up until it is 1/2 inch from the top edge of the document and crease at the fold. Bring the right edge two-thirds of the way across the width of the document and crease the paper. Then bring the left edge to the right edge and crease at the fold. Flip the document so the left edge is on the bottom and insert the letter into the envelope.	5			
12. File a copy of the letter in the paper medical record or upload an electronic copy of the letter to the electronic health record (EHR).	5			
Total Points	100			

Comments

CAAHEP Competencies	Step(s)
V.P.6. Using technology, compose clear and correct correspondence	Entire procedure
ABHES Competencies	**Step(s)**
7. Administrative Procedures g. Display professionalism through written and verbal communications	Entire procedure
7.h. Perform basic computer skills	Entire procedure

Procedure 7.4　Compose a Memorandum

Name _____　Date _____　Score _____

Task: Compose a professional memorandum.

Scenario: You are asked by the supervisor to compose a memo that can be posted in the department. You are to remind the staff about the department meeting next Tuesday at noon in the conference room. Staff can bring their lunches and beverages will be provided.

Equipment and Supplies:
- Computer with word processing software and printer
- Paper

Standard: Complete the procedure and all critical steps with a minimum score of 85% within two attempts *(or as indicated by the instructor).*

Scoring: Divide the points earned by the total possible points. Failure to perform a critical step, indicated by an asterisk (*), results in grade no higher than an 84% *(or as indicated by the instructor).*

Steps:	Point Value	Attempt 1	Attempt 2
1. Determine the message you want to convey. Using the computer and word processing software, compose the memo. Use 1-inch margins on all four sides, portrait orientation, and single line spacing throughout the memo. Use an easy to read font (e.g., Times New Roman or Calibri) in a 10- or 12-point size.	15		
2. Left-justify the headers and use boldface and capital letters, followed by a colon. Headers include TO, FROM, DATE, and SUBJECT. Leave one blank line between each header.	15		
3. Key (type) the information following the headers in regular font, using a mix of capital and lowercase letters. Using the tab tool, align the information vertically down the page. Key the date as indicated for professional letters.	15		
4. Add a centered black line between the headers and the body (optional). Leave two to three blank lines between the headers and the body of the memo.	15		
5. Key the message in the body of the memo. Left-justify the content in the body and use single line spacing. Use proper grammar and correct spelling and punctuation. With multiple paragraphs, skip a single line between paragraphs.	15		
6. Write the content of the message in the body of the memo clearly, concisely, and accurately. Add special notations as needed.	15		
7. Spell-check and proofread the document. Check for the proper tone, grammar, punctuation, capitalization, and sentence structure. Check for proper spacing between the parts of the memo. Make any final corrections. Print the document.	10		
Total Points	**100**		

Comments

CAAHEP Competencies	Step(s)
V.P.6. Using technology, compose clear and correct correspondence	Entire procedure
ABHES Competencies	**Step(s)**
7. Administrative Procedures g. Display professionalism through written and verbal communications	Entire procedure
7.h. Perform basic computer skills	Entire procedure

Procedure 7.5   Compose a Professional Email

Name _____ Date _____ Score _____

Task: Compose a professional email that conveys the message to the reader clearly, concisely, and accurately.

Scenario: Aaron Jackson (DOB: 10/17/20XX) has an appointment at 11 a.m. next Thursday. Send his guardian an appointment reminder via email. Aaron will be seeing David Kahn, MD. The guardian should bring in any medications Aaron is currently taking. You are working at Walden-Martin Family Medical Clinic. The healthcare facility's address is: 1234 Anystreet, Anytown, AL 12345. The phone number is 123-123-1234 and the fax number is 123-123-5678. Your instructor will supply you with the guardian's name and email address.

Equipment and Supplies:
- Patient's health record
- Computer with email software

Standard: Complete the procedure and all critical steps with a minimum score of 85% within two attempts *(or as indicated by the instructor).*

Scoring: Divide the points earned by the total possible points. Failure to perform a critical step, indicated by an asterisk (*), results in grade no higher than an 84% *(or as indicated by the instructor).*

Steps:	Point Value	Attempt 1	Attempt 2
1. Obtain the intended recipient's contact information and determine the message you want to convey.	5		
2. Using the computer and email software, key (type) the recipient's email address. If the email has two recipients, use a semicolon (;) after the name of the first recipient. Double-check the email addresses for accuracy.	5*		
3. Key a subject, keeping it simple but focused on the contents of the email.	10		
4. Key a formal greeting, using correct punctuation.	10		
5. Key the message in the body of the email using proper grammar, spelling, punctuation, capitalization, and sentence structure. Avoid abbreviations. The message should be clear, concise, and professional.	20		
6. Finish the email with closing remarks.	10		
7. Key a closing, followed by your name and title on the next line. Include the clinic's name and contact information below your name.	10		
8. Spell-check and proofread the email. Check for proper tone, grammar, punctuation, capitalization, and sentence structure. Check for proper spacing between the parts of the email.	10		
9. Make any final revisions, select any features to apply to the email, and then send it.	10		
10. Print a copy of the email to be filed in the paper medical record or upload an electronic copy of the email to the patient's electronic health record (EHR).	10		
Total Points	**100**		

Comments

CAAHEP Competencies	Step(s)
V.P.6. Using technology, compose clear and correct correspondence	Entire procedure
ABHES Competencies	**Step(s)**
7. Administrative Procedures g. Display professionalism through written and verbal communications	Entire procedure
7.h. Perform basic computer skills	Entire procedure

Procedure 7.6   Complete a Fax Cover Sheet

Name _____ Date _____ Score _____

Task: Complete a fax cover sheet clearly and accurately.

Scenario: Lisa Parker, mother of Johnny Parker (DOB: 06/15/20XX), requested his immunization history to be sent to Anytown School, attention: Susie Payne. The school's phone number is 123-123-5784, and the fax number will be supplied by your instructor. The release of medical records has been completed and signed by Lisa, Johnny's guardian/mother. Your phone number is the main clinic number listed on the header of the fax cover sheet.

Equipment and Supplies:
- Document to be faxed (optional)
- Fax machine and fax number (optional)
- Pen
- Fax cover sheet (Work Product 7.1, HIPAA-Compliant Fax Cover Sheet)

Standard: Complete the procedure and all critical steps with a minimum score of 85% within two attempts *(or as indicated by the instructor).*

Scoring: Divide the points earned by the total possible points. Failure to perform a critical step, indicated by an asterisk (*), results in grade no higher than an 84% *(or as indicated by the instructor).*

Steps:	Point Value	Attempt 1	Attempt 2
1. Using a pen and the fax cover sheet, clearly and accurately write your name, phone number, and the date.	20		
2. Clearly and accurately write the name of the person receiving the fax. Also include the company, fax number, and phone number.	20		
3. Write the number of pages. The cover sheet must be counted in the total.	20		
4. Complete Re: by indicating the subject of the fax. Be general with the subject and refrain from including anything confidential.	20		
5. Proofread the fax cover sheet. Verify the name, agency, and contact information of the recipient. Verify the document(s) being sent are correct. Optional: organize the documents so the coversheet is on top and fax to the recipient.	20		
Total Points	100		

Comments

ABHES Competencies	Step(s)
7. Administrative Procedures g. Display professionalism through written and verbal communications	Entire procedure

Work Product 7.1   HIPAA-Compliant Fax Cover Sheet

To be used with Procedure 7.6.

Name _____   Date _____   Score _____

WALDEN-MARTIN

FAMILY MEDICAL CLINIC

1234 ANYSTREET | ANYTOWN, ANYSTATE 12345

PHONE 123-123-1234 | FAX 123-123-5678

Fax

To: _____   From: _____

Company: _____   Phone: _____

Fax: _____   Date: _____

Phone: _____

Pages: _____

Re: _____

CONFIDENTIAL NOTICE

The material enclosed with this facsimile transmission is confidential and private. The material is the property of the sender and some or all of the information may be protected by the Health Insurance Portability & Accountability Act (HIPAA). This information is intended exclusively for the addressed person or agency indicated above. If you are not the intended individual or entity of this information, you are hereby notified that any use, duplication, circulation, or transmission of the information is strictly prohibited under state and federal law. Please notify the sender immediate using the telephone number indicated above.

Telephone Techniques

CAAHEP Competencies	Assessments
V.P.4. Demonstrate professional telephone techniques	Procedure 8.1
V.P.5. Document telephone messages accurately	Procedure 8.2
X.P.2.a. Apply HIPAA rules in regard to: privacy	Procedure 8.1
X.P.3. Document patient care accurately in the medical record	Procedures 8.1, 8.2
A.1 Demonstrate critical thinking skills	Procedure 8.2

ABHES Competencies	Assessments
7. Administrative Procedures g. Display professionalism through written and verbal communications	Procedures 8.1, 8.2

VOCABULARY REVIEW

Using the word pool on the right, find the correct word to match the definition. Write the word on the line after the definition.

Group A

1. A commercial service that answers telephone calls for its clients _____

2. An unexpected, life-threatening situation that requires immediate action _____

3. A business telephone system that allows more than one telephone line _____

4. A feature that states who the caller is and displays the telephone numbers of incoming calls made to a particular line _____

5. The depth of a tone or sound; a distinctive quality of sound _____

6. A telephone feature that allows calls made to one number to be sent to another specified number _____

Word Pool
- multiple line telephone system
- ergonomics
- speakerphone
- caller ID
- voice mail
- emergency
- call forwarding
- answering service
- intercom
- provider
- speed dialing
- pitch

7. An applied science concerned with designing and arranging things needed to do a job in an efficient and safe way

_____

8. An individual or company that supplies medical care and services to a patient or the public _____

9. A telephone with a loudspeaker and a microphone; it can be used without having to pick up and hold the handset

_____

10. A telephone function in which a selected stored number can be dialed by pressing only one key _____

11. An electronic system that allows messages from telephone callers to be recorded and stored _____

12. A two-way communication system with a microphone and loudspeaker at each station; often a feature of business telephones _____

Group B

1. Ability to communicate effectively in two languages

_____

2. A physician or other healthcare provider who enters into a contract with a specific insurance company or program and by doing so agrees to abide by certain rules and regulations set forth by that third-party payer _____

3. A set dollar amount that the patient must pay for each visit

_____

4. A system that distributes incoming calls to a specific group or person based on customer need; for example, the customer presses 1 for appointments, 2 for billing questions, and so on

_____

5. A succession of syllables, words, or sentences spoken in an unvaried key or pitch _____

6. The use of articulate, clear sounds when speaking

_____

7. The quality of having a sense of what to do or say to maintain good relations with others or to prevent offense

_____

8. The vocabulary of a particular profession as opposed to common, everyday terms _____

9. A system for examining and separating into different groups; in the healthcare facility, it means determining the severity of illness that patients experience and prioritizing appointments based on that severity _____

10. The process of assigning degrees of urgency to patients' conditions _____

11. An acute situation that requires immediate attention but is not life-threatening _____

12. The medical abbreviation for the Latin term *statum*, meaning immediately; at this moment _____

Word Pool
- monotone
- enunciation
- tactful
- jargon
- screen
- triage
- urgent
- copayment (copay)
- participating provider
- STAT
- bilingual
- automatic call routing

SKILLS AND CONCEPTS

Answer the following questions. Write your answer on the line or in the space provided.

A. Telephone Equipment

1. Give an example of when the following telephone features would be used.

   Speakerphone: _____

   _____

   _____

   _____

   _____

   Conference calls: _____

   _____

   _____

   _____

   _____

   Voice mail: _____

   _____

   _____

   _____

   _____

   Call forwarding: _____

   _____

   _____

   _____

   _____

   Intercom: _____

   _____

   _____

   _____

   _____

B. Effective Use of the Telephone

1. List three things involved in active listening.

   a. _____

   b. _____

   c. _____

2. If you are speaking clearly and distinctly, you are using good _____.

3. It is important to make sure that patients understand what we are saying to them. In healthcare, medical terminology or _____ can make things more difficult for patients to understand.

C. Managing Telephone Calls

1. List the supplies needed to be prepared to answer incoming telephone calls. _____

   _____

   _____

   _____

   _____

2. How should a second incoming call be handled when you are already answering another call?

   _____

   _____

   _____

   _____

3. How should callers who refuse to identify themselves be handled? _____

   _____

   _____

   _____

   _____

   _____

4. List the conditions and/or symptoms that would be considered an emergency call. _____

   _____

   _____

   _____

   _____

5. What questions should be asked of the patient who calls the healthcare facility to give the provider the information that they need?

_____

_____

_____

_____

D. Typical Incoming Calls

1. When a patient calls requesting a medication refill, what information is needed? _____

_____

_____

_____

_____

_____

_____

2. How should requests for directions be handled? _____

_____

_____

_____

3. When a patient calls and asks for a referral to another provider, what should the medical assistant do?

_____

_____

_____

_____

_____

E. Special Incoming Calls

1. If a patient refuses to discuss their symptoms over the phone with the medical assistant and the provider is not able to take the call, what should the medical assistant suggest the patient do?

_____

_____

2. What is the best policy when a patient calls for test results that are abnormal?_____

_____

_____

3. What documentation should be in place before a medical assistant can give information to a third party?

_____

_____

4. How should a caller with a complaint be handled? _____

_____

_____

_____

F. Handling Difficult Calls
Indicate how you would handle the following calls.

1. Angry callers _____

_____

_____

_____

_____

2. Aggressive callers _____

_____

_____

_____

_____

3. Unauthorized inquiry calls _____

_____

_____

_____

_____

4. Sales calls _____

_____

_____

_____

_____

5.   Callers who speak foreign languages or have heavy accents: _____

_____

_____

_____

_____

G. Typical Outgoing Calls

1.   Use Figure 8.4 in the textbook to answer the following questions.

   a.   You are in the Central time zone and need to call an insurance carrier in the Pacific time zone. It is 9:00 AM in your location. What time is it in the Pacific time zone?

   _____

   b.   You are in the Pacific time zone and your provider has asked you to contact another provider in the Eastern time zone. It is 10:00 AM in your time zone. What time is it in the Eastern time zone?

   _____

   c.   You are in the Eastern time zone and need to contact a patient who is vacationing in the Mountain time zone. It is 3:00 PM in your time zone. What time is it in the Mountain time zone?

   _____

H. Using Directory Assistance

1.   List options for locating a telephone number. _____

_____

_____

_____

_____

_____

I. Telephone Services

1.   Explain the difference between an answering machine and answering service. _____

_____

_____

_____

_____

_____

CERTIFICATION PREPARATION

Circle the correct answer.

1. Which best describes the primary goal of "screening" telephone calls?
   a. Preventing calls from reaching the provider
   b. Handling calls at the lowest level possible
   c. Selecting which calls should be forwarded to which staff members through an understanding of the purpose of the call
   d. Determining whether the calls are emergencies

2. Active listening involves
   a. giving the same attention to a person on the telephone as would be given to a person face to face.
   b. concentrating on the conversation at hand.
   c. discovering vital information.
   d. all of the above.

3. The medical assistant should be extremely careful when using a speakerphone because
   a. the service is expensive.
   b. it is distracting.
   c. the call can be traced.
   d. confidentiality can be violated.

4. Which term would be considered jargon?
   a. Encephalalgia
   b. Rash
   c. Dizziness
   d. Headache

5. The medical assistant may help an angry caller calm down by
   a. getting angry in return.
   b. speaking in a lower tone of voice.
   c. referring the situation to the office manager immediately.
   d. calling the provider into the situation.

6. If your office is in New York and you need to contact a supplier in Seattle, which New York time would be the earliest that you should call to place an order, assuming that the supplier opens at 8 AM?
   a. 8:00 AM
   b. 9:00 AM
   c. 10:00 AM
   d. 11:00 AM

7. Which types of calls should be limited in the professional setting?
   a. Local
   b. Long distance
   c. Toll free
   d. Personal

8. Enunciation is
   a. the choice of words.
   b. the highness or lowness of sound.
   c. articulation of clear sounds.
   d. a change in pitch.

9. Which is *not* required when a telephone message is taken?
   a. The caller's name and phone number
   b. The time and date
   c. The name of the person to whom the call is directed
   d. The caller's account number

10. When placing callers on hold, how often should you check back to make sure the caller still wants to remain on hold?
    a. No longer than 1 minute
    b. Every 2 minutes
    c. Until time is available to talk
    d. It is not necessary to check back; patients will hold until you return to the call

WORKPLACE APPLICATIONS

1. Mr. Ken Thomas calls to get his prescription for Ambien refilled. His pharmacy is Wolfe Drug, and the drugstore phone number is 214-555-4523. Mr. Thomas is allergic to penicillin. His phone number is 214-555-2377. Mr. Thomas' message was received on July 23 at 10:15 AM.

   a. Who should receive this message? _____

   _____

   b. Questions to ask the patient: _____

   _____

   _____

   c. What action should be taken after speaking with the patient? _____

   _____

   _____

   _____

   _____

2. Message retrieved from the answering machine, "This is Sarah at AnyTown Lab with a STAT laboratory report. It is 9:35 AM on November 16. The patient's name is Noemi Rodriguez, date of birth November 4, 19XX and her WBC count is 18,000. Please notify Dr. Walden immediately. The laboratory phone number is 800-555-3333 and my extension is 255. If she has any questions, please have her give me a call. Thanks."

   a. Who should receive this message? _____

   _____

   b. Questions to ask Sarah: _____

   _____

   _____

   c. What action should be taken? _____

   _____

   _____

   _____

   _____

   _____

3. Denise has been the receptionist for a moderately large clinic for the past 3 months. She replaced Dorothy, who retired. Denise has been overwhelmed with the calls to the clinic, and the office manager has spoken to her twice about missing calls. Denise insists that she is constantly on the phone answering and transferring calls. She is beginning to lose faith in herself, but as she considers why she is failing at her job, she realizes that two new physicians have joined the practice since Dorothy left, and numerous calls come to the clinic for those two providers. Denise wants to suggest to the office manager that perhaps the time has come for a second receptionist, but she is unsure how to broach the subject. How can Denise begin her conversation with the office manager? What should she not do or say?

_____

_____

_____

_____

_____

_____

INTERNET ACTIVITIES

1. Using online resources, locate the following telephone numbers for your city or community.

   a. Nonemergency number for the police department _____

   b. Local social security office _____

   c. American Red Cross office _____

   d. Acute care hospital _____

   e. Meals on Wheels _____

   f. American Cancer Society _____

   g. Local senior center _____

   h. Local food bank _____

   i. Poison control _____

   j. Local child protective services _____

Procedure 8.1 Demonstrate Professional Telephone Techniques

Name _____ Date _____ Score _____

Task: To answer the telephone in a provider's office in a professional manner and respond to a request for action.

Scenario: Charles Johnson, DOB 3/3/19XX, an established patient of Dr. Martin, has called to schedule an appointment to have his blood pressure checked. This will be a follow-up appointment that is 15 minutes long. He is requesting that the appointment be on a Friday during his lunchtime between 11:00 and 12:00.

Equipment and Supplies:
- Telephone
- Pen or pencil
- Computer
- Notepad

Standard: Complete the procedure and all critical steps in _____ minutes with a minimum score of 85% within two attempts (*or as indicated by the instructor*).

Scoring: Divide the points earned by the total possible points. Failure to perform a critical step, indicated by an asterisk (*), results in grade no higher than an 84% (*or as indicated by the instructor*).

Time: Began _____ Ended _____ Total minutes: _____

Steps:	Point Value	Attempt 1	Attempt 2
1. Demonstrate telephone techniques by answering the telephone by the third ring.	10		
2. Speak distinctly with a pleasant tone and expression, at a moderate rate, and with sufficient volume for the person to understand every word.	15*		
3. Identify the office and/or provider and yourself.	10		
4. Verify the identity of the caller, and if using an electronic health record, bring the patient's health record to the active screen of the computer.	15*		
5. Screen the call if necessary.	10		
6. Apply active listening skills to assess whether the caller is distressed or agitated and to determine the concern to be addressed.	10*		
7. Determine the needs of the caller and provide the requested information or service if possible. Provide the caller with excellent customer service. Be as helpful as possible. Check the appointment schedule and determine the first Friday that would have an open appointment between 11:00 and 12:00.	10		
8. Obtain sufficient patient information to schedule the appointment, including the patient's full name, DOB, insurance information, and preferred contact method. Repeat the date and time of the appointment to ensure that the patient has the correct information.	10		
9. Terminate the call in a pleasant manner and replace the receiver gently, always allowing the caller to hang up first.	10		
Total Points	**100**		

Comments

CAAHEP Competencies	Step(s)
V.P.4. Demonstrate professional telephone techniques	Entire procedure
X.P.2.a Apply HIPAA rules in regard to: privacy	4
X.P.3. Document patient care accurately in the medical record	Entire procedure
ABHES Competencies	**Step(s)**
7. Administrative Procedures g. Display professionalism through written and verbal communications	Entire procedure

Procedure 8.2 Document Telephone Messages and Report Relevant Information Concisely and Accurately

Name _____ Date _____ Score _____

Tasks: To take an accurate telephone message and follow up on the requests made by the caller.

Scenario: Norma Washington, DOB 8/1/19XX, an established patient of Dr. Martin, has called to report her blood pressure readings that she has been taking at home. Dr. Martin had made a recent change in her medication and wanted her to monitor her BP at home for 3 days and call in with the results. She has taken her blood pressure in the morning and in the evening for the past 3 days, with the following results: (Role play this scenario with a peer who is the patient.)
- Day 1: 144/92 in the AM, 156/94 in the PM
- Day 2: 136/84 in the AM, 142/86 in the PM
- Day 3: 132/80 in the AM, 138/82 in the PM

Equipment and Supplies:
- Telephone
- Computer or message pad
- Pen or pencil
- Health record

Standard: Complete the procedure and all critical steps in _____ minutes with a minimum score of 85% within two attempts (*or as indicated by the instructor*).

Scoring: Divide the points earned by the total possible points. Failure to perform a critical step, indicated by an asterisk (*), results in grade no higher than an 84% (*or as indicated by the instructor*).

Time: Began_____ Ended_____ Total minutes: _____

Steps:	Point Value	Attempt 1	Attempt 2
1. Demonstrate telephone techniques by answering the telephone using the guidelines in Procedure 8.1.	15		
2. Using a message pad or the computer, take the phone message (either on paper or by data entry into the computer) and obtain the following information: • Name of the person to whom the call is directed • Name of the person calling • Caller's telephone number • Reason for the call, using critical thinking skills to ask the appropriate questions (Refer to the Checklist for Affective Behaviors) • Action to be taken, using critical thinking skills to determine the correct action to be taken (Refer to the Checklist for Affective Behaviors) • Date and time of the call • Initials of the person taking the call	15*		
3. Apply active listening skills and repeat the information back to the caller after recording the message.	10		
4. End the call and wait for the caller to hang up first.	10		

5.	Document the telephone call with all pertinent information in the patient's health record.	**10***		
6.	Deliver the phone message to the appropriate person.	**10**		
7.	Follow up on important messages.	**10**		
8.	If using paper messaging, keep old message books for future reference. Carbonless copies allow the facility to keep a permanent record of phone messages. If using an electronic system, the message will be saved to the patient's record automatically.	**10**		
9.	File pertinent phone messages in the patient's health record. Make sure the computer record is closed after the documentation has been done.	**10**		
	Total Points	**100**		

Checklist for Affective Behaviors

Affective Behavior	Directions: *Check behaviors observed during the role-play.*					
Critical Thinking	**Negative, Unprofessional Behaviors**	**Attempt**		**Positive, Professional Behaviors**	**Attempt**	
		1	**2**		**1**	**2**
	Coached or told of an issue or problem			Independently identified the problem or issue		
	Failed to ask relevant questions related to the condition			Asked appropriate questions to obtain the information required		
	Failed to consider alternatives; failed to ask questions that demonstrate understanding of principles/concepts			Willing to consider other alternatives; asked appropriate questions that showed understanding of principles/concepts		
	Failed to make an educated, logical judgment/decision; actions or lack of actions demonstrated unsafe practices and/or do not follow the protocol			Made an educated, logical judgment/decision based on the protocol; actions reflected principles of safe practice		
	Other:			Other:		

Grading for Affective Behaviors		Point Value	Attempt 1	Attempt 2
Does not meet Expectation	• Response fails to show critical thinking. • Student demonstrated more than 2 negative, unprofessional behaviors during the interaction.	0		
Needs Improvement	• Response fails to show critical thinking. • Student demonstrated 1 or 2 negative, unprofessional behaviors during the interaction.	0		
Meets Expectation	• Response demonstrates critical thinking; no negative, unprofessional behaviors observed. • More practice is needed for behavior to appear natural and for student to appear comfortable and at ease.	15		
Occasionally Exceeds Expectation	• Response demonstrates critical thinking; no negative, unprofessional behaviors observed. • At times student appeared comfortable and at ease; but more practice is needed for behavior to become natural and consistent with a professional medical assistant.	15		
Always Exceeds Expectation	• Response demonstrates critical thinking; no negative, unprofessional behaviors observed. • Student's behaviors appeared natural and comfortable. Behaviors are consistent with a professional medical assistant.	15		

Comments

CAAHEP Competencies	Step(s)
V.P.4. Demonstrate professional telephone techniques	1, 3, 4
V.P.5. Document telephone messages accurately	2, 5
A.1 Demonstrate critical thinking skills	2
X.P.3. Document patient care accurately in the medical record	Entire procedure
ABHES Competencies	**Step(s)**
7. Administrative Procedures g. Display professionalism through written and verbal communications	Entire procedure

Scheduling Appointments and Patient Processing

chapter

9

CAAHEP Competencies	Assessments
VI.C.1. Identify different types of appointment scheduling methods	Skills and Concepts – C. 1-3
VI.C.2. Identify critical information required for scheduling patient procedures	Skills and Concepts – G. 1
VI.P.1. Manage appointment schedule using established priorities	Procedures 9.1, 9.2, 9.4
VI.P.2. Schedule a patient procedure	Procedure 9.5
VII.P.2. Input accurate patient billing information in Practice Management System (PMS)	Procedure 9.2
V.P.3.a. Coach patients regarding: office policies	Procedure 9.3
A.1. Demonstrate critical thinking skills	Procedures 9.2, 9.5
A.3. Demonstrate empathy for patients' concerns	Procedure 9.2
ABHES Competencies	**Assessments**
7. Administrative Procedures e. Apply scheduling principles	Procedures 9.1, 9.2, 9.4, 9.5

VOCABULARY REVIEW

Using the word pool on the right, find the correct word to match the definition. Write the word on the line after the definition.

Group A

1. Documentation in the medical record to track the patient's condition and progress _____

2. Space of time between events _____

3. An unexpected event that throws a plan into disorder; an interruption that prevents a system or process from continuing as usual or as expected _____

4. Skilled as a result of training or practice _____

5. A rule that controls how something should be done; guidelines or boundaries _____

6. An appointment type used when a patient needs to see the provider after a condition should have been resolved or to monitor an ongoing condition _____

7. The environment where something is created or takes shape; a base on which to build _____

8. Statistical data of a population; in healthcare, this includes patient name, address, date of birth, employment, and other details

   _____

9. A type of software that allows the user to enter demographic information, schedule appointments, maintain lists of insurance payers, perform billing tasks, and generate reports

   _____

10. Essential; being an indispensable part of a whole

    _____

Word Pool
- parameters
- demographics
- integral
- intervals
- matrix
- follow-up appointment
- proficiency
- practice management software
- progress notes
- disruption

Group B

1. A means of achieving a particular end, as in a situation requiring urgency or caution _____

2. The process of confirming health insurance coverage for the patient _____

3. A written document describing the healthcare facility's privacy practices _____

4. A system for examining and separating into different groups; in the healthcare facility, it means determining the severity of illness that patients experience and prioritizing appointments based on that severity _____

5. The process of determining if a procedure or service is covered by the insurance plan and what the reimbursement is for that procedure or service _____

Word Pool
- Notice of Privacy Practices
- preauthorization
- precertification
- established patients
- screening
- no-show
- expediency
- triage
- patient portal
- verification of eligibility

6. To sort out and classify the injured; used in the military and emergency settings to determine the priority of a patient to be treated _____

7. A patient who has been treated previously by the healthcare provider within the past 3 years _____

8. A secure online website that gives patients 24-hour access to personal health information using a username and password _____

9. When a patient fails to keep an appointment without giving advance notice _____

10. The process of determining if a procedure or service is covered by the insurance plan and what the reimbursement is for that procedure or service _____

ABBREVIATIONS
Write out what each of the following abbreviations stands for.

1. ECG _____

2. NPP _____

3. MRI _____

4. CT _____

5. EMT _____

6. EHR _____

7. HIPAA _____

8. CDC _____

SKILLS AND CONCEPTS
Answer the following questions. Write your answer on the line or in the space provided.

Scheduling Appointments

A. Establishing the Appointment Schedule

1. When developing an appointment schedule, _____ and _____ must be considered.

2. _____ information includes the patient's address, insurance information, and email address.

B. Creating the Appointment Matrix

1. Time would be blocked out in the schedule for what four reasons when setting up the appointment matrix?

   a. _____

   b. _____

   c. _____

   d. _____

2. How can the medical assistant handle a provider who habitually spends more than the allotted time with patients?

   _____

   _____

   _____

   _____

3. Using the appointment schedule page that follows, schedule these appointments, blocking out the appropriate amount of time:

   Recheck appointment   15 minutes

   Complete physical examination (PE)   45 minutes

   a. Jana Green; recheck appointment, prefers Wednesdays
   b. Pedro Gomez; complete physical examination, prefers Tuesdays
   c. Truong Tran; recheck, prefers Thursdays after 9:00 AM
   d. Walter Biller; complete physical examination, prefers Mondays as early as possible
   e. Reuven Ahmad; complete physical examination, prefers Fridays

	Monday	Tuesday	Wednesday	Thursday	Friday
8:00					
8:15					
8:30					
8:45					
9:00					
9:15					
9:30					
9:45					
10:00					

C. Methods of Scheduling Appointments

1. The two most common methods of appointment scheduling are _____ and _____.

2. Computerized scheduling utilizes _____ software.

3. The type of computerized scheduling that allows the patient to use secure links to find and select appointments is called _____.

D. Types of Appointment Scheduling
Briefly describe each type of scheduling and list one advantage and one disadvantage of each.

1. Time-specified (stream) scheduling _____

   _____

   _____

   _____

   _____

   _____

   _____

2. Open office hours _____

   _____

   _____

   _____

   _____

   _____

   _____

3. Wave scheduling _____

   _____

   _____

   _____

   _____

   _____

   _____

4. Modified wave scheduling _____

   _____

   _____

   _____

   _____

   _____

   _____

5. Double booking _____

_____

_____

_____

_____

_____

6. Grouping procedures _____

_____

_____

_____

_____

_____

_____

E. Telephone Scheduling

1. When scheduling an appointment over the telephone, what options are available to remind patients of the appointment?

_____

F. Scheduling Appointments for New Patients

1. To determine how much time to allow for an appointment, the medical assistant needs to obtain information about the _____.

2. New patients should be asked to arrive _____ minutes early to complete necessary paperwork.

3. An ideal tool to provide new patients with information is a(n) _____.

G. Scheduling Other Types of Appointments

1. Identify critical information required for scheduling patient procedures. _____

_____

_____

_____

_____

_____

2.   Identify the special requests that a provider may have for inpatient surgeries._____

_____

_____

_____

_____

H. Special Circumstances

1.   What is the difference between an emergency appointment and an urgent appointment? _____

_____

_____

_____

_____

2.   How does the medical assistant handle a patient who arrives at the clinic to see the provider but does not have an appointment?

_____

_____

_____

_____

I. Increasing Appointment Show Rates

Practice completing appointment reminder cards on the forms provided. Students should be able to fill out the appointment cards with the information provided without difficulty.

1.   Tai Yan has an appointment for August 23, 20XX, at 3:00 PM with Dr. Martin.

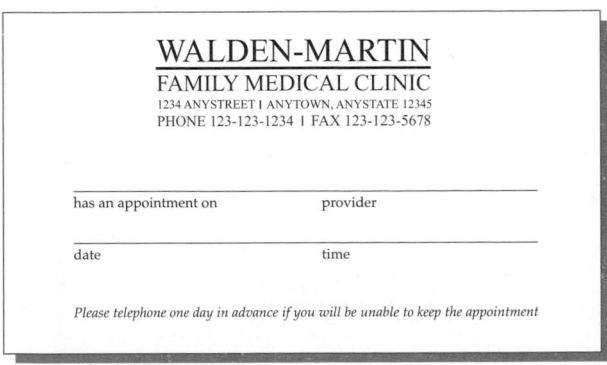

WALDEN-MARTIN
FAMILY MEDICAL CLINIC
1234 ANYSTREET I ANYTOWN, ANYSTATE 12345
PHONE 123-123-1234 I FAX 123-123-5678

has an appointment on   provider

date   time

Please telephone one day in advance if you will be unable to keep the appointment

2. Diego Lopez has an appointment for May 1, 20XX, at 9:00 AM with Dr. Walden.

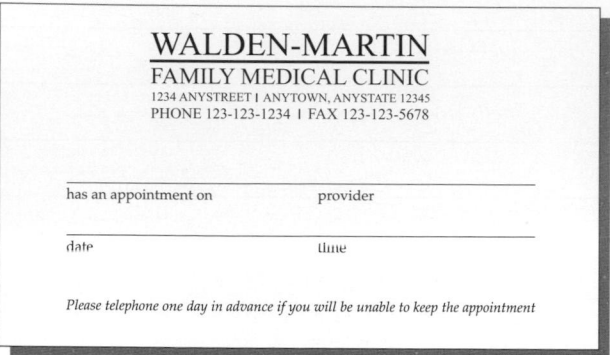

3. Julia Berkley has an appointment for June 13, 20XX, at 11:45 AM with Dr. Walden.

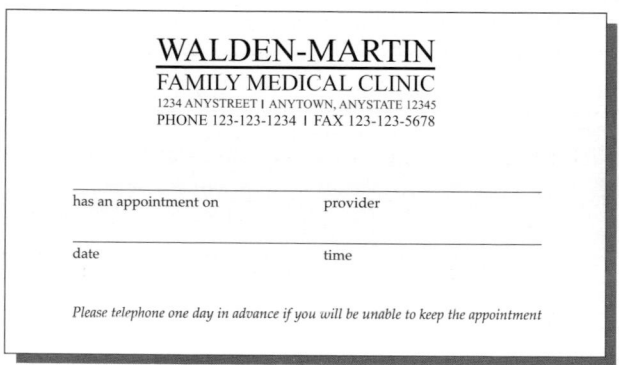

4. Monique Jones has an appointment for September 12, 20XX, at 2:40 PM with Jean Burke, N.P.

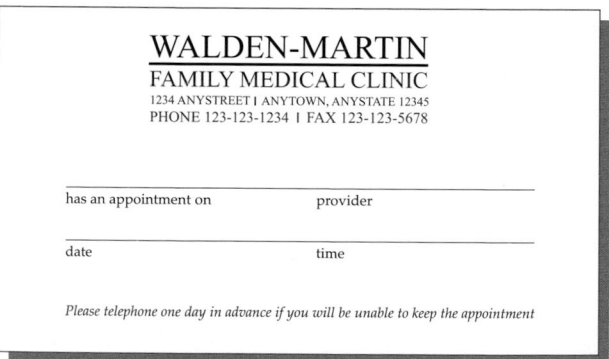

5. Ken Thomas has an appointment for December 15, 20XX, at 4:30 PM with Dr. Martin.

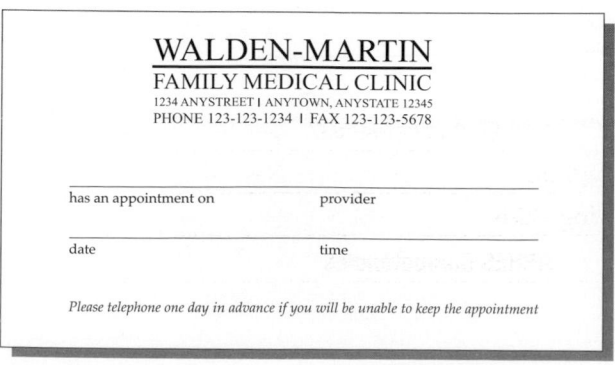

Patient Processing Tasks

1. When screening patients at the reception desk, what patient conditions require immediate action by the medical assistant?

   _____

   _____

2. What action should the medical assistant take when patients have emergent conditions? _____

   _____

   _____

   _____

   _____

3. If a medical assistant is unable to greet a patient at the reception desk, what actions can help acknowledge the person?

   _____

   _____

4. List six features of a HIPAA-appropriate sign-in register._____

   _____

   _____

   _____

   _____

   _____

   _____

5. List three features that would cause a HIPAA violation with sign-in registers._____

   _____

   _____

   _____

   _____

6. How does a medical assistant take steps to protect other patients in the reception area? _____

   _____

   _____

   _____

   _____

7. What must occur if a patient refuses to sign the NPP form? _____

_____

_____

_____

8. How should a medical assistant review a new patient brochure with a new patient? _____

_____

_____

_____

9. During the check-in process, what three things must the medical assistant do for all patients? _____

_____

_____

_____

_____

10. If the provider is delayed, what should the medical assistant do with the patients who are waiting?

_____

_____

_____

_____

11. How should a medical assistant handle a situation when a patient is angry? _____

_____

_____

_____

_____

12. What occurs during the checkout process?_____

_____

_____

_____

_____

CERTIFICATION PREPARATION

Circle the correct answer.

1. The medical assistant may help an angry caller to calm down by
   a. getting angry in return.
   b. speaking in a lower tone of voice.
   c. referring the situation to the office manager immediately.
   d. calling the provider into the situation.

2. Why is it necessary to include a note in the patient's chart when the person does not show up for a scheduled appointment?
   a. To bill the patient for the time
   b. To keep count of the number of no-shows for a possible drop in the future
   c. To be prepared for future legal consequences regarding the patient's care
   d. To provide the medical assistant with a reminder to call and reschedule

3. What is the appointment-setting method by which a patient logs onto the internet and views a facility's schedule to set his or her own appointment?
   a. Flexible office hours
   b. Self-scheduling
   c. Grouping procedures
   d. Advance booking

4. An obstetrician who devotes two afternoons a week to seeing pregnant patients is using an appointment scheduling method called
   a. wave scheduling.
   b. advance booking.
   c. grouping procedures.
   d. modified wave scheduling.

5. Which type of scheduling is an attempt to create short-term flexibility within each hour?
   a. Time-specified scheduling
   b. Wave scheduling
   c. Stream scheduling
   d. Modified wave scheduling

6. All patients want to be kept informed about how long they should expect to wait to see the provider. Any delay longer than _____ minutes should be explained.
   a. 15
   b. 20
   c. 30
   d. No explanation is necessary

7. When screening patients at the reception desk, which patient has an emergent condition and requires immediate care?
   a. Chest pain
   b. Sore throat
   c. Tick bite
   d. Ankle injury

8. When calling a patient from the reception room to escort him to an exam room, how should the medical assistant call the patient?
   a. "James Brown, Dr. Walden is ready for you."
   b. "James Brown with the sore throat"
   c. "James Brown with a birthdate of June 6"
   d. "James Brown"

9. The statistical characteristics of human populations are called
   a. numbers.
   b. perceptions.
   c. demographics.
   d. phonetics.

10. An effective way to deal with patients who are always late for appointments is to
    a. refuse to schedule them after this happens several times.
    b. have them wait until it is convenient for the physician.
    c. advise them that they disrupt the office schedule.
    d. give them the last appointment of the day.

WORKPLACE APPLICATIONS

1. Janie Haynes consistently arrives at the clinic between 15 and 45 minutes late. She always has a "good" excuse, but she could make her appointments on time if she had better time management skills. The office manager has mentioned to Paula, the receptionist, that Janie is to be scheduled at 4:45 PM and if she is late, she will not be seen by the provider. Paula books Janie's next three appointments at that time, and Janie actually arrives early. However, on the fourth appointment, Janie arrives at 5:50 PM, and Paula knows that it is her responsibility to tell Janie that she cannot see the provider. How does Paula handle this task? What are the options for Paula?

_____

_____

_____

_____

_____

2. Jill is the receptionist for Drs. Boles and Bailey, who are psychiatrists. Each week, Sara Ables comes to her appointments but brings her two children, Joey and Julie, ages 8 and 6 years, respectively. When Sara goes back for her appointment, the children are almost uncontrollable in the reception area. Although there are never more than two patients waiting, the kids are a serious disruption in the clinic. When Jill mentioned the problem to Dr. Boles, he said that Sara really needs the sessions and that Jill should try to work with Sara on this issue. What can Jill do to remedy the situation?

_____

_____

_____

_____

_____

INTERNET ACTIVITIES

1. Using online resources, research group appointments. Create a poster presentation, a PowerPoint presentation, or write a paper summarizing your research. Include the following points in your project:
   a. Description of a group appointment
   b. List the types of conditions that are best suited for group appointments
   c. Explain whose confidentiality is maintained with group appointments
   d. List the benefits for patients and providers when group appointments are used

Procedure 9.1   Establish the Appointment Matrix

Name _____ Date _____ Score _____

Task: To establish the matrix of the appointment schedule.

Scenario: You have been asked to set up the schedule matrix for Dr. Julie Walden, Dr. James Martin, and Dr. Angela Perez. Block off the following times in the appointment schedule:

Dr. Julie Walden:
- Lunch; daily from 11:30 AM to 12:30 PM
- Hospital Rounds; Mondays and Wednesday from 8:00 AM to 9:00 AM

Dr. James Martin:
- Lunch; daily from 12:00 PM to 1:00 PM
- Hospital Rounds; Tuesdays and Thursday from 8:00 AM to 9:00 AM

Dr. Angela Perez:
- Lunch; daily from 12:30 PM to 1:30 PM
- Hospital Rounds; Fridays from 8:00 AM to 9:00 AM

Equipment and Supplies:
- Appointment book or computer with scheduling software
- Office procedure manual (optional)
- Black pen, pencil, and highlighters
- Calendar

Standard: Complete the procedure and all critical steps in _____ minutes with a minimum score of 85% within two attempts (*or as indicated by the instructor*).

Scoring: Divide the points earned by the total possible points. Failure to perform a critical step, indicated by an asterisk (*), results in grade no higher than an 84% (*or as indicated by the instructor*).

Time: Began_____ Ended_____ Total minutes: _____

Steps:	Point Value	Attempt 1	Attempt 2
1. Using the calendar, determine when the office is not open (e.g., holidays, weekends, evenings). If using the appointment book and a black pen, draw an *X* through the times the office is not open. If using the scheduling software, block the times the office is not open.	25*		
2. Identify the times each provider is not available. If using the appointment book, write in the providers' names on each column and then draw an *X* through their unavailable times. If using the scheduling software, select each provider and block the times the provider is unavailable.	25*		
3. Using the office procedure manual or providers' preferences, determine when each provider performs certain types of examinations. In the appointment book, indicate these examinations either by writing the examination time or by highlighting the examination times. Follow the office's procedure on indicating these examination times in the appointment book. When using scheduling software, set up the times for the examinations or use the highlighting feature if available.	25*		

4.	Using the office procedure manual or the list of providers' preferences and availability, identify other times to block on the scheduling matrix. Some providers require catch-up times and these time slots are blocked. Some medical facilities save appointment times for same-day appointments. When saving time blocks for same-day appointments, make sure to use pencil so it can be erased and the patient's information entered on the day of the appointment. For the scheduling software, block those times when patients cannot be booked and indicate the times for the same-day appointments.	**25***		
	Total Points	**100**		

Comments

CAAHEP Competencies	Step(s)
VI.P.1. Manage appointment schedule using established priorities	Entire procedure
ABHES Competencies	**Step(s)**
7. Administrative Procedures e. Apply scheduling principles	Entire procedure

Procedure 9.2   Schedule a New Patient

Name _____   Date _____   Score _____

Task: To schedule a new patient for a first office visit and identify the urgency of the visit using established priorities.

Scenario: Patricia Black, a new patient, calls. She just moved to the area and her asthma has flared up over the last 24 hours, but her albuterol inhaler is empty, and she needs a new prescription for it. She states that she is doing okay, but without the albuterol she knows it will get worse within the next few days. According to your screening guidelines, she needs to be seen today and scheduling guidelines indicate she needs a 45-minute appointment.

Equipment and Supplies:
*   Appointment book or computer with scheduling software
*   Scheduling and screening guidelines
*   Pencil

Standard: Complete the procedure and all critical steps in _____ minutes with a minimum score of 85% within two attempts (*or as indicated by the instructor*).

Scoring: Divide the points earned by the total possible points. Failure to perform a critical step, indicated by an asterisk (*), results in grade no higher than an 84% (*or as indicated by the instructor*).

Time: Began_____ Ended_____ Total minutes: _____

Steps:	Point Value	Attempt 1	Attempt 2
1. Obtain the patient's demographic information (e.g., full name, birth date, address, and telephone number). Write this information down or enter it into the scheduling software. Verify the information.	15*		
2. Determine whether the patient was referred by another provider.	10		
3. Determine the patient's chief complaint and when the first symptoms occurred. Utilize the scheduling and screening guidelines as needed. (*Refer to the Checklist for Affective Behaviors*)	15*		
4. Search the appointment book or scheduling software for the first suitable appointment time and an alternate time. Offer the patient a choice of these dates and times. Be open to alternative times if the patient cannot make the initial options you gave. Provide additional appointment options as needed.	10*		
5. Enter the mutually agreeable time into the schedule. Enter the patient's name, telephone number, and add *NP* for new patient.	10		
6. Obtain the patient's insurance information. If new patients are expected to pay at the time of the visit, explain this financial arrangement when the appointment is made.	15*		
7. Provide the patient with directions to the healthcare facility and parking instructions if needed.	10		
8. Before ending the call, ask if the patient has any questions. Reinforce the date and time of the appointment. Politely and professionally end the call, making sure to thank the patient for calling. (*Refer to the Checklist for Affective Behaviors*)	15		
Total Points	**100**		

Checklist for Affective Behaviors

Affective Behavior	Directions: Check behaviors observed during the role-play.					
Critical Thinking	**Negative, Unprofessional Behaviors**	**Attempt**		**Positive, Professional Behaviors**	**Attempt**	
		1	**2**		**1**	**2**
	Coached or told of an issue or problem			Independently identified the problem or issue		
	Failed to ask relevant questions related to the condition			Asked appropriate questions to obtain the information required		
	Failed to consider alternatives; failed to ask questions that demonstrated understanding of principles/concepts			Willing to consider other alternatives; asked appropriate questions that showed understanding of principles/concepts		
	Failed to make an educated, logical judgment/decision; actions or lack of actions demonstrated unsafe practices and/or did not follow the protocol			Made an educated, logical judgment/decision based on the protocol; actions reflected principles of safe practice		
	Other:			Other:		
Empathy	Distracted; not focused on the other person			Focused full attention on the other person		
	Judgmental attitude; not accepting attitude			Nonjudgmental, accepting attitude		
	Failed to clarify what the person verbally or nonverbally communicated			Used summarizing or paraphrasing to clarify what the person verbally or nonverbally communicated		
	Failed to acknowledge what the person communicated			Acknowledged what the person communicated		
	Rude, discourteous			Pleasant and courteous		
	Disregarded the person's dignity and rights			Maintained the person's dignity and rights		
	Other:			Other:		

Grading for Affective Behaviors		Point Value	Attempt 1	Attempt 2
Does not meet Expectation	• Response was disrespectful and/or insensitive. • Student demonstrated more than 2 negative, unprofessional behaviors during the interaction.	0		
Needs Improvement	• Response was disrespectful and/or insensitive. • Student demonstrated 1 or 2 negative, unprofessional behaviors during the interaction.	0		
Meets Expectation	• Response was respectful and sensitive; no negative, unprofessional behaviors observed. • More practice is needed for behavior to appear natural and for student to appear comfortable and at ease.	15		
Occasionally Exceeds Expectation	• Response was respectful and sensitive; no negative, unprofessional behaviors observed. • At times student appeared comfortable and at ease; but more practice is needed for behavior to become natural and consistent with a professional medical assistant.	15		
Always Exceeds Expectation	• Response was respectful and sensitive; no negative, unprofessional behaviors observed. • Student's behaviors appeared natural and comfortable. Behaviors are consistent with a professional medical assistant.	15		

Comments

CAAHEP Competencies	Step(s)
VI.P.1. Manage appointment schedule using established priorities	1-7
VI.A.1. Display sensitivity when managing appointments	3, 8
VII.P.2. Obtain accurate patient billing information	6
A.1 Demonstrate critical thinking skills	3
A.3 Demonstrate empathy for patients' concerns	8
ABHES Competencies	**Step(s)**
7. Administrative Procedures e. Apply scheduling principles	1-7

Procedure 9.3   Coach Patients Regarding Office Policies

Name _____   Date _____   Score _____

Tasks: Create a new patient brochure and then role-play ways to coach patients regarding office policies.

Scenario: You work at Walden-Martin Family Medical Clinic. Your supervisor asks you to create a new patient brochure for the clinic. The healthcare facility's information is listed here. After you complete the brochure, you coach the following patients regarding office procedures:
- Mr. Charles Johnson (he has a question regarding the payment policy)
- Ms. Monique Jones (she has a question regarding the medication refill procedure)

Healthcare Facility	Providers
Walden-Martin Family Medical Clinic 1234 Anystreet Anytown, Anystate 12345 Phone: 123-123-1234 Fax: 123-123-5678	Julie Walden, M.D. James Martin, M.D. Angela Perez, M.D. David Kahn, M.D. Jean Burke, N.P.

Equipment and Supplies:
- Computer with word processing software and printer
- Office procedure manual (optional)

Standard: Complete the procedure and all critical steps with a minimum score of 85% within two attempts (*or as indicated by the instructor*).

Scoring: Divide the points earned by the total possible points. Failure to perform a critical step, indicated by an asterisk (*), results in grade no higher than an 84% (*or as indicated by the instructor*).

Steps:	Point Value	Attempt 1	Attempt 2

1. Using word processing software, design an informational brochure for patients that provides information about the healthcare facility and describes practice procedures. At a minimum, the information should include the following:
  a. Description of the healthcare facility (e.g., type of practice, mission statement)
  b. Location or a map of the facility
  c. Contact information (i.e., telephone numbers, emails, and website addresses)
  d. Providers' names and credentials
  e. Services offered
  f. Hours of operation
  g. How appointments can be scheduled
  h. Healthcare facility's policies and procedures (e.g., payment policies, appointment cancellations, medication refills, assistance after hours)
  i. Insurance plans accepted
	55		

2. Proofread the brochure. Revise as needed. Print the brochure.	5		
3. Using the scenario for the first patient, give a brief summary of the different parts of the brochure. Use words the patient will understand.	10*		

4.	Ask if the patient has any questions. Actively listen to the patient's concerns. Address those concerns.	**10***		
5.	Using the scenario for the second patient, give a brief summary of the different parts of the brochure. Use words that the patient understands.	**10***		
6.	Ask if the patient has any questions. Actively listen to the patient's concerns. Address those concerns.	**10***		
	Total Points	**100**		

Comments

CAAHEP Competencies	Step(s)
V.P.3.a. Coach patients regarding: office policies	3-6

Procedure 9.4   Schedule an Established Patient

Name _____ **Date** _____ **Score** _____

Task: To manage the provider's schedule by scheduling appointments for an established patient and handling rescheduling and a no-show appointment.

Scenario: Celia Tapia has just finished seeing Dr. Martin and is checking out at your desk. You see that she needs to schedule a follow-up appointment in 2 weeks. The scheduling guidelines indicate a follow-up appointment is 15 minutes long.

Equipment and Supplies:
- Appointment book or computer with scheduling software
- Scheduling guidelines
- Pencil, red pen
- Reminder card
- Patient's health record

Standard: Complete the procedure and all critical steps in _____ minutes with a minimum score of 85% within two attempts (*or as indicated by the instructor*).

Scoring: Divide the points earned by the total possible points. Failure to perform a critical step, indicated by an asterisk (*), results in grade no higher than an 84% (*or as indicated by the instructor*).

Time: Began_____ Ended_____ Total minutes: _____

Steps:	Point Value	Attempt 1	Attempt 2
1. Obtain the patient's name and information, purpose of the visit, the provider to be seen, and any scheduling preferences. If using the scheduling software, enter the patient's name and date of birth (DOB). Verify the correct patient is selected.	15		
2. Identify the length of the appointment by using the scheduling guidelines.	15*		
3. Search the appointment book or scheduling software for the first suitable appointment time and an alternate time. Offer the patient a choice of these dates and times. Be open to alternative times if the patient cannot make the initial options you gave. Provide additional appointment options as needed.	15		
4. Using a pencil, write the patient's name and phone number in the appointment book and block out the correct amount of time. Add in any other relevant information per the facility's procedures. If using the scheduling software, create the appointment per the facility's guidelines.	15*		
5. Complete the appointment reminder card and ensure the date and time on the card matches the appointment time. Give the card to the patient.	10		
Scenario continues: Later that day, Celica Tapia calls and needs to reschedule her appointment for the next day at the same time.			
6. When a patient calls to reschedule an appointment, follow steps #1 through #4. When the new appointment is made, make sure to erase the old appointment from the appointment log. With the scheduling software, ensure the old appointment time is removed from the schedule. Repeat the appointment date and time to the patient.	15		

Scenario continues: Celia Tapia no-shows for her follow-up appointment.

7. In the appointment book, using red pen, indicate the patient no-showed. Using the patient's health record, document that the patient failed to show for the follow-up examination with the provider. In an electronic system, change the appointment status to no-show and ensure that it is documented in the health record.	15		
Total Points	**100**		

Comments

CAAHEP Competencies	**Step(s)**
VI.P.1. Manage appointment schedule using established priorities	All
ABHES Competencies	**Step(s)**
7. Administrative Procedures e. Apply scheduling principles	All

Procedure 9.5   Schedule a Patient Procedure

Name _____   Date _____   Score _____

Task: To schedule a patient for a procedure within the time frame needed by the provider, confirm with the patient, and issue all required instructions.

Scenario: Monique Jones has just completed seeing Dr. Walden and is checking out at your desk. She gives you an order from the provider that states she needs to have a magnetic resonance image (MRI) of her left ankle within a week. The radiology department in your facility performs MRIs.

Equipment and Supplies:
- Provider's order detailing the procedure required
- Computer with order entry software (optional)
- Name, address, and telephone number of facility where procedure will take place
- Patient's demographic and insurance information
- Patient's health record
- Procedure preparation instructions
- Telephone
- Consent form (if required for procedure)

Standard: Complete the procedure and all critical steps in _____ minutes with a minimum score of 85% within two attempts (*or as indicated by the instructor*).

Scoring: Divide the points earned by the total possible points. Failure to perform a critical step, indicated by an asterisk (*), results in grade no higher than an 84% (*or as indicated by the instructor*).

Time: Began_____ Ended_____ Total minutes: _____

Steps:	Point Value	Attempt 1	Attempt 2
1. Obtain an oral or written order from the provider for the exact procedure to be performed.	15		
2. Gather the patient's demographic and insurance information. If using an electronic health record, verify you have the correct patient. *(Refer to the Checklist for Affective Behaviors)*	15		
3. Determine the patient's availability within the time frame provided by the provider for the procedure.	15		
4. Contact the diagnostic facility and schedule the patient's procedure. If you are using a computerized provider order entry (CPOE) system and your facility performs the procedure, you also need to enter the order using the CPOE system. • Provide the patient's diagnosis and provider's exact order, including the name of procedure and time frame. • Establish the date and time for the procedure. • Give the patient's name, age, address, telephone number, and insurance information (i.e., insurance policy numbers, precertification information, and addresses for filing claims). • Determine any special instructions for the patient or special anesthesia requirements. • Notify the facility of any urgency for test results.	20*		

5.	If a consent form is required for the procedure, ensure the provider has reviewed the form with the patient and the patient has signed the consent form. A copy of the consent form may be required by the diagnostic facility before the procedure. The consent form should be scanned and uploaded into the electronic health record or placed in the paper record.	15		
6.	Document the details of the scheduled procedure in the patient's health record. If applicable, create a reminder to check on the procedure results after the appointment date.	20*		
	Total Points	100		

Checklist for Affective Behaviors

Affective Behavior	Directions: Check behaviors observed during the role-play.					
Critical Thinking	**Negative, Unprofessional Behaviors**	**Attempt**		**Positive, Professional Behaviors**	**Attempt**	
		1	**2**		**1**	**2**
	Coached or told of an issue or problem			Independently identified the problem or issue		
	Failed to ask relevant questions related to the condition			Asked appropriate questions to obtain the information required		
	Failed to consider alternatives; failed to ask questions that demonstrated understanding of principles/concepts			Willing to consider other alternatives; asked appropriate questions that showed understanding of principles/concepts		
	Failed to make an educated, logical judgment/decision; actions or lack of actions demonstrated unsafe practices and/or did not follow the protocol			Made an educated, logical judgment/decision based on the protocol; actions reflected principles of safe practice		
	Other:			Other:		

Grading for Affective Behaviors		Point Value	Attempt 1	Attempt 2
Does not meet Expectation	• Response was disrespectful and/or insensitive. • Student demonstrated more than 2 negative, unprofessional behaviors during the interaction.	0		
Needs Improvement	• Response was disrespectful and/or insensitive. • Student demonstrated 1 or 2 negative, unprofessional behaviors during the interaction.	0		
Meets Expectation	• Response was respectful and sensitive; no negative, unprofessional behaviors observed. • More practice is needed for behavior to appear natural and for student to appear comfortable and at ease.	15		
Occasionally Exceeds Expectation	• Response was respectful and sensitive; no negative, unprofessional behaviors observed. • At times student appeared comfortable and at ease; but more practice is needed for behavior to become natural and consistent with a professional medical assistant.	15		
Always Exceeds Expectation	• Response was respectful and sensitive; no negative, unprofessional behaviors observed. • Student's behaviors appeared natural and comfortable. Behaviors are consistent with a professional medical assistant.	15		

Comments

CAAHEP Competencies	Step(s)
VI.P.2. Schedule a patient procedure	All
A.1 Demonstrate critical thinking skills	2
ABHES Competencies	**Step(s)**
7. Administrative Procedures e. Apply scheduling principles	All

Health Records

CAAHEP Competencies	Assessment
V.C.12. Identify subjective and objective information	Skills and Concepts – B. 7-16
VI.C.5. Identify the importance of data back-up	Skills and Concepts – C. 8.
VI.C.6. Identify the components of an Electronic Medical Record, Electronic Health Record, and Practice Management System	Skills and Concepts – A. 2-6
VI.P.3. Input patient data using an electronic system	Procedures 10.1, 10.2

ABHES Competencies	Assessment
1. General Orientation d. List the general responsibilities and skills of the medical assistant	Skills and Concepts – B. 17
4. Medical Law and Ethics a. Follow documentation guidelines	Skills and Concepts – C. 3-7
4. Medical Law and Ethics b. Institute federal and state guidelines when: 1) Releasing medical records or information 2) Entering orders in and utilizing electronic health records	Procedures 10.1, 10.2
7. Administrative Procedures a. Gather and process documents	Procedures 10.2, 10.5, 10.6
7. Administrative Procedures b. Navigate electronic health records systems and practice management software	Procedures 10.1, 10.2

VOCABULARY REVIEW

Using the word pool on the right, find the correct word to match the definition. Write the word on the line after the definition.

Group A

1. Data or information obtained from the patient
   _____

2. A process to ensure the reliability of test results
   _____

3. A computerized record that conforms to nationally recognized standards and contains health-related information about a specific patient _____

4. Data obtained through physical examination, laboratory and diagnostic testing, and measurable information
   _____

5. The likely outcome of a disease including chance of recovery
   _____

6. The ability to work with other systems _____

7. A rule that controls how something should be done; guidelines or boundaries _____

8. An interconnection between systems _____

9. A secure online website that gives patients 24-hour access to personal health information using a username and password
   _____

10. Meeting the standards and regulations of the practice's established policies and procedures _____

Word Pool
- electronic health record (EHR)
- quality control
- interoperability
- patient portal
- parameters
- interface
- compliance
- subjective information
- objective information
- prognosis

Group B

1. Occurring later or after _____
2. Granted or endowed with a particular authority, right, or property; to have a special interest in _____
3. Using as few words as possible to express the message
   _____
4. A temporary diagnosis made before all test results have been received _____
5. The smooth continuation of care from one provider to another that allows the patient to receive the most benefit and no interruption or duplication of care _____
6. Passed from parents to offspring through the genes
   _____
7. How often something happens _____
8. To remove or destroy all traces of; do away with
   _____
9. The most recent item is on top and oldest item is last
   _____
10. Pertaining to the measurement of the size and proportions of the human body _____

Word Pool
- continuity of care
- incidence
- hereditary
- concise
- anthropometric
- provisional diagnosis
- subsequent
- vested
- reverse chronologic order
- obliteration

Group C

1. The age at which a person is recognized by law to be an adult; it varies by state _____
2. A heading, title, or subtitle under which records are filed _____
3. To say something aloud for another person to write down _____
4. A chronologic file used as a reminder that something must be dealt with on a certain date _____
5. The filing of records, correspondence, or cards by number _____
6. To make a written copy of dictated material _____
7. A sturdy cardboard or plastic file-sized card used to replace a folder temporarily removed from the filing space _____
8. A system made up of combinations of the letters and numbers _____
9. A filing system where materials can be located without consulting another source of reference _____
10. Any system that arranges names or topics according to the sequence of the letters in the alphabet _____
11. A method or plan for retaining or keeping health records and for their movement from active to inactive to closed _____

Word Pool
- transcription
- dictation
- retention schedule
- age of majority
- out guides
- caption
- alphabetic filing
- direct filing system
- numeric filing
- alphanumeric
- tickler file

ABBREVIATIONS

Write out what each of the following abbreviations stands for.

1. AMA _____
2. CPT _____
3. EHR _____
4. HHS _____
5. HIE _____
6. HIPAA _____
7. HIV _____
8. ICD _____
9. NPP _____
10. ONC _____
11. PCP _____
12. PHI _____

13. PHR_____

14. POR_____

15. SOR _____

16. TPR _____

SKILLS AND CONCEPTS

Answer the following questions. Write your answer on the line or in the space provided.

A. Electronic Records

1. A(n) _____ is used to document patient care that is provided.

2. The health care facility's billing and accounting systems are part of the _____.

3. A(n) _____ can be accessed by more than one healthcare organization, while a(n) _____ can only be utilized by the healthcare organization that created it.

4. The legislation that provided financial incentives for providers to use an EHR in a meaningful way is
    a. HIPAA.
    b. ACA.
    c. HITECH.
    d. CMS.

5. The Promoting Interoperability program has _____ objectives that focus on patient health data access and interoperability.

B. Contents of the Health Record

1. Which of the following is a reason for having accurate health records?
    a. To provide legal protection for those who provided care to the patient
    b. To provide critical information for others
    c. To provide statistical information that is helpful to researchers
    d. To provide the best possible medical care for the patient
    e. All of the above

2. Patient's full name, email address, name of employer, and health insurance information are all examples of _____.

3. Previous illnesses, hospitalizations, and surgeries are considered _____.

4. The _____ contains health information about the patient's parents and siblings.

5. Lifestyle factors such as tobacco use, employment, and alcohol use are part of the _____.

6. The _____ is where information about the nature, location, frequency, and duration of pain of the patient's current condition are documented.

Match the description with the type of information. Answers can be used more than once.

7. _____ Patient's address
8. _____ Yellowed eyes
9. _____ Patient's email address
10. _____ Insurance information
11. _____ Elevated blood pressure
12. _____ Bloated stomach
13. _____ Complaint of headache
14. _____ Weight of 143 pounds
15. _____ Bruises on upper arms
16. _____ Patient's phone number

a.   subjective
b.   objective

17. Which of the following are the medical assistant's responsibilities when documenting in the health record?
    a.   Ensure patient privacy.
    b.   Use good interviewing techniques to obtain information.
    c.   Document only in the EHR.
    d.   All of the above
    e.   a and b

C. Working with Health Records

1. Which of the following is considered a category used for organizing information in a POR system?
   a.   Database
   b.   Problem list
   c.   Treatment plan
   d.   Progress notes
   e.   All of the above

2. Which of the following is an example category used in an SOR system?
   a.   Progress notes
   b.   Laboratory
   c.   Database
   d.   Radiology
   e.   a, b, and d

Correct the following entries as would be done in the health record. Then rewrite the entries correctly. Handwritten corrections are acceptable on these exercises.

3. The correct date of the appointment below was October 12, 20XX.

   10-21-20XX 1330 Patient did not arrive for scheduled appointment. P. Smith, RMA

   _____

   _____

   _____

   _____

4. The patient stated that the chest pain began 2 weeks ago.

    1-31-20XX 10:00 AM Patient complained of chest pain for the past 2 months. No pain noted in arms. No nausea. Desires ECG and bloodwork to check for heart problems. R. Smithee, CMA (AAMA)

    _____

    _____

    _____

    _____

Document the following exercises.

5. Eric Robertson canceled his surgical follow-up appointment today for the third time. Document this information.

    _____

    _____

    _____

    _____

6. Angela Adams called to report that she was not feeling any better since her office visit on Monday. She wants the doctor to call in a refill for her antibiotics. The chart says that she was to return to the clinic on Thursday if she was not feeling better. Today is Monday, and she says she cannot come into the clinic this week. The physician wants to see her before prescribing any other medication. Document this information.

    _____

    _____

    _____

    _____

    _____

    _____

7. Mary Elizabeth Smith called the physician's office to report redness around an injection site. She was in the office 3 hours ago and received an injection of penicillin. She says she also is itching quite a bit around the site and having trouble breathing. The doctor has left the office for the day. Office policy states that if the physician is out of the office and a patient presents or calls with an emergency, they are to be referred to the ER. Document the action that the medical assistant should take.

    _____

    _____

    _____

    _____

    _____

    _____

8. Explain the importance of data backup. _____

_____

_____

_____

9. If there is no rule to specify how long to retain records, it is best to keep them for _____ years.

10. According to HIPAA, which of the following has to be included on a release of information form?
    a. Who is releasing the information
    b. To whom the information is being released
    c. What specific information is to be released
    d. An expiration date for the release
    e. All of the above

D. Creating an Efficient Paper Health Records Management System

1. A(n) _____ have door locks to protect the contents and allows several individuals to have access to files at the same time.

2. _____ are used to replace a folder that has been temporarily removed.

3. Describe the indexing rules for alphabetic filing. _____

_____

_____

_____

_____

_____

_____

_____

_____

_____

E. Filing Methods

1. Using alphabetic filing, place the names below in correct alphabetic order with the last name first.

Cassidy Kay Hale

Candace Cassidy LeGrand

Taylor Ann Jackson

Anton Douglas Conn

Mitchel Michael Gibson

Lorienda Gaye Robison

LaNelle Elva Crumley

Allison Gaile Yarbrough

Sarah Kay Haile

Marie Gracelia Stuart

Karry Madge Chapmann

Randi Ann Perez

Cecelia Gayle Raglan

Sarah Sue Ragland

Riley Americus Belk

Starr Ellen Beall

Mitchell Thomas Gibson

George Scott Turner

Winston Roger Murchison

Sara Suzelle Montgomery

Tamika Noelle Frazier

Alisa Jordan Williams

Alisha Dawn Chapman

Bentley James Adams

Montana Skye Kizer

Dakota Marie LaRose

Robbie Sue Metzger

Thomas Charles Bruin

Percival "Butch" Adams

Carlos Perez Santos

1. _____
2. _____
3. _____
4. _____
5. _____
6. _____
7. _____
8. _____
9. _____
10. _____
11. _____
12. _____
13. _____
14. _____
15. _____
16. _____
17. _____
18. _____
19. _____
20. _____
21. _____
22. _____
23. _____
24. _____
25. _____
26. _____
27. _____
28. _____
29. _____
30. _____

2. Using terminal filing, place the numbers below in the correct order.

01-64-22	a.	_____
72-55-20	b.	_____
44-41-20	c.	_____
17-41-20	d.	_____
56-42-21	e.	_____
91-88-21	f.	_____
15-24-22	g.	_____
82-49-20	h.	_____
08-94-21	i.	_____
24-42-22	j.	_____

F. Organization of Files

1. Correspondence related to the operation of the of the office is considered _____ correspondence.

2. A filing system designed to remind you of something that needs to be done or followed up is a _____ file.

CERTIFICATION PREPARATION

Circle the correct answer.

1. Information that is obtained by questioning the patient or taken from a form is called _____ information.
   a. confidential
   b. subjective
   c. necessary
   d. objective

2. How would you properly index the name "Amanda M. Stiles-Duncan" for filing?
   a. Stilesduncan Amanda M.
   b. Stiles Duncan Amanda M.
   c. Duncanstiles Amanda M.
   d. Duncan Amanda M. Stiles

3. Who is the legal owner of the information stored in a patient's record?
   a. The patient
   b. The provider or agency where services were provided
   c. The patient's insurance company
   d. Both the patient and the provider

4. Which is *not* objective information?
   a. Progress notes
   b. Family history
   c. Diagnosis
   d. Physical examination and findings

5. Many healthcare facilities now use voice recognition software for transcription. The system can be used to dictate which types of reports?
   a. Progress notes
   b. Letters
   c. Emails
   d. All of the above

6. Perhaps the most essential action for the medical assistant working with a patient and using an electronic record is to
   a. type in every word the patient says.
   b. make sure the patient is not hiding any part of the health history.
   c. make frequent eye contact with patient and smile.
   d. sit in a chair across from the patient so that the person cannot see the screen.

7. Which EHR system backup requires the least amount of hardware?
    a. Online backup system
    b. External hard drives
    c. Full server backup
    d. Thumb drive backup

8. The concise account of symptoms in the patient's own words is the _____.
    a. objective information
    b. provisional diagnosis
    c. chief complaint
    d. caption

9. To completely remove all traces of an entry in a health record is _____.
    a. interface
    b. obliteration
    c. dictation
    d. compliance

10. The process of electronic data entry of a provider's instructions for the treatment of patients is called _____.
    a. progress notes
    b. computerized physician/provider order entry
    c. direct filing system
    d. continuity of care

WORKPLACE APPLICATIONS

1. Dr. Martin wants to be sure the Walden-Martin Family Medical (WMFM) Clinic is meeting all of the requirements for Promoting Interoperability. He has asked Susan to put together a list of what WMFM Clinic should be doing to meet those requirements. What would be on Susan's list?

    _____

    _____

    _____

    _____

2. Susan has been learning about the various EHR systems available. She has also been learning about the need to back up to protect the information stored in the EHR. Susan has asked the office manager at WMFM Clinic how the EHR is backed up at their facility. The office manager states that they currently use an external hard drive, but would like to look closer at other options. She asks Susan to determine what other options are available. Write a brief description of each of the options below.

    a. External hard drive _____

    _____

    b. Full server backup _____

    _____

    c. Online backup system _____

    _____

INTERNET ACTIVITIES

1. Using online resources, research EHR systems. Choose the one you think would be the best option and create a poster presentation, a PowerPoint presentation, or write a paper summarizing your research. Include the following points in your project:
   a. Description of the EHR
   b. Description of the practice management functions
   c. Does it include backup features?
   d. How does it meet the meaningful use requirements?

2. Using online resources, research a voice recognition software. Create a poster presentation, a PowerPoint presentation, or write a paper summarizing your research. Include the following points in your project:
   a. Description voice recognition software
   b. List the uses for voice recognition software
   c. Compare three different products
   d. Determine which one would be the best product

Procedure 10.1 Upload Documents to the Electronic Health Record

Name _____ Date _____ Score _____

Task: Scan paper records and upload digital files to the EHR.

Scenario: A new patient brings in a laboratory report and a radiology report that he would like to have added to his EHR. You need to scan in the original documents and upload them to the EHR.

Equipment and Supplies:
- Scanner
- Computer with SimChart for the Medical Office or EHR software
- Patient's laboratory and radiology reports (Figures 10.1 and 10.2)

Standard: Complete the procedure and all critical steps in _____ minutes with a minimum score of 85% within two attempts (*or as indicated by the instructor*).

Scoring: Divide the points earned by the total possible points. Failure to perform a critical step, indicated by an asterisk (*), results in grade no higher than an 84% (*or as indicated by the instructor*).

Time: Began_____ Ended_____ Total minutes: _____

Steps:	Point Value	Attempt 1	Attempt 2
1. Obtain the patient's name and date of birth if not on the reports.	10		
2. Using a scanner that is connected to the computer, scan each document, creating an individual digital image for each.	20		
3. Locate the file of the two scanned images in the computer drive. Open the files to ensure the images are clear.	15*		
4. To help ensure the integrity of the practice management and EHR systems, a search for the new patient's name must always be done. In the EHR, search for the patient, using the patient's last and first name. Verify the patient's date of birth.	15*		
5. Locate the window to upload diagnostic/laboratory results and add a new result. Enter the date of the test. Select the correct type of result. Browse for the image file of the laboratory file and attach it. Save the information.	15*		
6. Select the option to add a new result and repeat the steps to upload the second report.	10*		
7. To help ensure the integrity of the EHR system, verify that the correct documents were uploaded and specific headers (titles) were given to the document.	15*		
Total Points	100		

Comments

CAAHEP Competencies	Step(s)
VI.P.3. Input patient data using an electronic system	2-6
ABHES Competencies	**Step(s)**
7. Administrative Procedures a. Gather and process documents	2-5
7. Administrative Procedures b. Navigate electronic health records systems and practice management software	All

Figure 10.1 Laboratory Report

AnyTown Laboratory

Date Reported: 04/25/20XX
Patient Name: Jonathan S. Scott
Ordering Provider: George St. Cyr, MD
Date Collected: 04/15/20XX
Test Requested: Lipid Panel

Date Received: 04/25/20XX
DOB: 08/01/1990

Time Collected: 0830
Fasting?: Yes

Test	Result	Flag	Reference Range
Cholesterol, total	210	High	<200 mg/dL
HDL Cholesterol	26	Low	>40 mg/dL
LDL Cholesterol	142	High	<130 mg/dL
Triglycerides	236	High	<150 mg/dL
Total Cholesterol/HDL ratio	5.8	High	<4.5

Figure 10.2   Radiology Report

AnyTown Radiology

Date:	10/31/20XX	**Time:**	1430
Patient Name:	Jonathan S. Scott	**DOB:**	08/01/1990
Exam Type:	Chest x-ray 2 views	**Ordering Provider:**	George St. Cyr, MD

Final Report:
History: Cough and fever
Report: Frontal and lateral views of the chest
Comparison: None

Findings:
Lungs: The lungs are well inflated and clear. There is no evidence of pneumonia or pulmonary edema.
Pleura: There is no pleural effusion or pneumothorax.
Heart and mediastinum: The cardiomediastinal silhouette is normal.
Impression: Clear lungs without evidence of pneumonia.
Recommendation: None.
Provider: Bones, Seymore MD

Procedure 10.2 Register a New Patient in the Practice Management Software

Name _____ Date _____ Score _____

Task: Register a new patient in the practice management software, prepare a Notice of Privacy Practices (NPP) form and a Disclosure Authorization form for the new patient, and document this in the electronic health record (EHR).

Scenario: The patient received both documents and signed the Disclosure Authorization form.

Equipment and Supplies:
- Computer with SimChart for the Medical Office or practice management and EHR software
- Completed patient registration form (Figure 10.3)
- Scanner

Standard: Complete the procedure and all critical steps in _____ minutes with a minimum score of 85% within two attempts (*or as indicated by the instructor*).

Scoring: Divide the points earned by the total possible points. Failure to perform a critical step, indicated by an asterisk (*), results in grade no higher than an 84% (*or as indicated by the instructor*).

Time: Began_____ Ended_____ Total minutes: _____

Steps:	Point Value	Attempt 1	Attempt 2
1. Obtain the new patient's completed registration form. Log into the practice management software.	10		
2. To help ensure the integrity of the practice management and EHR systems, a search for the new patient's name must always be done before registering that patient. Using the patient's last and first names and date of birth, search the database for the patient. To help ensure the integrity of the practice management and EHR systems, a search for the new patient's name must always be done before registering that person. This prevents a double record from being created if the patient had been entered into the database earlier.	15*		
3. If the database does not contain the patient's name, add a new patient and enter the patient's demographics from the completed registration form.	10*		
4. Correctly spell the patient's name and accurately enter the patient's date of birth.	15*		
5. Verify that the information entered is correct and that all fields are completed before saving the data.	10		
6. Using the EHR software, prepare and print a copy of the NPP and a Disclosure Authorization form for the new patient. The Disclosure Authorization form should indicate the disclosure will be to the patient's insurance company.	15		
Scenario Update: The patient received both documents and signed the Disclosure Authorization form.			
7. Using the EHR, document that the patient received a copy of the NPP and signed the Disclosure Authorization form. Scan the Disclosure Authorization form and upload it into the EHR.	15*		
8. Log out of the software upon completion of the procedure.	10		
Total Points	100		

Comments

CAAHEP Competencies	Step(s)
VI.P.3. Input patient data using an electronic system	All
ABHES Competencies	**Step(s)**
7. Administrative Procedures a. Gather and process documents	All
7. Administrative Procedures b. Navigate electronic health records systems and practice management software	All

Figure 10.3   Patient Information Form

Patient Information:
Name: Jonathan S. Scott
Address: 922 Golf Road, Anytown, AK 12345
Date of Birth: 08/01/1990
Email: jscott16@anytown.mail
Sex: M
Home Phone: 123-123-3098
SSN: 987-66-1223
Emergency Contact Name: Callie Scott
Emergency Contact Phone: 123-123-0857

Guarantor Information:
Relationship of Guarantor to Patient: Self
Employer Name: Anytown Bank
Work Phone: 123-567-9012
Primary Provider: David Kahn, MD

Insurance Information:
  Primary Insurance:
      Insurance: Aetna
      Name of Policyholder: Jonathan S. Scott
      SSN of Policyholder: 987-66-1223
      Policy/ID Number: JS8884910
      Group Number: 66574W
      Claims Address: 1234 Insurance Way, Anytown, AL 12345-1234
      Claims Phone Number: 180-012-3222

Procedure 10.3 Protect the Integrity of the Medical Record

Name _____ Date _____ Score _____

Tasks: Protect the integrity of the medical record.

Scenario: You are mentoring a medical assistant student who is in practicum. You notice the student routinely does not sign out of the electronic health record before leaving the desk. The facility's policy is to sign out or lock the computer before leaving it.

Directions: Role-play the scenario with a peer, who plays the student. You, the medical assistant, must explain to the "student" the facility's policy. Also address the hazards of not protecting the medical record. If the student does not change the behavior, you will need to address the situation with the department supervisor.

Standard: Complete the procedure and all critical steps in _____ minutes with a minimum score of 85% within two attempts (*or as indicated by the instructor*).

Scoring: Divide the points earned by the total possible points. Failure to perform a critical step, indicated by an asterisk (*), results in grade no higher than an 84% (*or as indicated by the instructor*).

Time: Began_____ Ended_____ Total minutes: _____

Steps:	Point Value	Attempt 1	Attempt 2
1. Professionally and respectfully discuss the situation with the student.	25		
2. Inform the student about the facility's policy and the hazards of not protecting the electronic health record.	25		
3. Provide the student with strategies to protect the electronic health record.	25		
4. Inform the student what will occur if they do not protect the electronic record.	25		
Total Points	**100**		

Comments

CAAHEP Competencies	Step(s)
A.1. Demonstrate critical thinking skills	Entire procedure

Chapter 13

Procedure 13.2 Protect the Integrity of the Medical Record

Name _____ Date _____ Score _____

Procedure 10.4   Developing a Plan in the Event of Loss of EMR and PMS

Name _____ Date _____ Score _____

Task: To develop a plan to ensure information integrity and patient care when the access to the EMR and PMS is lost for more than 24 hours.

Scenario: Your supervisor at WMFM Clinic has asked you to develop a plan to protect patient information in case access is lost to the EHR and PMS.

Equipment and Supplies:
- Paper and pen, or word processing software

Standard: Complete the procedure and all critical steps in _____ minutes with a minimum score of 85% within two attempts (*or as indicated by the instructor*).

Scoring: Divide the points earned by the total possible points. Failure to perform a critical step, indicated by an asterisk (*), results in grade no higher than an 84% (*or as indicated by the instructor*).

Time: Began _____ Ended _____ Total minutes: _____

Steps:	Point Value	Attempt 1	Attempt 2
1. Using reliable internet resources, research ways to protect the information contained in the EMR and PMS.	25		
2. Develop a list of the top four options for protecting patient information and patient care.	20		
3. Develop a pros/cons list for each of the four options.	25		
4. Determine which option you would choose and create plan for implementing it at WMFM Clinic. Your plan should include how patients can still be seen and provided the same level of care.	30*		
Total Points	100		

Comments

CAAHEP Competencies	Step(s)
VI.C.5. Identify the importance of data back-up	All

Procedure 10.5   Create and Organize a Patient's Paper Health Record

Name _____ **Date** _____ **Score** _____

Task: Create a paper health record for a new patient. Organize health record documents in a paper health record.

Equipment and Supplies:
- End tab file folder
- Completed patient registration form
- Divider sheets with different color labels (4)
- Progress note sheet (1)
- Name label
- Color-coding labels (first two letters of the last name and first letter of the first name)
- Year label
- Allergy label
- Black pen or computer with word processing software to process labels
- Health record documents (i.e., prior records, laboratory reports)
- Hole puncher

Standard: Complete the procedure and all critical steps in _____ minutes with a minimum score of 85% within two attempts (*or as indicated by the instructor*).

Scoring: Divide the points earned by the total possible points. Failure to perform a critical step, indicated by an asterisk (*), results in grade no higher than an 84% (*or as indicated by the instructor*).

Time: Began_____ Ended_____ Total minutes: _____

Steps:	Point Value	Attempt 1	Attempt 2
1. Obtain the patient's first and last names.	**10**		
2. Neatly write or word-process the patient's name on the name label. Left-justify the last name, followed by a comma, the first name, middle initial, and a period (e.g., Smith, Mary J.).	**15***		
3. Adhere the name label to the bottom-left side of the record tab. When you hold the record by the main fold in your left hand, the writing should be easy to read. (For directional purposes, assume the record main fold is on the left and the tab is at the bottom.)	**10**		
4. Put the color-coding labels on the bottom-right edge of the folder. Start by placing the first letter of the last name at the farthest-right edge. Working left, place the second letter of the last name, then the first letter of the first name, and lastly the year label. The year label should be close to the name label.	**15***		
5. Place the allergy label on the front of the record. If allergies are known, clearly write the allergy on the label in red ink.	**15***		
6. Place the divider labels on the record divider sheets if they come separately. Ensure the labels on the divider sheets are staggered so they do not overlap. Print the name of the section on the front and back of the label. The print should be easy to read when the record is held by the main fold.	**15***		

7.	Using the prongs on the left-hand side of the record, secure the registration form.	**10**		
8.	Using the prongs on the right-hand side of the record, secure the index dividers with a progress note sheet under the progress note tab.	**10**		
	Total Points	**100**		

Comments

ABHES Competencies	Step(s)
7. Administrative Procedures a. Gather and process documents	All

Procedure 10.6 File Patient Health Records

Name _____ Date _____ Score _____

Task: File patient health records using two different filing systems: the alphabetic system and the numeric system.

Scenario: The agency utilizes the alphabetic system. You need to file health records in the correct location.

Equipment and Supplies:
- Paper health records using the alphabetic filing system
- Paper health records using the numeric filing system
- File box(es) or file cabinet

Standard: Complete the procedure and all critical steps in _____ minutes with a minimum score of 85% within two attempts (*or as indicated by the instructor*).

Scoring: Divide the points earned by the total possible points. Failure to perform a critical step, indicated by an asterisk (*), results in grade no higher than an 84% (*or as indicated by the instructor*).

Time: Began_____ Ended_____ Total minutes: _____

Steps:	Point Value	Attempt 1	Attempt 2
1. Using alphabetic guidelines, place the records to be filed in alphabetic order.	20		
2. Using the file box or file cabinet, locate the correct spot for the first file.	10		
3. Place the health record in the correct location. Continue these filing steps until all the health records are filed.	20*		
4. Using numeric guidelines, place the records to be filed in numeric order.	20		
5. Using the file box or file cabinet, locate the correct spot for the first file.	10		
6. Place the health record in the correct location. Continue these filing steps until all the health records are filed.	20*		
Total Points	100		

Comments

ABHES Competencies	Step(s)
7. Administrative Procedures a. Gather and process documents	All

Daily Operations and Safety

chapter

11

CAAHEP Competencies	Assessment
VI.C.3. Recognize the purpose of routine maintenance of equipment	Skills and Concepts – C. 5; Certification Preparation – 5
VI.C.4. Identify steps involved in completing an inventory	Skills and Concepts – D. 7-9
XII.C.3. Identify fire safety issues in a healthcare environment	Skills and Concepts – J. 2-3
XII.C.4. Identify emergency practices for evacuation of a healthcare setting	Skills and Concepts – K. 9-18; Internet Activities – 3
XII.C.7.a. Identify principles of: body mechanics	Skills and Concepts – H. 2-3; Certification Preparation – 6; Workplace Application – 2
XII.C.8. Identify critical elements of an emergency plan for response to a natural disaster or other emergency	Skills and Concepts – K. 1-5; Certification Preparation – 8; Internet Activities – 3
XII.C.9. Identify the physical manifestations and emotional behaviors of persons involved in an emergency	Skills and Concepts – L. 3; Certification Preparation – 10; Procedure 11.5 (Step 6)
VI.P.4. Perform an inventory of supplies.	Procedure 11.3
XII.P.2.b. Demonstrate proper use of: fire extinguishers	Procedure 11.6
XII.P.3. Use proper body mechanics	Procedure 11.3
XII.P.4. Evaluate an environment to identify unsafe conditions	Procedure 11.4
A.8. Demonstrate self-awareness	Procedure 11.5

ABHES Competencies	Assessment
7. Administrative Procedures f. Maintain inventory of equipment and supplies	Procedures 11.1, 11.3

VOCABULARY REVIEW

Using the word pool on the right, find the correct word to match the definition. Write the word on the line after the definition.

1. Doors made of fire-resistant materials; close manually or automatically during a fire to prevent the spread of the fire _____

2. A lack of similarity between what is stated and what is found; for instance, the computer inventory count is different than the physical count _____

3. Unforeseen situations that threaten employees and visitors; they can disrupt services provided _____

4. A document that accompanies purchased merchandise and shows what is in the box or package _____

5. Unique number assigned by the ordering facility that allows the facility to track or reference the order _____

6. Assistance (i.e., service) that is provided by a healthcare provider and can be billed to the insurance company or patient _____

7. To diminish in value (e.g., the value of an item) over a period of time; a concept used for tax purposes _____

8. Refers to how often an item is purchased; this depends on how frequently the item is used and the storage space available for it _____

9. Companies that sell supplies, equipment, or services to other companies or individuals _____

10. Billing statements that list the amount owed for goods or services purchased _____

11. An order placed for an item that is temporarily out of stock and will be sent later _____

12. Money owed by a company to other companies for services and goods; pertains to paying the bills of the facility _____

13. Reducing the level or intensity; bring down a person's anger or elevated emotions _____

Word Pool
- accounts payable
- backordered
- billable service
- buying cycle
- de-escalating
- depreciate
- discrepancy
- fire doors
- invoices
- packing slip
- purchase order number
- vendors
- workplace emergencies

ABBREVIATIONS

Write out what each of the following abbreviations stands for.

1. EHR _____

2. GPOs _____

3. PBGs _____

4. PO _____

5. OSH Act _____

6. OSHA _____

7. ADA _____

8. GAS _____

9. BTL _____

10. BX _____

11. CS _____

12. EA _____

13. PKG _____

14. DDL _____

15. PYMT _____

16. QTY _____

SKILLS AND CONCEPTS
Answer the following questions.

A. Opening Tasks for the Medical Assistant
Select the correct answer or fill in the blank.

1. Which is *not* an opening task for the clinical medical assistant?
   a. Preparing the exam rooms.
   b. Updating the voice mail message.
   c. Unlocking supply cabinets.
   d. Performing quality control tests on laboratory equipment.

2. The process to ensure the reliability of test results, often using manufactured samples with known values is called _____.

3. A commercial service that answers telephone calls for its clients is called a(n) _____.

4. Documentation in the medical record that can be used to track the patient's condition and progress is called the _____.

5. Which is *not* an opening task for the administrative medical assistant?
   a. Completing refrigerator and freezer temperature logs
   b. Checking the voice mail
   c. Turning on the computers
   d. Preparing the reception area
   e. Printing schedules of the day's appointments

6. For facilities with paper health records, what must the medical assistant do?
   a. Pull the paper health records, using a copy of the appointment schedule.
   b. Verify that the correct record was pulled for each patient.
   c. Check off the patient's name on the copy of the appointment schedule.
   d. All of the above

B. Closing Tasks for the Medical Assistant
Select the correct answer.

1. Which is *not* a closing task for the clinical medical assistant?
   a. Restock the rooms and organize any reading materials.
   b. Prepare the patient records and documents for the next day.
   c. Turn off computers and other devices.
   d. Sanitize, disinfect, or sterilize equipment and instruments.

2. Which is *not* a closing task for the administrative medical assistant?
   a. Turning off the computers, copy machine, and other office equipment.
   b. Lock supply and medication cabinets.
   c. Follow office procedures for handling money at the end of the day.
   d. Secure any confidential documents.

Match the description with the correct term.

3. _____ The ability to determine what needs to be done and take action on your own.

4. _____ The process of cleaning to destroy or prevent the growth of disease-causing microorganisms.

5. _____ The process of replacing the supplies that were used.

6. _____ The process of removing all microorganisms.

7. _____ Supplies and equipment stored in a cart and ready for an emergency.

8. _____ The process of cleaning equipment and instruments with detergent and water to remove debris and reduce the number of microorganisms.

a. Restock
b. Disinfect
c. Sanitize
d. Sterilize
e. Initiative
f. Crash cart

C. Equipment Management
Select the correct answer or fill in the blank.

1. A detailed list of equipment and supplies owned and stored is called a(n) _____.

2. A(n) _____ is the process of counting the supplies in stock.

3. How can an inventory be used?
   a. The information is used when preparing tax paperwork.
   b. The information is used to replace equipment lost in a disaster or theft.
   c. The information is used by the supervisors to identify equipment that needs to be replaced.
   d. All of the above

4. When creating an inventory list of equipment, what information is documented?
   a. Equipment name, manufacturer, and serial number
   b. Purchase date, cost, and supplier
   c. Warranty information
   d. All of the above

5. What is the purpose of routine maintenance of administrative and clinical equipment? _____

6. When performing routine maintenance, what must the medical assistant do?
   a. Check electrical cords on equipment for damage.
   b. Address any suspected overheating issues.
   c. Investigate any unusual noise or change in performance.
   d. Clean and maintain equipment routinely in accordance with the user's guide.
   e. All of the above

D. Supply Inventory
Select the correct answer or fill in the blank.

1. _____ involves ordering, tracking inventory, and identifying the quantity of product to purchase.

2. What is the goal of inventory management? _____

   _____

3. The amount of supplies that need to be ordered is called the _____.

4. The point at which low inventory requires the product to be ordered is called the

   _____.

5. Calculate the reorder point for this scenario. The practice uses 6 rolls of table paper per day. It takes 7 workdays to receive the order from the medical supply company. The medical practice wants 4 extra days' worth of supplies on hand to prevent issues related to running out of the item. What is the reorder point for the table paper rolls? _____

6. Calculate the reorder point for this scenario. The practice uses 12 vials of sterile normal saline per day. It takes 4 workdays to receive the order from the medical supply company. The medical practice wants 6 extra days' worth of supplies on hand to prevent issues related to running out of the item. What is the reorder point for the vials of sterile normal saline? _____

7. When a company uses an automated inventory control system:

   a. A hand-counted inventory must be done at least _____ a year.

   b. The hand inventory counts are compared to the computer counts and _____ are identified.

   c. The manual inventory procedure provides the company with information on the _____ of items in stock.

8. What type of information is found on a supply inventory list?
   a. Name, size, and quantity of the product
   b. Item number and supplier's name
   c. Cost, reorder point, and quantity to reorder
   d. All of the above

9. You have prepared supply inventory list and are ready to inventory the supplies in your department. Which of the following would be done when completing an inventory?
   a. Identify the correct item on the supply inventory list.
   b. Count the number of items and document the number on the supply inventory list.
   c. Neatly replace the supplies.
   d. Ensure the older supplies are in front of the new supplies.
   e. All of the above

E. Ordering Process
Fill in the blank.

1. Some medical facilities join _____, which combine orders from many different medical facilities and receive volume discounts.

2. _____ offer providers potential cost-saving pricing for vaccines.

3. Some medical facilities use _____, giving each order a unique reference number.

4. A(n) _____ is a preset borrowing limit.

F. Receiving Orders
Fill in the blank.

1. When an order arrives, the medical assistant must use the _____ and compare the items in the package to it.

2. The _____ stock should be placed in the front so it is used first.

3. Any items with expiration dates should be placed with the items _____ in front, so they are used first.

4. If you are removing expired stock, remember to _____ the quantity from the inventory system.

G. Vaccine Storage Requirements
Select the correct answer or fill in the blank.

1. How should vaccines be stored per the CDC?
   a. Each type of vaccine should be placed in its own tray.
   b. Allow space between the vials promote air circulation.
   c. Place newer vaccines behind older vaccines.
   d. Keep vaccine vials in their original boxes to prevent light exposure.
   e. All of the above

2. When storing vaccines, what is recommended by the CDC?
   a. The refrigerators should maintain temperatures between 36° F and 56° F.
   b. The freezer should maintain temperatures between -58° F and 25° F.
   c. Position vaccines and diluents 2 to 3 inches from the walls, ceiling, and floor.
   d. All of the above

3. All vaccine storage units must have a(n) _____, which should be placed in the center of the unit, with vaccines surrounding it.

4. The temperature of the refrigerator and freezer should be checked at the _____ of each workday.

5. The temperature monitoring log sheet should include which of the following?
   a. Date and time
   b. Current temperature or the maximum and minimum temperature record on the device
   c. Any action taken if the temperature is out of range
   d. Name or initials of person who checked and recorded the temperature
   e. All of the above

6. What do you do if the temperature log is missing a temperature check? _____

_____

_____

7. What should the medical assistant do if the temperature is out of range?
   a. Notify the vaccine coordinator and the supervisor.
   b. The vaccines should be labeled "DO NOT USE."
   c. Place vaccines in a separate container.
   d. All of the above

H. Personal Safety and Body Mechanics
Select the correct answer or fill in the blank.

1. The provisions of the Occupational Safety and Health Act of 1970 are enforced by the

   _____.

2. Which is a principle of proper body mechanics?
   a. To lift an object, maintain a wide, stable base with your feet.
   b. Your feet should be shoulder-width apart, and you should have good footing.
   c. Bend at the knees, keeping your back straight.
   d. Lift smoothly, using the major muscles in your arms and legs.
   e. All of the above

3. Which is a principle of proper body mechanics?
   a. When lifting and carrying heavy items, keep the item directly in front of you to avoid rotating your spine.
   b. Carry the item close to your body.
   c. Keep your movements smooth.
   d. When you reach for an object, your feet should face the object.
   e. All of the above

I. Providing a Safe Environment
Answer the question, select the correct answer, or fill in the blank.

1. How should cash drawers be stored? _____

_____

_____

2. Narcotic medications should always be in a(n) _____ cabinet.

3. What is an increased risk factor for violence in healthcare?
   a. Working with patients or family members who have a history of violence and abuse alcohol or other substances.
   b. Poorly designed work environments.
   c. Lack of emergency communication and training of employees.
   d. High employee turnover.
   e. All of the above

4. What is a strategy to secure the workplace environment?
   a. Physical barriers
   b. Bright, effective lighting and accessible exits
   c. Closed-circuit video
   d. De-escalating areas for patients and visitors
   e. All of the above

J. Evaluating the Work Environment
Select the correct answer or fill in the blank.

1. Which is *not* a high-risk situation that can result in an accident?
   a. Standing water on the floor
   b. Rugs and mats that are smooth and flat
   c. Cords, cables, and boxes in the walkway
   d. Heavy objects placed on high shelves

2. Which is *not* a way to prevent injuries and fires?
   a. Checking electrical cords and plugs for damage
   b. Turning off equipment that appears to be overheating
   c. Storing potentially flammable chemicals and supplies according to the manufacturer's guidelines
   d. Ensuring power strips are overloaded
   e. Not using electricity near water

3. Oxygen, other gases, and combustible chemicals should not be in the room when
   _____ equipment is used.

K. Emergency Response Plan
Match the description with the correct emergency response plan's critical element.

1. _____ Includes the reasons for evacuation, the methods for accounting for patients, meeting locations, and maps.

2. _____ How to alert employees, law enforcement, and the fire department of the emergency.

3. _____ Includes the names of specific employees who must turn off the water, gas, electricity, and oxygen.

4. _____ Includes the names of workers who need to perform rescue and medical duties.

5. _____ Includes the floor plan, workplace map, safe areas, and procedures.

a. methods to report a fire and other emergencies
b. evacuation policy and procedure
c. critical shutdown procedures
d. emergency escape/exit routes and procedures
e. rescue and medical duties

Fill in the blank.

6. Floor maps with _____ and _____ should be posted throughout the facility.

7. _____ must be clearly marked and well-lit.

8. Exit routes should be clear of _____ and _____ at all times.

Match the evacuation priority by location.

9. _____ First priority
10. _____ Second priority
11. _____ Third priority
12. _____ Fourth priority

   a. people on the rest of the floor
   b. people in immediate danger
   c. people on the floors immediately above and below the floor with the situation
   d. people located on the floor where the emergency is occurring

Fill in the blank.

13. Evacuation priority by people means the people _____ leave first, followed by the ambulatory people, and last the _____ people.

Match the description with the correct type of evacuation.

14. _____ Involves evacuating people who are located on the floors above and below the situation

15. _____ Involves evacuating everyone from the building to a safe location outside the building

16. _____ Involves moving one or more people out of immediate danger

17. _____ Evacuation to an interior room with no windows

18. _____ Involves evacuating people off the same floor as the emergency situation

   a. shelter-in-place evacuation
   b. local evacuation
   c. horizontal evacuation
   d. vertical evacuation
   e. building evacuation

Select the correct answer.

19. Which step is *not* part of the acronym RACE?
    a. Rescue individuals threatened by the fire.
    b. Activate the alarm if you discover the fire or respond if you hear the alarm.
    c. Confirm the location of the fire.
    d. Extinguish only small fires; otherwise evacuate individuals from the area.

20. Which step is *not* part of the PASS procedure for fire extinguishers?
    a. Pull the fire alarm.
    b. Aim the nozzle or hose at the base of the fire.
    c. Squeeze the handle to release the extinguishing agent.
    d. Sweep the nozzle or hose from side to side at the base of the fire until the fire is out.

Match the use with the correct class of fire extinguishers.

21. _____ Used on flammable liquids

22. _____ For fires involving combustible metals

23. _____ Used on ordinary combustibles

24. _____ Used on electrical equipment

25. _____ Used on ordinary combustibles, flammable liquids, or electrical equipment

a. Class C
b. Class A
c. Class B
d. Class ABC
e. Class D

L. Effects of Stress

Select the correct answer or fill in the blank.

1. _____ is a person's total response to environmental demands or pressures.

2. A(n) _____ is a stimulus that provokes a stress response.

3. Which are physical manifestations and emotional behaviors caused by the stress of being involved in an emergency?
    a. Shock, disbelief, irritability, crying, and anger
    b. Feelings of fear, anxiety, numbness, sadness, worry, powerlessness, or frustration
    c. Difficulty making decisions and trouble concentrating
    d. High blood pressure, high blood glucose levels
    e. All of the above

Match the description with the correct stage of the general adaptation syndrome.

4. _____ The body's resistance has been diminished by the continued stress.

5. _____ This is the immediate reaction to the stressor.

6. _____ If the stressor continues, the individual's body adapts to the stressor.

a. adaptation stage
b. alarm stage
c. exhaustion stage

Match the following strategies to indicate if they are either healthy or unhealthy. Answers can be used more than once.

7. _____ Lack of exercise and watching TV continuously

8. _____ Getting adequate sleep

9. _____ Eating healthy, well-balanced meals

10. _____ Using excessive amounts of alcohol and tobacco

a. healthy coping strategies
b. unhealthy coping strategies

CERTIFICATION PREPARATION

Circle the correct answer.

1. What is an opening task for the administrative medical assistant?
   a. Unlock supply cabinets.
   b. Perform quality-control tests on laboratory equipment.
   c. Update the voice mail message.
   d. Follow up on outstanding patient issues from the prior day.

2. What should be disinfected in the healthcare facility?
   a. Exam table
   b. Writing table
   c. Computer keyboard
   d. All of the above

3. How often do crash carts and other emergency supplies need to be inventoried?
   a. Every week
   b. Every other week
   c. Every month
   d. Every 6 months

4. What is *not* found on a routine maintenance log?
   a. Equipment name, serial number, and location of the machine
   b. Manufacturer's name and date of purchase
   c. Store name where the machine was purchased
   d. Warranty information and service provider information

5. What is the purpose of routine maintenance of administrative and clinical equipment?
   a. Prevent injury to the patients
   b. Prevent costly damage to the equipment
   c. Prevent injury to staff members
   d. All of the above

6. What is *not* a principle of proper body mechanics?
   a. When lifting an object, maintain a wide, stable base with your feet.
   b. Get help if the item is too heavy to lift by yourself.
   c. Keep your movements smooth.
   d. When reaching for an object, stand on tiptoes.

7. What is the correct way to operate most fire extinguishers?
   a. Pull the pin, squeeze the handle, aim the nozzle, and sweep the nozzle from side to side.
   b. Pull the pin, aim the nozzle, sweep the nozzle from side to side, and squeeze the handle.
   c. Pull the pin, sweep the nozzle from side to side, squeeze the handle, and aim the nozzle.
   d. Pull the pin, aim the nozzle, squeeze the handle, and sweep the nozzle from side to side.

8. What is a critical element of an emergency response plan?
   a. Evacuation policy and procedure
   b. Methods to report emergencies
   c. Critical shutdown procedures
   d. All of the above

9. Which is a dry chemical fire extinguisher that is used on fires related to electrical sources?
   a. Class A
   b. Class B
   c. Class C
   d. Class D

10. Which is *not* a symptom of stress?
    a. Anger
    b. Low blood pressure
    c. Anxiety
    d. Fear

WORKPLACE APPLICATION

1. Catherine is working at the reception desk and the procedure has been to place the cashbox on the receptionist's desk. Patients arrive, make payments, and the cashbox remains on the desk visible to all and in easy access to the public. How might Catherine safeguard the money in the cashbox?

   _____

   _____

2. Maria is lifting heavy boxes. Describe how she should lift and carry heavy boxes. _____

   _____

   _____

   _____

   _____

3. Maria sometimes needs to room patients who make her uncomfortable. Describe four ways she could keep safe in these situations.

   _____

   _____

   _____

INTERNET ACTIVITIES

1. Obtain a vaccine name from the instructor and research the storage directions for that medication.

2. Research guidelines for storing vaccines in the refrigerator. Create a poster that provides the key guidelines that must be followed for safe storage.

3. Using the OSHA website (https://www.osha.gov/), research emergency action plans. Create a poster, PowerPoint, or paper summarizing your research. Focus on these areas:
   - The minimum requirements for the emergency action plan
   - Evacuation elements
   - Shelter-in-place requirements and procedures

Procedure 11.1 Perform an Equipment Inventory with Documentation

Name _____ Date _____ Score _____

Tasks: Perform an equipment inventory. Document the inventory on the equipment inventory form.

Equipment and Supplies:
- Equipment inventory form (Work Product 11.1)
- Pens
- Administrative or clinical equipment
- Purchase information (e.g., date, cost, and supplier) and warranty information (e.g., start and end date, warranty coverage)

Standard: Complete the procedure and all critical steps with a minimum score of 85% within two attempts (*or as indicated by the instructor*).

Scoring: Divide the points earned by the total possible points. Failure to perform a critical step, indicated by an asterisk (*), results in grade no higher than an 84% (*or as indicated by the instructor*).

Steps:	Point Value	Attempt 1	Attempt 2
1. For each piece of equipment to be inventoried, gather the following information: a. Name of equipment, manufacturer, and serial number b. Location and facility number (if applicable) c. Purchase date, cost, supplier, and warranty information	20		
2. Complete an equipment inventory form (Work Product 11.1) by adding the gathered information for each item inventoried.	60		
3. Review the document created. Make any necessary revisions.	20		
Total Points	**100**		

Comments

ABHES Competencies	Step(s)
7. Administrative Procedures f. Maintain inventory of equipment and supplies	Entire procedure

Work Product 11.1   Equipment Inventory Form

Name _____ **Date** _____ **Score** _____

To be used with Procedure 11.1.

Equipment Name	Manufacturer/ Serial Number	Location/Facility Number	Purchase Date/ Supplier	Cost	Warranty Information

Procedure 11.2 Perform Routine Maintenance of Equipment

Name _____ Date _____ Score _____

Tasks: Perform routine maintenance of administrative or clinical equipment. Document the maintenance on the log.

Equipment and Supplies:
- Maintenance log(s) (Work Product 11.2)
- Pens
- Information regarding the equipment (i.e., name, serial number, location, facility number, manufacturer, purchase date, warranty information, frequency of inspections, and service provider)
- Administrative or clinical equipment (e.g., oral thermometers)
- Supplies for routine maintenance (e.g., battery)
- User's guide or owner's manual, if needed

Standard: Complete the procedure and all critical steps with a minimum score of 85% within two attempts (*or as indicated by the instructor*).

Scoring: Divide the points earned by the total possible points. Failure to perform a critical step, indicated by an asterisk (*), results in grade no higher than an 84% (*or as indicated by the instructor*).

Steps:	Point Value	Attempt 1	Attempt 2
1. Gather information on the piece of equipment identified for routine maintenance including name, serial number, location, facility number, manufacturer, purchase date, warranty information, frequency of inspections, and service provider.	20		
2. Fill in the equipment details on the log (Work Product 11.2).	20*		
3. To perform the maintenance activities, gather the required supplies. If you are not familiar with the procedure or the required supplies, refer to the user's guide.	10		
4. Perform the maintenance activities as directed in the user's guide. Take any required safety precautions necessary to protect yourself and others.	20*		
5. Clean up the work area.	10		
6. Using a pen, document the date, time, the maintenance activity performed, and include your signature on the log.	20		
Total Points	100		

Comments

Work Product 11.2 Maintenance Logs

Name _____ **Date** _____ **Score** _____

To be used with Procedure 11.2.

Maintenance Log

Equipment: _____ Serial #: _____ Location: _____

Facility #: _____ Manufacturer: _____ Purchased: _____

Warranty Information: _____

Frequency of Inspections: _____

Service Provider: _____

Date	Time	Maintenance Activities	Signature

Maintenance Log

Equipment: _____ Serial #: _____ Location: _____

Facility #: _____ Manufacturer: _____ Purchased: _____

Warranty Information: _____

Frequency of Inspections: _____

Service Provider: _____

Date	Time	Maintenance Activities	Signature

Maintenance Log

Equipment: _____ Serial #: _____ Location: _____

Facility #: _____ Manufacturer: _____ Purchased: _____

Warranty Information: _____

Frequency of Inspections: _____

Service Provider: _____

Date	Time	Maintenance Activities	Signature

Maintenance Log

Equipment: _____ Serial #: _____ Location: _____

Facility #: _____ Manufacturer: _____ Purchased: _____

Warranty Information: _____

Frequency of Inspections: _____

Service Provider: _____

Date	Time	Maintenance Activities	Signature

Procedure 11.3 Perform a Supply Inventory with Documentation While Using Proper Body Mechanics

Name _____ Date _____ Score _____

Tasks: Perform a supply inventory using correct body mechanics. Document the inventory on the supply inventory form.

Equipment and Supplies:
- Supply inventory form (Work Product 11.3)
- Pens
- Administrative or clinical supplies to be inventoried
- Purchase information (e.g., item number, cost, and supplier) for supplies in inventory
- Reorder point and quantity to reorder for each item in inventory

Standard: Complete the procedure and all critical steps with a minimum score of 85% within two attempts (*or as indicated by the instructor*).

Scoring: Divide the points earned by the total possible points. Failure to perform a critical step, indicated by an asterisk (*), results in grade no higher than an 84% (*or as indicated by the instructor*).

Steps:	Point Value	Attempt 1	Attempt 2
1. For the supplies in inventory, gather the following information for each item: • Name, size, quantity (e.g., purchased individually, 100 per box) • Item number, supplier's name, cost • Reorder point and quantity to reorder	5		
2. For each supply item, enter information on the inventory form (Work Product 11.3). Make sure the appropriate entry is in the right location. Note: The "Stock Available" column will be empty for now.	15*		
3. Review the document. Make any necessary revisions.	10		
4. Using the supply inventory list, inventory the supplies in the department. Identify how the supply should be counted (e.g., individually, by the box) and count the number of items in stock.	15		
5. Add the number in the appropriate row under the "Stock Available" header.	10		
6. Compare the reorder point number to the stock available number. If the stock available number is at or below the reorder point, indicate that the item needs to be reordered by checking the appropriate column.	10*		
7. Make sure the supplies are neatly arranged. The older stock should be in front of the newer stock.	5		
8. Repeat steps 5 through 7 until all supplies are inventoried.	10		
9. Use proper body mechanics when lifting and moving supplies by maintaining a wide, stable base with your feet. Your feet should be shoulder-width apart, and you should have good footing. Bend at the knees, keeping your back straight. Lift smoothly with the major muscles in your arms and legs. Use the same technique when putting the item down.	10*		

10. Use proper body mechanics when reaching for an object. Clear away barriers and use a step-stool if needed. Your feet should face the object. Avoid twisting or turning with a heavy load.	**10***			
Total Points	**100**			

Comments

CAAHEP Competencies	Step(s)
VI.P.4. Perform an inventory of supplies	1-8
XII.P.3. Use proper body mechanics	9, 10
ABHES Competencies	**Step(s)**
7. Administrative Procedures f. Maintain inventory of equipment and supplies	1-8

Work Product 11.3 Supply Inventory Form

Name _____ **Date** _____ **Score** _____

To be used with Procedure 11.3.

Item Name	Size	Quantity	Item Number	Supplier's Name	Reorder Point	Quantity to Reorder	Cost	Stock Available	Order (✓)

Procedure 11.4   Evaluate the Work Environment

Name _____   **Date** _____   **Score** _____

Tasks: Evaluate the work environment and identify unsafe working conditions.

Equipment and Supplies:
- Work environment evaluation form (Work Product 11.4)
- Pen

Standard: Complete the procedure and all critical steps with a minimum score of 85% within two attempts (*or as indicated by the instructor*).

Scoring: Divide the points earned by the total possible points. Failure to perform a critical step, indicated by an asterisk (*), results in grade no higher than an 84% (*or as indicated by the instructor*).

Steps:	Point Value	Attempt 1	Attempt 2
1. Observe the environment for slipping, tripping, or fall risks. Document your findings on the work environment evaluation form (Work Product 11.4).	20		
2. Observe the environment for safety and security issues. Document your findings.	20		
3. Observe the environment for fire risks and electrical issues. Document your findings.	20		
4. Observe the environment for fire containment and evacuation strategies. Document your findings.	20		
5. Based on your observations, summarize your findings. If risks are present, create a list of issues that need to be addressed. Describe what needs to be done for each risk.	20*		
Total Points	**100**		

Comments

CAAHEP Competencies	Step(s)
XII.P.4. Evaluate an environment to identify unsafe conditions	Entire procedure

Work Product 11.4   Work Environment Evaluation Form

Name _____   Date _____   Score _____
To be used with Procedure 11.4.

Directions: *Check either in the "Yes" or "No" column for each question. Check "NA" if it is not applicable. Include any issues in the comment column. Summarize your findings for each area, using the space indicated.*

Slipping, tripping, or fall risks	Yes	No	NA	Comments
• Is the lighting appropriate?				
• Are any lights burned out? Are any areas dim?				
• Is the flooring and carpeting ripped or pulled up?				
• If rugs/mats are present, are they folded?				
• Is water on the floor?				
• Is signage present warning of the water?				
• Are items cluttering the hallway, making walking difficult?				
• Are cords, cables, and other items in the walkway?				
• Is trash on the floor?				
• Are heavy items on high shelves?				
• Is a sturdy step stool available?				
Safety and security issues	**Yes**	**No**	**NA**	**Comments**
• Are rooms available that can be locked and used during workplace violence?				
• Is there limited visibility from the hallway into the room?				
• Are there areas in the building with limited visibility?				
• If the building is accessible to the public, are there any safe zones or areas for staff?				
• Are the emergency call lights in the exam rooms and bathrooms functioning?				
• Are the oxygen tanks (if available) checked per the facility's policy?				
Fire risks and electrical issues	**Yes**	**No**	**NA**	**Comments**
• Are electrical cords and plugs free from cracks, fraying, or other damage?				
• Are power strips overloaded?				
• Is electricity being used near a water source?				
• Are flammable chemicals and supplies stored according to manufacturers' guidelines?				
• Are combustibles (e.g., paper, cardboard, cloth, flammable chemicals) away from heat sources?				

Fire containment and evacuation strategies	Yes	No	NA	Comments
• Are building diagrams posted on walls indicating exit routes (two or more), fire alarms, and fire extinguishers?				
• Are exit routes uncluttered?				
• Are exit signs visible and lit?				
• Are fire doors unblocked and able to be closed in an emergency?				
• Are interior rooms available for severe storms?				
• Are smoke detectors located throughout the building?				
• Are fire alarms available?				
• Are fire extinguishers available and checked routinely (per the facility's policy)?				
• Are flammable products (e.g., oxygen tanks, chemicals) stored along the exit routes?				

Based on your observations, summarize your findings.

If risks are present, create a list of issues that need to be addressed. Describe what needs to be done for each risk.

Procedure 11.5 Participate in a Mock Exposure Event

Name _____ Date _____ Score _____

Tasks: Demonstrate self-awareness in an emergency situation. Participate in a mock exposure event and document specific steps taken. Recognize the physical and emotional effects on individuals involved in an emergency situation.

Scenario: You and Beth are in the autoclave room and two chemicals spill, creating toxic fumes. Beth is having trouble breathing. The following staff, patients, and visitors are present:

Rooms	Staff and Reception Areas
1—Teen and his mother	Reception Area A—Four people waiting
2—Older woman in a wheelchair	Reception Area B—Five people waiting
3—Mother with three little children	
4—Adult female	**Staff**
5—Empty	Tim—In MA station 3
6—An older couple	Rose—At the insurance desk
7—Adult male	Dave and Patty—At the reception desk
8—Empty	Julie Walden, MD—In provider office 1
Procedure room—Empty	Angela Perez, MD—In room 3
	Jean Burke, NP—In room 7

Directions: Using word processing software, write a paper and address the procedure steps. Use reliable Internet resources to research the physical manifestations and emotional behaviors of persons involved in an emergency. Include your findings in the paper as indicated in the procedure steps. Use 1-inch margins, double spacing, and 12-point font. Length should be at least two pages.

Equipment and Supplies:
- Paper
- Pen
- Floor map (see Figure 11.11 in the textbook)
- Computer with internet access

Standard: Complete the procedure and all critical steps with a minimum score of 85% within two attempts (*or as indicated by the instructor*).

Scoring: Divide the points earned by the total possible points. Failure to perform a critical step, indicated by an asterisk (*), results in grade no higher than an 84% (*or as indicated by the instructor*).

Steps:	Point Value	Attempt 1	Attempt 2
1. Using the scenario, describe how you would handle the emergency exposure situation with Beth. • Identify four steps a medical assistant could take to demonstrate self-awareness while responding to this emergency situation. • Describe exposure control mechanisms or how you might limit the exposure to other people once you remove Beth from the room.	15*		

Scenario continues: Dr. Walden informed the staff to evacuate from the building. The outdoor safe meeting location is at the back of the parking lot.
 2. Document the steps to handle the exposure event and evacuation from the building.
    • Describe what each staff member and provider should do to help with the evacuation procedure and notify 911.
    • Describe the steps (evacuations) in the order that they should occur.
    • Describe how the staff may ensure all individuals are out of the building.
	15*		

3. Dr. Walden is in charge during the emergency. Describe what her responsibilities include.	5		
4. Dave took the patient registry. Describe why the patient registry is important.	5		

Scenario continues: Two weeks after the event, Beth confides to you that she is not doing well. She recovered from the exposure, but since the event she has had difficulty sleeping. She is anxious when she goes into the autoclave room. She is having trouble concentrating on her job. She mentioned she has had two nightmares of emergencies occurring in the department in which she gets injured.
 5. *Do the following:*
    • Describe what might be occurring with Beth and the symptoms that relate to it.
    • Discuss what you might encourage her to do about the situation.
	15*		

6. Research the physical manifestations and emotional behaviors of persons involved in an emergency. Identify four physical signs and four emotional behaviors of stress in persons involved in an emergency situation. Cite your resources.	15*		
7. Describe how the physical and emotional effects of stress would be different for Beth, you, the providers, and the other employees present.	15		
8. Describe how a medical assistant could limit the physical and emotional effects of stress on each person/group: Beth, the providers, the other employees present in the facility, and yourself.	15		
Total Points	**100**		

Comments

CAAHEP Competencies	Step(s)
A.8. Demonstrate self-awareness	1

Procedure 11.6   Use a Fire Extinguisher

Name _____ Date _____ Score _____

Tasks: Select the correct fire extinguisher and demonstrate its use.

Equipment and Supplies:
• Fire extinguisher

Scenarios:
a. You are working in the medical laboratory, and an electrical fire starts.
b. You are working in the clinic, and a fire starts in a wastebasket.
c. You are working in the medical laboratory, and a chemical fire starts (combustible metal fire).

Standard: Complete the procedure and all critical steps with a minimum score of 85% within two attempts (*or as indicated by the instructor*).

Scoring: Divide the points earned by the total possible points. Failure to perform a critical step, indicated by an asterisk (*), results in grade no higher than an 84% (*or as indicated by the instructor*).

Steps:	Point Value	Attempt 1	Attempt 2
1. Using the scenario, identify the type of fire extinguisher required to put out the fire.	20		
2. Hold the extinguisher by the handle with the hose or nozzle pointing away from you. Pull out the pin that is located below the trigger.	20		
3. Stand about 10 feet from the fire. Aim the extinguisher hose or nozzle at the base of the fire. Keep the extinguisher in an upright position as you work.	20		
4. Squeeze the trigger slowly and evenly.	20		
5. Sweep from side to side until the fire is out.	20		
Total Points	100		

Comments

CAAHEP Competencies	Step(s)
XII.P.2.b. Demonstrate proper use of: fire extinguishers	Entire procedure

Health Insurance Essentials

chapter

12

CAAHEP Competencies	Assessment
VIII.C.1.a. Identify: types of third party plans	Skills and Concepts – B. 1
VIII.C.2. Identify managed care requirements for patient referral	Skills and Concepts – C. 4
VIII.C.3.a. Identify processes for: verification of eligibility for services	Skills and Concepts – D. 2
VIII.C.3.b. Identify processes for: precertification / preauthorization	Skills and Concepts – D. 3, 4
VIII.P.1. Interpret information on an insurance card	Procedure 12.1
ABHES Competencies	**Assessment**
5. Human Relations c. Assist the patient in navigating issues and concerns that may arise (i.e., insurance policy information, medical bills, and physician/ provider orders)	Case Scenario – 2
7. Administrative Procedures a. Gather and process documents	Procedure 12.1
7. Administrative Procedures c. Perform billing and collection procedures	Procedure 12.1

VOCABULARY REVIEW

Using the word pool on the right, find the correct word to match the definition. Write the word on the line after the definition.

Group A

1. A set dollar amount that the policyholder must pay before the insurance company starts to pay for services

   _____ _____

2. Poor, needy, impoverished _____

3. The amount paid or to be paid by the policyholder for coverage under the contract, usually in periodic installments

   _____

4. Services provided to help prevent certain illnesses or that lead to an early diagnosis _____

5. When the policyholder pays a certain percentage of the bill and the insurance company pays the rest _____

6. A formal request for payment from an insurance company for services provided _____

7. A written agreement between two parties, in which one party (the insurance company) agrees to pay another party (the patient) if certain specified circumstances occur _____

8. Services that are proper and needed for the diagnosis or treatment of the medical condition _____

9. A set dollar amount that the policyholder must pay for each office visit _____

10. The person responsible for the payment of the premium

    _____

Word Pool
- policy
- premium
- subscriber
- deductible
- coinsurance
- copayment
- claim
- medically necessary
- preventive care
- indigent

Group B

1. Government insurance plan for dependents of military personnel

   _____

2. Those covered by Medicare; a designated person who receives funds from an insurance policy _____

3. Insurance plan funded by a large company or organization for its own employees _____

4. Low-income Medicare patients who qualify for Medicaid for their secondary insurance _____

5. Government insurance plan for those age 65 or older

   _____

6. A list of fixed prices for services _____

7. Government insurance plan for surviving spouses and dependent children of veterans who died in the line of duty

   _____

Word Pool
- Medicare
- Medicaid
- TRICARE
- Civilian Health and Medical Program of the Veterans Administration
- beneficiary
- resource-based relative value scale
- explanation of benefits
- fee schedule
- Qualified Medicare Beneficiaries
- self-funded plan

8. A document sent by the insurance company to the provider and the patient explaining the allowed charge amount, the amount reimbursed for services, and the patient's financial responsibilities _____

9. Government insurance plan for those with low income _____

10. A system used to determine how much providers should be paid for services provided; used by Medicare and many other health insurance companies _____

Group C

1. In charge of coordinating the patient's care _____

2. When the patient has authorized the insurance company to make the payment directly to the provider _____

3. An organization that processes claims and provides administrative services for another organization _____

4. A process required by some insurance carriers in which the provider obtains permission to perform certain procedures or services _____

5. An online marketplace where you can compare and buy individual health insurance plans _____

6. The primary care provider who is in charge of a patient's treatment _____

7. The amount paid for a medical service in a geographic area based on what providers in the area usually charge for the same or similar service _____

8. Providers are contracted with the insurance plan and have agreed to accept the contracted fee schedule as payment in full _____

9. The maximum that the insurance plan will pay for a procedure or service _____

10. An order from a primary care provider for the patient to see a specialist or get certain medical services _____

Word Pool
- third-party administrator
- health insurance exchange
- participating provider
- allowable charge
- assignment of benefits
- usual, customary, and reasonable
- primary care provider
- referral
- preauthorization
- gatekeeper

Group D

1. Reviews individual cases to ensure that services are medically necessary _____

2. The provider is paid a set amount for each enrolled person assigned to him or her, per period of time, whether or not that person has received services _____

3. The length of time a patient waits for disability insurance to pay after the date of injury _____

4. Low- to middle-income Americans can compare plans and lower their costs for healthcare coverage _____

5. An approved list of physicians, hospitals, and other providers _____

6. A health problem that was present before new health insurance coverage started _____

7. A service provided by various insurance companies for providers to look up a patient's insurance benefits, eligibility, claims status, and explanation of benefits _____

8. A decision-making process used by managed care organizations to manage healthcare costs; involves case-by-case assessments of the appropriateness of care _____

9. Government insurance plan for employees who are injured or become ill due to work-related issues _____

Word Pool
- provider network
- capitation
- utilization management
- utilization review committee
- online insurance web portal
- workers' compensation
- waiting period
- preexisting condition
- health insurance marketplaces

ABBREVIATIONS
Write out what each of the following abbreviations stands for.

1. ACA _____

2. STI _____

3. CHAMPVA _____

4. ESRD _____

5. CMS _____

6. HHS _____

7. RBRVS _____

8. UCR _____

9. EOB _____

10. QMBs _____

11. CHIP _____

12. TPA _____

13. MCO _____

14. PCP _____

15. HMO _____

16. PPO _____

17. EPO _____

18. IPA _____

19. PAR _____

SKILLS AND CONCEPTS

Answer the following questions. Write your answer on the line or in the space provided.

A. Health Insurance Basics

1. Which of the following is *not* considered cost-sharing?
   a. Deductible
   b. Coinsurance
   c. Premium
   d. Copayment
   e. All of the above

2. A(n) _____ is submitted to the insurance carrier so the provider can be paid for services rendered.

3. The federal government requires all health plans cover _____ essential health benefits.

B. Health Insurance Plans

1. Match the following terms and definitions:

   _____ Medicaid
   _____ Medicare
   _____ Medigap

   a. A federally funded health insurance program for those older than 65 years or disabled individuals younger than 65 years
   b. A term sometimes applied to private insurance products that supplement Medicare insurance benefits
   c. A health insurance program that is funded by both federal and state governments for the medically indigent

2. List two different populations that qualify for Medicare. _____

   _____

3. The RBRVS includes the following three parts:

   a. _____

   b. _____

   c. _____

4. The intermediary and administrator who coordinates patients and providers and processes claims for self-funded plans is called a(n) _____.

5. Prescription drugs are covered by Medicare _____.

6. List four different populations that qualify for Medicaid. _____

_____

7. Active-duty military personnel, family members of active duty personnel, and military retirees and their eligible family members younger than age 65 are covered by _____.

8. The health benefits program run by the Department of Veterans Affairs (VA) that helps eligible beneficiaries pay the cost of specific healthcare services and supplies is the (give acronym) _____.

9. Private health insurance plans are obtained from which two sources? _____

_____

10. A(n) _____ is a healthcare provider who enters into a contract with a specific insurance company or program and agrees to accept the contracted fee schedule.

11. The _____ is the maximum that third-party payers will pay for a procedure or service.

C. Health Insurance Models

1. Traditional health insurance plans are also referred to as _____ plans.

2. For each of the following managed care plans, describe the deductible, coinsurance, and copayment requirements:

   a. Health maintenance organization (HMO): _____

   _____

   _____

   _____

   _____

   _____

   b. Preferred provider organization (PPO):_____

   _____

   _____

   _____

   _____

   _____

c. Exclusive provider organization (EPO):_____

_____

_____

_____

_____

_____

3. A(n) _____ is a review of individual cases by a committee to make sure services are medically necessary and to study how providers use medical care resources.

4. Describe the managed care requirements for a patient referral. _____

_____

_____

_____

_____

D. The Medical Assistant's Role

1. One of the medical assistant's responsibilities is verifying eligibility. Describe the processes available for the verification of eligibility for services.

_____

_____

_____

2. Describe how the patient's insurance eligibility is confirmed. _____

_____

_____

_____

3. What items should the medical assistant gather when using the paper method to obtain a precertification for a service or procedure?

_____

_____

_____

4. Describe the processes for precertification using the paper method. What does the medical assistant need to do?

_____

_____

_____

E. Other Types of Insurance

1. List the services covered by workers' compensation plans._____

   _____

   _____

   _____

2. Match the types of insurance benefits with their description.

   _____ Disability
   _____ Liability insurance
   _____ Life insurance
   _____ Long-term care insurance

   a. Provides payment of a specified amount upon the insured's death
   b. Covers a continuum of broad-range maintenance and health services to chronically ill, disabled, or mentally disabled individuals
   c. A form of insurance that provides income replacement if the patient has a non-work–related injury
   d. Often includes benefits for medical expenses related to traumatic injuries and lost wages payable to individuals who are injured in the insured person's home or in an automobile accident

CERTIFICATION PREPARATION

Circle the correct answer.

1. A policy that covers a number of people under a single master contract issued to the employer or to an association with which they are affiliated and that is not self-funded is usually called a(n)
   a. group policy.
   b. individual policy.
   c. government plan.
   d. self-insured plan.

2. The maximum amount of money third-party payers will pay for a specific procedure or service is called the
   a. benefit.
   b. allowed amount.
   c. allowable service.
   d. incurred amount.

3. A provider who enters into a contract with an insurance company and agrees to certain rules and regulations is called a _____ provider.
   a. paying
   b. physician
   c. participating
   d. none of the above

4. A review of individual cases by a committee to make sure that services are medically necessary and to study how providers use medical care resources is called a(n)
   a. credentialing committee review.
   b. peer review committee evaluation.
   c. utilization review.
   d. audit committee review.

5. Which type of HMO model consists of physicians with separately owned practices who formally organize into a group but continue to practice in their own offices?
   a. Staff model
   b. Independent practice association
   c. Group model
   d. None of the above

6. Which individuals would *not* normally be eligible for Medicare?
   a. A 66-year-old retired woman
   b. A blind teenager
   c. A 23-year-old recipient of Temporary Assistance for Needy Families (TANF)
   d. A person on dialysis

7. Which expenses would be paid by Medicare Part B?
    a. Inpatient hospital charges
    b. Hospice services
    c. Home healthcare charges
    d. Physician's office visits

8. A type of insurance that protects workers from loss of wages after an industrial accident that happened on the job is called
    a. an individual policy.
    b. workers' compensation.
    c. unemployment insurance.
    d. disability insurance.

9. A payment method in which providers are paid for each individual enrolled in a plan, regardless of whether the person sees the provider that month, is called a _____ plan.
    a. capitation
    b. self-insured
    c. managed care
    d. fee-for-service

10. What should the medical assistant always verify prior to the patient's appointment?
    a. Eligibility
    b. Benefits and exclusions
    c. Effective date of insurance
    d. All of the above

WORKPLACE APPLICATIONS

1. After reading the following paragraph, fill the blanks in the statements.

    The medical assistant's tasks related to health insurance processing are initiated when the patient encounters the provider by appointment, as a walk-in, or in the emergency department or hospital. To complete insurance billing and coding properly, the medical assistant must perform the following tasks:

    a. Obtain information from the patient and/or the guarantor, including _____ and _____ data.

    b. Verify the patient's _____ for insurance payment with the insurance carrier or carriers, as well as insurance _____, exclusions, and whether _____ is required to refer patients to specialists or to perform certain services or procedures such as surgery or diagnostic tests.

    c. Obtain _____ for referral of the patient to a specialist or for special services or procedures that require advance permission.

2. Julia Berkley has just gotten a new insurance policy and is struggling with all of the terminology she is seeing in her policy. She would like you to explain just what *premium, deductible, coinsurance,* and *copayment* really mean.

    _____

    _____

    _____

    _____

INTERNET ACTIVITIES

1. Using online resources, research TRICARE and CHAMPVA. Create a poster presentation, a PowerPoint presentation, or write a paper summarizing your research. Include the following points in your project:
   a. Describe both TRICARE and CHAMPVA.
   b. List who is eligible for TRICARE and who is eligible for CHAMPVA.
   c. Explain what is involved when a provider participates in TRICARE.

2. Using online resources, research preferred provider organizations (PPO). Create a poster presentation, a PowerPoint presentation, or write a paper summarizing your research. Include the following points in your project:
   a. Describe what a PPO is.
   b. List the ranges for deductibles and coinsurance amounts found.
   c. Explain how a PPO is different from an HMO.
   d. Describe why a patient might want to have a PPO policy instead of traditional insurance.

Procedure 12.1 Interpret Information on an Insurance Card

Name _____ Date _____ Score _____

Task: To identify essential information on the health insurance identification (ID) card to confirm copayment obligations and obtain accurate health insurance information for claims submission.

Equipment and Supplies:
- Patient's health insurance ID, both sides (Figure 12.1)

Standard: Complete the procedure and all critical steps in _____ minutes with a minimum score of 85% within two attempts (*or as indicated by the instructor*).

Scoring: Divide the points earned by the total possible points. Failure to perform a critical step, indicated by an asterisk (*), results in grade no higher than an 84% (*or as indicated by the instructor*).

Time: Began_____ Ended_____ Total minutes: _____

Steps:	Point Value	Attempt 1	Attempt 2
1. Review the patient's health insurance ID card and identify the insured on the health insurance ID card. If the patient is different than the insured, obtain the relationship with the insured and the insured's date of birth and gender.	20*		
2. Identify the insurance plan.	20		
3. Identify the insured's identification number and group number.	20		
4. Identify the patient's copayment, which is due before the appointment. Collect the correct amount.	20		
5. On the back of the health insurance ID card, ensure that a customer service phone number and medical claims address is present.	20		
Total Points	100		

Comments

CAAHEP Competencies	Step(s)
VIII.P.1. Interpret information on an insurance card	Entire procedure
ABHES Competencies	**Step(s)**
7. Administrative Procedures c. Perform billing and collection procedures	Entire procedure

Figure 12.1   Patient's Health Insurance ID Card

Front

AETNA

INSURED: Tapia, Arnold

IDENTIFICATION #: CH1197845   **DEPENDENTS:** Tapia, Celia B

GROUP #: 33347H   **EFFECTIVE DATE:** 06/26/2012

CO-PAY: $25   DRUG CO-PAY
SPECIALIST CO-PAY: $35   GENERIC: $10
EMERGENCY DEPT: $35   NAME BRAND: $50

Back

Submit claims to:

Aetna
1234 Insurance Way
Anytown, AK 12345

Member Services: 1-800-123-222

Insured: If a life threatening emergency exists, seek immediate attention.

Diagnostic Coding Essentials

chapter
13

CAAHEP Competencies	Assessments
IX.C.1. Identify the current procedural and diagnostic coding systems, including Healthcare Common Procedure Coding Systems II (HCPCS Level II)	Skills and Concepts – B. 1
IX.C.3. Define medical necessity	Skills and Concepts – A. 1
IX.P.2. Perform diagnostic coding	Procedure 13.1
ABHES Competencies	**Assessments**
1. General Orientation d. List the general responsibilities and skills of the medical assistant	Procedure 13.1

VOCABULARY REVIEW

Using the word pool on the right, find the correct word to match the definition. Write the word on the line after the definition.

Group A

1. The relative frequency of deaths in a specific population
   _____

2. Information about a patient's diagnosis or diagnoses that has been taken from the medical documentation _____

3. Any meeting between a patient and a healthcare provider
   _____

4. Radiology, pathology, and laboratory reports
   _____

5. The study of the causes or origin of diseases
   _____

6. The branch of medicine dealing with the incidence, distribution, and control of disease in a population _____

Word Pool
- diagnosis
- reimbursement
- mortality
- epidemiology
- encounter
- encoder
- diagnostic statement
- ancillary diagnostic services
- medically necessary
- etiology

7. Determining the cause of a condition, illness, disease, injury, or congenital defect _____

8. Accepted healthcare services that are appropriate for the evaluation and treatment of a disease, condition, illness, or injury and are consistent with the applicable standard of care

   _____

9. Software that will apply diagnostic or procedure codes to medical conditions or procedures _____

10. To make repayment for an expense or a loss incurred

    _____

Group B

1. A mental disorder in which the individual experiences a progressive loss of memory, personality alterations, confusion, loss of touch with reality, and stupor _____

2. Patient's chief complaint or statements about why the patient is seeking medical care _____

3. Developing slowly and lasting for a long time, generally 3 or more months _____

4. Suggest that it should not be used _____

5. An abnormal condition resulting from a previous disease

   _____

6. A document used to capture the services/procedures and diagnoses for a patient visit _____

7. The quality or state of being specific _____

8. A statement in the patient's own words that describes the reason for the visit _____

9. Abbreviations, punctuation, symbols, instructional notations, and related entities _____

10. Collecting important information from the health record

    _____

Word Pool
- specificity
- chronic
- conventions
- sequela
- dementia
- abstract
- encounter form
- chief complaint
- contraindicate
- subjective findings

Group C

1. Progressive loss of transparency of the lens of the eye

   _____

2. The signs and symptoms of a disease _____

3. The period from the last month of pregnancy to 5 months postpartum _____

4. Imminently threatening _____

5. First 6 weeks after delivery _____

6. The study of body tissues _____

Word Pool
- objective findings
- manifestation
- cataract
- myxedema
- impending
- histologic
- antepartum
- postpartum
- peripartum

7. Any measurable indicators found during the physical examination _____

8. Pregnancy _____

9. Advanced hypothyroidism in adulthood _____

ABBREVIATIONS

Write out what each of the following abbreviations stands for.

1. ICD-10-CM _____

2. CMS _____

3. WHO _____

4. EHR _____

5. HPI _____

6. H&P _____

7. CC _____

8. HIV _____

9. AIDS _____

10. DM _____

SKILLS AND CONCEPTS

Answer the following questions. Write your answer on the line or in the space provided.

A. Understanding Diagnostic Coding

1. Define *medically necessary* and explain how it applies to diagnostic coding. Give an example. _____

_____

_____

_____

_____

B. Getting to Know the ICD-10-CM

1. Fill in the blanks in the following statements with terms from the word bank to describe how to use the most current diagnostic coding classification system.

Word Bank:

code	coding guidelines	character
convention	diagnostic	diagnostic statements
essential modifier	exclusion	ICD-10-CM
main term	Tabular List	

a. Abstract the correct diagnosis from the _____ found in the patient health record.

b. Use the _____ to look up the diagnosis in the Alphabetic Index.

c. Review the _____ under the main term.

d. Choose the correct code based on the _____ statement.

e. Look up the code from the Alphabetic Index in the _____.

f. Check for any _____, _____, inclusion notes, _____ notes, or additional _____ symbol.

g. Assign the final _____ diagnosis code.

2. ICD-10-CM codes can have up to _____ characters. A(n) _____ "x" is used to fill in for positions that don't have characters.

3. What are the seventh characters used for encounter types and what do they indicate? _____

    _____

    _____

    _____

4. Four basic forms of punctuation are used in the Tabular Index. List them and what they are used for.

    _____

    _____

    _____

    _____

    _____

    _____

    _____

5. Match the following terms.

_____ Main terms

_____ Nonessential modifiers

_____ Subterms

_____ Essential modifiers

a. Indented under the main term; they change the description of the diagnosis in bold type

b. Appear in bold

c. Are found after the main term and are enclosed in parentheses

d. Indented under the essential modifier

6. Review the following diagnostic statements and determine the main term and essential modifier in the Alphabetic Index.

a. Morgan Smith had an acute myocardial infarction, commonly referred to as a *heart attack.*

Main Term: _____ Essential Modifier: _____

b. Georgia Summers went into anaphylactic shock after drinking milk.

Main Term: _____ Essential Modifier: _____

c. Roger Costen has benign essential hypertension.

Main Term: _____ Essential Modifier: _____

d. Raul Castro has been diagnosed with iron-deficiency anemia.

Main Term: _____ Essential Modifier: _____

e. Stephanie Thompson has a urinary tract infection.

Main Term: _____ Essential Modifier: _____

f. Mabel Johnson has rheumatoid arthritis.

Main Term: _____ Essential Modifier: _____

g. Amanda Smith was diagnosed with multiple sclerosis.

Main Term: _____ Essential Modifier: _____

h. Hudson Madison suffered a ruptured abdominal aneurysm.

Main Term: _____ Essential Modifier: _____

i. Don Julius died last week from congestive heart failure.

Main Term: _____ Essential Modifier: _____

j. Betty White has allergic gastroenteritis.

Main Term: _____ Essential Modifier: _____

C. Preparing for Diagnostic Coding

1. The SOAP notes system of documentation divides the information into what four areas?

    a. _____

    b. _____

    c. _____

    d. _____

2. To prepare for medical coding, the coder must analyze the patient's health record and
    _____ the diagnostic statement.

3. Information pertinent to code selection can be abstracted from a variety of medical documents. List the documents where the diagnostic statement may be found.

    _____

    _____

    _____

    _____

    _____

4. The _____ is the provider's health history evaluation and physical assessment of the patient.

5. The _____ is a statement in the patient's own words that describes why the person is seeking medical attention.

6. The _____ is used for extracting procedure and diagnostic information for patients who underwent surgery.

D. Steps in ICD-10-CM Coding

1. Code the following diagnoses to the highest level of specificity using either the ICD-10-CM coding manual or the TruCode encoder.

    a. Kayla Swift was diagnosed with infectious mononucleosis. _____

    b. Gerald Weaver has osteoarthritis in his right shoulder region. _____

    c. Jeffrey Rush has a personal history of alcoholism. _____

    d. Barry White's alcoholism has caused cirrhosis of the liver without ascites. _____

    e. Frank Emmett had atherosclerosis of the extremities with gangrene. _____

    f. Ginger Chan experienced dermatitis from using facial cosmetics. _____

    g. The Lewises' first child was born with Down syndrome. _____

    h. Lee Anna has experienced painful menstruation during her last three cycles. _____

    i.   Gary Stevens was diagnosed with cardiomegaly. _____

    j.   Jerry Stein developed Kaposi's sarcoma in his lymph nodes during the final stages of AIDS. _____

    k.   Terri Holden attempted suicide for the second time using a handful of lithium. _____

    l.   Susan French was stung by a jellyfish while swimming off the coast of Mexico. _____

   m.   Riley Brown has acute myocarditis. _____

    n.   Ordell Thompson has acute esophagitis. _____

    o.   Korney Ralphy was diagnosed with systemic lupus erythematosus. _____

    p.   Marcia Radson had a skin condition known as *bullous pemphigoid*, in which blisters form in patches all over her skin. _____

    q.   Osteomalacia caused by malnutrition made it impossible for Robbie Hernandez to walk. _____

    r.   Henry Casper has oral leukoplakia, which may have been caused by smoking a pipe. _____

    s.   Patricia Kielty has had uterine endometriosis for several years and may require a hysterectomy in the future. _____

    t.   Robert Bauer dislocated his right shoulder while playing baseball; it was a closed anterior dislocation. _____

E. Understanding Coding Guidelines

1.   If the provider note states _____, _____, or _____, the coder should code the documented signs and symptoms.

2.   _____ is the underlying cause of a disease. _____ are the signs and symptoms of a disease. The _____ code is always listed first.

3.   Coding of sequelae usually requires two codes with the _____ code sequenced second.

4.   Place of occurrence codes come from category _____.

5.   Category Y93 are _____ that define what the patient was doing at the time of injury or when the health condition developed.

F. Maximizing Third-Party Reimbursement

1.   When using ICD-10-CM codes it is important to code to the highest level of _____.

2.   Correct diagnostic coding can impact _____ for services provided, which in turn can impact the practice's _____.

CERTIFICATION PREPARATION

Circle the correct answer.

1. Which term defines a malignant neoplasm as the absence of invasion of surrounding tissues?
   a. Primary
   b. Secondary
   c. In situ
   d. Benign

2. Which code will be used for a patient with a history of myocardial infarction with no symptoms but diagnosed by means of an electrocardiogram?
   a. I21
   b. I25.2
   c. I21.3
   d. None of the above

3. Which term applies to the period from the last month of pregnancy to 5 months after giving birth?
   a. Antepartum
   b. Childbirth
   c. Postpartum
   d. Peripartum

4. The abbreviation that is the equivalent of "unspecified" is _____.
   a. NEC
   b. NOS
   c. NOW
   d. NCL

5. If the provider has documented "rule out" in the diagnostic statement, the medical assistant must code what?
   a. Whatever phrase follows "rule out"
   b. Lab results
   c. Signs/symptoms
   d. None of the above

6. A diagnosis is
   a. a third party's opinion of a patient's illness.
   b. determining the cause of a patient's illness.
   c. the process of finding a patient's past medical history.
   d. both b and c.

7. Currently in the United States, the source used for coding diagnoses in providers' offices is the
   a. *Diagnostic Guide for Medicare and Medicaid Services.*
   b. *Diagnostic Codes for Third-Party Payers.*
   c. *International Classification of Disease, 10th Revision, Clinical Modifications.*
   d. *AMA Manual of Essential Diagnostic Codes, Volume 1.*

8. Morbidity is the presence of illness or disease, whereas mortality is
   a. the determination of the nature of a disease.
   b. the deaths that occur from a disease.
   c. classification of a disease.
   d. All of the above.

9. In ICD-10, codes longer than three characters always have a decimal point between the
   a. fourth and fifth characters.
   b. fifth and sixth characters.
   c. third and fourth characters.
   d. sixth and seventh characters.

10. In the ICD-10-CM coding system, a lowercase "x" is used
    a. as a placeholder character within a code.
    b. to denote an obsolete code.
    c. as a cross-reference guide.
    d. to indicate the external causes of morbidity.

WORKPLACE APPLICATIONS

1. Dr. Martin has diagnosed Maude Crawford in the past with congestive heart failure and diabetes mellitus type 2 (insulin-dependent, long-term). She comes to the clinic today complaining of chest pain and has a fever of 101.8° F. Code all of these conditions. In which order should these codes be sequenced?

    a. _____

    b. _____

    c. _____

    d. _____

    e. _____

2. Dr. Perez has documented the following for Reuven Ahmad:

    CC: Shortness of breath, chest pain, nausea, and excessive sweating
    DX: 1. probable myocardial infarction, 2. rule out gastroesophageal reflux disease

    What are the correct diagnosis codes for this patient?

    Note to instructors: Remind students that codes may change with updated versions of ICD.

INTERNET ACTIVITIES

1. Using online resources, research diagnostic code encoders. Create a poster presentation, a PowerPoint presentation, or write a paper summarizing your research. Include the following points in your project:
    a. Describe the purpose of an encoder.
    b. List three reasons why a healthcare organization would want to use an encoder for diagnostic coding.
    c. Explain how using an encoder is different than using the ICD-10-CM coding manuals.

2. Using online resources, research the history and development of ICD. Create a poster presentation, a PowerPoint presentation, or write a paper summarizing your research. Include the following points in your project:
    a. Describe the ICD system.
    b. Explain how and why it was originally developed.
    c. List five reasons why ICD-10-CM was developed.

Procedure 13.1   Perform Coding Using the Current ICD-10-CM Manual or Encoder

Name _____ Date _____ Score _____

Task: To perform accurate diagnosis coding using the ICD-10-CM manual or encoder.

Scenario: The encounter form and progress notes both show that the diagnosis for this patient encounter is acute colitis. Locate the most accurate ICD-10-CM code for this diagnostic statement.

Equipment and Supplies:
- ICD-10-CM manual (current year) *or*
- Encoder software such as TruCode

Standard: Complete the procedure and all critical steps in _____ minutes with a minimum score of 85% within two attempts (*or as indicated by the instructor*).

Scoring: Divide the points earned by the total possible points. Failure to perform a critical step, indicated by an asterisk (*), results in grade no higher than an 84% (*or as indicated by the instructor*).

Time: Began_____ Ended_____ Total minutes: _____

Steps:	Point Value	Attempt 1	Attempt 2
Alphabetic Index			
1. Determine and locate the main terms from the diagnostic statement in the Alphabetic Index.	10		
2. Locate the essential modifiers listed under the main term in the Alphabetic Index.	10		
3. Review the conventions, punctuation, and notes in the Alphabetic Index.	10		
4. Choose a tentative code, codes, or code range from the Alphabetic Index that matches the diagnostic statement as closely as possible.	15*		
Tabular List			
5. Look up the codes chosen from the Alphabetic Index in the Tabular List.	10		
6. Review notes, conventions, and the Official Coding Guidelines associated with the code and code description in the Tabular List. a. Review conventions and punctuation. b. Review instructional notations: • *Includes* and *excludes* notes • *Code first, code also,* and *code additional* notes • *And, or,* and *with* statements	10		
7. Verify the accuracy of the tentative code in the Tabular List. a. Make sure all elements of the diagnostic statement are included in the codes selected. b. Make sure the code description does not include anything not documented in the diagnostic statement.	10		
8. Extend the codes to their highest level of specificity (up to the 7th character, if required). If a 7th character is required, and no codes are present for the 4th, 5th, or 6th characters, it is appropriate to use the dummy placeholder "x" for these positions.	10		

9.	Assign the code (or codes) selected from the Tabular List as the appropriate code for the patient's condition by documenting it in the patient's health record.	**15***		
	Total Points	**100**		
Alternate – Using the TruCode Encoder Software				
1.	Type in the main term from the diagnostic statement in the search box.	**20**		
2.	The software will provide a list of main terms that could be related to the diagnosis typed in the search box. The coder chooses the main term that best represents the diagnostic statement.	**20**		
3.	Based on the main term chosen, a list of essential modifiers is presented. The coder must review the diagnostic statement to ensure that all documented modifying terms are identified. If the provider does not document a modifying term, the coder should not assume that a modifying term was implied.	**20**		
4.	To determine the most accurate code, follow these coding guidelines.	**20**		
5.	Once all the menus of essential modifiers have been presented, choose the most accurate and specific code based on the diagnostic statement.	**20***		
	Total Points	**100**		

CAAHEP Competencies	Steps
IX.P.2. Perform diagnostic coding	Entire procedure

Procedural Coding Essentials

CAAHEP Competencies	Assessments
IX.C.1. Identify the current procedural and diagnostic coding systems, including Healthcare Common Procedure Coding Systems II (HCPCS Level II)	Skills and Concepts – A. 15, K. 1
IX.C.2.a. Identify the effects of: upcoding	Skills and Concepts – A. 11
IX.C.2.b. Identify the effects of: downcoding	Skills and Concepts – A. 12
IX.C.3. Define medical necessity	Skills and Concepts – A. 13
IX.P.1. Perform procedural coding	Procedures 14.1, 14.2
A.7. Demonstrate tactfulness	Procedure 14.3

ABHES Competencies	Assessments
1. General Orientation d. List the general responsibilities and skills of the medical assistant	Skills and Concepts – A. 9

VOCABULARY REVIEW

Using the word pool on the right, find the correct word to match the definition. Write the word on the line after the definition.

Group A

1. An online journal, supported by the AMA, that addresses subjects such as appealing insurance denials, validating coding to auditors, training staff members, and answering day-to-day coding questions _____

2. The use of a lower-level procedure code than is justified _____

3. Pertaining to, involving, or affecting two or both sides _____

4. The regular collection of data to assess whether the correct processes are being performed and desired results are being achieved _____

Word Pool
- performance measurement
- eponym
- specificity
- CPT Assistant
- débridement
- special report
- upcoding
- downcoding
- modifiers
- bilaterally

5. Additional medical documentation required to confirm the need for the use of unlisted, unusual, or newly adopted medical procedures code _____

6. Two-digit numeric codes that report or indicate specific criteria, specific condition, or special circumstance

   _____

7. The quality or state of being specific _____

8. The use of a higher-level procedure code than is supported in the documentation or by medical necessity _____

9. In medical terms, a medical diagnosis or procedure named for the person who discovered it _____

10. The surgical removal of dead, damaged, or infected tissue to improve the function of healthy tissue _____

Group B

1. A list of questions related to each organ system designed to uncover potential disease processes _____

2. The process of collecting pertinent medical information needed to assign the correct code _____

3. A statement in the patient's own words that describes the reason for the visit _____

4. The relative incidence of disease _____

5. Special symbols used to provide additional information about specific codes _____

6. Relates to the number of deaths from a given disease

   _____

7. Determine the amount of drug present _____

8. Each step of the procedure is listed separately

   _____

9. Medical services and procedures performed for the patient before, during, and after a surgical procedure _____

10. Based on the type of drug found _____

11. Includes services related to prepping the patient for the procedure, performing the procedure, and suturing to complete the procedure _____

12. A nursing healthcare professional who is certified to administer anesthesia _____

Word Pool
- conventions
- abstract
- chief complaint
- review of systems
- morbidity
- mortality
- Certified Registered Nurse Anesthetist
- global services
- bundled code
- unbundled code
- qualitative
- quantitative

ABBREVIATIONS
Write out what each of the following abbreviations stands for.

1. CPT _____

2. HCPCS _____

3. AMA _____

4. EHR_____

5. H&P _____

6. E/M_____

7. POS _____

8. NP _____

9. EP _____

10. ROS _____

11. CRNA _____

12. NCCI_____

13. MRI _____

14. TURP_____

15. ASA_____

16. RVG_____

SKILLS AND CONCEPTS
Answer the following questions. Write your answer on the line or in the space provided.

A. Introduction to the CPT Manual

1. The CPT system was developed and is maintained by the _____.

2. The CPT manual is updated every year on _____.

3. The CPT code is a five-digit code also known as a(n) _____ code.

4. Category II codes are primarily used for _____ and are optional.

5. Category _____ codes are for new experimental procedures or emerging technology.

6. The CPT coding manual organizes codes into the Alphabetic Index and the _____.

7. The six sections of the CPT manual include:

   a. _____

   b. _____

   c. _____

   d. _____

   e. _____

   f. _____

8. When using an unlisted procedure code, a(n) _____ must be sent with the insurance claim.

9. _____ are found at the beginning of each of the six sections of the CPT coding manual, and the medical assistant refers to them often when coding procedures.

10. Code additions that explain circumstances that alter a provided service or provide additional clarification or detail are called _____.

11. Define *upcoding* and discuss the effects. _____

    _____

12. Define *downcoding* and discuss the effects. _____

    _____

    _____

13. Define *medical necessity* as it applies to procedural coding. _____

    _____

    _____

B. Steps for Efficient CPT Procedural Coding

1. List the sources used for procedural coding. _____

   _____

   _____

2. Describe how to use the most current procedural coding system. _____

   _____

3. Describe the four primary classifications of main and modifying terms. _____

   _____

4. Explain the difference between "see" and "see also." _____

   _____

5. Provide the full description for CPT code 47563
   47562   Laparoscopy, surgical; cholecystectomy
      47363   Cholecystectomy with cholangiography

   _____

   _____

   _____

C. CPT Coding Guidelines: Evaluation and Management Section

1. _____ codes provide information on the healthcare facility where services were rendered.

2. When determining an evaluation and management code, you first need to identify the _____ and the _____.

3. _____ alone can be used to select the correct E/M code.

D. CPT Coding Guidelines: Anesthesia

1. CPT codes for anesthesia
   a. always start with a zero (0).
   b. identify the anatomic location of the surgery performed.
   c. are used for conscious and unconscious sedation.
   d. a and b.

2. Providing anesthesia services in an emergency situation is considered a(n) _____.

3. Which of the following are part of the formula for determining the fee for anesthesia services?
   a. Basic unit value
   b. Modifying unit
   c. Time unit
   d. Conversion unit
   e. All of the above

E. CPT Coding Guidelines: Surgical Section

1. Patient prep, surgical care, and postsurgical are considered _____ and the single code that is used is called a(n) _____.

2. Codes in which the components of a procedure are separated and reported separately are called _____ codes.

3. Code for the excision of benign lesions includes _____ and _____.

4. When coding fractures, a closed fracture is defined as the
   a. fracture is not surgically opened.
   b. fractured bone cuts through the skin layers and can be directly visualized.
   c. fractured bone does not protrude through the dermis or epidermis.
   d. none of the above.

5. Antepartum care includes which of the following?
   a. Monthly visits up to 28 weeks gestation.
   b. Management of uncomplicated labor.
   c. Hospital and office visits after vaginal or cesarean section delivery.
   d. All of the above

F. CPT Coding Guidelines: Radiology and Pathology and Laboratory Section

1. The radiology section of CPT includes codes for which of the following?
   a. Nuclear medicine procedures
   b. Radiation oncology
   c. MRIs
   d. X-ray studies
   e. All of the above

2. _____ codes are considered _____ codes and are billed under the single CPT code.

G. CPT Coding Guidelines: Medicine Section

1. Codes in the Medicine section of CPT include codes for which of the following?
   a. Therapeutic procedures
   b. Diagnostic testing
   c. Dialysis
   d. Acupuncture
   e. All of the above

2. When coding vaccinations, there should be one code for the _____ of the vaccine and one code for the actual _____.

H. HCPCS Code System

1. Describe how to use the most current HCPCS level II coding system. _____

   _____

   _____

   _____

   _____

   _____

   _____

CODING EXERCISES

Code the following procedures with modifiers if appropriate.

CPT Coding

1. Dr. Smith visits Eula Fairbanks, a patient with dementia, in the nursing home for less than 30 minutes and performs an expanded problem-focused examination with MDM of low complexity.

   _____

2. Jessica Lundy, a newborn, was admitted to the pediatric critical care unit after her birth, where Dr. Williams provided her initial care.

   _____

3. Dr. Partridge participated in a complex, lengthy telephone call lasting 30 minutes, regarding a patient who was scheduled for multiple surgeries.

   _____

4. When Terri Anderson was involved in a major car accident, the emergency department physician took a comprehensive history, performed a comprehensive examination, and then made highly complex decisions.

   _____

5. Tim Taylor is a new patient with a small cyst on his back. Dr. Young took a problem-focused history, performed a problem-focused examination, and then made straightforward medical decisions.

   _____

6. Jim Angelo, an established patient, saw the physician for a minor cut on the back of his hand. The physician spent approximately 10 minutes with Jim.

   _____

7. Because Lucille Westerman had multiple health problems, she was admitted for observation after a fainting spell. Dr. Adams took a comprehensive history and performed a comprehensive examination, then made medical decisions of high complexity regarding her care.

   _____

8. Dr. Wray saw Tammy Luttrell in the office as a new patient. He took a an appropriate history and examination, and then made medical decisions of low complexity. Total time spent with the patient was 30 minutes.

   _____

9. Dr. Tompkins visited a new patient at her home and spent about 20 minutes diagnosing and treating her for the flu. A problem-focused history and examination with straightforward MDM was performed.

   _____

10. Vera Carpenter was admitted to the hospital for diabetes mellitus, congestive heart failure, and an infection of unknown origin. Dr. Antonetti performed a consultation by doing a detailed history and examination, and MDM of low complexity that took about an hour, including the time spent writing orders in her medical record.

    _____

11. Sylvia Julius, an established patient, saw Dr. Bridges for her allergies. The physician took a medically appropriate history and examination and made straightforward decisions regarding her care. Total time spent with the patient was 15 minutes.

_____

12. Anesthesia for vaginal delivery

_____

13. Anesthesia was provided for a brain-dead patient whose organs were being harvested for donation.

_____

14. Laparoscopic biopsy of the left ovary

_____

15. Treatment of a clavicular fracture without manipulation

_____

16. Removal of nasal polyp, right nostril

_____

17. Tonsillectomy and adenoidectomy, younger than 12

_____

18. Left ectopic pregnancy

_____

19. Closed treatment of a coccygeal fracture

_____

20. A radiologic examination of mastoids, two views

_____

21. A chest x-ray examination, four views

_____

22. Magnetic resonance imaging (MRI) of spinal canal

_____

23. Computed tomography (CT) scan of abdomen with contrast medium

_____

24. Outpatient kidney imaging with vascular flow

_____

25. Creatine phosphokinase (CPK) total lab test

_____

26. Electrolyte panel

_____

27. Adrenocorticotropic hormone (ACTH) stimulation panel

_____

28. Obstetric panel

_____

29. Total protein urine test

_____

30. Blood alcohol level

_____

31. Acute hepatitis panel

_____

32. Urine pregnancy test

_____

33. Polio vaccine, intramuscular route

_____

34. Human papillomavirus (HPV) vaccine, nine types, three-dose schedule, intramuscular route

_____

35. Psychotherapy for crisis; first 60 minutes

_____

HCPCS Coding

1. Standard wheelchair

_____

2. Gradient compression stocking below-knee, 40-50 mm Hg each

_____

3. Above-knee, short prosthesis, no knee joint (stubbies), with articulated ankle/foot, dynamically aligned, right leg

_____

4. Disposable contact lens, per lens, one set

_____

5. Ambulance waiting time, 1 hour

_____

CERTIFICATION PREPARATION
Circle the correct answer.

1. The CPT coding manual is updated annually on
   a. January 1.
   b. December 1.
   c. October 1.
   d. June 1.

2. To find the most accurate code, coders use which progression?
   a. Categories, subcategories, sections, subsections
   b. Sections, subsections, categories, subcategories
   c. Sections, categories, subsections, subcategories
   d. Subsections, subcategories, sections, categories

3. The evaluation and management CPT codes are used for insurance reimbursement in the following healthcare settings *except*
   a. medical office.
   b. weight loss clinic.
   c. nursing home.
   d. hospital.

4. Which codes can be used to help measure performance?
   a. Category I codes
   b. Category II codes
   c. Category III codes
   d. Both a and b

5. Which section uses the code range between 70000 and 79999?
   a. Anesthesia section
   b. Surgery section
   c. Radiology section
   d. Medicine section

6. When searching the Alphabetic Index, "humerus" is an example of a(n)
   a. procedure or service.
   b. organ or anatomic site.
   c. condition, illness, or injury.
   d. eponym, synonym, abbreviation, or acronym.

7. Which level of history includes a review of the systems that relate to the chief complaint?
   a. Problem-focused history
   b. Expanded problem-focused history
   c. Detailed history
   d. Comprehensive history

8. Which HCPCS codes range from A4000 to A8999?
   a. Ambulance transport
   b. Medical supplies
   c. Surgical supplies
   d. Both b and c

9. Which modifier indicates a professional component and is used when a separate technician performs the service, but the provider reviews the report and makes a diagnosis?
   a. -50
   b. -62
   c. -26
   d. -RT, -LT

10. Which code is assigned to an urgent care facility as the place of service?
    a. 01
    b. 13
    c. 20
    d. 23

WORKPLACE APPLICATIONS

Identify all procedures that need to be coded for billing purposes in the following situations. Using the most current CPT manual or an encoder such as TruCode, determine the correct CPT codes.

1. Monique Jones is a new patient who saw Dr. Walden to report feeling tired all the time. She stated that she was exhausted even after a full 8 hours of sleep at night. Monique said that she did not have much of an appetite and that she had been eating mostly salads and chicken with a bowl of fruit as snacks. She is not overweight, and her blood pressure and other vital signs were normal. Dr. Walden decided to perform a complete blood count, an electrolyte panel, and a lipid panel. She also ordered a urinalysis, an iron-binding capacity, and a vitamin B_{12} test. The provider asked the patient if she had noticed any blood in her urine or stool, and she denied blood in the urine but did mention she had several episodes of diarrhea. Dr. Walden added an occult blood test and a stool culture to check for pathogens. The physician placed Monique on multivitamin therapy and told her to return in 1 week to discuss her laboratory test results. She spent approximately 30 minutes with Monique, taking a medically appropriate history and examination, making low-complexity medical decisions. Monique scheduled her appointment for the following week and left the clinic. Total time spent with the patient was 25 minutes.

   What are the appropriate CPT codes for Monique Jones' visit with Dr. Walden? _____

   _____

2. **Diagnosis:** Left cheek laceration

   Procedure: Repair left cheek laceration

   After the patient was prepped with local anesthetic to the left cheek area, the cheek was dressed and draped with Betadine. The 1.7-cm chin laceration of the skin was closed with three interrupted 6-0 silk sutures. Gentamicin ointment was applied to the lacerations and a dressing was placed on the left cheek. The patient tolerated the procedure well.

   What is the appropriate CPT code for this procedure? _____

   Can a modifier be used for this procedure? _____ If so, what would be the most appropriate? _____

   Because anesthesia was used, can an appropriate anesthesia CPT code be used?
   _____

3. **Diagnosis:** Abdominal pain

   Procedure: Esophagogastroduodenoscopy with biopsy

   The patient was premedicated and brought to the endoscopy suite where his throat was anesthetized with Cetacaine spray. He then was placed in the left lateral position and given 2 mg Versed, IV. An Olympus gastroscope was advanced into the esophagus, which was well visualized with no significant spasms. Subsequently the scope was advanced into the distal esophagus, which was essentially normal. Then the scope was advanced into the stomach, which showed evidence of erythema and gastritis. The pylorus was intubated, and the duodenal bulb visualized. The duodenal bulb showed severe erythema suggestive of duodenitis. Biopsies of both the duodenum and the stomach were obtained. The scope was withdrawn. The patient tolerated the procedure well.

   In the Alphabetic Index, which main term should be used to look up the correct CPT code?
   _____

   What is the appropriate CPT code for this procedure? _____

   CPT code 43236 is a similar code with submucosal injection. Can this be used if the physician usually performs it, but forgot to document? _____

INTERNET ACTIVITIES

1. Using online resources, research job postings on the Internet that relate to medical billing and coding. Review job qualifications and requirements to qualify for these positions. Create a poster presentation, a PowerPoint presentation, or write a paper summarizing your research. Include the following points in your project:
   a. List the qualifications and requirements for a position in the medical billing and coding field.
   b. Explain how a graduate from your program would meet the requirements.
   c. Explain what additional training would be beneficial for someone looking for a position in the medical billing and coding field.

2. Visit http://www.cms.gov/ and use the search words "CPT Coding" to explore the topics related to CPT and HCPCS coding. Create a poster presentation, a PowerPoint presentation, or write a paper summarizing your research. Include the following points in your project:
   a. Explain the differences between CPT coding and HCPCS coding.
   b. Explain when each would be used.
   c. Describe two things that you learned about CPT codes.
   d. Describe two things you learned about HCPCS codes.

Procedure 14.1   Perform Procedural Coding: Surgery

Name _____ Date _____ Score _____

Task: To use the steps for CPT procedural coding to find the most accurate and specific CPT surgery code.

Equipment and Supplies:
- CPT coding manual (current year) or TruCode encoder software
- Operative report (Figure 14.1)

Standard: Complete the procedure and all critical steps in _____ minutes with a minimum score of 85% within two attempts (*or as indicated by the instructor*).

Scoring: Divide the points earned by the total possible points. Failure to perform a critical step, indicated by an asterisk (*), results in grade no higher than an 84% (*or as indicated by the instructor*).

Time: Began_____ Ended_____ Total minutes: _____

Steps Using the CPT Coding Manual:	Point Value	Attempt 1	Attempt 2
1. Abstract the procedures and/or services from the procedural statement in the surgical report.	10		
2. Select the most appropriate main term to begin the search in the Alphabetic Index.	10		
3. Once the main term has been located in the Alphabetic Index, review and select the modifying term or terms if required. If the main term cannot be found in the Alphabetic Index, repeat steps 2 and 3 using a different main term, possibly based on the procedural statement.	10		
4. Once the CPT code or code range is identified in the Alphabetic Index, disregard any code or code range containing additional descriptions or modifying terms not found in the health record.	10		
5. Record the code or code ranges that best match the procedural statements in the surgical report.	10		
6. Turn to the Tabular List and find the first code or code range from your search of the Alphabetic Index. Compare the description of the code with the procedural statement in the surgical report. Verify that all or most of the health record documentation matches the code description and that there is no additional information in the code description that is not found in the documentation.	10		
7. Review the coding guidelines and notes for the section, subsection, and code to ensure that there are no contraindications to use of the code. Review the coding conventions and add-on codes, if any.	10		
8. Determine whether a modifier is needed.	10		
9. Determine whether a Special Report is required.	10		
10. Record the CPT code selected in the health record documentation next to the procedure or service performed and in the appropriate block of the insurance claim form.	10*		
Total Points	**100**		

Alternate Method **Steps Using the TruCode Software:**			
1. Abstract the procedures and/or services from the procedural statement in the surgical report.	**20**		
2. Type the main term into the encoder search box and select the CPT. Then click on Show All Results.	**20**		
3. If the main term cannot be found through the search, repeat steps 2 and 3 using a different main term based on the procedural statement.	**20**		
4. Choose the procedure description that is closest to the procedural statement in the surgical report.	**20***		
5. Record the CPT code that best matches the procedural statements in the surgical report in the patient's health record.	**20**		
Total Points	**100**		

Comments

CAAHEP Competencies	**Step(s)**
IX.P.1. Perform procedural coding	Entire procedure

Figure 14.1 Operative Report

Name _____ Date _____ Score _____

Operative Report

PATIENT NAME: Sonia Sample
ROOM NUMBER: 222 West
MR NUMBER: 12-34-56

DATE OF PROCEDURE: 04/22/00
PREOPERATIVE DIAGNOSIS: Acute cholecystitis
POSTOPERATIVE DIAGNOSIS: Acute cholecystitis
NAME OF PROCEDURE: 1. Laparoscopic cholecystectomy
2. Intraoperative cystic duct cholangiogram
SURGEON: Claude St. John, M.D.
ASSISTANT: Mark Weiss, D.O.
ANESTHESIOLOGIST: Angela Adams, M.D.
ANESTHESIA: General

DESCRIPTION OF THE OPERATION:
The patient was placed in the supine position under general anesthesia. The oral gastric tube was placed. The Foley catheter was placed. The patient received appropriate antibiotics. The abdomen was prepped with iodine and draped in the usual fashion. Using a midline subumbilical incision, we entered the subcutaneous fat to find the aponeurosis of the rectus abdominis. Two stay sutures were placed 0.5 cm from the midline bilaterally and we left on these sutures, creating an opening in the linea alba.

Under direct vision, the catheter was placed. The Hasson cannula was placed in the abdominal cavity and all was normal except an acute necrotizing and probably gangrenous gallbladder. There were multiple omental adhesions. Three other trocars were placed in the right subcostal plane in the midline, midclavicular line, and midaxillary line using a #10, #5, and #5 mm trocar, respectively. The gallbladder was punctured and emptied of clear white bile indicating a hydrops of the gallbladder. It was grasped at its fundus and at Hartmann's pouch retracted cephalad and to the right, respectively. We found the cystic duct and the cystic artery after circumferential dissection and isolated the cystic duct completely.

When we were sure that this structure was a deep cystic duct, the clip was placed at the most distal aspect to make an opening immediately proximally and we placed a Reddick cholangiocatheter into it via #14 gauge percutaneous catheter. The cholangiogram showed normal arborization of the liver radicals. Normal bifurcation of the common hepatic duct. Normal common hepatic duct. Long large cystic duct. The common bile duct had numerous stones within it. They could not be emptied from the common bile duct. There was good flow into the duodenum.

The impression was choledocholithiasis. This was corroborated by the radiologist. The decision was made to prepare the patient most probably for endoscopic retrograde cholangiopancreatography postoperatively, and no further intervention of the common bile duct was done in this setting.

The cholangiocatheter was removed. An attempt was made to milk the bile out, but no stones came out. Three clips were placed on the proximal aspect of the cystic duct and the duct was then cut distally. The artery was isolated and double clipped proximally and single clipped distally and cut in the intervening section. We then peeled the gallbladder off the gallbladder bed with some difficulty because of the intense edema and inflammation. It was then removed from the liver bed completely. Cautery, suctioning and irrigation were used copiously to create a bloodless field. A last check was made and there was no bleeding and no bile leaking. A #15 Jackson-Pratt type drain was placed into Morrison's pouch and brought out through the lateral most port. We then removed, with great difficulty, the gallbladder from the umbilicus. Because of its enormous size and a 3 cm stone within it that was very difficult to macerate, the opening of the umbilicus had to be enlarged.

As this was done, we removed the gallbladder completely and sent it for pathologic section. Two separate figure-of-eight 0 PDS were used to close the abdominal fascia. The Jackson-Pratt drain was then sutured in place with 2.0 nylon. The skin was closed throughout with subcuticular 3-0 PDS after copious irrigation of the subcutaneous plane. Mastisol and Steri-Strips were placed on the wound. The patient remained stable although she did have bigeminy during surgery and was on a Lidocaine drip. She will be going to the intensive care unit but as she left, she was extubated in the recovery room and was fully alert. She is moving all limbs.

I will discuss with the gastroenterologist postoperative endoscopic retrograde cholangiopancreatography.

SPECIMEN: Gallbladder.

Claude St. John, M.D.
CSJ/ld:
D: 04/22/00
T: 04/22/00 9:21 am
CC: Maria Acosta, M.D.

Procedure 14.2 Perform Procedural Coding: Office Visit and Immunizations

Name _____ Date _____ Score _____

Task: To use the steps for CPT Evaluation and Management coding and HCPCS coding to find the most accurate and specific CPT E/M and HCPCS codes using the coding manuals or the TruCode encoder.

Equipment and Supplies:
- CPT coding manual (current year)
- HCPCS coding manual (current year) or TruCode encoder software
- Progress note

Progress Note for Erma Willis (DOB 12/09/19XX):

04/08/20XX Mrs. Willis was seen today for a follow-up visit for a recent case of bronchitis. The infection has completely cleared, and she would like to get the influenza vaccine. The office visit involved a medically appropriate history and examination, and medical decision-making of straightforward complexity.

Standard: Complete the procedure and all critical steps in _____ minutes with a minimum score of 85% within two attempts (*or as indicated by the instructor*).

Scoring: Divide the points earned by the total possible points. Failure to perform a critical step, indicated by an asterisk (*), results in grade no higher than an 84% (*or as indicated by the instructor*).

Time: Began_____ Ended_____ Total minutes: _____

Steps Part A: CPT E/M Coding	Point Value	Attempt 1	Attempt 2
1. Determine the place of service from the progress note.	15		
2. Determine the patient's status.	15		
3. Identify the subsection, category, or subcategory of service in the E/M section.	10		
4. Determine the level of service: • Determine the complexity of medical decision-making. If necessary, compare the medical documentation against examples in Appendix C, Clinical Examples, of the CPT manual.	15		
5. Select the appropriate level of E/M service code, and document it in the patient's health record.	10		
Part B: HCPCS Coding with TruCode Encoder Software			
6. Review the provider documentation.	10		
7. Type the main term into the search box of the encoder and choose the HCPCS Tabular code set for accurate coding. If no modifying term produces an appropriate code or code range, review the documentation again and choose another main term.	10		
8. Compare the description of the code with the medical documentation. Select the appropriate HCPCS immunization code, and document it in the patient's health record.	15		
Total Points	**100**		

Comments

CAAHEP Competencies	Step(s)
IX.P.1. Perform procedural coding	Entire procedure

Procedure 14.3   Working with Providers to Ensure Accurate Code Selection

Name _____ **Date** _____ **Score** _____

Task: Communicate respectfully and tactfully with medical providers to ensure accurate code selection.

Background: Using tactful communication skills means using good manners as you provide truthful sensitive information to another person, while considering the person's feelings. Tactful communication skills include verbal and nonverbal communication that shows respect, discretion, compassion, honesty, diplomacy, and courtesy. When you use tactful behaviors, you demonstrate professionalism and you preserve relationships by avoiding conflicts and finding common ground.

Many times, the medical coder is the expert on the accurate CPT and ICD code selections. The highest level of specificity must be used when coding so that appropriate reimbursement can occur. It is not uncommon for the medical coder to interact with providers and assist them in understanding the coding process. During these interactions, it is crucial that the medical coder provides the information in a professional, organized, and logical manner. Using tactful communication skills is critical to maintaining a healthy working relationship with the providers.

Scenario: You are a new medical coder for the medical practice. You have been on the job for 6 weeks and have been seeing a trend that charges are being downcoded. The required documentation is present in the health records, but the providers have been selecting less specific codes for the appointment types. Your goal today is to explain to the providers accurate code selection for the appointment types.

Directions: Using the scenario, role-play with two peers, who will play the providers. You need to discuss the importance of selecting the correct code for reimbursement. You need to demonstrate respect during the conversation and utilize tactful communication skills.

Standard: Complete the role-play in _____ minutes with a minimum score of 100% within two attempts (*or as indicated by the instructor*).

Scoring: Divide the points earned by the total possible points. Met competency: 100% (10 points). Not met competency: 0% (0 points).

Time: Began_____ Ended_____ Total minutes: _____

Affective Behavior	**Directions:** *Check behaviors observed during the role-play.*					
Tactfulness	Improper and/or inappropriate			Proper and appropriate		
	Spoke and/or acted in a manner that was offensive to others; lacked compassion and/or courtesy			Spoke and acted without offending others; showed compassion and courtesy		
	Failed to be sensitive to others when explaining the situation			Explained the situation in a clear and diplomatic way		
	Failed to explain the downcoding issue and/or the importance of proper coding			Explained the issues with downcoding and the importance of accurate coding for reimbursement		
	Failed to offer a solution for the situation			Offered a solution for the situation		
	Failed to answer questions; or answers were inappropriate and/or inaccurate			Answered questions appropriately and accurately		
	Other:			Other:		

Grading		Point Value	Attempt 1	Attempt 2
Does not meet Expectation	• Response was disrespectful and/or not tactful. • Student demonstrated more than 2 negative, unprofessional behaviors during the interaction.	0		
Needs Improvement	• Response was disrespectful and/or not tactful. • Student demonstrated 1 or 2 negative, unprofessional behaviors during the interaction.	0		
Meets Expectation	• Response was respectful and tactful; no negative, unprofessional behaviors observed. • More practice is needed for behavior to appear natural and for student to appear comfortable and at ease.	10		
Occasionally Exceeds Expectation	• Response was respectful and tactful; no negative, unprofessional behaviors observed. • At times student appeared comfortable and at ease; but more practice is needed for behavior to become natural and consistent with a professional medical assistant.	10		
Always Exceeds Expectation	• Response was respectful and tactful; no negative, unprofessional behaviors observed. • Student's behaviors appeared natural and comfortable. Behaviors are consistent with a professional medical assistant.	10		

Comments

CAAHEP Competencies	Step(s)
A.7 Demonstrate tactfulness	Entire role-play

Medical Billing and Reimbursement Essentials

CAAHEP Competencies	Assessment
VII.C.4. Identify patient financial obligations for services rendered	Skills and Concepts – E. 1- 4
VII.P.3. Inform a patient of financial obligations for services rendered	Procedures 15.6, 15.7
VIII.C.1.b. Identify: the steps for filing a third-party claim	Skills and Concepts – B. 7, 8
VIII.C.2 Identify managed care requirements for patient referral	Skills and Concepts – A. 7
VIII.C.3.a. Identify processes for: verification of eligibility for services	Skills and Concepts – A. 3
VIII.C.3.b. Identify processes for: precertification/ preauthorization	Skills and Concepts – A. 5, 6
VIII.C.3.c. Identify processes for: tracking unpaid claims	Skills and Concepts – D. 1
VIII.C.3.d. Identify processes for: claim denials and appeals	Skills and Concepts - D. 9-12
VIII.C.4. Identify fraud and abuse as they relate to thrid-party reimbursement	Skills and Concepts – C. 1
VIII.C.5 b. Define the following: advanced beneficiary notice (ABN)	Skills and Concepts – E. 5
VIII.C.5.c. Define the following: allowed amount	Vocabulary Review – C. 5
VIII.C.5.d. Define the following: deductible	Vocabulary Review – D. 6
VIII.C.5.e. Define the following: co-insurance	Vocabulary Review – D. 3
VIII.C.5.f. Define the following: co-pay	Vocabulary Review – A. 8
VIII.C.6. Identify the purpose and components of the Explanation of Benefits (EOB) and Remittance Advice (RA) Statements	Skills and Concepts – D. 4-8
VIII.P.2. Verify eligibility for services	Procedures 15.1, 15.6
VIII.P.3. Obtain precertification or preauthorization with documentation	Procedure 15.1
VIII.P.4. Complete an insurance claim form	Procedures 15.2, 15.3
VIII.P.5. Assist a patient in understanding an Explanation of Benefits (EOB)	Procedure 15.5

CAAHEP Competencies	Assessment
IX.P.3. Utilize medical necessity guidelines	Procedure 15.4
A.1. Demonstrate critical thinking skills	Procedures 15.5, 15.6, 15.7
A.3. Demonstrate empathy for patient's concerns	Procedures 15.5, 15.6, 15.7
A.7. Demonstrate tactfulness	Procedures 15.5, 15.6, 15.7

ABHES Competencies	Assessment
7. Administrative Procedures c. Perform billing and collection procedures	Procedures 15.1-15.7
7. Administrative Procedures d. Process insurance claims	Procedures 15.2, 15.3

VOCABULARY REVIEW

Using the word pool on the right, find the correct word to match the definition. Write the word on the line after the definition.

Group A

1. The standard form used for all government and most commercial insurance companies _____

2. A document sent by the insurance company to the provider explaining the allowed charge amount, the amount reimbursed for services, and the patient's financial responsibilities _____

3. A document sent by the insurance company to the provider and the patient explaining the allowed charge amount, the amount reimbursed for services, and the patient's financial responsibilities _____

4. The process of determining if a procedure or service is covered by the insurance plan and what the reimbursement is for that procedure or service _____

5. Starts when a patient makes an appointment and is complete when payment for services has been received _____

6. Meeting the stipulated requirements to participate in the healthcare plan _____

7. A secure online website that gives contracted providers a single point of access to insurance companies. _____

8. A set dollar amount that the patient must pay for each office visit _____

9. A form completed by the patient that authorizes the medical office to release medical records to the insurance company for health insurance reimbursement _____

10. An organization that accepts the claim data from the provider, reformats the data to meet the specifications outlined by the insurance plan, and submits the claim _____

Word Pool
- provider web portals
- copayment
- explanation of benefits
- remittance advice
- medical billing process
- eligibility
- precertification
- CMS-1500 health insurance claim form
- claims clearinghouse
- release of information

Group B

1. Used when the provider believes that the patient must see a specialist to continue treatment. Usually takes 3 to 10 working days for review and approval _____

2. A process completed before claims submission in which claims are examined for accuracy and completeness

   _____

3. Gives the provider approval to render the medical service

   _____

4. Used in an emergency situation and can be approved online

   _____

5. The electronic transfer of data between two or more entities

   _____

6. When the provider is paid a set amount for each enrolled person assigned to him or her, per period of time, whether or not that person has received services _____

7. Nonsurgical procedure that uses an endoscope to view inside the body _____

8. The individual who is directly contracted with the insurance company _____

9. Used when an urgent but not life-threatening situation occurs

   _____

10. Used to determine primary and secondary insurance status

    _____

Word Pool
- preauthorization
- endoscopy
- regular referral
- urgent referral
- STAT referral
- capitation
- electronic data interchange
- audit
- birthday rule
- insured

Group C

1. Done on purpose_____
2. Agrees to accept the terms of the agreement with the insurance company, as well as accept what the plan states as an allowed amount for the services provided _____
3. Claims without errors_____
4. Knowingly and willfully attempting to execute a scheme to take from any healthcare benefit program _____
5. The maximum amount that an insurance company will pay for covered health services _____
6. To settle or determine judicially _____
7. Transfers the patient's legal right to collect benefits for medical expenses to the provider of those services, authorizing payment to be sent directly to the provider _____
8. Unintended action that directly or indirectly results in an overpayment to the healthcare provider _____
9. Software that finds common billing errors before the claim is sent to the insurance company _____
10. A number assigned by the Centers for Medicare and Medicaid Services (CMS) that classifies the healthcare provider by license and medical specialties _____

Word Pool
- adjudicate
- assignment of benefits
- National Provider Identifier
- participating provider
- allowed amount
- fraud
- abuse
- intentional
- claims scrubber
- clean claim

Group D

Word Pool
- dirty claim
- remark codes
- medical necessity
- deductible
- coinsurance
- guarantor
- advance beneficiary notice

1. Services or supplies that are used to treat the patient's diagnosis meet the accepted standard of medical practice
   _____

2. A document signed by the patient that authorizes a provider to bill the patient for services that Medicare may consider not medically necessary _____

3. When the insured and the insurance company share the cost of covered medical services after the deductible has been met
   _____

4. Claims with incorrect, missing, or insufficient data
   _____

5. The person legally responsible for the entire bill
   _____

6. A set dollar amount that the policyholder is responsible for each year before the insurance company begins to reimburse the healthcare provider _____

7. Where the insurance company indicates the conditions under which the claim was paid _____

ABBREVIATIONS

Write out what each of the following abbreviations stands for.

1. EOB _____

2. RA _____

3. H&P _____

4. CMS-1500 _____

5. HIPAA _____

6. MCOs _____

7. PCP _____

8. GI _____

9. NUCC _____

10. AMA _____

11. CMS _____

12. LMP _____

13. NPI _____

14. CPT _____

15. HCPCS _____

16. POS _____

17. EMG _____

18. EPSDT_____

19. CHAMPVA _____

20. FECA_____

21. SSN _____

22. EIN _____

23. PAR_____

24. CMPs_____

25. PPO _____

26. ABN _____

27. H&P _____

28. SSN _____

SKILLS AND CONCEPTS

Answer the following questions. Write your answer on the line or in the space provided.

A. Medical Billing Process

1. List four types of information collected when a patient calls to schedule an appointment.

    a. _____

    b. _____

    c. _____

    d. _____

2. At the time of the appointment, what two things are copied or scanned into the computer? _____

    _____

3. Describe how the patient's insurance eligibility is confirmed. _____

    _____

    _____

    _____

    _____

4. Referring to the information on the ID card, answer the following questions.

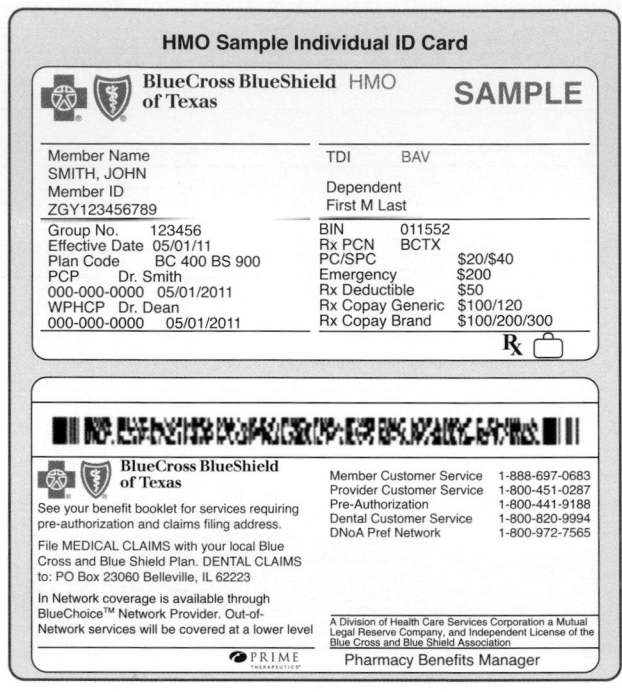

a. What is the member's name? _____

b. What is the member's ID number? _____

c. What is the group number? _____

d. Who is the member's primary care provider (PCP)? _____

e. What is the effective date of the plan? _____

f. What is the deductible for prescriptions (Rx)? _____

g. What is the copay for primary care (PC)? _____

h. What number should the patient call if he has a concern? _____

i. What number should you call if you need to get a preauthorization? _____

j. What number should a healthcare professional working with Dr. Smith call if there is a question about the coverage?

_____

5. The patient's billing record information is often found on the patient registration form. Using Figure 15.2 in the textbook, list the billing information found on the patient registration form.

_____

_____

_____

_____

_____

6. What items should the medical assistant gather when using the paper method to obtain a precertification for a service or procedure?

_____

_____

_____

_____

_____

7. Describe the processes for precertification using the paper method. What does the medical assistant need to do?

_____

_____

_____

_____

_____

8. Describe the managed care requirements for a patient referral. _____

_____

_____

_____

_____

_____

B. Submitting Claims to Third-Party Payers

1. In your own words, identify the steps for filing a third-party claim. _____

    _____

    _____

    _____

    _____

    _____

    _____

    _____

2. Describe the electronic claim form. _____

    _____

    _____

    _____

    _____

3. Describe two ways electronic claims can be submitted. _____

    _____

    _____

    _____

    _____

4. Describe direct billing. _____

    _____

    _____

    _____

    _____

    _____

    _____

    _____

5. Explain the role of a claims clearinghouse. _____

_____

_____

_____

_____

_____

6. The medical assistant obtained precertification for a procedure. After the procedure was completed, what are six items needed to complete the CMS-1500 health insurance claim form?

   a. _____

   b. _____

   c. _____

   d. _____

   e. _____

   f. _____

7. Name the three sections of the claim form.

   a. _____

   b. _____

   c. _____

8. Identify information required to file a third-party claim.

   a. What information must be included in Section 1 of the claim form? _____

   _____

   b. Name 13 pieces of information required in Section 2.

      1. _____

      2. _____

      3. _____

      4. _____

      5. _____

      6. _____

      7. _____

      8. _____

      9. _____

      10. _____

11. _____

12. _____

13. _____

c. Name 19 pieces of information required in Section 3.

1. _____

2. _____

3. _____

4. _____

5. _____

6. _____

7. _____

8. _____

9. _____

10. _____

11. _____

12. _____

13. _____

14. _____

15. _____

16. _____

17. _____

18. _____

19. _____

C. Impact of Accurate Coding

1. Differentiate between fraud and abuse. _____

_____

_____

_____

_____

_____

_____

_____

2.   What are the possible consequences of coding fraud and abuse?_____

   _____

   _____

   _____

   _____

3.   What is the purpose of "claim scrubbers"?_____

   _____

   _____

   _____

   _____

D. Claim Follow-up

1.   Which of the following are included in claims tracking?
   a.   Confirm that the claims submitted to the clearinghouse match the claims listed on the confirmation report.
   b.   Inquire about the status of claims that have not been paid within 10-14 days of submittal.
   c.   Resubmit the claim if not received by the insurance company.
   d.   All of the above

2.   Insurance companies will typically take _____ days to process insurance claims electronically.

3.   What information is needed to verify the claim status with insurance company?_____

   _____

   _____

   _____

   _____

Using the explanation below, answer the following questions:

01/20/20XX

XYZ Insurance Company Explanation of Benefits

Walden-Martin Family Medical Clinic
1234 Anystreet
Anytown, AK 12345-1234

Patient Name	Treatment Dates	CPT Code	Charge Amount	Reason Code	Covered Amount	Deductible Amount	Co-Pay Amount	Paid At	Payment Amount
Yan, Tai	01/06/20XX	99205	132.28	03	125.00	0.00	0.00	80%	100.00
	01/06/20XX	82947	15.00		15.00	0.00	0.00	80%	12.00
	01/06/20XX	86580	11.34		11.34	0.00	0.00	80%	9.07
	Totals		158.62		151.34				121.07
Gomez,	01/07/20XX	99212	28.55		28.55	0.00	0.00	80%	22.84
Pedro	Totals		28.55		28.55				22.84
Green,	01/04/20XX	99203	70.92	03	69.23	0.00	0.00	80%	55.38
Jana	01/04/20XX	71020	40.97	03	34.95	0.00	0.00	80%	27.96
	Totals		111.89		104.18				83.34

Reason Code: 03 Allowed amount per insurance contract

Check No: 56390 $227.25

4. For Tai Yan's office visit, 99205, there is a difference between the Charge Amount and Covered Amount. Based on the reason code supplied what will be done with the difference?

_____

_____

_____

_____

5. How much is Tai Yan responsible for? _____

_____

6. How much will be written off for Jana Green? _____

_____

7. How much is Jana Green responsible for? _____

_____

8. What is the covered amount services provided to Pedro Gomez? _____

_____

9. The process for claim denial starts with the review of _____ or _____.

10. When reviewing an EOB or RA, the _____ can identify why a claim was denied.

11. If a claim was denied due to medical necessity the medical assistant should
    a. talk to the business supervisor to determine if the patient can billed for the services.
    b. contact the patient to make sure that they understand that the procedure was not covered.
    c. review the documentation to determine if the correct diagnosis and procedure codes were submitted.
    d. obtain the correct insurance plan information.

12. When a claim has been denied and the provider feels that it was coded correctly, an appeal letter should be sent including which of the following?
    a. Identity of the denied claim.
    b. A statement from the provider detailing the medical reasoning for performing the procedure.
    c. Additional medical reports.
    d. All of the above

E. The Patient's Financial Responsibility

Calculating Coinsurance and Deductible
Use the following information as you answer the following questions.

> Patient: Zach Green
> Deductible: $750
> Coinsurance: 80/20
> Patient out-of-pocket expense maximum: $2000

1. During Zach's first visit of the year, he incurred a $500 bill. Who pays this bill?_____

   _____

   _____

2. During Zach's second visit of the year, he incurred a $450 bill. Describe how much is paid by Zach and the insurance carrier.

   _____

   _____

3. Zach had surgery, which was his third claim of the year. He had a bill of $5000. Considering the prior visits, what is Zach's portion of this bill and what is the responsibility of the insurance carrier?

   _____

   _____

   _____

4. How much is Zach responsible for so far this year considering his first three visits? _____

   _____

   _____

   _____

5. When services that a provider suggests are not covered by Medicare, the patient can sign a(n) _____ giving them the option to pay the provider's fee in full.

CERTIFICATION PREPARATION

Circle the correct answer.

1. To examine claims for accuracy and completeness before they are submitted is to _____ the claims.
   a. correct
   b. audit
   c. revise
   d. reject

2. Block 1 of the CMS-1500 form contains what information?
   a. Patient's name
   b. Insured's name
   c. Type of insurance coverage
   d. Carrier address

3. The patient's name is found in block
   a. 1.
   b. 2.
   c. 3.
   d. 4.

4. CPT codes are found in what block?
   a. 24a
   b. 24b
   c. 24d
   d. 24e

5. Claims with incorrect, missing, or insufficient data are called
   a. clean.
   b. dingy.
   c. incomplete.
   d. dirty.

6. Which is a common reason why insurance claims are rejected?
   a. When a procedure listed is not an insurance benefit
   b. Medical necessity
   c. Preauthorization not obtained
   d. All of the above

7. Which is a fixed amount per visit that is typically paid at the time of medical services?
   a. Copayment
   b. Deductible
   c. Coinsurance
   d. Both a and b

8. Patients sign a(n) _____ of benefits form so that the physician will receive payment for services directly.
   a. release
   b. assignment
   c. turning
   d. sending

9. Claims submitted to a _____ are forwarded to individual insurance carriers.
   a. direct biller
   b. third-party administrator
   c. clearinghouse
   d. post office

10. Electronic data interchange is
    a. transferring data back and forth between two or more entities.
    b. sending information to one insurance carrier.
    c. sending information to one clearinghouse for processing.
    d. None of the above

WORKPLACE APPLICATIONS

1. Sally is the only medical biller in her healthcare agency. One of the two providers orders and performs tests and procedures before getting the needed preauthorizations from the patients' insurance carriers. As a result, the insurance carriers are not covering the claims and the clinic has had to write off thousands of dollars. Discuss how Sally should deal with the situation.

   a. How might she display tactful behavior when communicating with the provider about the third-party requirements?

   _____

   _____

   _____

   b. How would you deal with this situation if you were Sally?_____

   _____

   _____

   _____

2. Christi Brown is meeting with you regarding the bill she received in the mail. When she called to make the appointment, she voiced her confusion about the bill, stating she thought her insurance covered everything. You check her record and see that she met her deductible and now needs to pay 20% of the billed amount. She owes $170. Explain what a deductible and coinsurance are.

   _____

   _____

   _____

INTERNET ACTIVITIES

1. Using online resources, research your insurance carrier or an insurance carrier popular in your area. Research the appeal process for denied claims. Create a poster presentation, a PowerPoint presentation, or write a paper summarizing your research. Include the following points in your project:
   a. Who can start the appeal process?
   b. What steps are involved in the appeal process?
   c. What is the time frame for getting a response to the appeal?

2. Visit http://www.nucc.org and research the resources available on this website. Create a poster presentation, a PowerPoint presentation, or write a paper summarizing your research. Include the following points in your project:
   a. What resources are available for a medical biller on this website?
   b. List three that you think would be most helpful to a medical assistant who does medical billing.
   c. What information is available about the CMS-1500 claim form?
   d. Describe two things you learned from this website.

3. Using online resources, research the most common errors that occur when submitting claims. Create a poster presentation, a PowerPoint presentation, or write a paper summarizing your research. Include the following points in your project:
   a. What are the most common errors?
   b. How can these errors be prevented?
   c. What can a medical assistant do to prevent those errors?

Procedure 15.1   Perform Precertification with Documentation

Name _____ Date _____ Score _____

Task: To obtain precertification from a patient's insurance carrier for requested services or procedures.

Equipment and Supplies:
- Paper method: Patient's health record, prior authorization (precertification) request form, copy of patient's health insurance ID card, a pen
- Electronic method: Electronic health record system such as SimChart for the Medical Office (SCMO)

Scenario: You are working with Dr. Julie Walden at Walden-Martin Family Medical Clinic. Erma Willis (DOB 12/09/19XX) was seen for excessive snoring and Dr. Walden ordered a sleep study. You need to complete a prior authorization/certification form for the sleep study, which will be conducted by Dr. Jim Sandman. You checked and there is a signed release of information form.

Insurance Information	Clinic and Provider Information
Aetna 1234 Insurance Way Anytown, AL 112345-1234 Member ID Number: EW8884910 Group Number: 66574W	Walden-Martin Family Medical Clinic 1234 Anystreet Anytown, AL 12345 Provider: Julie Walden, MD Fax: 123-123-5678 Phone: 123-123-1234 Provider Contact Name: (your name)
Service Information Place: Walden-Martin Family Medicine Clinic Service Requested: Sleep study Starting Service Date: 1 week from today Ending Service Date: 1 week from today Service Frequency: once ICD-10-CM code: R06.83 CPT code: 95807 Not related to an injury or workers' compensation	

Standard: Complete the procedure and all critical steps in _____ minutes with a minimum score of 85% within two attempts (*or as indicated by the instructor*).

Scoring: Divide the points earned by the total possible points. Failure to perform a critical step, indicated by an asterisk (*), results in grade no higher than an 84% (*or as indicated by the instructor*).

Time: Began_____ Ended_____ Total minutes: _____

Steps:	Point Value	Attempt 1	Attempt 2
1. For the paper method, gather the health record, precertification/prior authorization request form, copy of the health insurance ID card, and a pen. For the electronic method, access the Simulation Playground in SCMO.	20		
2. Using the health record, determine the service or procedure that requires precertification/preauthorization.	20*		

3.	For the paper method, complete the Precertification/Prior Authorization Request form. For the electronic method, click on the Form Repository icon in SCMO. Select Prior Authorization Request from the left INFO PANEL. Use the Patient Search button at the bottom to find the patient. Complete the remaining fields of the form.	20		
4.	Proofread the completed form and make any revisions needed.	20		
5.	Paper method: File the document in the health record after it is faxed to the insurance carrier. Electronic method: Print and fax or electronically send the form to the insurance company and save the form to the patient's record.	20		
	Total Points	100		

Comments

CAAHEP Competencies	Step(s)
VIII.P.2 Verify eligibility for services	Entire procedure
VIII.P.3. Obtain precertification or preauthorization with documentation	Entire procedure
ABHES Competencies	**Step(s)**
7. Administrative Procedures c. Perform billing and collection procedures	Entire procedure

Procedure 15.2   Generate an Insurance Claim

Name _____ Date _____ Score _____

Task: To accurately generate an insurance claim using NUCC guidelines.

Equipment and Supplies:
- Patient's health record
- Copy of patient's insurance ID card or cards
- Patient registration/intake form
- Encounter form
- Insurance claims processing guidelines
- Electronic claims software such as SimChart for the Medical Office

Scenario: Mr. Walter Biller had an appointment with Dr. Walden on November 16, 20XX. He came in for an influenza vaccination, and while he was there, he wanted Dr. Walden to look at his ear because he was having problems hearing. His right ear canal was impacted with cerumen; the ear canal was irrigated, and the cerumen was removed during the visit.

Patient Demographics	Clinic and Provider Information	
Walter B. Biller (patient and insured)	Walden-Martin Family Medical Clinic	
87 Willoughby Lane	1234 Anystreet	
Anytown, AL 12345-1234	Anytown, AL 12345	
Phone: 123-237-3748	123-123-1234	
DOB: 01/04/1970	POS – 11 Office	
SSN: 285-77-7796	Established patient of Julie Walden, MD	
HIPAA form on file: Yes – March 19, 20XX	Federal Tax ID# 651249831	
Signature on file: Yes – March 19, 20XX	NPI# 1467253823	
Insurance Information		
Account Number: 16611		
Aetna		
Policy/ID Number: CH8327753		
Group Number: 33347H		
Diagnosis:	**ICD-10-CM code**	
Impacted cerumen, right ear	H61.21	
Service	**CPT Code**	**Fee**
Est. minimal OV	99212	$24.00
Cerumen removal	69210	$46.00
Vaccine – Flu, 3 Y+	90658	$24.00
Preventive – Flu Administration	90471	$7.00

Standard: Complete the procedure and all critical steps in _____ minutes with a minimum score of 85% within two attempts (*or as indicated by the instructor*).

Scoring: Divide the points earned by the total possible points. Failure to perform a critical step, indicated by an asterisk (*), results in grade no higher than an 84% (*or as indicated by the instructor*).

Time: Began_____ Ended_____ Total minutes: _____

Steps:	Point Value	Attempt 1	Attempt 2
1. Gather the documents required to generate the claim.	5		
2. Perform a patient search to locate the correct patient. Verify name and date of birth.	15*		
3. Ensure that all of the demographic information has been entered into the practice management software accurately.	10		
4. Select the correct encounter needed for claim.	5		
5. Review the autopopulated patient information and document any additional information needed. Save this information.	10		
6. Review the autopopulated provider information and document any additional information that is needed. Save this information.	10		
7. Review the autopopulated payer information and document any additional information that is needed. Save this information.	10		
8. Review the patient claim information, including diagnoses, if the condition is related to employment, auto accident, other accident, disability information, release of information, assignment of benefits, and referring physician. Document any additional information needed. Save this information.	15*		
9. Verify or enter the date of service, CPT/HCPCS codes, POS codes, link the diagnoses to the correct charge, modifiers, fees, and units. Save this information.	15*		
10. Submit the claim.	5		
Total Points	100		

Comments

CAAHEP Competencies	**Step(s)**
VIII.P.4. Complete an insurance claim form	Entire procedure
ABHES Competencies	**Step(s)**
7. Administrative Procedures c. Perform billing and collection procedures	Entire procedure

Procedure 15.3   Complete an Insurance Claim Form

Name _____ Date _____ Score _____

Task: To accurately complete a CMS-1500 health insurance claim form using NUCC guidelines

Equipment and Supplies:
- Patient's health record
- Copy of patient's insurance ID card or cards
- Patient registration/intake form
- Encounter form
- Insurance claims processing guidelines (Table 15.2)
- Blank CMS-1500 health insurance claim form (Work Product 15.1)

Background: Almost all medical billing is done electronically through practice management billing software. The paper CMS-1500 health insurance claim form is provided only to help students practice and develop their medical billing skills.

Directions: Complete each block (as appropriate) of the CMS-1500 (see Table 15.2 for block descriptions).

Scenario: Kyle Reeves had an appointment with Dr. Walden on March 20, 20XX. He came in because he was experiencing extreme fatigue, fever, sore throat, head and body aches. On examination, Dr. Walden also discovered swollen lymph nodes in the neck and armpits along with a swollen liver and spleen. She ordered a CBC, mononucleosis test, and a urinalysis. The mononucleosis test came back positive.

Patient Demographics Kyle T. Reeves (patient) 8448 Washington Ave Anytown, AL 12345-1234 Phone: 123-255-6499 DOB: 01/01/2004 SSN: 933-35-3754 HIPAA form on file: Yes – March 19, 20XX Signature on file: Yes – March 19, 20XX	Clinic and Provider Information Walden-Martin Family Medical Clinic 1234 Anystreet Anytown, AL 12345 123-123-1234 POS – 11 Office Established patient of Julie Walden, MD Federal Tax ID# 651249831 NPI# 1467253823	
Insurance Information Account Number: 16611 Insured: Kim Reeves (mother) Blue Cross Blue Shield Policy/ID Number: K20568R Group Number: 21548R		
Diagnosis:	**ICD-10-CM code**	
Infectious mononucleosis	O75	
Service	**CPT Code**	**Fee**
Est. Expanded OV	99213	$43.00
CBC w/auto differential	85025	$35.00
Mononucleosis test	86663	$34.00
U/A, w/micro non-automated	81001	$27.00

Standard: Complete the procedure and all critical steps in _____ minutes with a minimum score of 85% within two attempts (*or as indicated by the instructor*).

Scoring: Divide the points earned by the total possible points. Failure to perform a critical step, indicated by an asterisk (*), results in grade no higher than an 84% (*or as indicated by the instructor*).

Time: Began_____ Ended_____ Total minutes: _____

Steps:	Point Value	Attempt 1	Attempt 2
1. Gather the documents required to complete the claim form.	10		
2. Complete the claim form using a pen. Use capital letters. Do not use punctuation (commas or dollar signs) unless indicated in the insurance manual or guidelines. Use a hyphen to hyphenate last names.	10		
3. Using the patient's health insurance ID card, determine the type of insurance, and the insurance ID number. Enter this information into block 1 and 1a.	10		
4. Using the ID card, the encounter form, and the registration/intake form, determine the patient's information and insured individual's information. Accurately complete blocks 2, 3, 5, 6, 9, and 10 a-c by entering in the patient's information. Complete 4, 7, and 11, a-d with the insured's information.	10		
5. Complete blocks 12 and 13 by entering "signature on file" and the date.	10		
6. Accurately enter the physician or supplier information by completing blocks 14 through 23. Use the eight (8)–digit format (MM/DD/YYYY) when needed.	10		
7. Using the encounter form, complete the appropriate blocks from 24A through 24H. **Note**: • Block 24A: Enter the dates of service, both From and To. For ambulatory services, enter the same date in the FROM and TO fields. Enter a date for each procedure, service, or supply in eight (8)–digit format (MM/DD/YYYY). • Block 24F: Enter the charge for the listed service or procedure. *Do not use commas when reporting dollar amounts.* The cents column is the small column to the right. • Block 24G: Enter the number of days or units. This block is usually used for multiple visits, units of supplies, anesthesia units or minutes, or oxygen volume. If only one service is performed, enter 1.0	10		
8. Complete blocks 24I through 27 by entering information on the provider's or healthcare facility where the service was provided and the patient's account number. Check the correct box to indicate acceptance of assignment of benefits.	10		
9. Complete blocks 28 through 29 by entering the total charges, total amount paid, and the total amount due. Complete blocks 31 through 33a by entering in the provider's and facility's information.	10		
10. Review the claim for accuracy and completeness before submitting. Correct any errors or missing information.	10*		
Total Points	**100**		

Comments

CAAHEP Competencies	Step(s)
VIII.P.4. Complete an insurance claim form	Entire procedure
ABHES Competencies	**Step(s)**
7. Administrative Procedures d. Process insurance claims	Entire procedure

Work Product 15.1   CMS-1500 Health Insurance Claim Form

HEALTH INSURANCE CLAIM FORM

APPROVED BY NATIONAL UNIFORM CLAIM COMMITTEE (NUCC) 02/12

| | PICA | | | | | | | PICA | |

1. MEDICARE (Medicare#) **MEDICAID** (Medicaid#) **TRICARE** (ID#/DoD#) **CHAMPVA** (Member ID#) **GROUP HEALTH PLAN** (ID#) **FECA BLK LUNG** (ID#) **OTHER** (ID#) | **1a. INSURED'S I.D. NUMBER** (For Program in Item 1)

2. PATIENT'S NAME (Last Name, First Name, Middle Initial)

3. PATIENT'S BIRTH DATE MM DD YY **SEX** M☐ F☐

4. INSURED'S NAME (Last Name, First Name, Middle Initial)

5. PATIENT'S ADDRESS (No., Street)

6. PATIENT RELATIONSHIP TO INSURED Self☐ Spouse☐ Child☐ Other☐

7. INSURED'S ADDRESS (No., Street)

CITY | STATE

8. RESERVED FOR NUCC USE

CITY | STATE

ZIP CODE | TELEPHONE (Include Area Code) (   )

ZIP CODE | TELEPHONE (Include Area Code) (   )

9. OTHER INSURED'S NAME (Last Name, First Name, Middle Initial)

10. IS PATIENT'S CONDITION RELATED TO:

11. INSURED'S POLICY GROUP OR FECA NUMBER

a. OTHER INSURED'S POLICY OR GROUP NUMBER

a. EMPLOYMENT? (Current or Previous) ☐YES ☐NO

a. INSURED'S DATE OF BIRTH MM DD YY **SEX** M☐ F☐

b. RESERVED FOR NUCC USE

b. AUTO ACCIDENT? ☐YES ☐NO PLACE (State)

b. OTHER CLAIM ID (Designated by NUCC)

c. RESERVED FOR NUCC USE

c. OTHER ACCIDENT? ☐YES ☐NO

c. INSURANCE PLAN NAME OR PROGRAM NAME

d. INSURANCE PLAN NAME OR PROGRAM NAME

10d. CLAIM CODES (Designated by NUCC)

d. IS THERE ANOTHER HEALTH BENEFIT PLAN? ☐YES ☐NO **If yes,** complete items 9, 9a, and 9d.

READ BACK OF FORM BEFORE COMPLETING & SIGNING THIS FORM.
12. PATIENT'S OR AUTHORIZED PERSON'S SIGNATURE I authorize the release of any medical or other information necessary to process this claim. I also request payment of government benefits either to myself or to the party who accepts assignment below.

SIGNED _____ DATE _____

13. INSURED'S OR AUTHORIZED PERSON'S SIGNATURE I authorize payment of medical benefits to the undersigned physician or supplier for services described below.

SIGNED _____

14. DATE OF CURRENT ILLNESS, INJURY, or PREGNANCY (LMP) MM DD YY QUAL.

15. OTHER DATE QUAL. MM DD YY

16. DATES PATIENT UNABLE TO WORK IN CURRENT OCCUPATION FROM MM DD YY TO MM DD YY

17. NAME OF REFERRING PROVIDER OR OTHER SOURCE 17a. 17b. NPI

18. HOSPITALIZATION DATES RELATED TO CURRENT SERVICES FROM MM DD YY TO MM DD YY

19. ADDITIONAL CLAIM INFORMATION (Designated by NUCC)

20. OUTSIDE LAB? ☐YES ☐NO $ CHARGES

21. DIAGNOSIS OR NATURE OF ILLNESS OR INJURY Relate A-L to service line below (24E) ICD Ind.

A. ___ B. ___ C. ___ D. ___
E. ___ F. ___ G. ___ H. ___
I. ___ J. ___ K. ___ L. ___

22. RESUBMISSION CODE ORIGINAL REF. NO.

23. PRIOR AUTHORIZATION NUMBER

24. A. DATE(S) OF SERVICE From MM DD YY To MM DD YY	B. PLACE OF SERVICE	C. EMG	D. PROCEDURES, SERVICES, OR SUPPLIES (Explain Unusual Circumstances) CPT/HCPCS	MODIFIER	E. DIAGNOSIS POINTER	F. $ CHARGES	G. DAYS OR UNITS	H. EPSDT Family Plan	I. ID. QUAL.	J. RENDERING PROVIDER ID. #
1									NPI	
2									NPI	
3									NPI	
4									NPI	
5									NPI	
6									NPI	

25. FEDERAL TAX I.D. NUMBER SSN☐ EIN☐

26. PATIENT'S ACCOUNT NO.

27. ACCEPT ASSIGNMENT? (For govt. claims, see back) ☐YES ☐NO

28. TOTAL CHARGE $

29. AMOUNT PAID $

30. Rsvd for NUCC Use

31. SIGNATURE OF PHYSICIAN OR SUPPLIER INCLUDING DEGREES OR CREDENTIALS (I certify that the statements on the reverse apply to this bill and are made a part thereof.)

SIGNED _____ DATE _____

32. SERVICE FACILITY LOCATION INFORMATION
a. NPI b.

33. BILLING PROVIDER INFO & PH # (   )
a. NPI b.

NUCC Instruction Manual available at: www.nucc.org | **PLEASE PRINT OR TYPE** | APPROVED OMB-0938-1197 FORM 1500 (02-12)

Procedure 15.4   Use Medical Necessity Guidelines: Respond to a "Medical Necessity Denied" Claim

Name _____   Date _____   Score _____

Task: To resolve the insurance company's denial of a claim for medical necessity by completing an accurate claim.

Equipment and Supplies:
- Paper method: Patient's health record, copy of patient's insurance ID card or cards, patient registration form, encounter form, blank CMS-1500 health insurance claim form (Work Product 15-2), and a pen
- Electronic method: SimChart for the Medical Office
- Insurance denial letter or scenario (see below)

Scenario: You are working at Walden-Martin Family Medical Clinic, 1234 Anystreet, Anytown, AL 12345 (phone: 123-123-1234). You receive a letter indicating that Medicare has denied the following claim for not being medically necessary:

Patient: Norma B. Washington   DOB: 08/07/19XX   Policy/ID Number: 847744144A

Date of Service: 06/13/20XX   ICD: G43.101 (Migraine)   CPT: J3420 (B-12 injection)

Provider: Julie Walden MD

You did some research and the information above was the only information sent to Medicare for that encounter. The following information was the correct information for the encounter:

Patient: Norma B. Washington   DOB: 08/01/19XX   Date of Service: 06/15/20XX

ICD: G43.101 (Migraine)   CPT: J1885 (Toradol 15 mg—$15.50) and 96372 (Injection, Ther/Proph/Diag—$25.00)

ICD: D51.0 (Vitamin B_{12} deficiency anemia)   CPT: J3420 (B_{12} injection—$24.00) and 96372 (Injection, Ther/Proph/Diag—$25.00)

To be billed to: Medicare, 1234 Insurance Road, Anytown, AL 12345-1234

Standard: Complete the procedure and all critical steps in _____ minutes with a minimum score of 85% within two attempts (*or as indicated by the instructor*).

Scoring: Divide the points earned by the total possible points. Failure to perform a critical step, indicated by an asterisk (*), results in grade no higher than an 84% (*or as indicated by the instructor*).

Time: Began_____ Ended_____ Total minutes: _____

Steps:	Point Value	Attempt 1	Attempt 2
1. Review the insurance denial letter (scenario) carefully. Compare the patient's information from the denial letter to the health record, claim, and encounter form. Look for errors in the patient's name and date of birth.	20*		
2. Compare the insurance denial letter (scenario) to the health record, claim, and encounter form. Look for errors in the date of service, the diagnosis, and the procedure codes. The procedure must be medically necessary for the diagnosis indicated.	20*		

3.	Complete a claim (either CMS-1500 or an electronic claim using SimChart) by entering in the information about the carrier, patient, and insured.	20		
4.	Enter the information regarding the physician, procedures, and diagnosis. Make sure to include all of the information from the encounter.	20		
5.	Proofread the claim form for accuracy before submitting the claim.	20		
	Total Points	100		

Comments

CAAHEP Competencies	Step(s)
IX.P.3. Utilize medical necessity guidelines	Entire procedure
ABHES Competencies	**Step(s)**
7. Administrative Procedures c. Perform billing and collection procedures	Entire procedure

Work Product 15.2 CMS-1500 Health Insurance Claim Form

CARRIER →

HEALTH INSURANCE CLAIM FORM

APPROVED BY NATIONAL UNIFORM CLAIM COMMITTEE (NUCC) 02/12

| | PICA | | | | | | | | PICA | | |

1. MEDICARE ☐ (Medicare#) MEDICAID ☐ (Medicaid#) TRICARE ☐ (ID#/DoD#) CHAMPVA ☐ (Member ID#) GROUP HEALTH PLAN ☐ (ID#) FECA BLK LUNG ☐ (ID#) OTHER ☐ (ID#)

1a. INSURED'S I.D. NUMBER (For Program in Item 1)

2. PATIENT'S NAME (Last Name, First Name, Middle Initial)

3. PATIENT'S BIRTH DATE MM DD YY SEX M ☐ F ☐

4. INSURED'S NAME (Last Name, First Name, Middle Initial)

5. PATIENT'S ADDRESS (No., Street)

6. PATIENT RELATIONSHIP TO INSURED Self ☐ Spouse ☐ Child ☐ Other ☐

7. INSURED'S ADDRESS (No., Street)

CITY STATE

8. RESERVED FOR NUCC USE

CITY STATE

ZIP CODE TELEPHONE (Include Area Code) ( )

ZIP CODE TELEPHONE (Include Area Code) ( )

9. OTHER INSURED'S NAME (Last Name, First Name, Middle Initial)

10. IS PATIENT'S CONDITION RELATED TO:

11. INSURED'S POLICY GROUP OR FECA NUMBER

a. OTHER INSURED'S POLICY OR GROUP NUMBER

a. EMPLOYMENT? (Current or Previous) ☐ YES ☐ NO

a. INSURED'S DATE OF BIRTH MM DD YY SEX M ☐ F ☐

b. RESERVED FOR NUCC USE

b. AUTO ACCIDENT? ☐ YES ☐ NO PLACE (State)

b. OTHER CLAIM ID (Designated by NUCC)

c. RESERVED FOR NUCC USE

c. OTHER ACCIDENT? ☐ YES ☐ NO

c. INSURANCE PLAN NAME OR PROGRAM NAME

d. INSURANCE PLAN NAME OR PROGRAM NAME

10d. CLAIM CODES (Designated by NUCC)

d. IS THERE ANOTHER HEALTH BENEFIT PLAN? ☐ YES ☐ NO *If yes*, complete items 9, 9a, and 9d.

READ BACK OF FORM BEFORE COMPLETING & SIGNING THIS FORM.
12. PATIENT'S OR AUTHORIZED PERSON'S SIGNATURE I authorize the release of any medical or other information necessary to process this claim. I also request payment of government benefits either to myself or to the party who accepts assignment below.

SIGNED _____ DATE _____

13. INSURED'S OR AUTHORIZED PERSON'S SIGNATURE I authorize payment of medical benefits to the undersigned physician or supplier for services described below.

SIGNED _____

PATIENT AND INSURED INFORMATION →

14. DATE OF CURRENT ILLNESS, INJURY, or PREGNANCY (LMP) MM DD YY QUAL.

15. OTHER DATE QUAL. MM DD YY

16. DATES PATIENT UNABLE TO WORK IN CURRENT OCCUPATION FROM MM DD YY TO MM DD YY

17. NAME OF REFERRING PROVIDER OR OTHER SOURCE
17a.
17b. NPI

18. HOSPITALIZATION DATES RELATED TO CURRENT SERVICES FROM MM DD YY TO MM DD YY

19. ADDITIONAL CLAIM INFORMATION (Designated by NUCC)

20. OUTSIDE LAB? ☐ YES ☐ NO $ CHARGES

21. DIAGNOSIS OR NATURE OF ILLNESS OR INJURY Relate A-L to service line below (24E) ICD Ind.

A. _____ B. _____ C. _____ D. _____
E. _____ F. _____ G. _____ H. _____
I. _____ J. _____ K. _____ L. _____

22. RESUBMISSION CODE ORIGINAL REF. NO.

23. PRIOR AUTHORIZATION NUMBER

24. A. DATE(S) OF SERVICE From MM DD YY To MM DD YY | **B. PLACE OF SERVICE** | **C. EMG** | **D. PROCEDURES, SERVICES, OR SUPPLIES** (Explain Unusual Circumstances) CPT/HCPCS MODIFIER | **E. DIAGNOSIS POINTER** | **F. $ CHARGES** | **G. DAYS OR UNITS** | **H. EPSDT Family Plan** | **I. ID. QUAL.** | **J. RENDERING PROVIDER ID. #**

1 | | | | | | | | | NPI
2 | | | | | | | | | NPI
3 | | | | | | | | | NPI
4 | | | | | | | | | NPI
5 | | | | | | | | | NPI
6 | | | | | | | | | NPI

25. FEDERAL TAX I.D. NUMBER SSN ☐ EIN ☐

26. PATIENT'S ACCOUNT NO.

27. ACCEPT ASSIGNMENT? (For govt. claims, see back) ☐ YES ☐ NO

28. TOTAL CHARGE $

29. AMOUNT PAID $

30. Rsvd for NUCC Use

31. SIGNATURE OF PHYSICIAN OR SUPPLIER INCLUDING DEGREES OR CREDENTIALS (I certify that the statements on the reverse apply to this bill and are made a part thereof.)

SIGNED _____ DATE _____

32. SERVICE FACILITY LOCATION INFORMATION
a. NPI b.

33. BILLING PROVIDER INFO & PH # ( )
a. NPI b.

PHYSICIAN OR SUPPLIER INFORMATION →

NUCC Instruction Manual available at: www.nucc.org   ***PLEASE PRINT OR TYPE***   APPROVED OMB-0938-1197 FORM 1500 (02-12)

Procedure 15.5   Assist a Patient in Understanding an Explanation of Benefits (EOB)

Name _____ Date _____ Score _____

Tasks: To explain an explanation of benefits (EOB) to a patient.

Equipment and Supplies:
• Explanation of benefits

Obtaining Payments – WMFM Clinic Policy
• For patients with copayments, all copayments must be collected before the patient leaves the clinic.
• For patients with balances overdue:
  • Patients must pay 20% of the balance before an appointment can be scheduled.
  • Or patients can establish a 6- or 12-month interest-free payment plan, making the first payment before the next visit can be scheduled.
• Payments can be made using VISA, MasterCard, personal check (no starter checks accepted), or cash. Payments can also be made online.

Scenario: Noemi Rodriguez has stopped in to WMFM Clinic with an explanation of benefits that she recently received from her insurance company (see next page). She states that her policy has a $1000 deductible and 80/20 coinsurance. She doesn't understand why the insurance company didn't pay the bill in full as she had services earlier in the year. She also is not clear on what she is financially responsible for.
WMFM Clinic is a participating provider with the Aetna Preferred Provider Plan that Ms. Rodriguez is part of.

Explanation of Benefits

Aetna
1234 Insurance Way
Anytown, AL 12345-
1234
800-333-444-5555
800-333-444-6666
(FAX)

Insured's Name: Noemi Rodriguez

Policy ID #   NR5006789

Date: 03/03/20XX

Patient Name: Noemi Rodriguez
441 Hyacinth Way
Anytown, AL 12345

Provider: Walden-Martin Family Medical Clinic
J.A. Martin NPI 1234567890
Claim No. 9885050333-XX
Check No. 2034422

Date of Service	CPT Code	Charge Amount	Allowable Charges	Applied to Deductible	Co-Pay	Total Benefit	Reason Code(s)
01/14/20XX	99205	225.00	200.00	150.00	0.00	40.00	01/42
01/14/20XX	85025	35.00	30.00	0.00	0.00	24.00	42
01/14/20XX	82272	7.00	7.00	0.00	0.00	5.60	
01/14/20XX	80061	47.00	45.00	0.00	0.00	36.00	42
01/14/20XX	80076	39.00	32.50	0.00	0.00	26.00	42
01/14/20XX	80069	41.50	40.00	0.00	0.00	32.00 42	
01/14/20XX	85652	16.00	16.00	0.00	0.00	12.80	
01/14/20XX	81001	27.00	25.00	0.00	0.00	20.00 42	
Total		437.50	395.50	150.00	0.00	236.40	

Reason Code:
01 Deductible amount
42 Charges exceed our fee schedule or maximum allowed amount

Standard: Complete the procedure and all critical steps in _____ minutes with a minimum score of 85% within two attempts (*or as indicated by the instructor*).

Scoring: Divide the points earned by the total possible points. Failure to perform a critical step, indicated by an asterisk (*), results in grade no higher than an 84% (*or as indicated by the instructor*).

Time: Began_____ Ended_____ Total minutes: _____

Steps:	Point Value	Attempt 1	Attempt 2
1. Review the each of the columns found on the explanation of benefits. Have a clear understanding how the insurance company came up with the patient's responsibility.	20		
2. Determine if any amount has been applied to Ms. Rodriguez's deductible. Explain to Ms. Rodriguez how that impacts how much the insurance company will pay and her financial responsibility.	20*		

3.	Compare the charge amount for each service to the allowed amount. Explain to Ms. Rodriguez how the difference between those two is taken care of. Inform the patient of the clinic policy regarding copayments and how the payment can be made.	20		
4.	Calculate what Ms. Rodriguez's financial responsibility is and explain to her how you came up with that amount.	20*		
5.	Ask if the patient has any further questions.	20*		
	Total Points	100		

Affective Behavior	Directions: Check behaviors observed during the role-play.					
	Negative, Unprofessional Behaviors	**Attempt**		**Positive, Professional Behaviors**	**Attempt**	
Tactfulness		**1**	**2**		**1**	**2**
	Rude, unkind			Courteous, professional; assertive as required		
	Disrespectful, impolite			Polite, patient		
	Negative verbal communication (e.g., harsh words, disrespectful comments)			Professional verbal communication (e.g., respectful and understanding communication)		
	Brief, abrupt			Took time with person		
	Unconcerned with person's dignity			Maintained person's dignity		
	Negative nonverbal behaviors			Positive nonverbal behaviors		
	Other:			Other:		
Empathy	Distracted; not focused on the other person			Focused full attention on the other person		
	Judgmental attitude; not accepting attitude			Nonjudgmental, accepting attitude		
	Failed to clarify what the person verbally or nonverbally communicated			Used summarizing or paraphrasing to clarify what the person verbally or nonverbally communicated		
	Failed to acknowledge what the person communicated			Acknowledged what the person communicated		
	Rude, discourteous			Pleasant and courteous		
	Disregarded the person's dignity and rights			Maintained the person's dignity and rights		
	Other:			Other:		

Critical Thinking	Coached or told of an issue or problem			Independently identified the problem or issue		
	Failed to ask relevant questions related to the condition			Asked appropriate questions to obtain the information required		
	Failed to consider alternatives; failed to ask questions that demonstrated understanding of principles/concepts			Willing to consider other alternatives; asked appropriate questions that showed understanding of principles/concepts		
	Failed to make an educated, logical judgment/decision; actions or lack of actions demonstrated unsafe practices and/or did not follow the protocol			Made an educated, logical judgment/decision based on the protocol; actions reflected principles of safe practice		
	Other:			Other:		

Grading for Affective Behaviors		Point Value	Attempt 1	Attempt 2
Does not meet Expectation	• Response was insensitive and/or disrespectful. • Student demonstrated more than 2 negative, unprofessional behaviors during the interaction.	0		
Needs Improvement	• Response was insensitive and/or disrespectful. • Student demonstrated 1 or 2 negative, unprofessional behaviors during the interaction.	0		
Meets Expectation	• Response was sensitive and respectful; no negative, unprofessional behaviors observed. • More practice is needed for behavior to appear natural and for student to appear comfortable and at ease.	15		
Occasionally Exceeds Expectation	• Response was sensitive and respectful; no negative, unprofessional behaviors observed. • At times student appeared comfortable and at ease; but more practice is needed for behavior to become natural and consistent with a professional medical assistant.	15		
Always Exceeds Expectation	• Response was sensitive and respectful; no negative, unprofessional behaviors observed. • Student's behaviors appeared natural and comfortable. Behaviors are consistent with a professional medical assistant.	15		

Comments

CAAHEP Competencies	Step(s)
VIII.P.5. Assist a patient in understanding an Explanation of Benefits (EOB)	Entire procedure
A.1. Demonstrate critical thinking skills	Entire procedure
A.3. Demonstrate empathy for patients' concerns	5
A.7. Demonstrate tactfulness	Entire procedure
ABHES Competencies	**Step(s)**
7. Administrative Procedures c. Perform billing and collection procedures	Entire procedure

Procedure 15.6 Inform a Patient of Financial Obligations for Services Rendered

Name _____ Date _____ Score _____

Tasks: Inform patient of his/her financial obligation and to demonstrate professionalism and sensitivity when discussing the patient's billing record.

Equipment and Supplies:
- Facility's payment policy
- Copy of patient's insurance card (or see information in the scenario)
- Patient's account record (or see information in the scenario)

Obtaining Payments – WMFM Clinic Policy
- For patients with copayments, all copayments must be collected before the patient leaves the clinic.
- For patients with balances overdue:
  - Patients must pay 20% of the balance before an appointment can be scheduled.
  - Or patients can establish a 6- or 12-month interest-free payment plan, making the first payment before the next visit can be scheduled.
- Payments can be made using VISA, MasterCard, personal check (no starter checks accepted), or cash. Payments can also be made online.

Scenario #1: Mr. Walter Biller arrives for his appointment. You need to check his eligibility for services and also if he has a copayment for today's visit. His insurance information: account number: 16611; Aetna, Policy/ID Number: CH8327753; and Group Number: 33347H

Scenario #2: Christi Brown is meeting with you regarding the bill she received in the mail. She called to make the appointment and she voiced her confusion about the bill. She stated that she thought her insurance covered everything. You check her record and see that she met her deductible and now needs to pay 20% of the billed amount. She owes $170.

Directions: Role-play the scenarios with a peer. The peer will be the insurance representative in Scenario #1, and then the patient in Scenario #2. You will be the medical assistant. You need to be professional and sensitive when working with patients regarding payments. You also need to follow the clinic's policy.

Standard: Complete the procedure and all critical steps in _____ minutes with a minimum score of 85% within two attempts (*or as indicated by the instructor*).

Scoring: Divide the points earned by the total possible points. Failure to perform a critical step, indicated by an asterisk (*), results in grade no higher than an 84% (*or as indicated by the instructor*).

Time: Began _____ Ended _____ Total minutes: _____

Steps:	Point Value	Attempt 1	Attempt 2
Scenario #1: Role-play with a peer who will be the insurance representative.			
1. Contact the patient's insurance company and verify the patient's eligibility for services. Provide the representative with the patient's information. Find out if the patient has a copayment for today's visit. Document the information obtained.	20*		
Scenario #1 update: You need to provide the patient with the information that he owes a copayment for today's visit.			
2. Inform the patient of his financial obligation of the copayment.	10*		

Scenario update: He states he does not have the cash with him.				
3. Inform the patient of the clinic policy regarding copayments and how the payment can be made.	**10**			
4. Demonstrate sensitivity and professionalism when discussing the payment.	**15***			
Scenario #2: Role-play with a peer who will be the patient.				
5. Determine the amount the patient owes by reviewing the patient's account record. Inform the patient the amount owed for services rendered.	**15***			
Scenario update: Patient stated she does not have the money to pay the entire bill today.				
6. Inform the patient of the clinic policy regarding overdue accounts and scheduling appointments. Provide the patient with options for the overdue amount based on the clinic policy.	**15**			
7. Demonstrate sensitivity and professionalism when discussing the payment and the situation.	**15***			
Total Points	**100**			

Affective Behavior	*Directions:* Check behaviors observed during the role-play.					
	Negative, Unprofessional Behaviors	**Attempt**		**Positive, Professional Behaviors**	**Attempt**	
Tactfulness		**1**	**2**		**1**	**2**
	Rude, unkind			Courteous, professional; assertive as required		
	Disrespectful, impolite			Polite, patient		
	Negative verbal communication (e.g., harsh words, disrespectful comments)			Professional verbal communication (e.g., respectful and understanding communication)		
	Brief, abrupt			Took time with person		
	Unconcerned with person's dignity			Maintained person's dignity		
	Negative nonverbal behaviors			Positive nonverbal behaviors		
	Other:			Other:		

Empathy	Distracted; not focused on the other person			Focused full attention on the other person		
	Judgmental attitude; not accepting attitude			Nonjudgmental, accepting attitude		
	Failed to clarify what the person verbally or nonverbally communicated			Used summarizing or paraphrasing to clarify what the person verbally or nonverbally communicated		
	Failed to acknowledge what the person communicated			Acknowledged what the person communicated		
	Rude, discourteous			Pleasant and courteous		
	Disregarded the person's dignity and rights			Maintained the person's dignity and rights		
	Other:			Other:		
Critical Thinking	Coached or told of an issue or problem			Independently identified the problem or issue		
	Failed to ask relevant questions related to the condition			Asked appropriate questions to obtain the information required		
	Failed to consider alternatives; failed to ask questions that demonstrated understanding of principles/concepts			Willing to consider other alternatives; asked appropriate questions that showed understanding of principles/concepts		
	Failed to make an educated, logical judgment/decision; actions or lack of actions demonstrated unsafe practices and/or did not follow the protocol			Made an educated, logical judgment/decision based on the protocol; actions reflected principles of safe practice		
	Other:			Other:		

Grading for Affective Behaviors		Point Value	Attempt 1	Attempt 2
Does not meet Expectation	• Response was insensitive and/or disrespectful. • Student demonstrated more than 2 negative, unprofessional behaviors during the interaction.	0		
Needs Improvement	• Response was insensitive and/or disrespectful. • Student demonstrated 1 or 2 negative, unprofessional behaviors during the interaction.	0		
Meets Expectation	• Response was sensitive and respectful; no negative, unprofessional behaviors observed. • More practice is needed for behavior to appear natural and for student to appear comfortable and at ease.	15		
Occasionally Exceeds Expectation	• Response was sensitive and respectful; no negative, unprofessional behaviors observed. • At times student appeared comfortable and at ease; but more practice is needed for behavior to become natural and consistent with a professional medical assistant.	15		
Always Exceeds Expectation	• Response was sensitive and respectful; no negative, unprofessional behaviors observed. • Student's behaviors appeared natural and comfortable. Behaviors are consistent with a professional medical assistant.	15		

Comments

CAAHEP Competencies	Step(s)
A.1. Demonstrate critical thinking skills	Entire procedure
A.3. Demonstrate empathy for patient's concerns.	4, 7
A.7. Demonstrate tactfulness	4, 7
VII.P.3. Inform a patient of financial obligations for services rendered	2, 5
VIII.P.2. Verify eligibility for services	1
ABHES Competencies	**Step(s)**
7. Administrative Procedures c. Perform billing and collection procedures	Entire procedure

Procedure 15.7   Show Sensitivity when Communicating with Patients Regarding Third-Party Requirements

Name _____ Date _____ Score _____

Tasks: Communicate in an assertive, professional manner with a third-party representative. Demonstrate sensitivity through verbal and nonverbal communication when discussing third-party requirements with a patient. Display tactful behavior when communicating with a provider regarding third-party requirements.

Equipment and Supplies:
- Copy of patient's health insurance ID card
- Prescription for new medication

Scenario: Ken Thomas saw Jean Burke N.P. for his asthma today. He was prescribed a fluticasone inhaler 220 mcg and a refill on his albuterol inhaler. When Ken stops at the checkout desk to make a follow-up appointment, he looks concerned. You inquire how you can help him and he states that he is wondering if his new insurance will pick up the fluticasone inhaler. He further explains that he has used it in the past with great results, but he recently switched insurance plans and he is finding it doesn't have the same coverage as his old plan.

- *Role-play #1:* You call the insurance company and discuss the coverage with the insurance carrier's representative. The representative tells you that the fluticasone inhaler is not covered for his condition. The representative gave you names of two other inhalers that would be covered.

  When you ask if the drug would be covered through the exceptions process, the representative indicated that the provider must send a letter indicating the drug is appropriate for the patient's condition because all other drugs covered by the plan have not been effective, those drugs have side effects that may be harmful to the patient, or the patient is allergic to the other drugs.
- *Role-play #2:* You must explain to Ken, who is upset with his insurance coverage, that he would have to cover the $250 inhaler.
- *Role-play #3:* Ken explains he does not have $250 for the inhaler. He asks what else he should do. You mention the exception process and Ken requests the provider to send a letter. You need to role-play notifying the provider of the third-party requirements.

Directions: Role-play the scenarios with a peer. The peer will play the part of the insurance representative, the patient, and the provider. You need to be professional and assertive with the insurance representative. When working with the patient, you need to show sensitivity. When communicating with the provider, you need to be professional and tactful.

Standard: Complete the procedure and all critical steps in _____ minutes with a minimum score of 85% within two attempts (*or as indicated by the instructor*).

Scoring: Divide the points earned by the total possible points. Failure to perform a critical step, indicated by an asterisk (*), results in grade no higher than an 84% (*or as indicated by the instructor*).

Time: Began_____ **Ended**_____ **Total minutes:** _____

Steps:	Point Value	Attempt 1	Attempt 2
1. Obtain a copy of the patient's health insurance ID card and the prescription for the new medication.	10		
2. Review the insurance card for coverage information and the phone number for providers.	20		

3.	*Scenario: Role-play #1 with a peer. The peer will be the insurance representative.* Contact the insurance company and clearly state the patient's information, the patient's question, and the new medication. Write down information provided by the representative.	10*		
4.	Demonstrate professionalism through verbal communication skills, by stating a respectful, assertive, clear, organized message while pronouncing medical terminology and medications correctly.	10*		
5.	*Scenario: Role-play #2 with a peer. The peer will be the patient.* Explain to the patient the message from the insurance representative using language that can be understood by the patient. *(Refer to the Checklist for Affective Behaviors - Respect and Sensitivity)*	10*		
6.	Demonstrate sensitivity to the patient by paying attention to and responding appropriately to the patient's nonverbal body language and verbal message.	10*		
7.	Demonstrate sensitivity to the patient by showing empathy and clarifying that you understand what the patient is stating. Give the patient your full attention during the conversation and reserve judgment.	10*		
8.	Demonstrate sensitivity to the patient by using a pleasant, courteous tone of voice. Use body language to communicate respect (e.g., eye contact if culturally appropriate, keep arms uncrossed and relaxed).	10*		
9.	*Scenario: Role-play #3 with a peer. The peer will be the provider.* Demonstrate tactful behavior when explaining the third-party requirements to the provider. *(Refer to the Checklist for Affective Behaviors - Tactful)*	10*		
	Total Points	100		

Affective Behavior	**Directions:** *Check behaviors observed during the role-play.*					
Tactfulness	**Negative, Unprofessional Behaviors**	**Attempt**		**Positive, Professional Behaviors**	**Attempt**	
		1	**2**		**1**	**2**
	Rude, unkind			Courteous, professional; assertive as required		
	Disrespectful, impolite			Polite, patient		
	Negative verbal communication (e.g., harsh words, disrespectful comments)			Professional verbal communication (e.g., respectful and understanding communication)		
	Brief, abrupt			Took time with person		
	Unconcerned with person's dignity			Maintained person's dignity		
	Negative nonverbal behaviors			Positive nonverbal behaviors		
	Other:			Other:		

Empathy	Distracted; not focused on the other person			Focused full attention on the other person		
	Judgmental attitude; not accepting attitude			Nonjudgmental, accepting attitude		
	Failed to clarify what the person verbally or nonverbally communicated			Used summarizing or paraphrasing to clarify what the person verbally or nonverbally communicated		
	Failed to acknowledge what the person communicated			Acknowledged what the person communicated		
	Rude, discourteous			Pleasant and courteous		
	Disregarded the person's dignity and rights			Maintained the person's dignity and rights		
	Other:			Other:		
Critical Thinking	Coached or told of an issue or problem			Independently identified the problem or issue		
	Failed to ask relevant questions related to the condition			Asked appropriate questions to obtain the information required		
	Failed to consider alternatives; failed to ask questions that demonstrated understanding of principles/concepts			Willing to consider other alternatives; asked appropriate questions that showed understanding of principles/concepts		
	Failed to make an educated, logical judgment/decision; actions or lack of actions demonstrated unsafe practices and/or did not follow the protocol			Made an educated, logical judgment/decision based on the protocol; actions reflected principles of safe practice		
	Other:			Other:		

Grading for Affective Behaviors		Point Value	Attempt 1	Attempt 2
Does not meet Expectation	• Response was insensitive and/or disrespectful. • Student demonstrated more than 2 negative, unprofessional behaviors during the interaction.	0		
Needs Improvement	• Response was insensitive and/or disrespectful. • Student demonstrated 1 or 2 negative, unprofessional behaviors during the interaction.	0		
Meets Expectation	• Response was sensitive and respectful; no negative, unprofessional behaviors observed. • More practice is needed for behavior to appear natural and for student to appear comfortable and at ease.	10		
Occasionally Exceeds Expectation	• Response was sensitive and respectful; no negative, unprofessional behaviors observed. • At times student appeared comfortable and at ease; but more practice is needed for behavior to become natural and consistent with a professional medical assistant.	10		
Always Exceeds Expectation	• Response was sensitive and respectful; no negative, unprofessional behaviors observed. • Student's behaviors appeared natural and comfortable. Behaviors are consistent with a professional medical assistant.	10		

Comments

CAAHEP Competencies	Step(s)
VII.P.3. Inform a patient of financial obligations for services rendered	5
A.1. Demonstrate critical thinking skills	Entire procedure
A.3. Demonstrate empathy for patients' concerns	7
A.7. Demonstrate tactfulness	9
ABHES Competencies	**Step(s)**
7. Administrative Procedures c. Perform billing and collection procedures	Entire procedure

Patient Accounts and Practice Management

CAAHEP Competencies	Assessment
VII.C.1.a. Define the following bookkeeping terms: charges	Skills and Concepts – A. 5
VII.C.1.b. Define the following bookkeeping terms: payments	Skills and Concepts – A. 6
VII.C.1.c. Define the following bookkeeping terms: accounts receivable	Skills and Concepts – A. 3
VII.C.1.d. Define the following bookkeeping terms: accounts payable	Skills and Concepts – A. 2
VII.C.1.e. Define the following bookkeeping terms: adjustments	Skills and Concepts – A. 4
VII.C.1.f. Define the following bookkeeping terms: end of day reconciliation	Procedure 16.4
VII.C.2.a. Identify precautions for accepting the following types of payments: cash	Skills and Concepts – B. 2
VII.C.2.b. Identify precautions for accepting the following types of payments: check	Skills and Concepts – B. 1
VII.C.2.c. Identify precautions for accepting the following types of payments: credit card	Skills and Concepts – B. 3
VII.C.2.d. Identify precautions for accepting the following types of payments: debit card	Skills and Concepts – B. 3
VII.C.3.a. Identify types of adjustments made to patient accounts including: non-sufficient funds (NSF) check	Skills and Concepts – A. 10
VII.C.3.b. Identify types of adjustments made to patient accounts including: collection agency transaction	Skills and Concepts – C. 4
VII.C.3.c. Identify types of adjustments made to patient accounts including: credit balance	Skills and Concepts – A. 9
VII.C.3.d. Identify types of adjustments made to patient accounts including: third party	Skills and Concepts – A. 8
VII.C.4. Identify patient financial obligations for services rendered	Workplace Applications – 1

CAAHEP Competencies	Assessment
VII.P.1.a. Perform accounts receivable procedures to patient accounts including posting: charges	Procedure 16.1
VII.P.1.b. Perform accounts receivable procedures to patient accounts including posting: payments	Procedures 16.1, 16.3
VII.P.1.c. Perform accounts receivable procedures to patient accounts including posting: adjustments	Procedure 16.3
VII.P.2. Input accurate patient billing information in Practice Management Systems (PMS)	Procedures 16.1, 16.3
VII.P.3. Inform a patient of financial obligations for services rendered	Procedure 16.2
A.3. Demonstrate empathy for patients' concerns	Procedure 16.2
A.7. Demonstrate tactfulness	Procedure 16.2

ABHES Competencies	Assessment
7. Administrative Procedures c. Perform billing and collection procedures	Procedures 16.1, 16.2, 16.3, 16.4

VOCABULARY REVIEW

Using the word pool on the right, find the correct word to match the definition. Write the word on the line after the definition.

Group A

1. The person legally responsible for the entire bill
   _____

2. A document sent by the insurance company to the provider and the patient explaining the allowed charge amount, the amount reimbursed for services, and the patient's financial responsibilities
   _____

3. The process of recording financial transactions
   _____

4. A manual bookkeeping system that uses a day sheet to record all financial transactions for the date of service and maintains patient account balances by using physical ledger cards
   _____

5. Poor, needy, impoverished _____

6. To come into or acquire _____

7. A list of fixed fees for services _____

8. A minor who has been granted emancipation by the court; the minor can assume the rights and responsibilities of adulthood
   _____

9. The amount of money the healthcare facility has in the bank that can be withdrawn as cash _____

10. A running balance of all financial transactions for a specific patient
    _____

Word Pool
- patient account
- bookkeeping
- cash on hand
- incurred
- pegboard system
- fee schedule
- explanation of benefits
- emancipated minor
- guarantor
- indigent

Group B

1. Something of value that cannot be touched physically
   _____

2. Hostile and aggressive _____

3. An imitation intended to be passed off fraudulently or deceptively as genuine; forgery _____

4. A chronologic file used as a reminder that something must be dealt with on a certain date _____

5. All property available for the payment of debts
   _____

6. An oath or swear word _____

7. Global technology that includes imbedded microchips that store and protect cardholder data; also called *chip and PIN* and *chip and signature* _____

8. Debt that is not guaranteed by something of value; credit card debt is the most common type _____

9. An individual assigned to make financial decisions about the estate of a deceased patient _____

10. The misuse of a healthcare facility's funds for personal gain _____embezzlement

Word Pool
- counterfeit
- EMV chip technology
- belligerent
- expletive
- embezzlement
- tickler file
- intangible
- executor
- assets
- unsecured debt

Group C

1. Money the bank pays the account holder on the amount in their account for using the money in the account
   _____

2. A special court established to handle small claims or debts, without the services of lawyers _____

3. Money in a bank account that is not assigned to pay for any office expenses _____

4. An individual or party who brings the suit to court
   _____

5. A fixed compensation periodically paid to a person for regular work _____

6. The central bank of the United States _____

7. The coordinator of financial resources assigned by the court during a bankruptcy case _____

8. An individual or business against whom a lawsuit is filed
   _____

9. To bring into agreement _____

10. A document guaranteeing payment of a specific amount of money to the payer named on the document _____

Word Pool
- trustee
- small claims court
- plaintiff
- defendant
- salaried
- reconciliation
- interest
- Federal Reserve Bank
- discretionary income
- negotiable instrument

ABBREVIATIONS

Write out what each of the following abbreviations stands for.

1. EOB _____

2. A/R _____

3. A/P _____

4. NSF _____

5. TILA _____

6. FTC _____

7. APR _____

8. PIN _____

9. POS _____

10. EFT _____

11. RTN _____

12. ACH _____

SKILLS AND CONCEPTS

Answer the following questions. Write your answer on the line or in the space provided.

A. Accounts Receivable

1. Examine the fee schedule and answer the following questions.

FEE SCHEDULE

BLACKBURN PRIMARY CARE ASSOCIATES, PC
1990 Turquiose Drive
Blackburn, WI 54937
608-459-8857

Federal Tax ID Number: 00-0000000   **BCBS Group Number: 14982**
                                                                  Medicare Group Number: 14982

OFFICE VISIT, NEW PATIENT

Focused, 99201	$45.00
Expanded, 99202	$55.00
Intermediate, 99203	$60.00
Extended, 99204	$95.00
Comprehensive, 99205	$195.00

Consultation, 99245	$250.00

OFFICE VISIT, ESTABLISHED PATIENT

Minimal, 99211	$40.00
Focused, 99212	$48.00
Intermediate, 99213	$55.00
Extended, 99214	$65.00
Comprehensive, 99215	$195.00

OFFICE PROCEDURES

ECG, 12 lead, 93000	$55.00
Stress ECG, Treadmill, 93015	$295.00
Sigmoidoscopy, Flex; 45330	$145.00
Spirometry, 94010	$50.00
Cerumen Removal, 69210	$40.00

Collection & Handling	
Lab Specimen, 99000	$9.00
Venipuncture, 35415	$9.00
Urinalysis, 81000	$20.00
Urinalysis, 81002 (Dip Only)	$12.00

Influenza Injection, 90724	$20.00
Pneumococcal Injection, 90732	$20.00
Oral Polio, 90712	$15.00
DTaP, 90700	$20.00
Tetanus Toxoid, 90703	$15.00
MMR, 90707	$25.00
HIB, 90737	$20.00
Hepatitis B, newborn to	
age 11 years, 90744	$60.00
Hepatitis B, 11-19 years, 90745	$60.00
Hepatitis B, 20 years and above	
90746	$60.00
Intramuscular Injection, 90788	
Penicillin	$30.00
Cephtriaxone	$25.00
Solu-Medrol	$23.00
Vitamin B-12	$13.00
Subcutaneous Injection, 90782	
Epinephrine	$18.00
Susphrine	$25.00
Insulin, U-100	$15.00

COMMON DIAGNOSTIC CODES

Acute coronary thrombosis without
   myocardial infarction I24.0
Other forms of acute ischemic heart
   disease I24.8
Chronic ischemic heart disease I25.9
Essential hypertension (arterial)(benign)
   (essential)(malignant)(primary)(systemic) I10
Hypertensive heart disease with heart failure I11.0
Unspecified asthma, uncomplicated J45.909
Asthma with COPD J44.9
Other asthma J45.998
Unspecified asthma with status asthmaticus
   J45.902
Postural kyphosis M40.00
Osteoporosis M81.0
Acute otitis media H66.0
Chronic otittis media H66.3

---

   a.   What is the charge for a consultation? _____

   b.   What is the charge for CPT code 99203? _____

   c.   What is the most expensive procedure on the list? _____

   d.   Which injection is more expensive, insulin or vitamin B_{12}? _____

Match the following terms with the correct definition:

2. _____ Accounts payable

3. _____ Accounts receivable

4. _____ Adjustments

5. _____ Charges

6. _____ Payments

a. Money that is expected but has not yet been received

b. Fees applied to the patient account when services are rendered

c. The management of debt incurred and not yet paid

d. Money given to the provider in exchange for services

e. Credits posted to the patient account when the provider's fee exceeds the amount allowed stated on the EOB

7. What are the pitfalls of fee adjustments? _____

_____

_____

_____

_____

8. When a provider's fee exceeds the allowed amount stated on the explanation of benefits from the insurance company, a(n) _____ is posted to the patient account record for that difference.

9. When a patient has a credit balance on their account, what adjustment is posted to the account?

_____

_____

_____

_____

10. Describe the adjustments that are made to the patient's account when an NSF check is received by the healthcare facility.

_____

_____

_____

_____

11. What information should be included on the patient ledger? _____

_____

_____

_____

_____

B. Patient Payment Management

1. Describe five precautions for accepting checks in the healthcare facility.

   a. _____

   b. _____

   c. _____

   d. _____

   e. _____

2. Describe four precautions to take if a patient is paying with cash.

   a. _____

   b. _____

   c. _____

   d. _____

3. Describe precautions to take when a patient pays with a debit card or a credit card. _____

   _____

   _____

   _____

   _____

   _____

C. Collection Procedures

1. Briefly explain how "skips" can be traced. _____

   _____

   _____

   _____

   _____

   _____

2. When a patient account is turned over to a collection agency, what adjustment is posted to the account?

   _____

   _____

D. Accounts Payable

1. Vendors supply which of the following?
    a. Parking lot maintenance
    b. Office supplies
    c. Cleaning services
    d. Utilities
    e. All of the above

2. If an employee is paid with a(n) _____ , their _____ paycheck will always be the same dollar amount.

3. Each employee must complete a W-4 form. What information is indicated on that form? _____

    _____

    _____

    _____

    _____

E. Banking Procedures in the Ambulatory Care Setting

1. Describe the banking procedures as related to the ambulatory care setting and include the medical assistant's role with each procedure.

    a. Making bank deposits: _____

        _____

        _____

        _____

    b. Preparing a bank deposit:_____

        _____

        _____

        _____

    c. Endorsing checks: _____

        _____

        _____

        _____

    d. Writing checks:_____

        _____

        _____

        _____

2. Describe three ways to do a mobile deposit of a check.

   a. _____

   b. _____

   c. _____

3. Describe each type of endorsement.

   a. Blank endorsement: _____

   _____

   _____

   _____

   b. Restrictive endorsement: _____

   _____

   _____

   _____

   c. Special endorsement: _____

   _____

   _____

   _____

4. List three reasons a stop-payment would be done.

   a. _____

   b. _____

   c. _____

5. When preparing the bank deposit, you have the following in cash:

   (3) $50 bills
   (22) $20 bills
   (20) $10 bills
   (46) $5 bills
   (68) $1 bills

   What is the total for currency that you would record on the deposit slip? _____

F. Banking in Today's Business World

1. In the ambulatory care setting, what is the checking account used for? _____

   _____

   _____

2. In the ambulatory care setting, what is a savings account used for? _____

   _____

   _____

3. You are a medical assistant in a small practice and have been told that you now have the responsibility for paying the bills by writing out and signing the checks. What is the first action you need to take before writing out the first check?

   _____

   _____

4. Name six activities that can be done with basic online banking services.

   a. _____

   b. _____

   c. _____

   d. _____

   e. _____

   f. _____

5. List the four requirements for a check to be negotiable.

   a. _____

   b. _____

   c. _____

   d. _____

CERTIFICATION PREPARATION

Circle the correct answer.

1. Which agreement for payment plans is *not* subject to Truth in Lending Act and does *not* require a signed Truth in Lending statement?
   a. Specific agreement for fewer than four installments and finance charge
   b. Specific agreement with more than four installments and finance charge
   c. Credit card or loan specifically for health-care treatment
   d. All of the above

2. What should be considered when using a collection agency?
   a. Net back
   b. Fee percentage
   c. Fee charged by the collection agency
   d. Both a and b

3. Accounts _____ are debts incurred but not yet paid.
   a. receivable
   b. delinquent
   c. payable
   d. bookkeeping

4. The recording of business and accounting transactions is called _____.
   a. receivables
   b. payables
   c. accounting
   d. bookkeeping

5. Which does *not* conform to the general rules for telephone collections?
   a. Call only between 8 AM and 9 PM.
   b. Assume a positive attitude.
   c. Leave a message at work revealing the nature of the call.
   d. Keep the conversation brief and to the point.

6. When should checks from patients and other sources be deposited?
   a. At the same time bills are paid
   b. The same day that they are received
   c. When the bank statement is reconciled each month
   d. At the end of the week

7. Which is *not* one of the four types of endorsements?
   a. Blank
   b. Quality
   c. Restrictive
   d. Special

8. A check drawn on the bank's own account and signed by an authorized bank official is called a _____.
   a. bank draft
   b. voucher check
   c. cashier's check
   d. certified check

9. The country is divided into how many Federal Reserve districts?
   a. 8
   b. 10
   c. 12
   d. 14

10. Which endorsement includes words specifying the person to whom the endorser makes the check payable?
    a. Blank endorsement
    b. Restrictive endorsement
    c. Qualified endorsement
    d. Special endorsement

WORKPLACE APPLICATIONS

1. Mr. Sanchez comes to the desk to check out after seeing the provider. When Laura tells him that his bill is $95, he complains that he only saw the provider for 10 minutes. The fee is in accordance with evaluation and management guidelines. Explain the fees to Mr. Sanchez.

   _____

   _____

   _____

   _____

2. In Laura's new role at Walden-Martin Family Medical Clinic, she will be writing checks to take care of the accounts payable for the clinic. A practicum student has just started at the clinic and will be working with Laura for the next several days. How should Laura describe this aspect of her job?

   _____

   _____

   _____

   _____

INTERNET ACTIVITIES

1. Using online resources, research the role of an accountant. Create a poster presentation, a PowerPoint presentation, or write a paper summarizing your research. Include the following points in your project:
   a. Why most healthcare providers employ one to handle financials for the office
   b. What an accountant does for the provider
   c. How a medical assistant helps the accountant do their job

2. Using online resources, research mobile deposit technology. Create a poster presentation, a PowerPoint presentation, or write a paper summarizing your research. Include the following points in your project:
   a. Describe three different mobile deposit technologies available for healthcare facilities.
   b. Describe which technology would work best for a small provider's office, large provider's office, and physical therapy rehabilitation facility.

Procedure 16.1 Post Charges and Payments to Patient Accounts

Name _____ Date _____ Score _____

Task: To enter charges into the patient account record manually and electronically.

Equipment and Supplies:
- Patient account ledger card (Work Product 16.1)
- SimChart for the Medical Office software
- Encounter form/superbill
- Provider's fee schedule

Scenario: Ken Thomas is a returning patient of Dr. Martin. He makes his $50 copayment at the time of the office visit.

Standard: Complete the procedure and all critical steps in _____ minutes with a minimum score of 85% within two attempts (*or as indicated by the instructor*).

Scoring: Divide the points earned by the total possible points. Failure to perform a critical step, indicated by an asterisk (*), results in grade no higher than an 84% (*or as indicated by the instructor*).

Time: Began_____ Ended_____ Total minutes: _____

Steps for Posting Charges Manually:	Point Value	Attempt 1	Attempt 2
1. For new patients, create the patient account by entering the following information on a patient account ledger card: • Patient's full name, address, and at least two contact phone numbers • Date of birth • Health insurance information, including the subscriber number, group number, and effective date • Subscriber's name and date of birth (if the subscriber is not the patient) For returning patients, review the account record to see whether a balance is due. If there is a balance, bring this to the patient's attention when they come for the appointment. Respectfully explain that the provider would appreciate a payment on the previous balance before they can care for the patient.	50		
2. After seeing the patient, the provider completes the encounter form, which includes all procedures and the associated fee schedule. Using the completed encounter form (see Figure 16.1 in textbook), enter the charges manually on the ledger card for the patient's account record. Total all the charges on the encounter form for the services rendered. Then subtract the copayment made from the total charges. The previous balance, if any, is added to this new total. Use the following worksheet to calculate the new balance. The new balance due amount should be presented to the patient before they leave the healthcare facility.<table><tr><td>TOTAL CHARGES</td><td>$_____</td></tr><tr><td>Amount paid (copayment)</td><td>$_____</td></tr><tr><td>+ Previous balance (if any)</td><td>$_____</td></tr><tr><td>= New Balance Due</td><td>$_____</td></tr></table>	50*		
Total Points	100		

Steps for Posting Charges in SimChart for the Medical Office			
1. After logging into SimChart, locate the established patient by clicking on Find Patient, enter the patient's name, verify DOB, and click on the radio button. This will bring you to the Clinical Care tab. If there is no encounter shown, create an encounter by clicking on Office Visit under Info Panel on the left, select a visit type, and click on Save. Once an encounter has been created, return to the Patient Dashboard and click on the Superbill link on the right (or click on the Coding and Billing tab).	20		
2. From the Superbill area, in the Encounters Not Coded section, click on the encounter (in blue). On page 1, enter the diagnosis in the Diagnosis field and document the services provided (additional services are found on pages 2-3 of the Superbill).	20		
3. Complete the information needed on page 4 of the Superbill and submit.	20*		
4. Click on Ledger on the left and search for your patient. Once your patient has been located, click on the arrow across from the name in the ledger.	20		
5. Enter the payment received. The balance will be auto-calculated for you.	20		
Total Points	100		

Comments

CAAHEP Competencies	Step(s)
VII.P.1.a. Perform accounts receivable procedures to patient accounts including posting: charges	Manual: 2 SimChart: 2
VII.P.1.b. Perform accounts receivable procedures to patient accounts including posting: payments	Manual: 2 SimChart: 5
VII.P.2. Input accurate patient billing information in Practice Management Systems (PMS)	SimChart: 2-5
ABHES Competencies	**Step(s)**
7. Administrative Procedures c. Perform billing and collection procedures	Entire procedure

Work Product 16.1 Ledger

Ledger:

Blue Cross Blue Shield					
ID # KT4496785					
Group # 55124T					
Subscriber: Ken Thomas	Ken Thomas				
	398 Larkin Avenue				
DOB: 10/25/1961	Anytown, Anystate 12345-1234				

Date	Service Description	Charges	Payments	Adjustments	Balance

Procedure 16.2   Inform a Patient of Financial Obligations for Services Rendered

Name _____ Date _____ Score _____

Tasks: Inform a patient of his/her financial obligation and demonstrate professionalism and sensitivity when discussing the patient's billing record.

Equipment and Supplies:
- Copy of patient's insurance card (or see information in the scenario)
- Patient's account record (or see information in the scenario)

Scenario: Christi Brown is meeting with you regarding the bill she received in the mail. She called to make the appointment and she voiced her confusion about the bill. She stated that she thought her insurance covered everything. You check her record and see that she met her deductible and now needs to pay 20% of the billed amount. She owes $170.

Standard: Complete the procedure and all critical steps in _____ minutes with a minimum score of 85% within two attempts (*or as indicated by the instructor*).

Scoring: Divide the points earned by the total possible points. Failure to perform a critical step, indicated by an asterisk (*), results in grade no higher than an 84% (*or as indicated by the instructor*).

Time: Began_____ Ended_____ Total minutes: _____

Steps:	Point Value	Attempt 1	Attempt 2
1. Determine the patient's financial responsibility under the insurance plan by reviewing the copy of the patient's insurance card.	20*		
2. Determine the amount the patient owes by reviewing the patient's account record.	20*		
3. Discuss the situation with the patient. (Role-play the above scenario.)	20		
4. Demonstrate professionalism when discussing the situation with the patient. Verbal and nonverbal communication should demonstrate patience, understanding, and sensitivity. The medical assistant should refrain from inappropriate and unprofessional behavior, including eye rolling, harsh words, disrespectful comments, and similar behaviors.	20*		
5. Demonstrate professionalism by respectfully providing the patient with payment options based on the clinic's policies and what the patient can pay on a monthly basis.	20*		
Total Points	100		

Affective Behavior	Directions: Check behaviors observed during the role-play.					
	Negative, Unprofessional Behaviors	**Attempt**		**Positive, Professional Behaviors**	**Attempt**	
Tactfulness		**1**	**2**		**1**	**2**
	Rude, unkind			Courteous, professional; assertive as required		
	Disrespectful, impolite			Polite, patient		
	Negative verbal communication (e.g., harsh words, disrespectful comments)			Professional verbal communication (e.g., respectful and understanding communication)		
	Brief, abrupt			Took time with person		
	Unconcerned with person's dignity			Maintained person's dignity		
	Negative nonverbal behaviors			Positive nonverbal behaviors		
	Other:			Other:		
Empathy	Distracted; not focused on the other person			Focused full attention on the other person		
	Judgmental attitude; not accepting attitude			Nonjudgmental, accepting attitude		
	Failed to clarify what the person verbally or nonverbally communicated			Used summarizing or paraphrasing to clarify what the person verbally or nonverbally communicated		
	Failed to acknowledge what the person communicated			Acknowledged what the person communicated		
	Rude, discourteous			Pleasant and courteous		
	Disregarded the person's dignity and rights			Maintained the person's dignity and rights		
	Other:			Other:		

Grading for Affective Behaviors		Point Value	Attempt 1	Attempt 2
Does not meet Expectation	• Response was insensitive and/or disrespectful. • Student demonstrated more than 2 negative, unprofessional behaviors during the interaction.	0		
Needs Improvement	• Response was insensitive and/or disrespectful. • Student demonstrated 1 or 2 negative, unprofessional behaviors during the interaction.	0		
Meets Expectation	• Response was sensitive and respectful; no negative, unprofessional behaviors observed. • More practice is needed for behavior to appear natural and for student to appear comfortable and at ease.	15		
Occasionally Exceeds Expectation	• Response was sensitive and respectful; no negative, unprofessional behaviors observed. • At times student appeared comfortable and at ease; but more practice is needed for behavior to become natural and consistent with a professional medical assistant.	15		
Always Exceeds Expectation	• Response was sensitive and respectful; no negative, unprofessional behaviors observed. • Student's behaviors appeared natural and comfortable. Behaviors are consistent with a professional medical assistant.	15		

Comments

CAAHEP Competencies	Step(s)
VII.P.3. Inform a patient of financial obligations for services rendered	3
A.7. Demonstrate tactfulness	5
A.3. Demonstrate empathy for patients' concerns	4
ABHES Competencies	**Step(s)**
7. Administrative Procedures c. Perform billing and collection procedures	Entire procedure

Procedure 16.3   Post Payments and Adjustments to Patient Account

Name _____   **Date** _____   **Score** _____

Task: To post payments and adjustments to patient accounts accurately.

Equipment and Supplies:
- Patient account ledger card or SimChart for the Medical Office software

Scenario: Monique Jones (06/23/1985) was seen 6 months ago for a wellness visit and lab work. Her insurance had lapsed, and she is completely responsible for the bill. She did not make any payments and resisted all attempts at collection of the balance of $172.00. Her account was turned over to the collection agency and they were able to collect the balance in full. The collection agency retains 50% of what they collect as payment. Post the collection agency payment and adjustment to her account.

Standard: Complete the procedure and all critical steps in _____ minutes with a minimum score of 85% within two attempts (*or as indicated by the instructor*).

Scoring: Divide the points earned by the total possible points. Failure to perform a critical step, indicated by an asterisk (*), results in grade no higher than an 84% (*or as indicated by the instructor*).

Time: Began_____ Ended_____ Total minutes: _____

Steps:	Point Value	Attempt 1	Attempt 2
1. Look up the ledger card for the patient account (or the patient ledger in SimChart). Confirm that you have the correct patient account.	30		
2. Post an adjustment to reverse the adjustment done when the account was turned over to the collection agency.	30		
3. Post the payment and adjustment that reflects the actual dollar amount received from the collection agency and the amount that was retained as payment.	40*		
Total Points	100		

Comments

CAAHEP Competencies	Step(s)
VII.P.1.b. Perform accounts receivable procedures to patient accounts including posting: payments	3
VII.P.1.c. Perform accounts receivable procedures to patient accounts including posting: adjustments	2, 3
VII.P.2. Input accurate patient billing information in Practice Management Systems (PMS)	2, 3
ABHES Competencies	**Step(s)**
7. Administrative Procedures c. Perform billing and collection procedures	Entire procedure

Procedure 16.4 End-of-Day Reconciliation

Name _____ Date _____ Score _____

Task: To complete the end-of-day reconciliation including preparing a bank deposit for currency and checks.

Equipment and Supplies:
- Daily transaction report (see scenario)
- Checks and currency for deposit (see scenario)
- Check for endorsement
- Calculator
- Paper method: bank deposit slip (Work Product 16.2)
- Electronic method: SimChart for the Medical Office (SCMO)

Scenario:
The following payments were received today at Walden-Martin Family Medical Clinic:

Cash:
Reuven Ahmad - $25.00
Amma Patel - $15.00
Ken Thomas - $40.00
Maude Crawford - $25.00
Al Neviaser - $30.00

At the start of the day, the cash drawer had 10 - $1 bills, 10 - $5 bills, 10 - $10 bills, 10 - $20 bills for a total of $360.00. At the end of the day, there is a total of $495.00.

Checks:
Julia Berkley - #3456 for $89.00
Jana Green - #6954 for $136.00
Kyle Reeves - #9854 for $1366.65
Truong Tran - #8546 for $653.36
Quinton Brown - #9865 for $890.22

The healthcare facility's name is Walden-Martin Family Medical Clinic, account number 123-456-78910, and the bank is Clear Water Bank, Anytown, Anystate.

Credit Cards:
Tai Yan - $150.00
Ella Rainwater - $300.00
Diego Miller - $75.00
Carl Bowden - $25.00
Noemi Rodriguez – $45.00

Daily Transaction Report:

Date	Patient	Account	Cash	Check	Debit/Credit
11/6/20XX	Reuven Ahmad	11872534	$25.00		
11/6/20XX	Amma Patel	12156063	$15.00		
11/6/20XX	Ken Thomas	11644627	$40.00		
11/6/20XX	Maude Crawford	12568850	$25.00		
11/6/20XX	Al Neviaser	11279412	$30.00		
11/6/20XX	Julia Berkley	12062515		$89.00	
11/6/20XX	Jana Green	10944532		$136.00	
11/6/20XX	Kyle Reeves	12073635		$1366.65	
11/6/20XX	Truong Tran	11726005		$650.36	
11/6/20XX	Quinton Brown	11272882		$890.22	
11/6/20XX	Tai Yan	12658901			$150.00
11/6/20XX	Ella Rainwater	11885104			$300.00
11/6/20XX	Diego Lupez	12530423			$75.00
11/6/20XX	Carl Bowden	11265329			$25.00
11/6/20XX	Noemi Rodriquez	11766543			$45.00
Total			$135.00	$3132.23	$595.00

Standard: Complete the procedure and all critical steps in _____ minutes with a minimum score of 85% within two attempts (*or as indicated by the instructor*).

Scoring: Divide the points earned by the total possible points. Failure to perform a critical step, indicated by an asterisk (*), results in grade no higher than an 84% (*or as indicated by the instructor*).

Time: Began_____ Ended_____ Total minutes: _____

Steps:	Point Value	Attempt 1	Attempt 2
1. Complete the starting cash portion of the cash reconciliation form (see Figure 16.12) using the information from the scenario.	5		
2. Complete the ending cash portion of the cash reconciliation form using the information from the scenario.	5		
3. Compare the cash taken in from the cash reconciliation form to the cash total from the daily transaction report. If the totals do not match, compare the individual transactions and determine where the error occurred.	10*		
4. Compare the total from the credit card processing terminal and the debit/credit card total from the daily transaction report. if the totals do not match compare the individual transactions and determine where the error occurred.	10*		
5. Gather the documents to be used to prepare the bank deposit. For the electronic method, enter the Simulation Playground in SCMO. Click on the Form Repository icon. On the INFO PANEL, click on Office Forms and then select Bank Deposit Slip.	5		

6.	Enter the date on the deposit slip.	**5**		
7.	Using the calculator, calculate the amount of currency to be deposited. Enter the amount in the CURRENCY line, completing the dollar and cent boxes.	**5**		
8.	Enter the total amount in the TOTAL CASH line.	**5**		
9.	For each check to be deposited, enter the check number, the dollars, and cents. List each check on a separate line.	**10***		
10.	Calculate the total to be deposited and enter the number in the TOTAL FROM ATTACHED LIST box.	**10***		
11.	Enter the number of items deposited in the TOTAL ITEMS box.	**5**		
12.	Before completing the deposit slip, verify the check amounts listed and recalculate the totals. For the electronic method, click on SAVE.	**10***		
13.	Place a restrictive endorsement on the check(s).	**5**		
14.	Compare the total from the deposit slip to the total for checks from the daily transaction report. If the totals do not match, compare the individual transactions and determine where the error occurred.	**10***		
	Total Points	**100**		

Comments

CAAHEP Competencies	Step(s)
VII.C.1.f. Define the following bookkeeping terms: end of day reconciliation	Entire procedure
ABHES Competencies	**Step(s)**
7. Administrative Procedures c. Perform billing and collection procedures	Entire procedure

Work Product 16.2   Bank Deposit Slip

DEPOSIT TICKET

WALDEN-MARTIN FAMLY MEDICAL CLINIC
1234 ANYSTREET
ANYTOWN, ANYSTATE 12345

DEPOSITS MAY NOT BE AVAILABLE FOR
IMMEDIATE WITHDRAWAL

Clear Water Bank
Anytown, Anystate

ACCOUNT NUMBER: 123-456-78910

Endorse & List Checks Separately

DATE _____	Dollars	Cents
CURRENCY		
COIN		
TOTAL CASH		
1.		
2.		
3.		
4.		
5.		
6.		
7.		
8.		
9.		
10.		
11.		
12.		
Less Cash Returned		
Total Items	Total Deposit	

Advanced Roles in Administration

chapter

17

CAAHEP Competencies	Assessments
V.C.2 Identify communication barriers	Skills and Concepts – D. 4
X.C.7.i. Define: risk management	Skills and Concepts – B. 2
X.C.10a Identify: Health Information Technology for Economic and Clinical Health (HITECH) Act	Skills and Concepts – F. 1

VOCABULARY REVIEW

Using the word pool on the right, find the correct word to match the definition. Write the word on the line after the definition.

1. The environment where something is created or takes shape; a base on which to build _____

2. Obeying, obliging, or yielding _____

3. Sticking together tightly _____

4. Evidence of authority, status, rights, entitlement to privileges _____

5. Contains all documents related to an individual's employment _____

6. A relationship of harmony and accord between the patient and the healthcare professional _____

7. To appoint a person as a representative _____

8. A term referring to actions taken by management to keep good employees _____

9. General agreement _____

10. A steady employee whom a new staff member can approach with questions and concerns _____

11. Things that incite or spur to action; rewards or reasons for performing a task _____

12. Slighting; having a negative or degrading tone _____

13. Able to pay all debts _____

Word Pool
- consensus
- credential
- solvent
- matrix
- delegate
- incentive
- cohesive
- disparaging
- mentor
- retention
- human resources file
- compliant
- rapport

ABBREVIATIONS

Write out what each of the following abbreviations stands for.

1. HR _____

2. EHR _____

3. OCR _____

4. HITECH _____

5. PHI _____

6. ePHI _____

7. OSHA _____

SKILLS AND CONCEPTS

Answer the following questions. Write your answer on the line or in the space provided.

A. Medical Office Management

1. Describe the traits of a successful medical office manager. _____

_____

_____

_____

_____

_____

_____

2. Describe a good relationship between a manager and their employees. _____

_____

_____

_____

_____

_____

_____

B. Office Management Responsibilities

1. List five office management responsibilities.

   a. _____

   b. _____

   c. _____

   d. _____

   e. _____

2. Risk management involves which of the following?
   a. Identifying, planning, and implementing strategies to minimize the risk of a lawsuit
   b. Creating policies and procedures
   c. Reviewing incident reports
   d. All of the above

C. Office Management Skills
There are 5 Cs of good communication. Match the C with the correct definition.

1. _____ Get to the point and do not wonder off topic.
2. _____ Be friendly, open, and honest.
3. _____ Use terms in the right way and use proper grammar.
4. _____ Use words that accurately convey your meaning.
5. _____ Provide the same message day to day.

   a. clear
   b. concise
   c. consistent
   d. correct
   e. courteous

6. Characteristics of a good listener include all of the following *except*
   a. remain nonjudgmental and neutral.
   b. do not allow for silence.
   c. use appropriate eye contact.
   d. avoid distractions.
   e. all of the above.

7. When using the ABC method of time management, a(n) _____ is given to the most urgent or important task, a(n) _____ is given to less urgent or important tasks, and a(n) _____ is given those tasks that are the least important.

8. When staff members collaborate as a team in the healthcare workplace, communication _____ .

9. When communication improves in the healthcare workplace, medical errors are _____ and patient satisfaction _____ .

10. Employee morale can be improved when an office manager communicates openly and honestly through
    a. staff meetings.
    b. emails.
    c. memos.
    d. all of the above.

Match the following barriers with the way to overcome them.

11. _____ Physical separation barrier

12. _____ Language barriers

13. _____ Status barriers

14. _____ Gender difference barriers

15. _____ Cultural diversity barriers

a. Know that all employees, regardless of gender, feel empowered to communicate openly with others.

b. Encourage awareness and acceptance of everyone's language and culture differences will strengthen the team's communication

c. To help the team embrace the cultural differences among the members and educating the team on the differences can help promote understanding and cohesion.

d. Using technology (e.g., videoconferencing and webcams) can help employees interact and strengthen communication.

e. Promote awareness and acceptance that everyone counts and every position on the team is important

D. Finding the Right Employee for the Job

1. Effective methods for finding new employees include which of the following?
   a. Have medical assistants complete their practicum at the healthcare facility.
   b. Advertise on the local job boards.
   c. Post the job on the facility's website and link to other job boards.
   d. All of the above
   e. Only a and c

2. Which of the following is an illegal interview question?
   a. What motivates you to succeed?
   b. Why did you leave your last job?
   c. Do you have any children?
   d. Are you willing to work more than 40 hours a week?

3. Laws that affect employment include which of the following?
   a. Fair Labor Standards Act
   b. HIPAA
   c. Occupational Safety and Health Act
   d. Only a and c
   e. All of the above

4. State standards for minimum wage and overtime pay were established in the _____ Act.

5. Conditions affecting employees' safety and health in the workplace were established in the _____ Act.

6. _____ Act requires employers of 50 or more employees to offer up to 12 weeks of unpaid, job-protected leave to eligible employees for the birth of a child, an adoption, or a personal or family illness.

7. Follow-up activities after the interview include checking _____.

E: Working with New and Established Employees

1. Documentation for new employees would include which of the following?
   a. Form I-9
   b. W-4
   c. W-2
   d. a and b

2. A critical error with new employees is failing to provide them with a fair _____ and _____.

3. One type of benefit often offered to employees, where the employer pays a percentage of the employee's health insurance _____ premium is _____.

4. When providing remote/virtual training, the employer need to keep which of the following in mind?
   a. Equipment needs
   b. Internet access
   c. Learning styles
   d. All of the above

F. Policies and Procedures

1. List five items that should be included in a personnel policy manual.

   a. _____

   b. _____

   c. _____

   d. _____

   e. _____

2. _____ is defined by the U.S. Equal Employment Opportunity Commission as unwelcome sexual advances, requests for sexual favors, and other verbal and physical harassment of sexual nature.

3. The act that expanded on HIPAA is _____.

G. Generating and Using Reports

1. _____ is used to generate reports used to ensure that patients are getting all of the care that they need, and that the health care facility remains healthy financially.

2. Clinical reports that can be generated include
   a. symptoms of disease/illness.
   b. medications.
   c. laboratory tests.
   d. encounter summary.
   e. all of the above

3. _____ are used to make administrative decisions within a healthcare facility.

4. Part of _____ is when the practice management software uses claim scrubbers to evaluate the data entered for claim submission.

5. The process of extracting usable data from a larger set of raw data is referred to as _____.

CERTIFICATION PREPARATION
Circle the correct answer.

1. Which is a quality of an effective leader or office manager?
   a. Has a sense of fairness
   b. Has good communication skills
   c. Uses good judgment
   d. All of the above

2. Something that spurs an individual to action or rewards an individual for performing a task is called
   a. morale.
   b. incentive.
   c. appraisal.
   d. circumvention.

3. Which of the following protects the employee against unsafe workplaces?
   a. Fair Labor Standards Act
   b. Family and Medical Leave Act
   c. Occupational Safety and Health Act
   d. Age Discrimination Act

4. Some managers assign a person to assist new employees during the initial probationary period; this person is called a
   a. mentor.
   b. supervisor.
   c. coworker.
   d. subordinate.

5. A group of employees who stick together during difficult times could be called
   a. cohesive.
   b. adaptive.
   c. affable.
   d. meticulous.

6. Which subjects *cannot* be discussed in a job interview?
   a. Religion
   b. Work history
   c. Previous terminations of employment
   d. None of the above

7. The process of inciting a person to some action or behavior is called
   a. a reprimand.
   b. motivation.
   c. circumvention.
   d. an appraisal.

8. Which is a strong method of improving employee morale and encouraging outstanding performance?
   a. Incentives
   b. Recognition
   c. Fraternizing with subordinates outside work
   d. All of the above

9. Which is critical for good communication and smooth operation of a medical facility?
   a. Scheduling activities that involve the families of employees
   b. Holding regular staff meetings and sending regular emails and memos
   c. Shielding employees from negative information
   d. All of the above

10. Which employee behavior is grounds for immediate dismissal without warning?
   a. Embezzlement
   b. Insubordination
   c. Violation of patient confidentiality
   d. All of the above

WORKPLACE APPLICATIONS

1. Create a job description or job posting for a "dream" job of your choice. Make sure to include the duties, required education, and other details typically found in postings.

   _____

   _____

   _____

   _____

   _____

   _____

2. Create a plan of how to screen applications and résumés for a medical assistant job in a family practice department. Describe the process you would use to evidentially identify the few applicants who should be interviewed.

   _____

   _____

   _____

   _____

   _____

   _____

   _____

   _____

   _____

   _____

INTERNET ACTIVITIES

1. Using online resources, research team-building exercises designed to promote and build teamwork for a group of employees. Create a poster presentation, a PowerPoint presentation, or write a paper summarizing your research. Include the following points in your project:
   a. Describe three team-building activities.
   b. Why do you think each of these activities will promote and build teamwork?
   c. How would you make sure that these activities are relevant to working in healthcare?

2. Using online resources, research the I-9 form. Create a poster presentation, a PowerPoint presentation, or write a paper summarizing your research. Include the following points in your project:
   a. Describe the purpose of the form.
   b. Summarize the process for completing the I-9 form.
   c. Describe acceptable documentation used to complete the form.

Introduction to Medical Terminology and Anatomy

chapter

18

CAAHEP Competencies	Assessment
I.C.1. Identify structural organization of the human body	Skills and Concepts D. 11-14; Certification Preparation – 6; Case Scenario – 4
I.C.2. Identify body systems	Skills and Concepts – B. 14-25
I.C.3.a. Identify: body planes	Skills and Concepts – E. 2-5; Certification Preparation – 7
I.C.3.b. Identify: directional terms	Skills and Concepts – E. 6-15; Certification Preparation – 8
I.C.3.c. Identify: quadrants	Skills and Concepts – E. 25-28; Certification Preparation – 9
I.C.3.d. Identify: body cavities	Skills and Concepts – E. 17-24; Certification Preparation – 10
I.C.4. Identify major organs in each body system	Skills and Concepts – B. 1-13
V.C.8.a. Identify the following related to body systems: medical terms	Skills and Concepts – B. 26-36; C. 1-70

ABHES Competencies	Assessment
3. Medical Terminology a. Define and use the entire basic structure of medical terminology and be able to accurately identify the correct context (i.e., root, prefix, suffix, combinations, spelling and definitions)	Skills and Concepts – A. 1-61; B. 26-36; C. 1-70; Certification Preparation – 1-5; Workplace Applications – 1-2; Internet Activities – 1-2
3b. Build and dissect medical terminology from roots and suffixes to understand the word element combinations	Skills and Concepts – C. 1-48
3c. Apply medical terminology for each specialty	Skills and Concepts – B. 26-36; C. 1-70; Certification Preparation – 3, 5; Workplace Applications – 2; Internet Activities – 2
3d. Define and use medical abbreviations when appropriate and acceptable	Abbreviations – 1-6

VOCABULARY REVIEW

Using the word pool on the right, find the correct word to match the definition. Write the word on the line after the definition.

Group A

1. An abbreviation formed from the first letter of each word of a phrase and pronounced as a word _____

2. A word that come from the name of a person, place, or thing associated with the word _____

3. A shortened version of a word or phrase _____

4. Picture that represents a word or phrase _____

5. A word part found at the beginning of the word _____

6. A word part found at the end of the word _____

7. A word part that is the foundation of the term _____

8. A vowel that links the root to the suffix or a root to a root _____

9. A root and a combining vowel _____

10. A steady state that is created by all the body systems working together to provide a consistent and unvarying internal environment _____

Word Pool
- abbreviation
- acronym
- combining form
- combining vowel
- eponym
- homeostasis
- prefix
- root
- suffix
- symbol

Group B

1. Outer covering surrounding the cell that allows certain substances to enter the cell and blocks other substances _____

2. Study of disease _____

3. Wavelike motion _____

4. The microscopic study of body tissues _____

5. Rod-shaped structures found in the cell's nucleus; contain genetic information _____

6. Tests and procedures used to help diagnose or monitor a condition _____

7. A group of similar cells from the same source that together carry out a specific function _____

8. Structures inside of the cell _____

9. Jelly-like substance the surrounds the nucleus and fills the cells _____

10. A cell division process by which two daughter cells are formed from one parent cell _____

Word Pool
- chromosomes
- cytoplasm
- diagnostic procedures
- histology
- mitosis
- organelles
- pathology
- peristalsis
- plasma membrane
- tissue

Group C

1. A broad, dome-shaped muscle used for breathing that separates the thoracic and abdominopelvic cavities
   _____

2. Work to prevent changes in the pH _____

3. Reflects the number of newly diagnosed people with the disease
   _____

4. The cause of the disorder or disease _____

5. How often the disease occurs _____

6. A severe, sudden onset of a disease _____

7. Something that is only perceived by the patient; called *subjective data* _____

8. Substances that stimulate the production of an antibody when introduced into the body _____

9. A disease-causing organism _____

10. Something that is measured or observed by others; called *objective data* _____

Word Pool
- acute
- antigens
- buffers
- diaphragm
- etiology
- incidence
- pathogen
- prevalence
- signs
- symptoms

Group D

1. Substances created by microorganisms, plants, or animals and poisonous to humans _____

2. A rapidly dividing cancer cell that has little to no similarity to normal cells _____

3. A physician specially trained in the nature and cause of disease
   _____

4. Process of viewing living tissue that has been removed for the purpose of diagnosis or treatment _____

5. To spread from one part of the body (the primary tumor) to another part of the body forming a secondary tumor
   _____

6. Protein substances produced in the blood or tissues in response to a specific antigen that destroy or weaken the antigen
   _____

7. Describes how malignant tissue or cells looks like the normal tissue or cells it came from _____

8. A specially trained physician who diagnoses and treats cancer
   _____

9. Refers to how abnormal the malignant cells look
   _____

10. Refers to the extent of the cancer, including the size and if it has spread _____

Word Pool
- anaplastic
- antibodies
- biopsy
- differentiated
- grade
- metastasize
- oncologist
- pathologist
- toxins
- stage

ABBREVIATIONS

Write out what each of the following abbreviations stands for.

1. BP _____

2. CBC _____

3. HTN _____

4. AIDS _____

5. HIPAA _____

6. SIDS_____

SKILLS AND CONCEPTS

Answer the following questions.

A. Medical Terminology

1. Write the meaning of the following symbols.

    a. $\bar{s}$ _____

    b. $\bar{p}$ _____

    c. $\bar{a}$ _____

For the following word parts, write the definition.

2. ec- _____

3. contra-_____

4. end- _____

5. brady- _____

6. endo-_____

7. anti- _____

8. dia- _____

9. epi-_____

10. ante- _____

11. ana- _____

12. dys- _____

13. macro-_____

14. per- _____

15. hypo- _____

16. supra- _____

17. hyper- _____

18. megalo- _____

19. micro- _____

20. tachy- _____

21. mal- _____

22. -ac _____

23. -is _____

24. -stasis _____

25. -ary _____

26. -tension _____

27. -phagia _____

28. -al _____

29. -ism _____

30. -pathy _____

31. -plegia _____

32. -ent _____

33. -osis _____

34. -pnea _____

35. -ic _____

36. -dipsia _____

For the following definitions, write the medical terminology word part.

37. out _____

38. within _____

39. outside of _____

40. between _____

41. near, beside _____

42. four _____

43. together, with _____

44. beyond _____

45. one _____

46. through, across _____

47. instrument to record _____

48. instrument to view _____

49. tumor, mass _____

50. abnormal condition of hardening _____

51. process of, condition _____

52. process of recording _____

53. process of viewing _____

54. surgical fixation _____

55. to cut _____

56. new opening _____

57. one who specializes _____

58. study of _____

59. towards _____

60. crushing _____

61. suture repair _____

B. Combining Forms
Match the body system to the correct major organs and structures it includes.

1. _____ Mouth, tongue, teeth, pharynx, esophagus, stomach, small intestine, large intestine, liver, gallbladder, pancreas, and appendix

2. _____ Ovaries, fallopian tubes, uterus, vagina, vulva, mammary glands, and ovum

3. _____ Brain, spinal cord, neurons, neuroglia cells, peripheral nerves, and autonomic nerves

4. _____ Heart, valves, arteries, arterioles, veins, and venules

5. _____ Lymph, lymph vessels, lymph nodes, thymus, tonsils, spleen, lymphocytes, and antibodies

6. _____ Skin, subcutaneous tissue, sweat and sebaceous glands, hair, nails, and sense receptors

7. _____ Pituitary gland, pineal gland, hypothalamus, thyroid gland, pancreas, adrenal cortex and medulla, parathyroid gland, thymus gland, ovaries, and testes

8. _____ Bones, joints, tendons, ligaments, and cartilage

9. _____ Epididymis vas deferens, prostate gland, testes, scrotum, penis, urethra, and sperm

10. _____ Nephron unit, kidneys, ureters, bladder, and urethra

11. _____ Nose, sinuses, pharynx, larynx, trachea, bronchi, lungs, bronchioles, and alveoli

12. _____ Eyes, ears, taste buds, olfactory receptors, and sensory receptors

13. _____ Muscles

a. cardiovascular system
b. endocrine system
c. gastrointestinal system
d. integumentary system
e. lymphatic and immune system
f. muscular system
g. nervous system
h. reproductive system (female)
i. reproductive system (male)
j. respiratory system
k. sensory system
l. urinary system
m. skeletal system

Match the description of the body system to the correct body system.

14. _____ Produces hormones and is involved with reproduction.

15. _____ Produces hormones that circulate in the blood to target tissues that stimulate a particular action.

16. _____ Protects the body, acts as a sense organ, helps to retain body fluids, protects against infection, and helps regulate the body temperature.

17. _____ Involved with movement, regulation of blood calcium, and the formation of blood cells.

18. _____ Transport materials in the blood through the body. The components in the blood also fight infections and form clots.

19. _____ Breaks down, digests, and absorbs nutrients from food eaten.

20. _____ Controls body structures to maintain homeostasis and receives and processes information from other body structures.

21. _____ Eliminates nitrogenous waste and maintains the electrolyte, water, and acid-base balances.

22. _____ Delivers oxygen to the cells and removes carbon dioxide from the body.

23. _____ Gathers information through the sense of vision, hearing, balance, taste, and smell.

24. _____ Involved with heat production, and muscle contraction, tone, and posture.

25. _____ Maintains fluid balance, provides immunity to some diseases, and protects the internal environment of the body.

a. cardiovascular system
b. endocrine system
c. gastrointestinal system
d. integumentary system
e. lymphatic and immune system
f. skeletal system
g. nervous system
h. reproductive system
i. respiratory system
j. sensory system
k. urinary system
l. muscular system

For the following questions, write your answer on the line.

26. For the following cardiovascular system word parts, write the definition.

   a. aort/o _____

   b. arteri/o _____

   c. coron/o _____

   d. phleb/o _____

   e. plasm/o _____

27. For the following endocrine system word parts, write the definition.

   a. hypophys/o _____

   b. oophor/o _____

   c. pancreat/o _____

   d. parathyroid/o _____

   e. thyroid/o _____

28. For the following gastrointestinal system word parts, write the definition.

    a. col/o _____

    b. esophag/o_____

    c. gastr/o_____

    d. hepat/o _____

    e. pancreat/o _____

29. For the following integumentary system word parts, write the definition.

    a. cutane/o _____

    b. derm/o _____

    c. onych/o_____

    d. pil/o_____

    e. seb/o _____

30. For the following lymphatic system and immune system word parts, write the definition.

    a. lymph/o _____

    b. lymphangi/o _____

    c. myel/o_____

    d. splen/o _____

    e. thym/o _____

31. For the following musculoskeletal system word parts, write the definition.

    a. arthr/o_____

    b. crani/o_____

    c. ligament/o _____

    d. lumb/o _____

    e. my/o _____

    f. oste/o _____

    g. stern/o_____

    h. ten/o _____

    i. thorac/o _____

    j. vertebr/o_____

32. For the following nervous system word parts, write the definition.

    a. cerebell/o _____

    b. cerebr/o _____

    c. encephal/o _____

    d. myel/o _____

    e. neur/o _____

33. For the following reproductive system word parts, write the definition.

    a. cervic/o _____

    b. colp/o _____

    c. mamm/o _____

    d. orch/o _____

    e. uter/o _____

34. For the following respiratory system word parts, write the definition.

    a. bronch/o _____

    b. cyan/o _____

    c. nas/o _____

    d. pulmon/o _____

    e. sin/o _____

35. For the following sensory system word parts, write the definition.

    a. audi/o _____

    b. blephar/o _____

    c. corne/o _____

    d. ot/o _____

    e. scler/o _____

36. For the following urinary system word parts, write the definition.

    a. cyst/o _____

    b. vesic/o _____

    c. nephr/o _____

    d. ren/o _____

    e. ureter/o _____

C. Building, Defining, and Pronouncing Medical Terms

In the table, combine the word parts and write in the new word and its definition.

	Combining Form	Suffix	New Word	Definition
1.	arteri/o	-stenosis		
2.	cardi/o	-megaly		
3.	angi/o	-oma		
4.	angi/o	-graphy		
5.	phleb/o	-itis		
6.	epiglott/o	-itis		
7.	valv/o	-itis		
8.	arteri/o	-ole		
9.	pneumon/o	-ia		
10.	blephar/o	-itis		
11.	mast/o	-itis		
12.	an/o	-plasty		
13.	col/o	-stomy		
14.	col/o	-scopy		
15.	thorac/o	-algia		
16.	myel/o	-oma		
17.	trache/o	-stenosis		
18.	cyst/o	-itis		
19.	enter/o	-rrhaphy		
20.	glycos/o	-uria		
21.	chondr/o	-malacia		
22.	ankyl/o	-osis		
23.	scler/o	-malacia		
24.	appendic/o	-itis		

Combining Form	Suffix	New Word	Definition
25. irid/o	-plegia		
26. abdomen/o	-centesis		
27. col/o	-ectomy		
28. gastr/o	-stomy		
29. gingiv/o	-ectomy		
30. nephr/o	-oma		
31. rhin/o	-rrhagia		

Prefix	Combining Form	Suffix	New Word	Definition
32. endo-	cardi/o	-tis		
33. dys-	men/o	-rrhea		
34. brady-	cardi/o	-ia		
35. tachy-	cardi/o	-ia		
36. a-	men/o	-rrhea		
37. inter-	ventricul/o	-ar		

Combining Form	Combining Form	Suffix	New Word	Definition
38. my/o	cardi/o	-tis		
39. rhin/o	myc/o	-osis		
40. gastr/o	enter/o	-tis		

For the following words, split the word apart into word parts. Label each word part (e.g., prefix, suffix, and combining form). Define each word part.

41. efferent _____

42. proximal _____

43. unilateral _____

44. ventral _____

45. popliteal _____

46. gluteal _____

47. antecubital _____

48. ocular _____

For each of the following words, write the pluralized word on the line.

49. septum _____

50. ruga _____

51. fimbria _____

52. testis _____

53. alveolus _____

54. sulcus _____

55. canthus _____

56. conjunctiva _____

57. bacterium _____

58. labium _____

59. coccus _____

60. embolus _____

61. prognosis _____

62. scapula _____

63. acetabulum _____

64. diverticulum _____

65. axilla _____

66. glomerulus _____

67. phalanx _____

68. meniscus _____

69. verruca vulgaris _____

70. stratum _____

D. Structural Organization of the Body

1. The _____ is the basic unit of life.

2. Relate each of the parts of a cell to something found in a city. For instance, the plasma membrane would be the city limits or the walls of the city. In the space provided, draw the "Cell City" and label the structures. Use the cell parts listed in the textbook.

3. _____ is the process where one cell splits into two identical daughter cells.

4. At what stage of mitosis is the genetic information replicated?_____

Match the phases of mitosis with the correct description.

5. _____ Spindle fibers pull the sister chromatids apart.

6. _____ The membrane around the nucleus starts to break down. Centrioles produce spindle fibers and start to move toward opposite sides of the cell.

7. _____ The nucleus reforms around each set of chromosomes. The cell continues to separate into two daughter cells.

8. _____ Each pair of chromatids lines up, and each chromatid is attached to a spindle fiber.

a. prophase
b. metaphase
c. anaphase
d. telophase

Write your answer on the line.

9. _____ is the jelly-like substance that surrounds the organelles and fills the cell.

10. _____ attach to the endoplasmic reticulum, giving the ER a rough appearance.

11. _____ are a group of similar cells from the same source that together carry out a specific function.

12. _____ is a structure composed of two or more types of tissue.

13. A(n) _____ is composed of several organs and their related structures.

14. Put the following in order from the simplest to the most complex: organism, organs, cells, body systems, tissue

_____

E. Anatomical Position, Planes, Cavities and Quadrants

1. The _____ is a standard frame of reference. This means the body stands erect with the face forward, arms at the sides, palms forward, and toes pointed forward.

2. _____ are imaginary cuts or sections through the body.

3. The _____ or frontal plane divides the body into front and back portions.

4. The _____ or median plane divides the body into equal right and left halves.

5. The _____ or horizontal plane divides the body horizontally into an upper part and a lower part.

Match the following terms with the correct definition.

6. _____ Opposite of anterior and refers to the back
7. _____ Pertains to the midline
8. _____ Carrying toward a structure
9. _____ Front of body
10. _____ Far from the origin or farthest from the trunk of the body
11. _____ Towards the surface of the body
12. _____ Near the origin or toward the trunk of the body
13. _____ Away from the surface of the body
14. _____ Downward
15. _____ Opposite side

a. deep
b. anterior or ventral
c. interior
d. posterior or dorsal
e. afferent
f. distal
g. contralateral
h. medial
i. proximal
j. superficial

Write your answers on the line.

16. Using the directional and positional terms listed in this chapter, write four sentences that use a term in reference to the body. Use four different terms. Example: The fingers are distal to the elbows.

_____

_____

_____

_____

Match the cavity with the correct description.

17. _____ Contains the heart, lungs, esophagus, and trachea
18. _____ Contains the abdominal and pelvic cavities
19. _____ Contains the spinal cord
20. _____ Contains the thoracic and abdominopelvic cavities
21. _____ Contains the brain
22. _____ Contains the cranial and spinal cavities
23. _____ Contains the stomach, liver, gallbladder, and intestines
24. _____ Contains the urinary bladder and the reproductive organs

a. dorsal body cavity
b. ventral body cavity
c. cranial cavity
d. spinal cavity
e. thoracic cavity
f. abdominopelvic cavity
g. pelvic cavity
h. abdominal cavity

Match the quadrant with the organs found within the quadrant.

25. _____ The appendix, cecum, right ovary, right ureter, right spermatic cord, large intestine (ascending colon), right kidney
26. _____ The stomach, spleen, left lobe of liver, pancreas, left kidney, and large intestine (transverse and descending colon)
27. _____ The small intestine, large intestine (descending and sigmoid colon), left ovary, left ureter, left spermatic cord, and left kidney
28. _____ The right lobe of liver, gallbladder, right kidney, small intestine (duodenum), large intestine (ascending and transverse colon), head of pancreas

a. left upper quadrant
b. right upper quadrant
c. left lower quadrant
d. right lower quadrant

F. Acid-Base Balance

1. A solution with a pH under 7 is a(n) _____ solution.

2. A solution with a pH over 7 is a(n) _____ solution.

3. For the body to maintain homeostasis, a pH between _____ and _____ must be maintained in the blood.

4. Which of the following helps maintain the acid-base balance in the body?
   a. Urinary system
   b. Respiratory system
   c. Chemical buffers
   d. All of the above

G. Pathology Basics
Match the definition with the correct term.

1. _____ Something that is measured or observed by others; called *objective data*
2. _____ How often the disease occurs
3. _____ A severe, sudden onset of a disease
4. _____ Something that is only perceived by the patient; called *subjective data*
5. _____ A disease, disorder, or syndrome that lasts longer than 6 months
6. _____ Death
7. _____ Reflects the number of newly diagnosed people with the disease
8. _____ Illness

a. prevalence
b. incidence
c. morbidity
d. mortality
e. acute
f. chronic
g. sign
h. symptom

H. Causes of Disease
Match the definition with the correct term.

1. _____ Cellular structure is the same as the surrounding tissue. The tumor is encapsulated and grows slowly.
2. _____ Have anaplastic changes and are poorly differentiated; infiltrates and metastasizes. May grow at a slow, rapid, or very rapid rate.
3. _____ Refers to how abnormal the malignant cells look.
4. _____ A disease that cannot be transmitted from one person to another.
5. _____ Refers to the extent of the cancer, including the size and if it has spread.
6. _____ A disease that can be transmitted from one person to another.

a. grade
b. communicable disease
c. stage
d. benign tumor
e. malignant tumor
f. noncommunicable disease

CERTIFICATION PREPARATION
Circle the correct answer.

1. What does the prefix "sub-" mean?
   a. Forward, before
   b. Before, in front of
   c. Upward, above
   d. Under, less than

2. What does the suffix "-osis" mean?
   a. Tumor, mass
   b. Softening
   c. Abnormal condition
   d. Disease condition

3. What does the combining form "thromb/o" mean?
   a. Blood
   b. Clot
   c. Artery
   d. Blood cell

4. What does the combining form "olig/o" mean?
   a. Night
   b. Water
   c. Pain
   d. Scanty

5. What does the combining form "hemat/o" mean?
   a. Vein
   b. Blood
   c. Plasma
   d. Valve

6. What is the structural organization of the body from the simplest to the most complex?
   a. Organism, body system, tissues, organs, and cells
   b. Cells, organs, tissues, and body systems
   c. Cells, tissues, organs, body systems, and organism
   d. Cells, tissues, body systems, organs, and organism

7. Which plane divides the body horizontally into upper and lower sections?
   a. Frontal plane
   b. Median plane
   c. Midsagittal plane
   d. Transverse plane

8. _____ pertains to closer to the midline and _____ pertains to farther away from the midline.
   a. Anterior, posterior
   b. Superior, inferior
   c. Ipsilateral, contralateral
   d. Medial, lateral

9. Which quadrant contains the stomach, spleen, left lobe of the liver, pancreas, and left kidney?
   a. RUQ
   b. LUQ
   c. RLQ
   d. LLQ

10. Which cavity is part of the ventral body cavity and contains the heart and lungs?
    a. Spinal cavity
    b. Thoracic cavity
    c. Abdominopelvic cavity
    d. Cranial cavity

WORKPLACE APPLICATIONS

1. Daniela is learning suffixes. List ten suffixes that mean "pertaining to." _____

   _____

   _____

   _____

2. Daniela has floated to cardiology. Using the word parts in this chapter, create five medical terms for diseases a person might hear if working in a cardiology department.

   _____

   _____

   _____

3. Daniela was discussing directional terms with a peer in her class. She was explaining the importance of using directional terms in healthcare. Describe why directional terms are useful when documenting healthcare information.

   _____

   _____

   _____

   _____

4. Describe the organizational structure of the body from simple to complex._____

_____

_____

_____

_____

_____

_____

_____

INTERNET ACTIVITIES

1. Using a reliable internet site, research healthcare related acronyms. Make a list of five acronyms.

2. Using a reliable internet site, identify 10 diseases that can be broken down into word parts. Make a list of the disease, then break down each disease name into word parts. Label each word part (e.g., prefix, suffix, root, combining vowel, and combining form). Define each word part.

3. Select one of the causes of disease (e.g., genetics, infectious pathogen). Using online resources, find four diseases that are caused by it. Research each disease and the cause of the disease. Create a paper, poster presentation, PowerPoint presentation, or storyboard based on your research.

4. Using online resources, research grading and staging of cancers. Create a short paper or PowerPoint presentation describing the difference between grading and staging.

Infection Control

CAAHEP Competencies	Assessment
III.C.1. Identify major types of infectious agents	Skills and Concepts – A. 12-16
III.C.2.a. Identify the infection cycle including: the infectious agent	Skills and Concepts – A. 5, 6
III.C.2.b. Identify the infection cycle including: reservoir	Skills and Concepts – A. 5, 7
III.C.2.c. Identify the infection cycle including: susceptible host	Skills and Concepts – A. 5, 11
III.C.2.d. Identify the infection cycle including: means of transmission	Skills and Concepts – A. 5, 9
III.C.2.e. Identify the infection cycle including: portals of entry	Skills and Concepts – A. 5, 10
III.C.2.f. Identify the infection cycle including: portals of exit	Skills and Concepts – A. 5, 8
III.C.3.a. Identify the following as practiced within an ambulatory care setting: medical asepsis	Skills and Concepts – E. 4
III.C.3.b. Identify the following as practiced within an ambulatory care setting: surgical asepsis	Skills and Concepts – E. 9
III.C.4. Identify methods of controlling the growth of microorganisms	Skills and Concepts – A. 13
III.C.5. Identify the principles of standard precautions	Skills and Concepts – E. 1
III.C.6.a. Identify personal protective equipment (PPE)	Skills and Concepts – E. 3
III.C.7. Identify the implications for failure to comply with Centers for Disease Control (CDC) regulations in health care settings	Internet Activities – 1
III.P.1. Participate in bloodborne pathogen training	Procedure 19.1
III.P.2. Select appropriate barrier/personal protective equipment (PPE)	Procedure 19.3
III.P.3. Perform handwashing	Procedure 19.2
ABHES Competencies	**Assessment**
8.a. Practice standard precautions and perform disinfection/sterilization techniques	Procedures 19.1, 19.2, 19.3

VOCABULARY REVIEW

Using the word pool on the right, find the correct word to match the definition. Write the word on the line after the definition.

Group A

1. Substances that inhibit the growth of microorganisms on living tissue; they are used to cleanse the skin, wounds, and so on

   _____

2. A thick-walled, dormant form of bacteria that is very resistant to disinfection measures _____

3. Passed from parents to offspring through the genes

   _____

4. Capable of producing disease _____

5. A disease where the body produces antibodies that attack its own tissues, leading to the deterioration of tissue

   _____

6. Diseases spread from person to person either by direct or indirect contact _____

7. To take, as food, into the body _____

8. An illness resulting from the deterioration of tissues and organs

   _____

9. Free from all microorganisms, pathogenic and nonpathogenic

   _____

10. A protein formed when a cell is exposed to a virus; the protein blocks viral action on the cell and protects against viral invasion

    _____

Word Pool
- sterile
- hereditary
- autoimmune
- degenerative
- communicable
- pathogenic
- ingested
- antiseptics
- interferon
- spore

Group B

1. Protein substances produced in the blood or tissues in response to a specific antigen that destroys or weakens the antigen

   _____

2. The presence of pus-forming organisms in the blood

   _____

3. To pass or spread disease _____

4. Animals or insects (e.g., ticks) that transmit a pathogen

   _____

5. To void waste from the bowels through the anus; have a bowel movement _____

6. An infection caused by a yeast, *Candida albicans*, that typically affects the vaginal mucosa and skin _____

7. Not animate; lifeless _____

8. Any fungal skin disease that results in scaling, itching, and inflammation; examples are ringworm, athlete's foot

   _____

9. Agents that destroy pathogenic organisms

   _____

10. To breathe in _____

Word Pool
- candidiasis
- tinea
- vectors
- transmission
- inanimate
- inhalation
- germicides
- defecation
- antibodies
- pyemia

Group C

1. The partial or complete disappearance of the clinical and subjective characteristics of a chronic or malignant disease

   _____

2. Not permitting penetration _____

3. To take into the body by any route other than the digestive tract

   _____

4. Infections that are acquired in a healthcare setting

   _____

5. Any chemical agent used on nonliving objects to destroy or inhibit the growth of harmful organisms; not effective against bacterial spores _____

6. Condition of general bodily weakness or discomfort

   _____

7. Those procedures that do not penetrate human tissue

   _____

8. The recurrence of the symptoms of a disease after apparent recovery _____

9. A set of infection control practices used to prevent transmission of diseases that can be acquired by contact with blood, body fluids, nonintact skin, and mucous membranes _____

10. Extreme tiredness _____

Word Pool
- fatigue
- malaise
- relapse
- remission
- Standard Precautions
- parenteral
- disinfectant
- impervious
- noninvasive procedures
- nosocomial infections

ABBREVIATIONS

Write out what each of the following abbreviations stands for.

1. OSHA _____

2. DNA _____

3. RNA _____

4. AIDS _____

5. HIV _____

6. COVID-19_____

7. CDC_____

8. WBCs _____

9. HSV_____

10. HBV_____

11. OPIM_____

12. CSF _____

13. IV _____

14. PPE _____

15. EPA _____

16. HCV _____

SKILLS AND CONCEPTS

Answer the following questions. Write your answer on the line or in the space provided.

A. Chain of Infection

1. A(n) _____ disease is one that is passed from one generation to another.

2. A(n) _____ disease is one in which a person's antibodies attack his or her own tissues.

3. A(n) _____ disease results from a deterioration of the tissues and/or organs.

4. A(n) _____ disease is one that is spread from person to person.

5. Label the chain of infection diagram with the following terms. Place the correct letter in the chain of infection next to the corresponding letters that follow.

Portal of entry _____

Portal of exit _____

Infectious agent _____

Mode of transmission _____

Reservoir host _____

Susceptible host _____

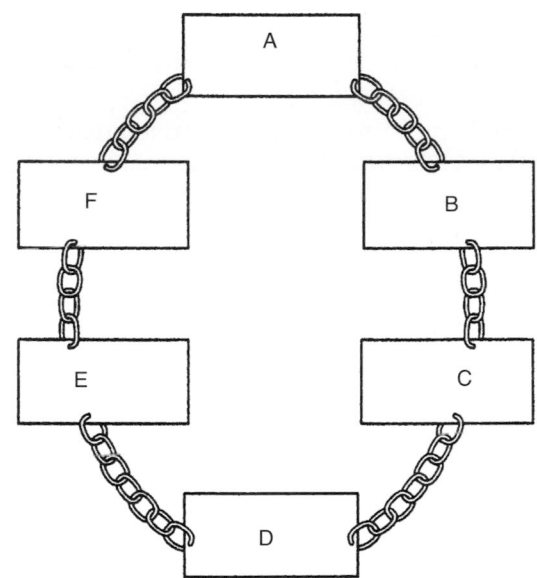

Match the links in the chain of infection with the example of the link. Some answers may be used more than once.

6. _____ Infectious agent

7. _____ Reservoir host

8. _____ Portal of exit

9. _____ Mode of transmission

10. _____ Portal of entry

11. _____ Susceptible host

a. mouth, eyes, intestines, reproductive tract, nose, ears, urinary tract, open wounds

b. capable of supporting the growth of the infection organism

c. viruses, bacteria, fungi, protozoa, helminths

d. sneezing, coughing, contaminated objects, animals, insects

e. people, insects, animals, water, food, contaminated instruments, equipment

Match the characteristic with correct pathogen.

12. _____ Viruses

13. _____ Bacteria

14. _____ Fungi

15. _____ Protozoa

16. _____ Helminths

a. May be unicellular or multicellular; they include molds and yeasts and cause tinea infections.

b. Bacteria are tiny, simple cells that produce disease by secreting toxins, act as parasites inside human cells, or grow on body surfaces, disrupting normal human functions.

c. Multicellular parasites and include tapeworms, roundworms, and flatworms (flukes).

d. The smallest of all pathogens, lead the list of important disease-causing agents. Particles insert their own deoxyribonucleic acid (DNA) or ribonucleic acid (RNA) into a host cell and then use the host cell to help reproduce more particles.

e. Unicellular parasites that can replicate and multiply rapidly once inside the host.

17. Describe the infection cycle and identify three methods you can use to control the growth of microorganisms in a medical facility.

_____

_____

_____

_____

_____

_____

18. _____ serves as a natural barrier to disease.

19. _____ linking the openings of the body help protect underlying tissues and trap foreign substances.

20. Tiny, hairlike projections, called _____, line the respiratory tract and move in a coordinated upward motion to expel trapped foreign substances.

21. Trapped substances can be expelled with _____ before the organisms invade underlying tissue.

22. Some body secretions, such as _____, have antimicrobial properties that help destroy invading pathogens.

23. The natural _____ of many of the body's organs discourage the growth of microbes.

B. How Does the Body Defend Itself?

1. The inflammatory response helps prevent the invasion of microorganisms after trauma or limits the number of these invaders. The four classic symptoms of the inflammatory response include which of the following?
    a. Erythema
    b. Pain
    c. Edema
    d. Heat
    e. All of the above

2. The first line of defense includes which of the following anatomic defense mechanisms?
    a. Tears
    b. Phagocytic cells
    c. Mucous membranes
    d. Antibodies
    e. a and c

3. The second line of defense is made up of _____ chemical and _____ responses.

4. The third line of defense involves _____ and production of _____.

C. Types of Infection

Match the stage of an acute infection with the correct description.

1. _____ Incubation
2. _____ Prodromal
3. _____ Acute
4. _____ Declining
5. _____ Convalescent

a. The symptoms of the disease start to subside. If patients have been prescribed antibiotics, this when they may decide to stop taking them. It is important to stress to patients that they must take all of the medication. With mononucleosis, this stage can take several weeks or even months.

b. The period of time between exposure to the pathogen and the appearance of the first symptoms. It can be from a few days to a few months. This period for mononucleosis is 4 to 6 weeks.

c. The disease is at its peak and symptoms are fully developed. With mononucleosis, pharyngitis, tonsillitis, and lymphadenopathy are common symptoms.

d. In this stage, patients will regain their strength and return to a state of good health.

e. The short period of time when the first symptoms appear. With mononucleosis, the patient may have 1 to 2 weeks of fatigue, malaise, myalgia, and a low-grade fever.

6. An infection that cycles through periods of relapse and remission, such as herpes simplex virus and shingles, is a(n) _____ infection.

7. A(n) _____ infection is one that is caused by organisms that are not typically pathogenic but cause disease under certain circumstances.

D. Occupational Safety and Health Administration Standards for the Healthcare Setting

1. The five major areas included in the OSHA compliance guidelines include which of the following?
   a. Barrier protection devices
   b. Housekeeping controls
   c. Hepatitis B immunizations
   d. Post exposure follow-up
   e. All of the above

2. Which of the following is not considered OPIM?
   a. Vaginal secretions
   b. Urine
   c. Wound drainage
   d. Saliva in dental procedures
   e. Cerebrospinal fluid

3. Medical assistants should routinely use appropriate _____ precautions when contact with blood or other body fluids is expected.

4. Immediately after use, syringe, needle, and scalpel blades should be disposed of in a labeled, leakproof, puncture-resistant _____ container.

5. After accidental spills of blood or body fluids, work surfaces must be immediately cleaned and then disinfected with a disinfectant registered with the _____.

6. Identify four safety rules that should be followed in the ambulatory care setting to comply with the OSHA environmental protection guidelines.

   a. _____

   b. _____

   c. _____

   d. _____

E. Aseptic Techniques: Preventing Disease Transmission

1. Which of the following is considered an infection control practice as specified in Standard Precautions?
   a. Correct disposal of contaminated products
   b. Handwashing
   c. Proper wound care
   d. Gloves and masks
   e. All of the above

2. Place a check mark beside the procedures that require the use of disposable gloves.
   a. _____ Assisting with a vaginal examination
   b. _____ Performing a routine urinalysis
   c. _____ Measuring a patient's temperature, pulse, and respirations
   d. _____ Performing a patient interview
   e. _____ Drawing blood from a 6-year-old child

3. Which of the following is considered PPE?
   a. Face mask, face shields
   b. Laboratory coats, barrier gowns
   c. Gloves
   d. Protective glasses
   e. All of the above

Match the following terms with the correct definition.

4. _____ Disinfection
5. _____ Medical asepsis
6. _____ Surgical asepsis
7. _____ Sanitization
8. _____ Sterilization

a. Removal of disease-causing organisms or destruction of the organisms
b. Destruction of all microorganisms
c. Destruction of all organisms
d. A cleansing process that reduces the number of microorganisms to a safe level
e. The process of killing pathogenic organisms or rendering them inactive

9. _____ is essential for achieving surgical asepsis.

CERTIFICATION PREPARATION
Circle the correct answer.

1. What are the two important factors in performing an effective hand wash?
   a. Friction and running warm water
   b. Antibacterial soap and hot water
   c. Length of time spent and type of soap
   d. Position of the hands and temperature of the water

2. The process used to wash and remove blood and tissue from medical instruments is called
   a. asepsis.
   b. disinfection.
   c. sanitization.
   d. sterilization.

3. The method that completely destroys microorganisms is
   a. disinfection.
   b. sterilization.
   c. sanitization.
   d. boiling.

4. Based on the chain of infection, what would be the most effective method of controlling the spread of conjunctivitis in a day care center?
   a. Conjunctivitis is not contagious.
   b. Close the day care center until all children are symptom-free.
   c. Sanitize hands thoroughly after each contact with a symptomatic child.
   d. Immediately send the child home to prevent the spread of the disease.

5. Inflammation mediators that are released at the site of cellular damage perform which function?
   a. Increase blood flow to the site
   b. Increase the permeability of blood vessel walls
   c. Cause more RBCs to be attracted to the site of injury
   d. Both a and b

6. Relapse and remission are seen frequently in what types of infections?
   a. Chronic infections
   b. Latent infections
   c. Infections with rapid onset
   d. Infections that cause fever

7. Viral infections
   a. are treated effectively with antibiotics.
   b. include malaria and gonorrhea.
   c. are treated with a focus on palliative care.
   d. may form spores.

8. The immune system response called *humoral immunity* is
   a. cellular immune reactions.
   b. production of antibodies in response to a foreign substance in the body.
   c. the inflammatory process.
   d. natural protection against disease.

9. Rosa is responsible for training a new employee in medical aseptic handwashing. Which should Rosa emphasize?
   a. Using hot running water
   b. Carefully washing around all rings
   c. Using an adequate amount of soap and rubbing in a circular motion around all fingers
   d. Carefully drying the hands with a sterile disposable drape

10. The key to reducing the prevalence of antibiotic resistance is to
   a. prescribe antibiotics for all cases of the flu.
   b. order antibiotics for a minimum of 2 days.
   c. use an antibiotic that is specific to the pathogen.
   d. all of the above.

WORKPLACE APPLICATIONS

1. Rosa is explaining the signs and symptoms of inflammation to a patient. List the four classic symptoms.

   a. _____

   b. _____

   c. _____

   d. _____

2. A patient asks Rosa why the provider did not prescribe an antibiotic for her viral illness. What should Rosa say to the patient? Include in your discussion the provider's concerns about antibiotic resistance.

   _____

   _____

   _____

   _____

3. While performing venipuncture, Rosa has an accidental needlestick. Describe postexposure actions and follow-up procedures.

   _____

   _____

   _____

   _____

INTERNET ACTIVITIES

1. Visit www.osha.gov. Review the OSHA Bloodborne Pathogens Standards. Create a poster presentation, a PowerPoint presentation, or write a paper summarizing your research. Include the following points in your project:
   a. What can you do in your workplace to prevent accidental exposure to blood-borne pathogens?
   b. What types of equipment can be used to prevent accidental exposure to blood-borne pathogens?
   c. What are the implications for failure to comply with the CDC's regulations in healthcare settings?

2. Visit the Infection Control area of the CDC site at https://www.cdc.gov/hai/. Investigate the material on healthcare-associated infections. Create a poster presentation, a PowerPoint presentation, or write a paper summarizing your research. Include the following points in your project:
   a. Define *healthcare-associated infection*.
   b. What are the most common healthcare-associated infections?
   c. How can a medical assistant prevent healthcare-associated infections?

Procedure 19.1 Remove Contaminated Gloves and Discard Biohazardous Material

Name _____ Date _____ Score _____

Task: To minimize exposure to pathogens by aseptically removing and discarding contaminated gloves.

Equipment and Supplies:
- Disposable gloves
- Biohazard waste container with labeled red biohazard bag

Standard: Complete the procedure and all critical steps in _____ minutes with a minimum score of 85% within two attempts (*or as indicated by the instructor*).

Scoring: Divide the points earned by the total possible points. Failure to perform a critical step, indicated by an asterisk (*), results in grade no higher than an 84% (*or as indicated by the instructor*).

Time: Began_____ Ended_____ Total minutes: _____

Steps:	Point Value	Attempt 1	Attempt 2
1. With the dominant hand, grasp the glove of the opposite hand near the palm and begin removing the first glove. The arms should be held away from the body with the hands pointed down.	15		
2. Pull the glove inside out. After removal, ball it into the palm of the remaining gloved hand.	15		
3. Insert two fingers of the ungloved hand between the edge of the cuff of the other contaminated glove and the hand.	15		
4. Push the glove down the hand, inside out, over the contaminated glove being held, leaving the contaminated side of both gloves on the inside.	15		
5. Properly dispose of the inside-out, contaminated gloves in a biohazard waste container.	20*		
6. Perform a medical aseptic hand wash as described in Procedure 19.2 or sanitize the hands with an alcohol-based sanitizer.	20		
Total Points	100		

Comments

CAAHEP Competencies	Step(s)
III.P.1. Participate in bloodborne pathogen training	Entire procedure
ABHES Competencies	**Step(s)**
8.a. Practice standard precautions and perform disinfection/sterilization techniques	Entire procedure

Procedure 19.2   Perform Hand Hygiene

Name _____   Date _____   Score _____

Task: To minimize the number of pathogens on the hands, thus reducing the risk of transmission of pathogens.

Equipment and Supplies:
- Sink with warm running water
- Liquid soap in a dispenser (bar soap is not acceptable)
- Disposable nail brush or orange stick
- Paper towels in a dispenser
- Water-based lotion
- Covered waste container with foot pedal
- Alcohol-based hand sanitizer

Standard: Complete the procedure and all critical steps in _____ minutes with a minimum score of 85% within two attempts (*or as indicated by the instructor*).

Scoring: Divide the points earned by the total possible points. Failure to perform a critical step, indicated by an asterisk (*), results in grade no higher than an 84% (*or as indicated by the instructor*).

Time: Began_____ Ended_____ Total minutes: _____

Steps:	Point Value	Attempt 1	Attempt 2
1. Remove all jewelry except your wristwatch, if it can be pulled up above your wrist, and a plain wedding ring.	10		
2. Turn on the faucet and regulate the water temperature to lukewarm.	5		
3. Wet your hands, apply soap, and lather using a circular motion with friction while holding your fingertips downward. Rub well between your fingers. If this is the first hand wash of the day, use a nail brush or an orange stick and clean under every fingernail. Inspect your nails thoroughly.	10*		
4. Rinse well, holding your hands so that the water flows from your wrists downward to your fingertips.	10		
5. If this is the first hand wash of the day or if your hands are obviously contaminated, wet your hands again and repeat the scrubbing procedure using a vigorous, circular motion over the wrists and hands for at least 1-2 minutes.	10		
6. Rinse your hands a second time, keeping the fingers lower than your wrists.	10		
7. Dry your hands with paper towels. Do not touch the paper towel dispenser as you are obtaining towels.	10		
8. If the faucet is not foot-operated, turn it off with a dry paper towel.	10		
9. After you finish drying your hands and turning off the faucet, place used towels into a covered waste container.	10		
10. If needed, apply a water-based antibacterial hand lotion to prevent chapped or dry skin.	10		
11. Repeat the procedure as indicated throughout the day.	5		
Total Points	100		

Comments

CAAHEP Competencies	Step(s)
III.P.3. Perform handwashing	Entire procedure
ABHES Competencies	**Step(s)**
8.a. Practice standard precautions and perform disinfection/sterilization techniques	Entire procedure

Procedure 19.3   Sanitizing Soiled Instruments

Name _____ Date _____ Score _____

Task: Remove all contaminated matter from instruments in preparation for disinfection or sterilization while following Standard Precautions and wearing appropriate personal protective equipment (PPE).

Equipment and Supplies:
- Sink with cold and hot running water
- Sanitizing agent or low-sudsing soap with enzymatic action
- Decontaminated utility gloves that show no signs of deterioration
- Chin-length face shield or goggles and face mask if contamination with blood-borne pathogens is possible
- Impermeable gown
- Disposable brush
- Disposable paper towels
- Instruments for sanitization
- Disinfectant cleaner prepared according to manufacturer's directions
- Covered waste container with foot pedal
- Biohazard waste container with labeled red biohazard bag

Standard: Complete the procedure and all critical steps in _____ minutes with a minimum score of 85% within two attempts (*or as indicated by the instructor*).

Scoring: Divide the points earned by the total possible points. Failure to perform a critical step, indicated by an asterisk (*), results in grade no higher than an 84% (*or as indicated by the instructor*).

Time: Began_____ Ended_____ Total minutes: _____

Steps:	Point Value	Attempt 1	Attempt 2
1. Put on an impermeable gown and face shield or goggles and mask if potential for splashing of infectious material exists.	10		
2. Put on utility gloves.	5		
3. Separate the sharp instruments from other instruments to be sanitized.	10		
4. Rinse the instruments under cold running water.	5		
5. Open hinged instruments and scrub all grooves, crevices, and serrations with a disposable brush.	10*		
6. Rinse well with hot water.	5		
7. Towel-dry all instruments thoroughly and dispose of contaminated towels and disposable brush in a biohazard waste container. Do not touch the paper towel dispenser as you are obtaining towels.	10		
8. Remove the utility gloves and wash your hands according to Procedure 19.2.	10		
9. Towel-dry your hands and put on gloves. Decontaminate the utility gloves and work surfaces using disinfectant cleaner.	10		
10. Dispose of the contaminated towels in a covered waste container.	5		
11. Place sanitized instruments in a designated area for disinfection or sterilization.	10		

12. Remove the gloves according to Procedure 19.1. Dispose of the gloves in a biohazard waste container. Sanitize hands.	**10**		
Total Points	**100**		

Comments

CAAHEP Competencies	Step(s)
III.P.2. Select appropriate barrier/personal protective equipment	Entire procedure
ABHES Competencies	**Step(s)**
8.a. Practice standard precautions and perform disinfection/sterilization techniques	Entire procedure

Vital Signs

chapter

20

CAAHEP Competencies	Assessment
I.P.1.a. Accurately measure and record: blood pressure	Procedure 20.9
I.P.1.b. Accurately measure and record: temperature	Procedures 20.1, 20.2, 20.3, 20.4, 20.5, 20.6
I.P.1.c. Accurately measure and record: pulse	Procedures 20.7, 20.8
I.P.1.d. Accurately measure and record: respirations	Procedure 20.8
I.P.1.e. Accurately measure and record: height	Procedure 20.11
I.P.1.f. Accurately measure and record: weight (adult)	Procedure 20.11
I.P.1.i. Accurately measure and record: oxygen saturation	Procedure 20.10

ABHES Competencies	Assessment
8. Clinical Procedures b. Obtain vital signs, obtain patient history, and formulate chief complaint	Procedures 20.1 through 20.10

VOCABULARY REVIEW

Using the word pool on the right, find the correct word to match the definition. Write the word on the line after the definition.

Group A

1. A waxy secretion in the ear canal; commonly called *ear wax*
   _____

2. To shift back and forth _____

3. Voice box _____

4. The internal environment of the body that is compatible with life; a steady state that is created by all the body systems working together to provide a consistent and unvarying internal environment _____

5. A term that refers to an area outside of or away from an organ or structure _____

6. Pertaining to an elevated body temperature
   _____

7. A condition of general bodily weakness or discomfort, often marking the onset of a disease _____

8. Inflammation or infection of the external auditory canal; commonly called *swimmer's ear* _____

9. A febrile condition or fever _____

10. Fluctuations that occur during each day _____

Word Pool
- homeostasis
- diurnal variation
- febrile
- pyrexia
- fluctuate
- malaise
- otitis externa
- cerumen
- peripheral
- larynx

Group B

1. A slow heartbeat; a pulse below 60 beats per minute
   _____

2. To close, shut, or stop up _____

3. A term used to describe a pulse that feels full because of increased power of cardiac contraction or as a result of increased blood volume _____

4. An irregular heartbeat that originates in the sinoatrial node (pacemaker) _____

5. To listen with a stethoscope _____

6. A rapid but regular heart rate; one that exceeds 100 beats per minute _____

7. Difficult and/or painful breathing _____

8. A condition in which the radial pulse is less than the apical pulse; it may indicate a peripheral vascular abnormality
   _____

9. A term describing a pulse that is thin and feeble
   _____

10. A pulse in which beats occasionally are skipped
    _____

Word Pool
- bradycardia
- tachycardia
- pulse deficit
- intermittent pulse
- sinus arrhythmia
- bounding
- thready
- occlude
- auscultated
- dyspnea

Group C

1. Abnormally rapid breathing _____
2. Abnormally slow breathing _____
3. Whistling sound made during breathing
   _____
4. Excessively deep breathing _____
5. An abnormal lung sound heard on auscultation, characterized by discontinuous bubbling noises _____
6. A progressive, irreversible lung condition that results in diminished lung capacity _____
7. Condition of difficult breathing unless in an upright position
   _____
8. Abnormal, periodic cessation of breathing
   _____
9. Rapid, shallow breathing _____
10. Deep, rapid breathing followed by a period of apnea
    _____

Word Pool
- chronic obstructive pulmonary disease (COPD)
- bradypnea
- apnea
- tachypnea
- hyperpnea
- hyperventilation
- orthopnea
- wheezing
- Cheyne-Stokes respiration
- rales

Group D

1. Elevated blood pressure of unknown cause that develops for no apparent reason; sometimes called *primary hypertension*
   _____
2. Heavy snoring _____
3. A temporary fall in blood pressure when a person rapidly changes from a recumbent position to a standing position
   _____
4. To determine or check readings with those of a standard
   _____
5. Abnormal rumbling sound heard on auscultation, caused by airways blocked by secretions or muscle contractions
   _____
6. A condition in which extra lymph fluid builds up in tissues and causes swelling _____
7. The difference between the systolic and diastolic blood pressures
   _____
8. Middle layer and the thickest layer of the heart; composed of cardiac muscles _____
9. Of unknown cause _____
10. Thickening, decreased elasticity, and calcification of arterial walls
    _____
11. Fainting; a brief lapse in consciousness _____
12. Dizziness; abnormal sensation of movement when there is none
    _____
13. Blood pressure that is below normal (systolic pressure below 90 mm Hg and diastolic pressure below 50 mm Hg)
    _____

Word Pool
- rhonchi
- stertorous
- vertigo
- pulse pressure
- arteriosclerosis
- myocardium
- essential hypertension
- idiopathic
- hypotension
- orthostatic (postural) hypotension
- syncope
- calibrated
- lymphedema

ABBREVIATIONS
Write out what each of the following abbreviations stands for.

1. Pap_____

2. F_____

3. C_____

4. T_____

5. A_____

6. R_____

7. TA_____

8. IFR_____

9. CPR_____

10. COPD_____

11. AHA_____

12. CNS_____

13. SpO$_2$_____

14. BMI_____

SKILLS AND CONCEPTS
Answer the following questions. Write your answer on the line or in the space provided.

A. Temperature

1. Vital signs can be influenced by _____ and _____ factors.

2. A medical assistant should be aware of _____ that could indicate discomfort or pain.

3. A(n) _____ fever rises and falls only slightly during a 24-hour period. It remains above the patient's average normal range.

4. A(n) _____ fever comes and goes, or it spikes and then returns to the average range.

5. A(n) _____ fever fluctuates greatly (more than 3° F) but does not return to the average range.

6. _____ temperatures are approximately 1° F lower than accurate oral readings.

7. _____ thermometers are an accurate means of taking temperatures in adults and older children because of the closeness to the hypothalamus.

8. _____ temperatures are an easy, noninvasive, and accurate alternative to taking rectal temperatures in infants.

9. Medication to reduce a fever is called a(n) _____.

10. Tympanic thermometers should not be used if the patient has _____ or
    _____.

11. Temperatures considered febrile include the following:

    a. Aural (ear) temperatures higher than _____ ° F (38° C)

    b. Oral temperatures higher than _____° F (37.8° C)

    c. Axillary temperatures higher than _____ ° F (37.2° C)

12. Use the following formulas to convert the temperatures in the chart from one system to the other.
    Round answers to the nearest tenth.

    Fahrenheit to Celsius: Celsius to Fahrenheit:

    $°C = (°F − 32) / 1.8$ $°F = (°C × 1.8) + 32$

    a. 98.6° F =   _____ °C
    b. 39.5° C =   _____ °F
    c. 97.6° F =   _____ °C
    d. 99.4° F =   _____ °C
    e. 40° C =   _____ °F
    f. 36° C =   _____ °F
    g. 38.5° C =   _____ °F
    h. 41° C =   _____ °F
    i. 102° F =   _____ °C
    j. 37.5° C =   _____ °F

13. Which of the following factors can affect body temperature?
    a. Age
    b. Stress
    c. Gender
    d. External factors
    e. All of the above

14. When taking an oral temperature, the medical assistant should ask the patient about which of the
    following?
    a. Have they had anything to eat or drink in the last 15 minutes.
    b. Have they smoked in the last 15 minutes.
    c. Have they spoken to anyone in the last 15 minutes.
    d. Both a and b

15. A(n) _____ probe is used to take an oral temperature and a(n)
    _____ probe is used to take a rectal temperature.

16. To expose the tympanic membrane in a child younger than 3 years, the earlobe should be pulled
    _____ and back; for patients older than age 3, the pinna should be pulled
    _____ and back.

17. When taking a temperature using a temporal artery thermometer, which of the following statements is *not* true?
    a. The forehead should be exposed by moving bangs to the side.
    b. The probe is placed near the temple on one side of the forehead, halfway between the eyebrows and the hairline.
    c. Depress the button and move the thermometer across the forehead to the hairline.
    d. Keeping the button depressed, lift the thermometer and place behind the earlobe.

B. Pulse

1. List eight pulse sites and label their correct locations on the figure.

    a. _____

    b. _____

    c. _____

    d. _____

    e. _____

    f. _____

    g. _____

    h. _____

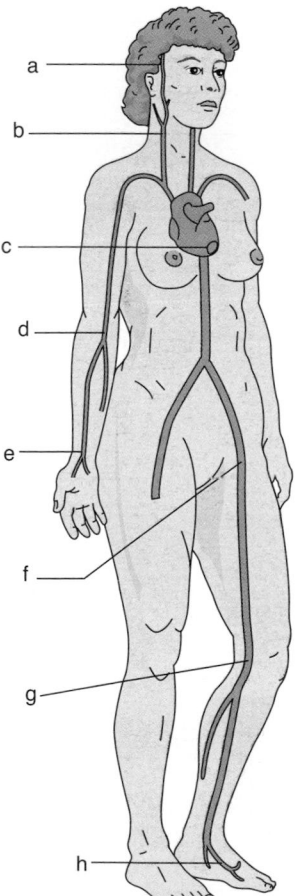

2. Which of the following are characteristics that should be noted when taking a patient's pulse?
    a. Rate
    b. Rhythm
    c. Volume
    d. All of the above

3. A patient with a significant difference between the apical and brachial pulse counts has a(n) _____.

4. A patient who is anxious or in pain may have an increase in the pulse rate, which is called _____.

5. The brachial pulse, which is palpated before the blood pressure is taken, is located in the _____ of the elbow.

6. _____ is when the heart rate varies with respirations.

7. The _____ pulse is the most accurate method of taking the pulse of infants and of patients with an arrhythmia.

Match the pulse volume measurement with correct description.

8. _____ 1+   a.   Full, bounding; pulsation is very strong and does not disappear with moderate
9. _____ 2+   pressure.
10. _____ 3+   b.   Weak, thready; pulsation is not easily felt and disappears with slight pressure.
              c.   Normal; pulsation is easily felt but disappears with moderate pressure.

11. A(n) _____ pulse should be done when irregularities are noted when taking a(n) _____ pulse.

12. The proper placement of the stethoscope for taking an apical pulse is
    a.   the antecubital space on the left.
    b.   2-3 inches above the nipple on the left.
    c.   the fifth intercostal space at the left midclavicular line.
    d.   none of the above.

C. Respiration

1. One full respiration includes both _____ and _____.

2. The exchange of oxygen and carbon dioxide in the lungs is called _____.

3. Carlos counts eight respirations for 30 seconds. The rate is _____ respirations per minute.

4. Breathing rates are controlled by the respiratory center, which is located in the _____ of the brain.

5. When assessing a patient's respiration, what characteristics are should be noted?
    a.   Rate
    b.   Rhythm
    c.   Depth
    d.   All of the above

D. Blood Pressure

1. Blood pressure reflects the pressure of the blood against the walls of the _____.

2. Blood pressure is recorded as a fraction; the _____ reading is the numerator (top number), and the _____ reading is the denominator (bottom number).

3. When you subtract the diastolic pressure from the systolic pressure, you get the
   _____.

4. _____ is the contraction of the heart.

5. _____ reflects the relaxation of the heart.

6. The most common type of hypertension is _____. It is _____, but can be associated with obesity, high blood level of sodium, elevated cholesterol levels, family history, and race.

7. Hypertension that develops from another condition such as kidney disease is _____.

Match the Korotkoff sound phase with the correct description.

8. _____ Phase 1

9. _____ Phase 2

10. _____ Phase 3

11. _____ Phase 4

12. _____ Phase 5

a. Blood is flowing easily, and the sound changes to a soft tapping, which becomes muffled and begins to grow fainter.

b. Movement of the blood makes a swishing sound as the blood rushes through the artery.

c. All sounds disappear. Note the gauge reading when the last sound is heard.

d. First sound heard as the cuff deflates. The blood is resurging into the patient's artery and can be heard clearly as a sharp, tapping sound. Note the gauge reading when the first sound is heard.

e. Distinct, sharp tapping sounds return and continue rhythmically; the beginning of phase III may be incorrectly interpreted as the systolic blood pressure.

13. When a blood pressure cuff is too large, the blood pressure reading may be _____. If the blood pressure cuff is too small, the blood pressure reading may be _____.

14. Factors that determine blood pressure include which of the following?
    a. Blood volume
    b. Peripheral resistance created by blood viscosity
    c. Vessel elasticity
    d. The condition of the heart muscle and arterial walls
    e. All of the above

E. Oxygen Saturation

1. List conditions for which a pulse oximetry may be used to assess a patient's oxygenation status.

   _____

   _____

2. A normal pulse oximetry reading would be _____ or higher.

F. Anthropometric Measurements

1. Use the formulas below to convert the following weights from one system to the other.

To Convert Kilograms to Pounds
1 kg = 2.2 lb
Multiply the number of kilograms by 2.2.

To Convert Pounds to Kilograms
1 lb = 0.45 kg
Multiply the number of pounds by 0.45, or divide the number of pounds by 2.2 kg.

a. 145 lb = _____ kg

b. 54 kg = _____ lb

c. 60 kg = _____ lb

d. 112 lb = _____ kg

e. 50 lb = _____ kg

CERTIFICATION PREPARATION

Circle the correct answer.

1. How long should the pulse be counted for the most accurate results?
    a. 15 seconds
    b. 30 seconds
    c. 45 seconds
    d. 1 minute

2. What would be considered a normal pulse for an average-sized 37-year-old patient in good health?
    a. 45 beats per minute
    b. 52 beats per minute
    c. 66 beats per minute
    d. 110 beats per minute

3. Which pulse is palpated on the wrist?
    a. Apical
    b. Brachial
    c. Carotid
    d. Radial

4. If a patient is diagnosed with secondary hypertension, this means that the
    a. patient has the most severe form of hypertension.
    b. hypertension is associated with another disease.
    c. patient has the most common form of hypertension.
    d. condition has worsened from essential hypertension.

5. As a blood pressure cuff is deflated, the first tapping sound is the _____ pressure.
    a. mean arterial
    b. systolic
    c. diastolic
    d. pulse

6. The diastolic BP is heard during which Korotkoff phase?
    a. I
    b. II
    c. IV
    d. V

7. How can you help patients feel comfortable about having their weight measured in the office?
    a. Place the scale in a private area of the office.
    b. Reassure them that their weight is at a healthy level.
    c. Have them remain in their shoes and outer clothing.
    d. Allow them to weigh themselves at home and bring in the results.

8. In a healthy adult at rest, the ratio of respirations to pulse beats is typically
    a. 1:3.
    b. 1:4.
    c. 1:5.
    d. 1:8.

9. Mr. Garcia weighs 250 pounds. You are expected to record this weight in kilograms. It is equal to _____ kg.
   a. 113.6
   b. 550.0
   c. 56.8
   d. 226.0

10. Which respiration characteristic frequently occurs in patients with congestive heart failure and COPD?
    a. Orthopnea
    b. Wheezing
    c. Hyperventilation
    d. Hyperpnea

WORKPLACE APPLICATIONS

1. Mrs. Parker stops at the clinic on her way home from work. She does not have an appointment to see the provider but asks if Carlos can take her blood pressure because she hasn't been "feeling herself" the last few days.

   a. Carlos is not sure whether he should use a normal adult-size blood pressure cuff or a large adult cuff. How would he be able to tell if he needs the large adult cuff? Why is this important?

   _____

   _____

   _____

   _____

   b. Carlos has obtained a blood pressure reading of 150/94 mm Hg in the left arm and 160/98 mm Hg in the right arm. Should Carlos wait for a few minutes and then take the pressures again? Why or why not? Concerned about the readings, Carlos decides the patient should see the provider. What type of questions might Carlos want to ask Mrs. Parker?

   _____

   _____

   _____

   _____

2. Sarah, an 18-month-old patient, is being seen today for a possible ear infection. The best method of taking her temperature is _____. Her mother is concerned because Sarah's temperature has been fluctuating between normal and high levels for 2 days; this is called a(n) _____ fever. Carlos should take Sarah's pulse using the _____ method. Sarah's mother has a digital thermometer at home.

   a. What would be the best method she could use to take the baby's temperature and why? _____

   _____

   _____

   _____

b. What patient education should Carlos give Sarah's mother about taking axillary temperatures accurately?

_____

_____

_____

3. Carlos is responsible for training a new medical assistant in the Occupational Safety and Health Administration (OSHA) guidelines for preventing disease transmission when taking vital signs. What important factors should Carlos include?

_____

_____

_____

INTERNET ACTIVITIES

1. Visit www.heart.org/HBP. Review the links found on this page. Create a poster presentation, a PowerPoint presentation, or write a paper summarizing your research. Include the following points in your project:
   a. What are the blood pressure categories? List the name of the category as well as the systolic and diastolic numbers.
   b. Why is high blood pressure considered the "silent killer"?
   c. How can high blood pressure harm your health?
   d. List tools and resources available for patients.

2. Investigate the patient education materials available at the American Lung Association site (www.lung.org/lung-disease/copd) for individuals with COPD. Create a poster presentation, a PowerPoint presentation, or write a paper summarizing your research. Include the following points in your project:
   a. Describe COPD, including symptoms, causes, risk factors, and examples.
   b. How is COPD diagnosed and treated?
   c. What assistance is available for those patients living with COPD?

Procedure 20.1   Accurately Measure and Record a Temperature Using a Temporal Artery Thermometer

Name _____ Date _____ Score _____

Task: To accurately measure and record a patient's temperature using a temporal artery thermometer.

Equipment and Supplies:
- Patient's record
- Professional temporal artery thermometer with probe covers
- Alcohol wipes
- Waste container

Standard: Complete the procedure and all critical steps in _____ minutes with a minimum score of 85% within two attempts (*or as indicated by the instructor*).

Scoring: Divide the points earned by the total possible points. Failure to perform a critical step, indicated by an asterisk (*), results in grade no higher than an 84% (*or as indicated by the instructor*).

Time: Began _____ Ended _____ Total minutes: _____

Steps:	Point Value	Attempt 1	Attempt 2
1. Wash hands or use hand sanitizer.	10*		
2. Gather the necessary equipment and supplies.	5		
3. Greet the patient. Identify yourself. Verify the patient's identity with full name and date of birth. Explain the procedure to be performed in a manner that is understood by the patient. Answer any questions the patient may have on the procedure.	5		
4. Remove the protective cap on the probe. Depending on the facility's infection control procedures, disposable covers can be used on the scanner, or it can be cleaned by lightly wiping the surface with an alcohol wipe.	10		
5. Push the patient's hair up off the forehead to expose the site. Gently place the probe on the patient's forehead, halfway between the edge of the eyebrows and the hairline, at the center of the face (just above the nose).	10*		
6. Depress and hold the SCAN button and lightly glide the probe sideways across the patient's forehead to the hairline just above the ear. As you move the sensor across the forehead, you will hear a beep, and a red light will flash.	10		
7. Keeping the button depressed, lift the thermometer, and place the probe behind the ear lobe. The thermometer may continue to beep, indicating that the temperature is rising.	10		
8. When scanning is complete, release the button and lift the probe. Note the temperature recorded on the digital display. The scanner automatically turns off 15-30 seconds after release of the button.	10		
9. If a probe cover was used, eject it directly into a biohazard waste container. Disinfect the thermometer if indicated and replace the protective cap.	10		
10. Wash hands or use hand sanitizer.	10*		
11. Document the reading in the patient's health record.	10*		
Total Points	100		

Documentation

Comments

CAAHEP Competencies	Step(s)
I.P.1.b. Accurately measure and record: temperature	Entire procedure
ABHES Competencies	**Step(s)**
8.b. Obtain vital signs, obtain patient history, and formulate chief complaint	Entire procedure

Procedure 20.2 Accurately Measure and Record a Temperature Using a Tympanic Thermometer

Name _____ Date _____ Score _____

Task: To accurately measure and record a patient's temperature using a tympanic thermometer.

Equipment and Supplies:
- Patient's record
- Alcohol wipes (optional)
- Tympanic thermometer and probe covers

Standard: Complete the procedure and all critical steps in _____ minutes with a minimum score of 85% within two attempts (*or as indicated by the instructor*).

Scoring: Divide the points earned by the total possible points. Failure to perform a critical step, indicated by an asterisk (*), results in grade no higher than an 84% (*or as indicated by the instructor*).

Time: Began_____ Ended_____ Total minutes: _____

Steps:	Point Value	Attempt 1	Attempt 2
1. Wash hands or use hand sanitizer.	15*		
2. Gather the necessary equipment and supplies.	10		
3. Greet the patient. Identify yourself. Verify the patient's identity with full name and date of birth. Explain the procedure to be performed in a manner that is understood by the patient. Answer any questions the patient may have on the procedure.	10		
4. Clean the probe with an alcohol wipe if indicated. Place a disposable cover on the probe.	10		
5. Insert the probe into the ear canal far enough to seal the opening. Do not apply pressure. For children younger than age 3, gently pull the earlobe down and back; for patients older than age 3, gently pull the top of the ear (pinna) up and back.	15*		
6. Press the button on the probe as directed. The temperature will appear on the display screen in 1-2 seconds.	10		
7. Remove the probe, note the reading, and discard the probe cover into a biohazard waste container without touching it.	10		
8. Wash hands or use hand sanitizer and disinfect the equipment if indicated.	10*		
9. Document the reading in the patient's health record.	10*		
Total Points	100		

Documentation

Comments

CAAHEP Competencies	Step(s)
I.P.1.b. Accurately measure and record: temperature	Entire procedure
ABHES Competencies	**Step(s)**
8.b. Obtain vital signs, obtain patient history, and formulate chief complaint	Entire procedure

Procedure 20.3 Accurately Measure and Record an Oral Temperature Using a Digital Thermometer

Name _____ Date _____ Score _____

Task: To accurately measure and record a patient's oral temperature using a digital thermometer.

Equipment and Supplies:
- Patient's record
- Digital thermometer and probe covers
- Biohazard waste container

Standard: Complete the procedure and all critical steps in _____ minutes with a minimum score of 85% within two attempts (*or as indicated by the instructor*).

Scoring: Divide the points earned by the total possible points. Failure to perform a critical step, indicated by an asterisk (*), results in grade no higher than an 84% (*or as indicated by the instructor*).

Time: Began_____ Ended_____ Total minutes: _____

Steps:	Point Value	Attempt 1	Attempt 2
1. Wash hands or use hand sanitizer.	15*		
2. Assemble the needed equipment and supplies.	10		
3. Greet the patient. Identify yourself. Verify the patient's identity with full name and date of birth. Explain the procedure to be performed in a manner that is understood by the patient. Answer any questions the patient may have on the procedure. Make sure the patient has not eaten, consumed any hot or cold fluids, smoked, or exercised during the 15 minutes before the temperature is measured.	10		
4. Prepare the probe for use as described in the directions. Make sure probe covers are always used.	10		
5. Place the probe under the patient's tongue and instruct the patient to close the mouth tightly without biting down on the thermometer. Help the patient by holding the probe end, or the patient can hold the probe end if that is more comfortable.	15*		
6. When a beep is heard, remove the probe from the patient's mouth and immediately eject the probe cover into an appropriate biohazard waste container.	10		
7. Note the reading on the display screen of the thermometer.	10		
8. Wash hands or use hand sanitizer and disinfect the equipment as indicated.	10		
9. Document the reading in the patient's health record.	10*		
Total Points	100		

Documentation

Comments

CAAHEP Competencies	Step(s)
I.P.1.b. Accurately measure and record: temperature	Entire procedure
ABHES Competencies	**Step(s)**
8.b. Obtain vital signs, obtain patient history, and formulate chief complaint	Entire procedure

Procedure 20.4 Accurately Measure and Record an Axillary Temperature Using a Digital Thermometer

Name _____ Date _____ Score _____

Task: To accurately measure and record a patient's axillary temperature using a digital thermometer.

Equipment and Supplies:
- Patient's record
- Digital thermometer and probe cover
- Supply of tissues
- Patient gown as needed
- Biohazard waste container

Standard: Complete the procedure and all critical steps in _____ minutes with a minimum score of 85% within two attempts (*or as indicated by the instructor*).

Scoring: Divide the points earned by the total possible points. Failure to perform a critical step, indicated by an asterisk (*), results in grade no higher than an 84% (*or as indicated by the instructor*).

Time: Began_____ Ended_____ Total minutes: _____

Steps:	Point Value	Attempt 1	Attempt 2
1. Wash hands or use hand sanitizer.	10*		
2. Gather the needed equipment and supplies.	5		
3. Greet the patient. Identify yourself. Verify the patient's identity with full name and date of birth. Explain the procedure to be performed in a manner that is understood by the patient. Answer any questions the patient may have on the procedure.	10		
4. Prepare the thermometer in the same manner as for oral use.	5		
5. Expose the axillary region. If necessary, provide the patient with a gown for privacy.	5		
6. Pat the patient's axillary area dry with tissues if needed.	5		
7. Place the probe tip into the center of the armpit. Making sure the thermometer is touching only skin, not clothing.	10*		
8. Instruct the patient to hold the arm snugly across the chest or abdomen until the thermometer beeps.	10		
9. Remove the thermometer, note the digital reading, and dispose of the cover in the biohazard waste container.	10		
10. Disinfect the thermometer if indicated.	10		
11. Wash hands or use hand sanitizer.	10*		
12. Document the reading in the patient's health record.	10*		
Total Points	100		

Documentation

Comments

CAAHEP Competencies	Step(s)
I.P.1.b. Accurately measure and record: temperature	Entire procedure
ABHES Competencies	**Step(s)**
8.b. Obtain vital signs, obtain patient history, and formulate chief complaint	Entire procedure

Procedure 20.5   Accurately Measure and Record a Rectal Temperature of an Infant Using a Digital Thermometer

Name _____   Date _____   Score _____

Task: To accurately measure and record a patient's rectal temperature using a digital thermometer.

Equipment and Supplies:
- Patient's record
- Digital thermometer and probe covers
- Gloves
- Water-soluble lubricant (KY Jelly)
- Biohazard waste container

Standard: Complete the procedure and all critical steps in _____ minutes with a minimum score of 85% within two attempts (*or as indicated by the instructor*).

Scoring: Divide the points earned by the total possible points. Failure to perform a critical step, indicated by an asterisk (*), results in grade no higher than an 84% (*or as indicated by the instructor*).

Time: Began_____ Ended_____ Total minutes: _____

Steps:	Point Value	Attempt 1	Attempt 2
1. Wash hands or use hand sanitizer.	10*		
2. Assemble the needed equipment and supplies. Make sure that the red probe is used.	5		
3. Greet the patient. Identify yourself. Verify the patient's identity with full name and date of birth. Explain the procedure to be performed in a manner that is understood by the patient. Answer any questions the patient may have on the procedure.	10		
4. Have the parent or caregiver undress the infant.	5		
5. Put on gloves.	5		
6. Prepare the probe for use as described in the directions. Make sure probe covers are always used. Lubricate first two inches of probe.	5		
7. Gently insert the thermometer probe 1/2 inch for infants, 5/8 inch for children, 1 inch for adults. Remain with the patient at all times and hold the thermometer in place until a beep is heard.	10*		
8. Remove the probe and immediately eject the probe cover into an appropriate biohazard waste container.	10		
9. Note the reading on the display screen of the thermometer.	10		
10. Remove soiled gloves and discard into an appropriate biohazard waste container.	10		
11. Wash hands or use hand sanitizer and disinfect the equipment as indicated.	10*		
12. Document the reading in the patient's health record.	10*		
Total Points	100		

Documentation

Comments

CAAHEP Competencies	Step(s)
I.P.1.b. Accurately measure and record: temperature	Entire procedure
ABHES Competencies	**Step(s)**
8.b. Obtain vital signs, obtain patient history, and formulate chief complaint	Entire procedure

Procedure 20.6 Accurately Measure and Record a Temperature Using an Infrared Thermometer

Name _____ **Date** _____ **Score** _____

Task: To accurately measure and record a patient's temperature using an infrared thermometer.

Equipment and Supplies:
- Patient's record
- Infrared thermometer

Standard: Complete the procedure and all critical steps in _____ minutes with a minimum score of 85% within two attempts (*or as indicated by the instructor*).

Scoring: Divide the points earned by the total possible points. Failure to perform a critical step, indicated by an asterisk (*), results in grade no higher than an 84% (*or as indicated by the instructor*).

Time: Began_____ Ended_____ Total minutes: _____

Steps:	Point Value	Attempt 1	Attempt 2
1. Wash hands or use hand sanitizer.	15*		
2. Gather the necessary equipment and supplies.	10		
3. Greet the patient. Identify yourself. Verify the patient's identity with full name and date of birth. Explain the procedure to be performed in a manner that is understood by the patient. Answer any questions the patient may have on the procedure.	10		
4. Check the sensor. If dirty, gently wipe the sensor with an alcohol wipe and allow to dry.	10		
5. Se the measurement mode to Body.	10		
6. From a distance of 3-5 cm, aim the thermometer at the patient's forehead and depress the button until you hear one beep.	15*		
7. Read the temperature from the display screen.	10		
8. Wash hands or use hand sanitizer and disinfect the equipment as indicated.	10		
9. Document the reading in the patient's health record.	10*		
Total Points	100		

Documentation

Comments

CAAHEP Competencies	Step(s)
I.P.1.b. Accurately measure and record: temperature	Entire procedure
ABHES Competencies	**Step(s)**
8.b. Obtain vital signs, obtain patient history, and formulate chief complaint	Entire procedure

Procedure 20.7 Accurately Measure and Record an Apical Pulse

Name _____ Date _____ Score _____

Task: To accurately measure and record the patient's apical heart rate.

Equipment and Supplies:
- Patient's record
- Watch with a second hand
- Patient gown as needed
- Stethoscope
- Alcohol wipes

Standard: Complete the procedure and all critical steps in _____ minutes with a minimum score of 85% within two attempts (*or as indicated by the instructor*).

Scoring: Divide the points earned by the total possible points. Failure to perform a critical step, indicated by an asterisk (*), results in grade no higher than an 84% (*or as indicated by the instructor*).

Time: Began _____ Ended _____ Total minutes: _____

Steps:	Point Value	Attempt 1	Attempt 2
1. Wash hands or use hand sanitizer and clean the stethoscope earpieces and diaphragm with alcohol wipes.	10*		
2. Greet the patient. Identify yourself. Verify the patient's identity with full name and date of birth. Explain the procedure to be performed in a manner that is understood by the patient. Answer any questions the patient may have on the procedure.	10		
3. If necessary, assist the patient in disrobing from the waist up and provide the patient with a gown that opens in the front.	5		
4. Assist the patient into the sitting or supine position.	5		
5. Hold the stethoscope's diaphragm against the palm of your hand for a few seconds.	10		
6. Place the stethoscope at the left midclavicular line at the fifth intercostal space over the apex of the heart. Do not touch the bell end of the stethoscope.	10*		
7. Listen carefully for the heartbeat. Count the pulse for 1 full minute. Note any irregularities in rhythm and volume.	10*		
8. Help the patient sit up and dress.	10		
9. Disinfect the stethoscope with an alcohol wipe.	10		
10. Wash hands or use hand sanitizer.	10*		
11. Document the reading in the patient's health record.	10*		
Total Points	100		

Documentation

Comments

CAAHEP Competencies	Step(s)
I.P.1.c. Accurately measure and record: pulse	Entire procedure
ABHES Competencies	**Step(s)**
8.b. Obtain vital signs, obtain patient history, and formulate chief complaint	Entire procedure

Procedure 20.8 Accurately Measure and Record the Patient's Radial Pulse and Respiratory Rate

Name _____ Date _____ Score _____

Task: To accurately measure and record a patient's radial pulse rate, rhythm, and volume; and respiratory rate, rhythm, and depth.

Equipment and Supplies:
- Patient's record
- Watch with a second hand

Standard: Complete the procedure and all critical steps in _____ minutes with a minimum score of 85% within two attempts (*or as indicated by the instructor*).

Scoring: Divide the points earned by the total possible points. Failure to perform a critical step, indicated by an asterisk (*), results in grade no higher than an 84% (*or as indicated by the instructor*).

Time: Began_____ Ended_____ Total minutes: _____

Steps:	Point Value	Attempt 1	Attempt 2
1. Wash hands or use hand sanitizer.	10*		
2. Greet the patient. Identify yourself. Verify the patient's identity with full name and date of birth. Explain the procedure to be performed in a manner that is understood by the patient. Answer any questions the patient may have on the procedure.	10		
3. Place the patient's arm in a relaxed position, palm at or below the level of the heart.	5		
4. Gently grasp the palm side of the patient's wrist with your first two or three fingertips approximately 1 inch below the base of the thumb.	5		
5. Count the beats for 1 full minute using a watch with a second hand.	10*		
6. While counting the beats, also assess the rhythm and volume of the patient's pulse.	10*		
7. While continuing to hold the patient's arm in the same position used to count the radial pulse, observe the rise and fall of the patient's chest. If you have difficulty noticing the patient's breathing, place the arm across the chest to detect movement.	5		
8. Inhalation and exhalation make up one complete breathing cycle or respiration. Count the respirations for 30 seconds and multiply by 2.	10*		
9. While counting the respirations, also assess the rhythm and depth of the patient's respirations.	10*		
10. Release the patient's wrist.	5		
11. Wash hands or use hand sanitizer.	10*		
12. Document the readings in the patient's health record.	10*		
Total Points	**100**		

Documentation

Comments

CAAHEP Competencies	Step(s)
I.P.1.c. Accurately measure and record: pulse	Entire procedure
I.P.1.d. Measure and record: respirations	Entire procedure
ABHES Competencies	**Step(s)**
8.b. Obtain vital signs, obtain patient history, and formulate chief complaint	Entire procedure

Procedure 20.9   Accurately Measure and Record a Patient's Blood Pressure

Name _____ **Date** _____ **Score** _____

Task: Accurately measure and record a blood pressure measurement.

Equipment and Supplies:
- Patient's record
- Sphygmomanometer
- Stethoscope
- Antiseptic wipes/alcohol wipes

Standard: Complete the procedure and all critical steps in _____ minutes with a minimum score of 85% within two attempts (*or as indicated by the instructor*).

Scoring: Divide the points earned by the total possible points. Failure to perform a critical step, indicated by an asterisk (*), results in grade no higher than an 84% (*or as indicated by the instructor*).

Time: Began_____ Ended_____ Total minutes: _____

Steps:	Point Value	Attempt 1	Attempt 2
1. Wash hands or use hand sanitizer.	5*		
2. Assemble the equipment and supplies needed. Clean the earpieces and diaphragm of the stethoscope with alcohol wipes.	5*		
3. Greet the patient. Identify yourself. Verify the patient's identity with full name and date of birth. Explain the procedure to be performed in a manner that is understood by the patient. Answer any questions the patient may have on the procedure.	3		
4. Select the appropriate arm for application of the cuff (no mastectomy on that side, no injury or disease). If the patient has had a bilateral mastectomy, the blood pressure should be taken using a large thigh cuff with the stethoscope over the popliteal artery.	3		
5. Seat the patient in a comfortable position with the legs uncrossed and the arm resting, palm up, at heart level on the arm of a chair or a table next to where the patient is seated.	2		
6. Roll up the sleeve to about 5 inches above the elbow or have the patient remove the arm from the sleeve.	2		
7. Select the correct cuff size.	5*		
8. Palpate the brachial artery at the antecubital space in both arms. If one arm has a stronger pulse, use that arm. If the pulses are equal, select the right arm.	5		
9. Center the cuff bladder over the brachial artery with the connecting tube away from the patient's body and the tube to the bulb close to the body.	5		
10. Place the lower edge of the cuff about 1 inch above the palpable brachial pulse, normally located in the natural crease of the inner elbow, and wrap it snugly and smoothly.	3		
11. Position the gauge of the sphygmomanometer so that it is easily seen.	2		

12. Palpate the radial pulse, tighten the screw valve on the air pump, and inflate the cuff until the pulse can no longer be felt. Make a note at the point on the gauge where the pulse could no longer be felt. Mentally add 30 mm Hg to the reading. Deflate the cuff and wait 15 seconds.	**5**		
13. Insert the earpieces of the stethoscope turned forward into the ear canals.	**5**		
14. Place the stethoscope's diaphragm over the palpated brachial artery for an adult patient or the bell for a pediatric patient. Press firmly enough to obtain a seal but not so tightly that the artery is constricted. Only touch the edges of the stethoscope head.	**5**		
15. Close the valve and squeeze the bulb to inflate the cuff, rapidly but smoothly, to 30 mm above the palpated systolic level, which was previously determined.	**5**		
16. Open the valve slightly and deflate the cuff at a constant rate of 2 to 3 mm Hg per heartbeat.	**5**		
17. Listen throughout the entire deflation; note the point on the gauge at which you hear the first sound (systolic), the last sound (diastolic) and until the sounds have stopped for at least 10 mm Hg.	**5**		
18. Do not reinflate the cuff once the air has been released. Wait 30-60 seconds to repeat the procedure if needed.	**5**		
19. Remove the cuff from the patient's arm.	**5**		
20. Remove the stethoscope from your ears and document the systolic and diastolic readings and the arm used as BP systolic/diastolic.	**5**		
21. Clean the earpieces and the head of the stethoscope with an alcohol wipe and return both the cuff and the stethoscope to storage.	**5**		
22. Wash hands or use hand sanitizer.	**5***		
23. Document the readings in the patient's health record.	**5***		
Total Points	**100**		

Documentation

Comments

CAAHEP Competencies	Step(s)
I.P.1.a. Accurately measure and record: blood pressure	Entire procedure
ABHES Competencies	**Step(s)**
8.b. Obtain vital signs, obtain patient history, and formulate chief complaint	Entire procedure

Procedure 20.10   Accurately Measure and Record Oxygen Saturation

Name _____   **Date** _____   **Score** _____

Task: Accurately measure and record the adequacy of oxygen levels (or oxygen saturation) in the blood using a pulse oximeter.

Equipment and Supplies:
- Patient's health record
- Pulse oximeter and appropriately sized probe

Standard: Complete the procedure and all critical steps in _____ minutes with a minimum score of 85% within two attempts (*or as indicated by the instructor*).

Scoring: Divide the points earned by the total possible points. Failure to perform a critical step, indicated by an asterisk (*), results in grade no higher than an 84% (*or as indicated by the instructor*).

Time: Began_____ Ended_____ Total minutes: _____

Steps:	Point Value	Attempt 1	Attempt 2
1. Wash hands or use hand sanitizer.	15*		
2. Assemble the equipment.	10		
3. Greet the patient. Identify yourself. Verify the patient's identity with full name and date of birth. Explain the procedure to be performed in a manner that is understood by the patient. Answer any questions the patient may have on the procedure.	10		
4. Turn on the monitor and attach the probe to the finger (preferred) or ear lobe so it is flush with the skin.	10		
5. The light-emitting diode (LED) should be placed on top of the nail. If the patient is wearing nail polish or has artificial nails, these may have to be removed to get a strong pulse signal.	15*		
6. Sanitize the patient probe and the external portion of the monitor with an aseptic cleaner.	10*		
7. Wash hands or use hand sanitizer.	15*		
8. Document the oxygen saturation percentage and pulse in patient's health record. Include date, time, and if the patient is receiving supplemental oxygen record the amount in liters.	15*		
Total Points	100		

Documentation

Comments

CAAHEP Competencies	Step(s)
I.P.1.i. Accurately measure and record: oxygen saturation	Entire procedure
ABHES Competencies	**Step(s)**
8.b. Obtain vital signs, obtain patient history, and formulate chief complaint	Entire procedure

Procedure 20.11   Accurately Measure and Record a Patient's Weight and Height

Name _____   Date _____   Score _____

Task: Accurately measure and record the weight and height of a patient as part of the physical assessment procedure.

Equipment and Supplies:
• Balance beam scale with a measuring bar
• Paper towel
• Patient record

Standard: Complete the procedure and all critical steps in _____ minutes with a minimum score of 85% within two attempts (*or as indicated by the instructor*).

Scoring: Divide the points earned by the total possible points. Failure to perform a critical step, indicated by an asterisk (*), results in grade no higher than an 84% (*or as indicated by the instructor*).

Time: Began_____ Ended_____ Total minutes: _____

Steps:	Point Value	Attempt 1	Attempt 2
1. Wash hands or use hand sanitizer.	5*		
2. Greet the patient. Identify yourself. Verify the patient's identity with full name and date of birth. Explain the procedure to be performed in a manner that is understood by the patient. Answer any questions the patient may have on the procedure.	5		
3. Have the patient remove his or her shoes. Place a paper towel on the scale platform. Check to see that the balance bar pointer floats in the middle of the balance frame when all weights are at zero.	5		
4. Help the patient onto the scale. Make sure the patient has removed any heavy objects from pockets and is not holding anything such as a jacket or purse.	5		
5. Move the large weight into the groove closest to the patient's estimated weight.	5		
6. While the patient is standing still, slide the small upper weight to the right along the pound markers until the pointer balances in the middle of the balance frame.	10*		
7. Leave the weights in place.	5		
8. Ask the patient to step off the scale and move the height bar to a point above the patient's height. Extend the bar and ask the patient step back on the scale.	5		
9. Adjust the height bar so that it just touches the top of the patient's head.	5		
10. Leave the elevation bar set.	5		
11. Assist the patient off the scale. Make sure all items that were removed for weighing are given back to the patient.	5		
12. Read the weight scale. Add the numbers at the markers of the large and small weights and document the total to the nearest 1/4 lb in the patient's health record.	10*		

13. Read the height. Read the marker at the movable point of the ruler and document the measurement to the nearest 1/4 inch on the patient's health record.	**10***		
14. Use the patient's weight and height to determine the BMI if it is not automatically done by the EHR program.	**5**		
15. Return the weights and the measuring bar to zero.	**5**		
16. Remove the paper towel and dispose of in the waste container. Wash hands or use hand sanitizer.	**5**		
17. Document the results in the patient's health record.	**5**		
Total Points	**100**		

Documentation

Comments

CAAHEP Competencies	Step(s)
I.P.1.e. Accurately measure and record: height	9-17
I.P.1.f. Accurately measure and record: weight	3-8
ABHES Competencies	**Step(s)**
8.b. Obtain vital signs, obtain patient history, and formulate chief complaint	Entire procedure

Physical Examination

CAAHEP Competencies	Assessment
V.C.9. Identify principles of self-boundaries	Skills and Concepts – B. 3
V.C.12. Identify subjective and objective information	Skills and Concepts – D. 1.
V.C.15. Identify the medical assistant's role in telehealth	Skills and Concepts – C.2
XII.C.7.a. Identify principles of: body mechanics	Skills and Concepts – F. 3
I.P.9. Assist provider with a patient exam	Procedures 21.4 through 21.9, 21.11
V.P.1. Respond to nonverbal communication	Procedure 21.2
V.P.2. Correctly use and pronounce medical terminology in health care interactions	Procedure 21.1
V.P.8. Participate in a telehealth interaction with a patient	Procedure 21.3
X.P.3. Document patient care accurately in the medical record	Procedures 21.1. 21.3
XII.P.3. Use proper body mechanics	Procedure 21.10
A.3. Demonstrate empathy for patients' concerns	Procedure 21.1
A.4. Demonstrate active listening	Procedure 21.1
A.6. Recognize personal boundaries	Procedure 21.1
ABHES Competencies	Assessment
4. Medical Law and Ethics a. Follow documentation guidelines	Procedure 21.1
8.b. Obtain vital signs, obtain patient history, and formulate chief complaint	Procedures 21.1, 21.2
8.c. Assist provider with general/physical examination	Procedures 21.4 through 21.9, 21.11

VOCABULARY REVIEW

Using the word pool on the right, find the correct word to match the definition. Write the word on the line after the definition.

Group A

1. Arranged in the order of time _____
2. Considering the patient as a whole; includes the physical, emotional, social, economic, and spiritual needs of the person _____
3. Statistical data of a population; in healthcare, this includes the patient's name, address, date of birth, employment, and other details _____
4. Allows the listener to get additional information _____
5. A secure online website that gives patients 24-hour access to personal health information using a username and password _____
6. A procedure in which a fiberoptic scope is used to examine the large intestine _____
7. Describes the signs and symptoms from the time of onset _____
8. A statement in the patient's own words that describes the reason for the visit _____
9. Occurring in or affecting members of a family more than would be expected by chance _____
10. To establish an orderly relationship or connection _____

Word Pool
- chief complaint
- holistic
- patient portal
- correlates
- demographic
- history of present illness
- chronologic
- familial
- clarification
- colonoscopy

Group B

1. Subjective complaints reported by the patient, such as pain or nausea _____
2. A record or recording of electrical impulses of the heart produced by an electrocardiograph _____
3. A problem with the function of the nerves outside the spinal cord _____
4. A relationship of harmony and accord between the patient and the healthcare professional _____
5. Pertaining to the area between the vaginal opening and the rectum _____
6. Using good judgment; being discreet, sensible _____
7. A physical injury or wound caused by external force or violence _____
8. Agreement; the state that occurs when the verbal expression of the message matches the sender's nonverbal body language _____
9. To listen with a stethoscope _____
10. Objective findings determined by a clinician such as a fever, hypertension, or rash _____

Word Pool
- congruence
- rapport
- judicious
- symptoms
- signs
- electrocardiogram
- auscultate
- peripheral neuropathy
- trauma
- perineal

Group C

1. An abnormal sound heard during auscultation of the heart that may or may not have a pathologic origin

_____

2. Referring to normal skin tension; the resistance of the skin to being grasped between the fingers and released

_____

3. Movement or exercise of a body part by means of an externally applied force _____
4. Not noticeable or prominent _____
5. An abnormal sound or murmur heard on auscultation of an organ, vessel, or gland _____
6. The manner or style of walking _____
7. The process of stretching out; increasing the angle of a joint

_____

8. Similarity in size, form, and arrangement of parts on opposite sides of the body _____
9. The process of decreasing the angle of a joint

_____

10. The use of touch during the physical examination to assess the size, consistency, and location of certain body parts

_____

Word Pool
- palpation
- manipulation
- gait
- symmetry
- murmur
- bruit
- flexion
- extension
- inconspicuous
- turgor

Group D

1. The white part of the eye that forms the orbit

_____

2. Abnormal enlargement of the distal phalanges (fingers and toes) associated with cyanotic heart disease or advanced chronic pulmonary disease _____
3. Thinning and eventual destruction of the alveoli

_____

4. Small lumps, lesions, or swellings that are felt when the skin is palpated _____
5. Inspection of a cavity or organ by passing light through its walls

_____

Word Pool
- clubbing
- nodules
- sclera
- transillumination
- emphysema

ABBREVIATIONS
Write out what each of the following abbreviations stands for.

1. MRI _____
2. EHR_____
3. HIPAA _____
4. CC _____
5. VS _____
6. HPI _____

7. PH _____

8. PMH _____

9. UCD _____

10. UCHD _____

11. OTC _____

12. FH _____

13. SH _____

14. SR _____

15. ROS _____

16. HIV _____

17. RPM _____

18. BMI _____

19. ECG _____

20. EKG _____

21. ROM _____

22. CVA _____

23. EOM _____

24. BSE _____

25. TSE _____

26. GI _____

SKILLS AND CONCEPTS

Answer the following questions. Write your answer on the line or in the space provided.

A. Health History

1. A(n) _____ considers which of several diseases may be producing the patient's symptoms. A(n) _____ is arrived at after taking a detailed history and doing a comprehensive examination and considering all of the possible factors.

Match the components of the health history to the correct definition.

2. _____ Database
3. _____ Chief complaint
4. _____ Past history or past medical history
5. _____ Family history
6. _____ Social history
7. _____ Systems review of review of systems

   a. Summary of patient's previous health including the dates and details of the patient's usual childhood diseases, major illnesses, surgeries, allergies, accidents, and immunization record

   b. Logical sequence of examinations to determine the body systems' state of health

   c. The record of the patient's name, address, date of birth, insurance information, personal data, history, physical examination, and initial laboratory findings

   d. Includes information about the patient's lifestyle including feeling safe at home; use of tobacco, alcohol, or recreational drugs; sleeping and exercise habits; typical diet; education and occupation; dental care history

   e. Details about the patient's parents and siblings and their health; if they are deceased, the age and cause of death

   f. Present illness or purpose of the patient's visit

B. Understanding and Communicating with the Patient

Match the process of active listening to the correct definition.

1. _____ Restatement
2. _____ Reflection
3. _____ Clarification

   a. summarize or simplify the sender's thoughts and feelings as well as resolve any confusion in the message

   b. paraphrasing, or repeating, the patient's statements with phrases such as "You are saying…" or "You are telling me the problem is…"

   c. repeating the main idea of the conversation while also identifying the sender's feelings

4. Label the following questions as either open-ended or closed.

   a. How have you been feeling? _____

   b. Do you have a headache? _____

   c. Have you ever broken a bone? _____

   d. What brings you to the provider? _____

   e. Are you feeling better? _____

   f. Do you have high blood pressure? _____

   g. Tell me about your back pain. _____

   h. When did the nausea start? _____

   i. Did your mother have a history of cancer? _____

   j. Do you smoke? _____

5. When demonstrating self-boundaries, the focus is kept on the patient. Developing a friendship with a patient is an example of self-boundaries.
   a. The first statement is true, and the second statement is false.
   b. The first statement is false and the second statement if true.
   c. Both statements are true.
   d. Both statements are false.

C. Interviewing the Patient

1. Identify the defense mechanism displayed by the following patients.

   a. A patient who refuses to believe she has breast cancer _____

   _____

   _____

   b. A 5-year-old child who starts to suck his thumb again when he is ill_____

   _____

   _____

   c. A patient who accuses you of being disrespectful when he has acted that way himself _____

   _____

   _____

   d. A patient who explains that she missed her appointment because she was so busy, and she really didn't need to follow up on the biopsy results anyway

   _____

   _____

2. The medical assistant's role in telehealth involves updating patient _____,
   _____, _____, and _____.

D. Patient Assessment and Documentation

1. Label the following as "subjective" (symptom) or "objective" (sign).

   a. Pain _____

   b. Nausea_____

   c. Dizziness _____

   d. Elevated blood pressure _____

   e. Labored respirations _____

   f. Headache _____

   g. Temperature of the skin _____

   h. Back pain_____

   i. Color of the skin_____

   j. Abdominal pain_____

2. Complete the following table.

Abbreviation	Definition
	abdomen
	before eating
ASHD	
bid	
	blood urea nitrogen
CAD	
CHF	
DM	
	fever of unknown origin
hs	
	no known allergies
	rule out
SOB	
STI	
	upper respiratory infection

E. Physical Examination

1. Preparing the examination room includes which of the following?
   a. Checking the expiration dates on all of the packages and supplies
   b. Cleaning and disinfecting the area daily and between patients
   c. Prepare the instruments and equipment needed for the examination
   d. Replacing sharps containers when they are two-thirds full
   e. All of the above

2. The medical assistant's responsibilities for preparing the patient for in examination include which of the following?
   a. Measure and record the patient's height, weight, BMI, and vital signs.
   b. Obtain specimens, such as urine and blood, if they have been preordered by the provider.
   c. Make sure that the health record is complete and any needed consent forms have been signed.
   d. Document current medications and allergies.
   e. All of the above.

3. When assisting the provider, the medical assistant should position and drape the patient during the
    different phases of the examination. The medical assistant may also hand instruments and equipment to
    the provider as requested.
    a. The first statement is true and the second statement is false.
    b. The first statement is false and the second statement is true.
    c. Both statements are true.
    d. Both statements are false.

Match the method of assessment to the correct definition.

1. _____ Inspection
2. _____ Palpation
3. _____ Percussion
4. _____ Auscultation
5. _____ Mensuration
6. _____ Manipulation

a. Involves tapping or striking the body, usually with the fingers
    or a small hammer, to elicit sounds or vibratory sensations.
b. The examiner uses the sense of touch.
c. The forceful, passive movement of a joint to determine the
    range of extension or flexion of a part of the body.
d. Use of a stethoscope to listen to sounds arising from the body.
e. The examiner uses observation to detect significant physical
    features or objective data.
f. The process of measuring.

F. Assisting with the Physical Examination

1. Identify the instruments needed for the physical examination that are shown in the following figures
    and describe their purpose.

a. _____

    _____

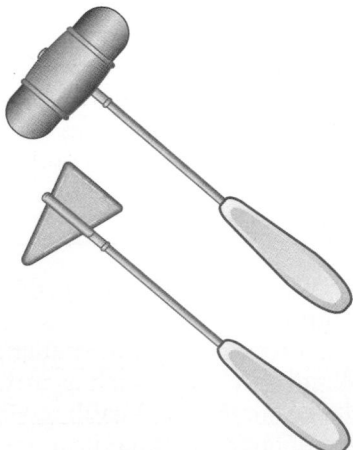

b. _____

    _____

c. _____

_____

d. _____

_____

e. _____

_____

f. _____

_____

2. Label the positions for examination shown in the following figures and give an example of a physical examination that is appropriate for each.

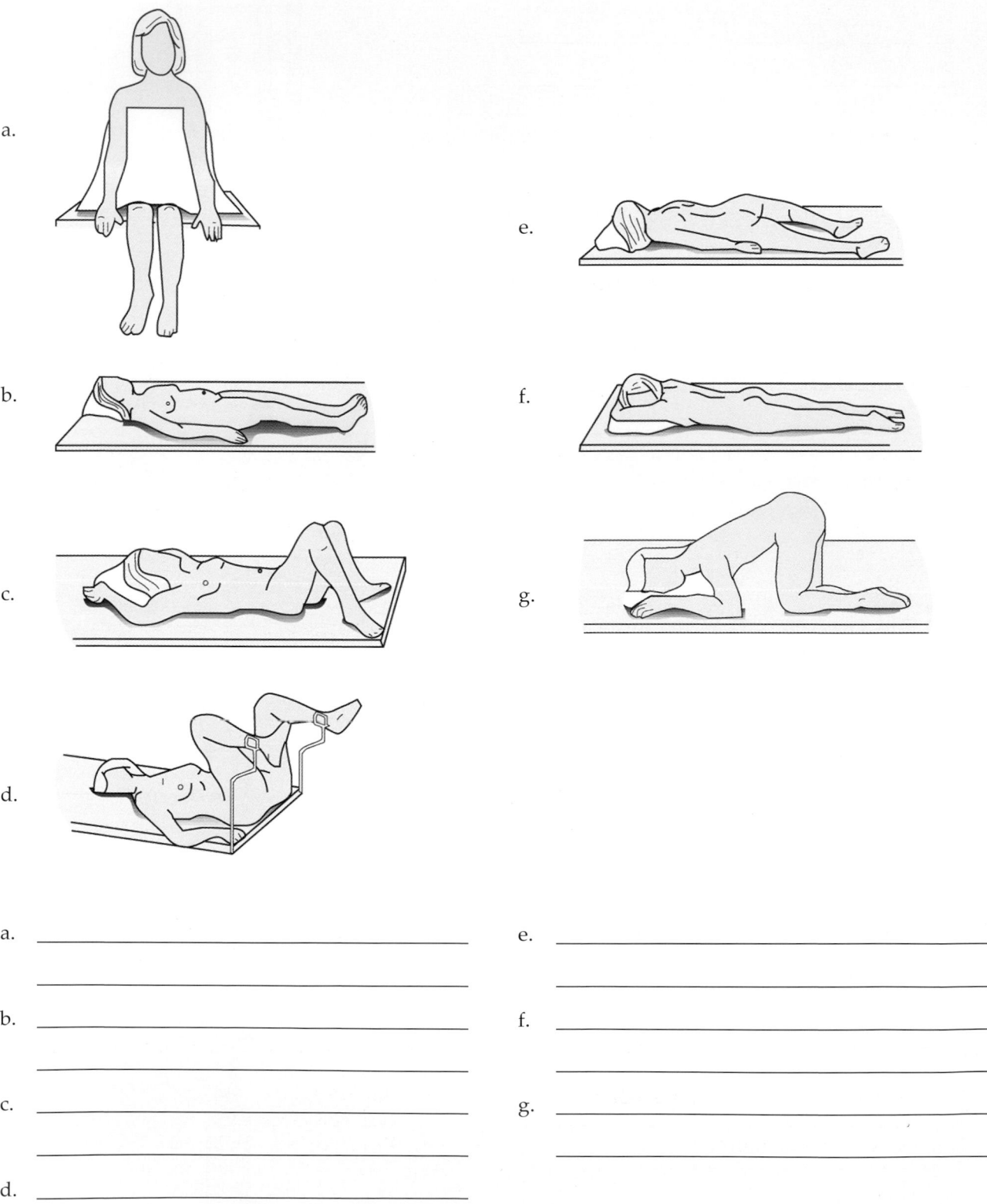

a.
a.

b.
b.

c.
c.

d.
d.

e.
e.

f.
f.

g.
g.

a. _____

b. _____

c. _____

d. _____

e. _____

f. _____

g. _____

3. Proper body mechanics include which of the following?
   a. Maintain good posture.
   b. Avoid twisting or turning when reaching for an object.
   c. Do not cross legs while sitting.
   d. All of the above.
   e. None of the above.

4. Proper lifting techniques include which of the following?
   a. Bend at the knees with the feet shoulder-width apart and keep the back straight.
   b. When carrying a heavy item, keep the weight as close to the body as possible.
   c. Move feet in the direction of the lift. Do not twist or turn on fixed feet.
   d. If possible, slide, roll, or push a heavy item rather than lifting or pulling.
   e. All of the above.

5. A(n) _____ should be used when transferring patients to prevent injury to yourself and safeguard patients from falling.

CERTIFICATION PREPARATION

Circle the correct answer.

1. What does it mean when medical assistants display *empathy* when dealing with patients?
   a. They feel sorry for patients who have serious health problems.
   b. They are able to hear what patients say without judging the content.
   c. The can detach themselves emotionally from the problems of their patients.
   d. They truly like and care about each of their patients.

2. Which factor is likely to have the most influence on the accuracy and completeness of the information obtained from the patient during the medical history?
   a. The comfort of the chairs in the meeting area.
   b. The medical assistant's ability to take complete and detailed notes.
   c. The privacy of the area in which the interview takes place.
   d. The efficiency of the medical assistant in conducting the interview.

3. Which is an open-ended question?
   a. How old are you?
   b. What brings you to the office today?
   c. Do you smoke?
   d. Does your head hurt?

4. Which is an example of objective data?
   a. Complaints of pain
   b. Social history
   c. Past medical history
   d. Blood pressure recordings

5. During a physical examination, the provider discovers a bruit. What method would she be using to make this discovery?
   a. Auscultation
   b. Palpation
   c. Manipulation
   d. Percussion

6. The provider asks the medical assistant to position a patient on the examination table so that the patient can breathe easier. The most appropriate position is
   a. dorsal recumbent.
   b. lithotomy.
   c. semi-Fowler's.
   d. left lateral.

7. Which defense mechanism is a patient using when they completely reject the information?
   a. Denial
   b. Suppression
   c. Reaction formation
   d. Projection

8. Which defense mechanism is a patient using when they express their feelings as the opposite of what they really feel?
   a. Denial
   b. Suppression
   c. Reaction formation
   d. Projection

9. What type of telehealth involves the transmission of medical data to providers?
   a. Store-and-forward
   b. Remote patient monitoring
   c. Virtual visits
   d. None of the above

10. The position used primarily for Pap tests is
    a. supine.
    b. left lateral.
    c. lithotomy.
    d. dorsal recumbent.

WORKPLACE APPLICATIONS

In the following scenarios, what types of interview barriers are indicated? Explain how these statements are problematic and may interfere with the patient interview.

1. Mrs. Miller is expressing her concern about a changing mole in her left axillary region. Chris, the medical assistant obtaining her health history, makes the statement, "Mrs. Miller, the dysplastic nevus found in the left axillary region looks as if it could be malignant. You haven't been using sunscreen, have you?"

   _____

   _____

   _____

   _____

2. Mr. Sunsari is being seen today for a suspicious mass in his left lung. The physician has recommended a biopsy of the mass; however, Mr. Sunsari prefers to postpone the procedure. He asks Chris what he should do about scheduling the procedure. Chris states, "I would do it right away."

   _____

   _____

   _____

   _____

3. Carmen Largosi is a diabetic patient who is very concerned about her blood glucose levels. Her mother had diabetes and had to have her left leg amputated. When Carmen expresses her fears, Chris responds with, "I wouldn't worry about that. The doctor is very good with diabetic patients."

   _____

   _____

   _____

   _____

4. Mrs. Xu Nyguen will not establish eye contact with you during the patient interview. Do you think this means Mrs. Nyguen is not telling the truth?

_____

_____

_____

_____

5. Carl Worth, a 78-year-old patient, is hard of hearing and does not appear to be paying attention when you ask questions for the patient history. His daughter is in the examination room with him, so would it be better to gather patient information from her? Why or why not?

_____

_____

_____

_____

6. Theo Lang is being seen today for a surgical follow-up visit. He asks that his partner, David, accompany him into the examination room. What should you do?

_____

_____

_____

_____

INTERNET ACTIVITIES

1. Using online resources, research a culture other than your own in your area. Research the healthcare and communication practices. Create a poster presentation, a PowerPoint presentation, or write a paper summarizing your research. Include the following points in your project:
   a. How does this culture feel about eye contact?
   b. How does this culture view personal space?
   c. Are there any beliefs that would impact how care is provided in the healthcare setting?

2. Using online resources, research the use of chaperones in the healthcare setting. Create a poster presentation, a PowerPoint presentation, or write a paper summarizing your research. Include the following points in your project:
   a. What are the patient's rights when it comes to having a chaperone in the examination room?
   b. What are the responsibilities of the chaperone?
   c. What should the healthcare facility have in place when using chaperones?

Procedure 21.1   Obtain and Document Patient Information

Name _____   **Date** _____   **Score** _____

Task: To use restatement, reflection, and clarification to obtain patient information and document patient care accurately.

Equipment and Supplies:
- History form (Work Product 21.1) or EHR system with the patient history window opened
- If using a paper form—a red pen for recording the patient's allergies, and a black pen to meet legal documentation guidelines
- Quiet, private area

Directions: Complete this procedure with another student playing the role of the patient. To make the experience more realistic, choose a student about whom you know very little. To maintain the student's privacy, he or she does not have to share any confidential information.

Standard: Complete the procedure and all critical steps in _____ minutes with a minimum score of 85% within two attempts (*or as indicated by the instructor*).

Scoring: Divide the points earned by the total possible points. Failure to perform a critical step, indicated by an asterisk (*), results in grade no higher than an 84% (*or as indicated by the instructor*).

Time: Began_____ Ended_____ Total minutes: _____

Steps:	Point Value	Attempt 1	Attempt 2
1. Greet the patient. Identify yourself. Verify the patient's identity with full name and date of birth. Explain your role.	5		
2. Take the patient to a quiet, private area for the interview and explain why the information is needed.	5		
3. Complete the history form by using therapeutic communication techniques, including restatement, reflection, and clarification. Use active listening. Correctly use and pronounce medical terminology. Make sure all medical terminology is adequately explained. (*Refer to the Checklist for Affective Behaviors - Active Listening*)	10*		
4. Speak in a pleasant, distinct manner, remembering to maintain eye contact with your patient.	10*		
5. Demonstrate empathy and remain sensitive to the diverse needs of your patient throughout the interview process. (*Refer to the Checklist for Affective Behaviors - Empathy*)	10*		
6. Record the following statistical information: • Patient's full name, including middle initial • Address, including apartment number and ZIP code • Marital status • Sex (gender) • Age and date of birth • Telephone numbers for home, cell, and work • Insurance information if not already available • Employer's name, address, and telephone number	10		

7. Record the following medical history: • Chief complaint • Present illness • Past medical history • Family history • Social history	**10**			
8. Ask about allergies to drugs and any other substances and record any allergies in red ink on every page of the history form, on the front of the patient record, and on each progress note page; in the EHR, enter allergy information where designated.	**10**			
9. If using a paper form, record all information legibly and neatly and spell words correctly.	**5**			
10. Thank the patient for cooperating and direct him or her back to the reception area.	**5**			
11. Review the record for errors before you pass it to the provider or exit the EHR health history area.	**10**			
12. Protect the integrity of the health record and the confidentiality of patient information. Safeguards mandated by the Health Insurance Portability and Accountability Act (HIPAA) include: • Passwords to secure access to all EHRs • Computer monitor shields to protect patient information if data are left on the screen • Turning monitors away from patient traffic areas to prevent accidental release of information • Securing all medical records	**10**			
Total Points	**100**			

Affective Behavior	*Affective Behaviors Checklist* **Directions:** Check behaviors observed during the role-play.					
Empathy	**Negative, Unprofessional Behaviors**	**Attempt**		**Positive, Professional Behaviors**	**Attempt**	
		1	**2**		**1**	**2**
	Unsupportive, uninterested, or uncaring			Demonstrated supportive, caring behaviors		
	Did not acknowledge or respond appropriately to the patient's emotional responses; cold, aloof, insensitive, indifferent, or unfeeling			Acknowledged and responded appropriately to the patient's emotional responses; showed sensitivity		
	Failed to reassure patient; did not respond to the patient's concerns			Reassured patient by repeating and responding to the patient's concerns		
	Used language that is hard to understand (e.g., slang, generational terms, medical terminology, too scientific)			Used language that the patient can understand		
	Other:			Other:		

Active Listening	Failed to use therapeutic communication techniques			Asked appropriate open-ended questions; repeated back (paraphrased) and clarified important information; responded to patient's emotional responses		
	Did not listen to the patient, interrupted patient			Allowed patient to talk; listened without interrupting		
	Responded with bias; judgmental and/or condescending to the patient			Responded without bias or judgment; refrained from condescending attitude		
	Failed to address the patient's questions; or answers to patient's questions were inappropriate			Answered the patient's questions appropriately		
	Other:			Other:		

Grading Rubric for the Affective Behaviors Checklist **Directions:** *Based on checklist results, identify the points received for the procedure checklist. Indicate how the behaviors demonstrated met the expectations.*		**Point Value**	**Attempt 1**	**Attempt 2**
Does not meet Expectation	• Response demonstrated lack of active listening and/or lacks empathy. • Student demonstrated more than 2 negative, unprofessional behaviors during the interaction.	0		
Needs Improvement	• Response demonstrated lack of active listening and/or lacks empathy. • Student demonstrated 1 or 2 negative, unprofessional behaviors during the interaction.	0		
Meets Expectation	• Response demonstrated active listening skills and empathy; no negative, unprofessional behaviors observed. • More practice is needed for behavior to appear natural and for student to appear comfortable and at ease.	10		
Occasionally Exceeds Expectation	• Response demonstrated active listening skills and empathy; no negative, unprofessional behaviors observed. • At times student appeared comfortable and at ease; but more practice is needed for behavior to become natural and consistent with a professional medical assistant.	10		
Always Exceeds Expectation	• Response demonstrated active listening skills and empathy; no negative, unprofessional behaviors observed. • Student's behaviors appeared natural and comfortable. Behaviors are consistent with a professional medical assistant.	10		

Comments

CAAHEP Competencies	Step(s)
V.P.2. Correctly use and pronounce medical terminology in health care interactions	3
A.3. Demonstrate empathy for patients' concerns	3
A.4. Demonstrate active listening	5
A.6. Recognize personal boundaries	3, 4, 5
ABHES Competencies	**Step(s)**
8.b. Obtain vital signs, obtain patient history, and formulate chief complaint	7

Work Product 21.1   History Form

Name _____ Date _____ Score _____

MEDICAL RECORD		
NAME	AGE	SEX S / M / D / W
ADDRESS	PHONE	DATE
SPONSOR	ADDRESS	
OCCUPATION	REF BY	ACKN

CHIEF COMPLAINT
PRESENT ILLNESS

FAMILY HISTORY

MOTHER   FATHER   SIBLING(S)

TB   DIAB   MALIG   HT DIS   NEPH   EPILEP   PSYCH

PAST HISTORY — GENERAL HEALTH	**GASTROINTESTINAL**		
CHILDHOOD DISEASES	APPETITE	BOWEL HABITS	VOMITING
SC FEV RHEUM FEV ASTHMA	INDIGESTION	HEMORRHOIDS	BLEEDING
OTHER _____	NAUSEA	DIET	ITCHING
SOCIAL HISTORY	JAUNDICE	PAIN	PAIN WITH STOOL
COFFEE TOBACCO ALCOHOL DRUG USE	OTHER		

WEIGHT	**URINARY TRACT**		
USUAL WEIGHT	NOCTURIA	INCONTINENCE	INFECTION
RECENT WEIGHT FLUCTUATIONS	PAIN	FREQUENCY	
HX OF EATING DISORDER	BLEEDING	BURNING	

REVIEW OF SYSTEMS	**GENITAL TRACT**	
E E N T	AGE AT MENST	TYPE PERIOD
EYES EARS NOSE THROAT NECK	PAINFUL PERIOD	INTERMITTENT BLEEDING
NEUROMUSCULAR	AMENORRHEA	DYSMENORRHEA
STRENGTH ANXIETY	VAG DISCH	IRRITATION
SLEEP DEPRESSION	BREAST EXAM	PROSTATE EXAM
MUSCULAR PAIN PERIPHERAL NEUROPATHY	TESTICULAR EXAM	
JOINT PAIN	**L M P**	
CARDIOVASCULAR	AGES OF CHILDREN	CONTRACEPTION TYPE
HEART DISEASE MI	LMP DATE	NO. OF PREGNANCIES
CONGENITAL HEART DEFECTS TIAS	NO. OF LIVE BIRTHS	AGES OF CHILDREN
HYPERTENSION STROKE	**OTHER**	
EDEMA	_____	

LUNGS	**ACCIDENTS**
PAIN DYSPNEA	_____
COUGHING UP BLOOD COUGH	_____
IRREG BREATHING	_____

OPERATIONS	**CURRENT MEDICATIONS AND TREATMENTS**
_____	_____
_____	_____
_____	_____

COMMENTS
_____
_____
_____

Procedure 21.2 Respond to Nonverbal Communication

Name _____ Date _____ Score _____

Task: To observe the patient and respond appropriately to nonverbal communication.

Equipment and Supplies:
- Patient's record

Scenario: Monique Jones is a new patient with the chief complaint of intermittent abdominal pain with alternating diarrhea and constipation. Ms. Jones has experienced this discomfort for several months and appears very frustrated. She is sitting on the end of the exam table with her arms wrapped around her abdomen. She sighs frequently and refuses to maintain eye contact. What is her nonverbal behavior telling you, and how can you establish therapeutic communication with this patient?

Directions: Complete this procedure with another student playing the role of the patient. To make the experience more realistic, choose a student about whom you know very little. To maintain the student's privacy, he or she does not have to share any confidential information.

Standard: Complete the procedure and all critical steps in _____ minutes with a minimum score of 85% within two attempts (*or as indicated by the instructor*).

Scoring: Divide the points earned by the total possible points. Failure to perform a critical step, indicated by an asterisk (*), results in grade no higher than an 84% (*or as indicated by the instructor*).

Time: Began_____ Ended_____ Total minutes: _____

Steps:	Point Value	Attempt 1	Attempt 2
1. Greet the patient. Identify yourself. Verify the patient's identity with full name and date of birth. Explain your role.	20		
2. Ask the patient the purpose of her visit and the onset, duration, and frequency of her symptoms. Pay close attention to her body language to determine whether what she is telling you is congruent with her body language.	20*		
3. Use restatement, reflection, and clarification to gather as much information as possible about the patient's chief complaint. Make sure all medical terminology is adequately explained.	20		
4. Speak in a pleasant, distinct manner, remembering to maintain eye contact with your patient.	20		
5. Continue to observe nonverbal patient behaviors and select the appropriate verbal response to demonstrate your sensitivity to her discomfort, frustration, and anxiety.	20		
Total Points	100		

Comments

CAAHEP Competencies	Step(s)
V.P.1. Respond to nonverbal communication	Entire procedure
ABHES Competencies	**Step(s)**
8. b. Obtain vital signs, obtain patient history, and formulate chief complaint	Entire procedure

Procedure 21.3 Participate in a Telehealth Interaction with a Patient

Name _____ Date _____ Score _____

Task: Using interactive technology, participate in a telehealth interaction with a patient.

Scenario: Dr. Perez has been using interactive telehealth visits to follow-up certain patients. She has asked you to update the patient demographics and health history information prior to Dr. Perez joining the visit. The patient is Jana Green (DOB 05/01/19XX). Mrs. Green was seen 2 weeks ago by Dr. Perez at WMFM Clinic and was diagnosed with rheumatoid arthritis. Dr. Perez prescribed hydroxychloroquine and prednisone at that time and wanted a follow-up visit with Mrs. Green to see how she was tolerating the medication. At that visit, she mentioned that is getting harder for her to come into the office as she and her husband no longer drive. Dr. Perez offered the option of an interactive telehealth visit that would utilize the WMFM Clinic patient portal. Mrs. Green is quite familiar with the portal and thought that would be wonderful option for this visit. It was confirmed that Mrs. Green had the appropriate equipment to be able to access the portal for telehealth visit. Today is the day for this visit.

Directions: Using the scenario, role-play the medical assistant's interaction with Mrs. Green via a virtual environment. Verify her address, phone number, and insurance information. Review her allergies and medication list. The partner (patient) should make up any information required.

Equipment and Supplies:
- Patient's record
- Access to a virtual environment such as Zoom

Standard: Complete the procedure and all critical steps in _____ minutes with a minimum score of 85% within two attempts (*or as indicated by the instructor*).

Scoring: Divide the points earned by the total possible points. Failure to perform a critical step, indicated by an asterisk (*), results in grade no higher than an 84% (*or as indicated by the instructor*).

Time: Began_____ Ended_____ Total minutes: _____

Steps:	Point Value	Attempt 1	Attempt 2
1. Log into the virtual environment and connect with your patient. Make sure that you are not on mute and that your patient can hear and see you.	15		
2. Greet the patient. Identify yourself. Verify the patient's identity with full name and date of birth. Explain what will be happening during the medical assistant's portion of the interactive telehealth visit. Demonstrate respect for the patient. Be sincere, courteous, polite, and welcoming.	15		
3. Using appropriate closed and open-ended questions to verify the patient's demographic information. Document any changes in the patient's health record.	15*		
4. Using appropriate closed and open-ended questions and statements, review the patient's allergies. Document any changes in the patient's health record.	15*		
5. Using appropriate closed and open-ended questions and statements, review the patient's medication list. Document any changes in the patient's health record.	15*		

6.	Using appropriate closed and open-ended questions and statements, obtain information about the patient's health, family, and social history. Document any changes in the patient's health record.	15*		
7.	Thank the patient for their time and ask if they have any questions about the next stage of the interactive telehealth visit.	10		
	Total Points	100		

Comments

CAAHEP Competencies	Step(s)
V.P.8. Participate in a telehealth interaction with a patient	Entire procedure
X.P.3. Document patient care accurately in the medical record	3, 4, 5, 6
ABHES Competencies	**Step(s)**
8.c. Assist provider with general/physical examination	Entire procedure

Procedure 21.4 Fowler's and Semi-Fowler's Positions

Name _____ Date _____ Score _____

Task: To position and drape the patient for examinations of the head, neck, and chest, or patients who have difficulty breathing when lying flat.

Equipment and Supplies:
- Patient's record
- Examination table
- Table paper
- Patient gown
- Drape
- Disinfectant wipes
- Gloves

Standard: Complete the procedure and all critical steps in _____ minutes with a minimum score of 85% within two attempts (*or as indicated by the instructor*).

Scoring: Divide the points earned by the total possible points. Failure to perform a critical step, indicated by an asterisk (*), results in grade no higher than an 84% (*or as indicated by the instructor*).

Time: Began_____ Ended_____ Total minutes: _____

Steps:	Point Value	Attempt 1	Attempt 2
1. Wash hands or use hand sanitizer.	10		
2. Greet the patient. Identify yourself. Verify the patient's identity with full name and date of birth. Explain the procedure to be performed in a manner that is understood by the patient. Answer any questions the patient may have on the procedure.	10		
3. Give the patient a gown. Explain what clothing must be removed for the particular examination being done and whether the gown should open in the front or the back. Provide assistance as needed. Give the patient privacy while changing. Knock on the examination room door before re-entering to make sure the patient has completed undressing and gowning.	10		
4. For Fowler's position, elevate the head of the bed 90 degrees. If the patient feels more comfortable, she can sit at the end of the table. Extend the footrest as needed for patient comfort. The patient may be more comfortable in semi-Fowler's position. In this modification of Fowler's position, the head of the table is elevated 45 degrees.	15*		
5. Drape the patient according to the type of examination and the required patient exposure.	10		
6. After the examination has been completed, assist the patient as needed to get off the table and get dressed.	10		
7. Put on gloves and use disinfectant wipes to clean the exam table and all potentially contaminated surfaces. Dispose of used gloves and examination table paper according to facility policies. Pull clean paper over the table.	15		
8. Wash hands or use hand sanitizer.	10		

9.	Follow up with the provider's orders regarding scheduling of diagnostic studies, collection of specimens, and/or scheduling of future appointments.	10		
	Total Points	100		

Comments

CAAHEP Competencies		**Step(s)**
I.P.9. Assist provider with a patient exam		Entire procedure
ABHES Competencies		**Step(s)**
8.c. Assist provider with general/physical examination		Entire procedure

Procedure 21.5 Supine (Horizontal Recumbent) and Dorsal Recumbent Positions

Name _____ Date _____ Score _____

Task: To position and drape the patient for examinations of the abdomen, heart, and breasts in the horizontal recumbent (supine) position, and exams of the rectal, vaginal, and perineal areas in the dorsal recumbent position.

Equipment and Supplies:
- Patient's record
- Examination table
- Table paper
- Patient gown
- Drape
- Disinfectant wipes
- Gloves

Standard: Complete the procedure and all critical steps in _____ minutes with a minimum score of 85% within two attempts (*or as indicated by the instructor*).

Scoring: Divide the points earned by the total possible points. Failure to perform a critical step, indicated by an asterisk (*), results in grade no higher than an 84% (*or as indicated by the instructor*).

Time: Began _____ Ended _____ Total minutes: _____

Steps:	Point Value	Attempt 1	Attempt 2
1. Wash hands or use hand sanitizer.	10		
2. Greet the patient. Identify yourself. Verify the patient's identity with full name and date of birth. Explain the procedure to be performed in a manner that is understood by the patient. Answer any questions the patient may have on the procedure.	10		
3. Give the patient a gown. Explain the clothing that must be removed for the particular examination being done and whether the gown should open in the front or in the back. Provide assistance as needed. For the horizontal recumbent position, the gown should be open in the front. Give the patient privacy while changing. Knock on the examination room door before re-entering to make sure the patient has completed undressing and gowning.	10		
4. Do not place the patient in the necessary positions until the provider is ready for that part of the examination.	10		
5. Pull out the table extension that supports the patient's legs. For the horizontal recumbent (supine) position, help the patient lie flat on the table with the face upward. For the dorsal recumbent position, have the patient lie flat on the back and flex the knees so the feet are flat on the table. If needed, help the patient move down toward the foot of the table for the examination.	10*		
6. Drape the patient from nipple line to feet in the supine position, and diagonally with the point of the drape between the feet for the dorsal recumbent position.	10		
7. After the examination has been completed, assist the patient as needed to get off the table and get dressed.	10		

8.	Put on gloves and use disinfectant wipes to clean the exam table and all potentially contaminated surfaces. Dispose of used gloves and examination table paper according to facility policies. Pull clean paper over the table.	10		
9.	Wash hands or use hand sanitizer.	10		
10.	Follow up with the provider's orders regarding scheduling of diagnostic studies, collection of specimens, and/or scheduling of future appointments.	10		
	Total Points	100		

Comments

CAAHEP Competencies	Step(s)
I.P.9. Assist provider with a patient exam	Entire procedure
ABHES Competencies	**Step(s)**
8.c. Assist provider with general/physical examination	Entire procedure

Procedure 21.6   Lithotomy Position

Name _____ **Date** _____ **Score** _____

Task: To position and drape the patient primarily for vaginal and pelvic examinations and Pap tests.

Equipment and Supplies:
- Patient's record
- Examination table
- Table paper
- Patient gown
- Drape
- Disinfectant wipes
- Gloves

Standard: Complete the procedure and all critical steps in _____ minutes with a minimum score of 85% within two attempts (*or as indicated by the instructor*).

Scoring: Divide the points earned by the total possible points. Failure to perform a critical step, indicated by an asterisk (*), results in grade no higher than an 84% (*or as indicated by the instructor*).

Time: Began_____ Ended_____ Total minutes: _____

Steps:	Point Value	Attempt 1	Attempt 2
1. Wash hands or use hand sanitizer.	5		
2. Greet the patient. Identify yourself. Verify the patient's identity with full name and date of birth. Explain the procedure to be performed in a manner that is understood by the patient. Answer any questions the patient may have on the procedure.	5		
3. Give the patient a gown. Instruct the patient to undress from the waist down with the gown open in the back. If the provider also will be doing a breast examination, the patient should undress completely and put on the gown so that it opens in the front. Provide assistance as needed. Give the patient privacy while changing. Knock on the examination room door before re-entering to make sure the patient has completed undressing and gowning.	10		
4. Do not place the patient in the lithotomy position until the provider is ready for that part of the examination.	10		
5. Pull out the table extension that supports the patient's legs and help the patient lie face upward on the table. Pull out the stirrups, adjust their extension length for the patient's comfort, and lock them in place.	10*		
6. Reinsert the table extension and have the patient move toward the foot of the table with her buttocks on the bottom table edge. Gently place the patient's legs in the stirrups, checking for comfort. Some offices may stock cloth or paper stirrup covers to protect the patient and make the position more comfortable. The patient's arms can be placed alongside the body or across the chest.	10*		
7. Drape the patient diagonally, with the point of the drape between the feet. The drape should be large enough to cover the patient from the nipple line to the ankles and wide enough so the patient's thighs are not exposed.	10		

8.	After the examination has been completed, assist the patient as needed to get off the table and get dressed.	**10**		
9.	Put on gloves and use disinfectant wipes to clean the exam table and all potentially contaminated surfaces. Dispose of used gloves and examination table paper according to facility policies. Pull clean paper over the table.	**10**		
10.	Wash hands or use hand sanitizer.	**10**		
11.	Follow up with the provider's orders regarding scheduling of diagnostic studies, collection of specimens, and/or scheduling of future appointments.	**10**		
	Total Points	**100**		

Comments

CAAHEP Competencies	**Step(s)**
I.P.9. Assist provider with a patient exam	Entire procedure
ABHES Competencies	**Step(s)**
8.c. Assist provider with general/physical examination	Entire procedure

Procedure 21.7   Left Lateral Position

Name _____ **Date** _____ **Score** _____

Task: To position and drape the patient for examination of the rectum, instillation of rectal medication, perineal examination, and some pelvic examinations.

Equipment and Supplies:
- Patient's record
- Examination table
- Patient gown
- Table paper
- Drape
- Disinfectant wipes
- Gloves

Standard: Complete the procedure and all critical steps in _____ minutes with a minimum score of 85% within two attempts (*or as indicated by the instructor*).

Scoring: Divide the points earned by the total possible points. Failure to perform a critical step, indicated by an asterisk (*), results in grade no higher than an 84% (*or as indicated by the instructor*).

Time: Began _____ Ended _____ Total minutes: _____

Steps:	Point Value	Attempt 1	Attempt 2
1. Wash hands or use hand sanitizer.	10		
2. Greet the patient. Identify yourself. Verify the patient's identity with full name and date of birth. Explain the procedure to be performed in a manner that is understood by the patient. Answer any questions the patient may have on the procedure.	10		
3. Give the patient a gown and explain what clothing must be removed for the particular examination being done. Tell the patient that the gown should open in the back. Provide assistance as needed. Give the patient privacy while changing. Knock on the examination room door before re-entering to make sure the patient has completed undressing and gowning.	10		
4. Do not place the patient in the left lateral position until the provider is ready for that part of the examination.	10		
5. Help the patient turn onto the left side; the left arm and shoulder should be drawn back behind the body so that the patient is tilted onto the chest. Flex the right arm upward for support, slightly flex the left leg, and sharply flex the right leg upward. Help the patient move the buttocks to the side edge of the table.	10*		
6. Drape the patient over an exposed area that is not included in the examination. The drape should cover from the shoulders to the feet so that the patient is not exposed accidentally.	10*		
7. After the examination has been completed, assist the patient as needed to get off the table and get dressed.	10		

8.	Put on gloves and use disinfectant wipes to clean the exam table and all potentially contaminated surfaces. Dispose of used gloves and examination table paper according to facility policies. Pull clean paper over the table.	**10**		
9.	Wash hands or use hand sanitizer.	**10**		
10.	Follow up with the provider's orders regarding scheduling of diagnostic studies, collection of specimens, and/or scheduling of future appointments.	**10**		
	Total Points	**100**		

Comments

CAAHEP Competencies	**Step(s)**
I.P.9. Assist provider with a patient exam	Entire procedure
ABHES Competencies	**Step(s)**
8.c. Assist provider with general/physical examination	Entire procedure

Procedure 21.8   Prone Position

Name _____ Date _____ Score _____

Task: To position and drape the patient for examination of the back and for certain surgical procedures.

Equipment and Supplies:
- Patient's record
- Examination table
- Patient gown
- Table paper
- Drape
- Disinfectant wipes
- Gloves

Standard: Complete the procedure and all critical steps in _____ minutes with a minimum score of 85% within two attempts (*or as indicated by the instructor*).

Scoring: Divide the points earned by the total possible points. Failure to perform a critical step, indicated by an asterisk (*), results in grade no higher than an 84% (*or as indicated by the instructor*).

Time: Began_____ Ended_____ Total minutes: _____

Steps:	Point Value	Attempt 1	Attempt 2
1. Wash hands or use hand sanitizer.	5		
2. Greet the patient. Identify yourself. Verify the patient's identity with full name and date of birth. Explain the procedure to be performed in a manner that is understood by the patient. Answer any questions the patient may have on the procedure.	5		
3. Give the patient a gown and explain what clothing must be removed for the particular examination being done. Tell the patient that the gown should open in the back. Provide assistance as needed. Give the patient privacy while changing. Knock on the examination room door before re-entering to make sure the patient has completed undressing and gowning.	10		
4. Do not place the patient in the prone position until the provider is ready for that part of the examination.	10		
5. Pull out the table extension and help the patient lie down on his or her stomach.	15*		
6. Drape the patient over any exposed area that is not included in the examination. For female patients, the drape should be large enough to cover from the breasts to the feet so that the patient is not exposed accidentally if she is asked to roll over.	15		
7. After the examination has been completed, assist the patient as needed to get off the table and get dressed.	10		
8. Put on gloves and use disinfectant wipes to clean the exam table and all potentially contaminated surfaces. Dispose of used gloves and examination table paper according to facility policies. Pull clean paper over the table.	10		
9. Wash hands or use hand sanitizer.	10		

10. Follow up with the provider's orders regarding scheduling of diagnostic studies, collection of specimens, and/or scheduling of future appointments.	10		
Total Points	100		

Comments

CAAHEP Competencies	Step(s)
I.P.9. Assist provider with a patient exam	Entire procedure
ABHES Competencies	**Step(s)**
8.c. Assist provider with general/physical examination	Entire procedure

Procedure 21.9 Knee-Chest Position

Name _____ Date _____ Score _____

Task: To position and drape the patient for examinations of the back and rectum and for certain surgical procedures.

Equipment and Supplies:
- Examination table
- Table paper
- Patient gown
- Drape
- Disinfectant wipes
- Gloves

Standard: Complete the procedure and all critical steps in _____ minutes with a minimum score of 85% within two attempts (*or as indicated by the instructor*).

Scoring: Divide the points earned by the total possible points. Failure to perform a critical step, indicated by an asterisk (*), results in grade no higher than an 84% (*or as indicated by the instructor*).

Time: Began_____ Ended_____ Total minutes: _____

Steps:	Point Value	Attempt 1	Attempt 2
1. Wash hands or use hand sanitizer.	5		
2. Greet the patient. Identify yourself. Verify the patient's identity with full name and date of birth. Explain the procedure to be performed in a manner that is understood by the patient. Answer any questions the patient may have on the procedure.	5		
3. Give the patient a gown and explain what clothing must be removed for the particular examination being done. Tell the patient that the gown should open in the back. Provide assistance as needed. Give the patient privacy while changing. Knock on the examination room door before re-entering to make sure the patient has completed undressing and gowning.	10		
4. Do not place the patient in the knee-chest position until the provider is ready for that part of the examination.	10		
5. Pull out the table extension if necessary. Help the patient lie down on his or her back and then turn over into the prone position. Ask the patient to move up onto the knees, spread the knees apart, and lean forward onto the head so that the buttocks are raised. Tell the patient to keep the back straight and turn the face to either side. The patient should rest his or her weight on the chest and shoulders.	10*		
6. If the patient has difficulty maintaining this position, an alternative is to place weight on bent elbows with the head off the table.	10		
7. Drape the patient diagonally in a diamond shape, with the point of the diamond dropping below the buttocks. Make sure the drape is large enough to prevent exposure of the patient.	10		
8. After the examination has been completed, assist the patient as needed to get off the table and get dressed.	10		

9. Put on gloves and use disinfectant wipes to clean the exam table and all potentially contaminated surfaces. Dispose of used gloves and examination table paper according to facility policies. Pull clean paper over the table.	**10**		
10. Wash hands or use hand sanitizer.	**10**		
11. Follow up with the provider's orders regarding scheduling of diagnostic studies, collection of specimens, and/or scheduling of future appointments.	**10**		
Total Points	**100**		

Comments

CAAHEP Competencies	Step(s)
I.P.9. Assist provider with a patient exam	Entire procedure
ABHES Competencies	**Step(s)**
8.c. Assist provider with general/physical examination	Entire procedure

Procedure 21.10 Use Proper Body Mechanics

Name _____ Date _____ Score _____

Task: To safely transfer a patient from a wheelchair to an examination table using proper body mechanics.

Equipment and Supplies:
- Patient's record
- Wheelchair
- Examination table with pull-out foot rest
- Gait belt

Standard: Complete the procedure and all critical steps in _____ minutes with a minimum score of 85% within two attempts (*or as indicated by the instructor*).

Scoring: Divide the points earned by the total possible points. Failure to perform a critical step, indicated by an asterisk (*), results in grade no higher than an 84% (*or as indicated by the instructor*).

Time: Began_____ Ended_____ Total minutes: _____

Steps:	Point Value	Attempt 1	Attempt 2
1. Wash hands or use hand sanitizer.	5		
2. Greet the patient. Identify yourself. Verify the patient's identity with full name and date of birth. Explain the procedure to be performed in a manner that is understood by the patient. Determine how much assistance the patient will need to transfer from the wheelchair to the examination table. Do not proceed if you think you will need additional help.	5		
3. Place the wheelchair at a 45-degree angle toward the foot rest at the base of the examination table.	5		
4. Lock the brakes on the wheelchair and move the foot rests of the wheelchair out of the way.	10*		
5. Place the gait belt around the patient's waist over clothing with the buckle in front. Insert the belt through the teeth of the buckle and pull it tight to lock it. The belt should be tight with just enough room to place your fingers under it.	10*		
6. Request that the patient place both feet flat on the floor with the hands on the armrests.	5		
7. Stand directly in front of the patient with your feet apart, back straight, and knees bent.	5		
8. Slide your fingers under the gait belt on opposite sides of the patient's waist.	5		
9. Instruct the patient at the count of three to push off from the armrests while you at the same time grasp the gait belt and, using your leg muscles, straighten your knees so that the patient is in a standing position.	10*		
10. Ask the patient to step up onto the footrest at the bottom of the exam table and assist the person in pivoting and sitting down on the examination table. Remove the gait belt until the provider has completed the examination.	5		

11. After the examination is complete, place the wheelchair at an angle next to the exam table and lock the wheels. Replace the gait belt. Make sure the patient is positioned at the edge of the table.	10*			
12. Place yourself directly in front of the patient with your back straight and your knees bent. Slide your fingers under the gait belt on opposite sides of the patient's waist.	5			
13. Grasp the gait belt on both sides at the waist. Instruct the patient at the count of three to push off from the examination table and, using your leg muscles, straighten your knees so that the patient is in a standing position on the footrest.	10*			
14. Maintaining your hold on the gait belt, ask the patient to step down. Pivot the person so that she can slowly sit in the wheelchair; at the same time, bend your knees but keep your back straight.	5			
15. Remove the gait belt. Replace the wheelchair footrests and unlock the brakes on the wheelchair.	5			
Total Points	100			

Comments

CAAHEP Competencies	**Step(s)**
I.P.9. Assist provider with a patient exam	Entire procedure
XII.P.3. Use proper body mechanics	12-14
ABHES Competencies	**Step(s)**
8.c. Assist provider with general/physical examination	Entire procedure

Procedure 21.11   Assist Provider with a Patient Exam

Name _____ Date _____ Score _____

Task: To aid the provider in the examination of a patient by preparing the patient and the necessary equipment and ensuring the patient's safety and comfort during the examination.

Equipment and Supplies:
- Patient's record
- Stethoscope
- Gauze
- Ophthalmoscope
- Pen light
- Scale with height measurement bar
- Tuning fork
- Tongue depressor
- Biohazard waste container
- Cotton balls
- Examination light
- Laboratory request forms
- Percussion hammer
- Specimen bottles and laboratory requisitions
- Lubricating gel
- Gloves
- Patient gown
- Sphygmomanometer
- Drapes
- Otoscope with disposable speculum
- Thermometer
- Cotton-tipped applicators
- Tape measure
- Fecal occult blood test supplies
- Disinfectant wipes
- Table paper

Standard: Complete the procedure and all critical steps in _____ minutes with a minimum score of 85% within two attempts (*or as indicated by the instructor*).

Scoring: Divide the points earned by the total possible points. Failure to perform a critical step, indicated by an asterisk (*), results in grade no higher than an 84% (*or as indicated by the instructor*).

Time: Began _____ Ended _____ Total minutes: _____

Steps:	Point Value	Attempt 1	Attempt 2
1. Check the examination room at the beginning of each day and between patients to make sure it is completely stocked with equipment and supplies and that the equipment functions properly.	5		
2. Check expiration dates on all packages and supplies regularly and discard expired materials.	5		
3. Prepare the examination room before and between patients according to acceptable medical rules of asepsis.	5		

4.	Wash hands or use hand sanitizer.	**5**		
5.	Locate the instruments for the procedure. Set them out in order of use within reach of the provider and cover them until the provider enters the examination room.	**10***		
6.	Greet and identify the patient, introduce yourself, and determine whether the patient understands the procedure. If the patient does not, explain what to expect. Refer any unanswered questions to the provider.	**5**		
7.	Review the medical history with the patient and investigate the purpose of the visit. Review current medications and document any changes or prescription refills needed. Document the interview results.	**5**		
8.	Measure and record the patient's vital signs, height, weight, and body mass index (BMI). Instruct the patient on how to collect a urine specimen, if ordered, and hand the patient a properly labeled specimen container. Obtain blood samples for any tests ordered.	**10***		
9.	Hand the patient a gown and drape. Explain what clothes should be removed for the examination and whether the gown should open in the front or the back. Help the patient undress as needed (most patients prefer to undress in privacy). Knock on the door before re-entering the room to protect the patient's privacy.	**5**		
10.	Assist the patient as needed in sitting at the foot of the examination table; place the drape over the patient's lap and legs. If the patient is elderly, confused, or feeling faint or dizzy, do not leave him or her alone.	**5**		
11.	Place the patient's paper health record in the designated area or make sure the computer is ready for the provider to log in and access the patient's electronic health record (EHR). Be careful to safeguard patient confidentiality during this step of the procedure.	**5**		
12.	Assist during the examination by handing the provider instruments as needed and by positioning and draping the patient.	**10**		
13.	When the provider has completed the examination, allow the patient to rest for a moment, then help the patient from the table. Assist with dressing, if necessary. Use proper body mechanics if assistance in transfer is needed.	**5**		
14.	Return to the patient and ask whether he or she has any questions. Give the patient any final instructions, and schedule tests as ordered by the provider and/or the next appointment.	**5**		
15.	Put on gloves and dispose of used supplies and linens in designated biohazard waste containers. Dispose of exam table paper. Use disinfectant wipes to clean the examination table and any other potentially contaminated surface. Disinfect all equipment.	**5**		
16.	Remove the gloves, discard them in the biohazard waste container, and wash hands or use hand sanitizer.	**5**		
17.	Cover the exam table with fresh paper, replace used supplies, and prepare the room for the next patient.	**5**		
	Total Points	**100**		

Comments

CAAHEP Competencies		Step(s)
I.P.9. Assist provider with a patient exam		Entire procedure
ABHES Competencies		**Step(s)**
8.c. Assist provider with general/physical examination		Entire procedure

Patient Coaching

CAAHEP Competencies	Assessments
V.C.5. Identify challenges in communication with different age groups	Skills and Concepts – C. 10-16
V.C.6. Identify techniques for coaching a patient related to specific needs	Skills and Concepts – C. 10-16; D. 1-6
V.C.10. Identify the role of the medical assistant as a patient navigator	Skills and Concepts – K. 4-5
V.C.13.b. Identify the basic concepts of the following theories: Erikson	Skills and Concepts – C. 2-9; Certification Preparation – 6; Workplace Applications – 1a-h.
V.C.13.c. Identify the basic concepts of the following theories: Kübler-Ross	Skills and Concepts – A. 1-10; Certification Preparation – 4
V.P.3.b. Coach patients regarding: medical encounters	Procedure 22.1
V.P.7. Use a list of community resources to facilitate referrals.	Procedure 22.2
X.P.3. Document patient care accurately in the medical record	Procedures 22.1, 22.2
A.4. Demonstrate active listening.	Procedure 22.1
ABHES Competencies	**Assessments**
5. Human Relations b. 3) List organizations and support groups that can assist patients and family members of patients experiencing terminal illnesses	Procedure 22.2
5.d. Adapt care to address the developmental stages of life	Procedure 22.1
8.h. Teach self-examination, disease management and health promotion	Procedure 22.1
8.i. Identify community resources and Complementary and Alternative Medicine practices (CAM)	Procedure 22.2
8.j. Make adaptations for patients with special needs (psychological or physical limitations)	Procedure 22.1
8.k. Make adaptations to care for patients across their lifespan	Procedure 22.1

VOCABULARY REVIEW

Using the word pool on the right, find the correct word to match the definition. Write the word on the line after the definition.

1. The act of sticking to something _____

2. The process of gaining new knowledge or skills through instruction, experience, or study _____

3. Patients are taking the right dose at the right times as prescribed by the provider _____

4. Bringing to an end _____

5. Provides personalized patient- and family-centered care in a team-based environment _____

6. The act of following through on a request or demand _____

7. The inability to feel or experience pleasure during a pleasurable activity _____

8. A person who identifies patients' barriers, works closely with the healthcare team and patients, and guides the patients through the healthcare system _____

9. The set of behaviors, ideas, and customs shared by a specific group of people, which distinguishes the members from other people _____

10. Focuses on the interrelationship among the physical, mental, social, and spiritual aspects of the person's life _____

Word Pool

- adherence
- anhedonia
- care coordination
- cessation
- compliance
- culture
- holistic approach
- learning
- medication adherence
- patient navigator

ABBREVIATIONS

Write out what each of the following abbreviations stands for.

1. Td _____

2. RZV _____

3. PCV13 _____

4. Tdap _____

5. PPSV23 _____

6. BSE _____

7. TSE _____

8. UV _____

9. PSA _____

10. DRE _____

11. AAA _____

12. PHQ-9 _____

13. NIH _____

14. CDC _____

15. ADA _____

16. AHA _____

17. HPV _____

18. DEA _____

19. FDA _____

20. gFOBT _____

21. FIT _____

SKILLS AND CONCEPTS

Answer the following questions.

A. Making Changes for Health

Match the description and adaptive interactions with the correct stage of Kübler-Ross's theory. Answers can be used more than once.

1. _____ Person feels sad, fearful, and uncertain. They may grieve the loss of their health or independence.

2. _____ Refuse to accept the fact. May refuse to discuss the diagnosis.

3. _____ Has come to terms with situation.

4. _____ This emotion can be directed at self or others and surface at unrelated times.

5. _____ Attempts to negotiate with the higher power the person believes in (e.g., God).

6. _____ For this stage, provide handouts that explain the disease and treatment and encourage family support.

7. _____ For this stage, provide coaching on aspects of the disease and self-care management.

8. _____ For this stage, use therapeutic communication techniques to acknowledge the patient's feeling about the issue.

9. _____ For this stage, work with the healthcare team regarding the patient's requests.

10. _____ For this stage, encourage the patient to use the community and healthcare resources to help ease the change process.

a. denial
b. anger
c. bargaining
d. depression
e. acceptance

Select the correct answer.

11. The health belief model
    a. deals with a person's perception of their chance of developing a disease.
    b. deals with a person's perception of the severity of the disease.
    c. focuses on whether the person will take preventive action.
    d. all of the above

B. Domains of Learning

Match the domain of learning with the description of the domain. Answers can be used more than once.

1. _____ The "doing" domain
2. _____ The "feeling" domain
3. _____ Involves the mental processes of recall, application, and evaluation

a. cognitive domain
b. psychomotor domain
c. affective domain

Match the domain of learning with the tips that a medical assistant can use. Answers can be used more than once.

4. _____ Make sure that you address any barriers (e.g., pain) prior to educating a patient.
5. _____ Have the patient teach back the skill or do a return demonstration to check for accuracy.
6. _____ Have a family member present during the teaching.
7. _____ Present the information at an appropriate level for the patient.
8. _____ Present information in small chunks in a clear, well-organized manner.
9. _____ Build on the patient's prior knowledge about the topic.
10. _____ Repeated practice doing the skill helps with recall and retention of the steps.
11. _____ Provide the information in two different ways.
12. _____ Make sure to use the equipment and supplies the patient will be using at home.

a. cognitive domain
b. psychomotor domain
c. affective domain

Match the domain of learning with barriers to the domain and the strategies for adapting to barriers. Answers can be used more than once.

13. _____ Barriers include memory or cognitive issues.
14. _____ Barriers include anxiety, denial, fatigue, and stress.
15. _____ Barriers include cultural customs and previous experience.
16. _____ Barriers include language barriers.
17. _____ Barriers include tremors and paralysis.
18. _____ Barriers include visual and hearing impairments.
19. _____ Use adaptive equipment.
20. _____ Use an interpreter and provide handouts in the patient's primary language.

a. cognitive domain
b. psychomotor domain
c. affective domain

C. The Medical Assistant's Role in Coaching

1. When a medical assistant coaches a patient, it is important to
    a. recognize the patient is an individual.
    b. remember the patient has unique concerns.
    c. consider the barriers to learning.
    d. all of the above

Match the goal of the stage with the correct psychosocial developmental stages.

2. _____ Encourage to try new activities. Must assume responsibilities and learn new skills.

3. _____ To know who you are as a person and how you fit into the world around you. Creates a meaningful self-image.

4. _____ Must develop trust, with the ability to mistrust should the need arise.

5. _____ Must seek to finish tasks. Recognition for accomplishments is important.

6. _____ Must explore and manipulate things in their "world" to develop autonomy and self-esteem.

7. _____ Develops friendships; takes on commitments.

8. _____ Reflect on one's life and come to terms with it, instead of regretting the past.

9. _____ Achieve a balance between the concern for the next generation (having a family) and being self-absorbed.

a. Trust versus Mistrust
b. Autonomy versus Shame and Doubt
c. Initiative versus Guilt
d. Industry versus Inferiority
e. Identity versus Role Confusion
f. Intimacy versus Isolation
g. Generativity versus Stagnation
h. Ego Integrity versus Despair

Match the age group with the coaching strategies to use.

10. _____ Use engaging simple tools to communicate information.

11. _____ Provide privacy and independence. Promote responsible decision making and an honest discussion on lifestyle issues.

12. _____ Use a calm, soothing voice and hold patient securely.

13. _____ Use familiar words and simple explanations and demonstrations. Explain how the patient would sense the procedure.

14. _____ Use simple, familiar words, allow the patient to handle equipment, and make choices.

15. _____ Important to identify the patient's motivating factor to learn the new content.

16. _____ Communicate with dignity and respect; speak clearly and allow time for the patient to respond.

a. infants
b. toddlers
c. preschoolers
d. school-age children
e. adolescents
f. young and middle adults
g. older adults

D. Adapting Coaching for Communication Barriers
Match the communication barriers with the coaching strategies to use.

1. _____ Use a low-pitched voice and speak clearly, slowly, and distinctly. Pause between sentences or phrases. Speak naturally; do not shout.
2. _____ Use an interpreter or an interpretation service. Focus on the patient and not on the interpreter.
3. _____ Use translated materials.
4. _____ Face the patient directly. Make eye contact, if culturally appropriate. Use a normal tone of voice.
5. _____ Speak louder if you are wearing a mask.
6. _____ Provide the patient with large-print directions or brochures.

a. impaired vision
b. impaired hearing
c. language barriers

E. Cultural Diversity

1. What are factors affected by a person's culture that can impact healthcare?
   a. Role of the family and community
   b. Religion and beliefs regarding sexuality, fertility, and childbirth
   c. Views on health, wellness, death, dying, and complementary therapies
   d. All of the above

2. _____ involves applying suction to the skin, which can leave marks.

3. _____ involves applying firm pressure on specific points on the body.

4. _____ involves inserting fine needles into specific sites on the body.

F. Teaching-Learning Process
Match the steps in coaching a patient relevant to an individual patient's need with the description. Answers can be used more than once.

1. _____ First step in the teaching-learning process.
2. _____ Second step in the teaching-learning process.
3. _____ Third step in the teaching-learning process.
4. _____ Fourth step in the teaching-learning process.
5. _____ Fifth step in the teaching-learning process.
6. _____ Summarize the coaching provided in the patient's health record.
7. _____ Start with the basics and build from there. Keep the information simple and focused.
8. _____ After coaching on the topic, have the patient summarize what was stated. Obtain feedback from the patient during the coaching to determine if they understand the content.
9. _____ Consider the patient's individual needs and identify strategies to overcome issues that may impact the coaching.
10. _____ Identify what the patient needs to learn, the patient's motivation and concerns, and the patient's learning styles.

a. evaluating the patient's learning
b. identifying barriers to learning
c. identifying the patient's educational needs
d. documenting the coaching
e. coaching the patient on the topic

G. Coaching on Disease Prevention

1. Tetanus and diphtheria (Td) is given every _____ years.

2. Recombinant zoster vaccine schedule includes _____ doses for adults age 50 or older.

3. 13-valent pneumococcal conjugate vaccine (PCV13) involves _____ dose(s) usually after age 65 unless given before based on the patient's health.

4. What is incorrect regarding the CDC's respiratory hygiene/cough etiquette?
   a. Cover your mouth and nose with your sleeve when coughing or sneezing.
   b. Discard any tissues used in the nearest waste container.
   c. Wash your hands or use hand sanitizer.
   d. All of the above

5. _____ is the most reliable way to prevent STIs.

6. _____ tobacco includes chewing tobacco, moist snuff, snus, and moist powder tobacco.

7. Which statement is incorrect regarding nicotine?
   a. Nicotine is readily absorbed into the blood.
   b. Nicotine triggers the release of epinephrine, which stimulates the central nervous system.
   c. Epinephrine will lower the blood pressure and respiration and pulse rates.
   d. Nicotine increases the level of dopamine in the brain, helping the person feel happy and focused.

8. _____ causes lung cancer, strokes, low-birth-weight babies, and heart disease.

9. _____ is the residue or chemicals from the smoke that gets on skin, clothing, furniture, carpeting, and so on.

H. Coaching on Self-Exams for Health Maintenance and Wellness

1. Women with an average risk of breast cancer should have yearly mammograms between age _____ and _____.

2. _____ is the most dangerous type of skin cancer.

3. What is *not* a risk factor for skin cancer?
   a. Family or personal history of skin cancer
   b. Exposure to sun through work or play
   c. Brown eyes
   d. Skin that is lighter than normal color with freckles

4. What is not a sign or symptom of oral cancer?
   a. White or red patches in the mouth or on the gums
   b. Numbness or pain in the mouth
   c. Short-term hoarseness or sore throat
   d. Swelling in the jaw area or constant earache

I. Coaching on Screening for Health Maintenance and Wellness

1. People age 18-39 years should have a blood pressure check every _____ to _____ years.

2. Adults with no history of high cholesterol should have it checked every _____ to _____ years.

3. Adults 45 years and older with normal risk should have a fecal stool test (e.g., gFOBT) every _____ or a stool DNA test (Cologuard) every _____ years.

4. Adults 45 years and older with normal risk should have a colonoscopy every _____ years.

5. A dental exam and cleaning are recommended _____.

6. For women ages 30-65, a Pap test is recommended every 5 years if the _____ _____ test is also done.

7. Type 2 diabetes mellitus screening should be done every _____ years starting at age 18.

8. What is *not* a risk factor for hepatitis C?
   a. Born between 1935 and 1965
   b. History of a blood transfusion or organ transplantation before 1992
   c. Use of injected illegal drugs
   d. Chronic liver disease, HIV, or AIDS

9. An alcoholic drink is classified as a(n) _____ of beer, a(n) _____ of wine, or a(n) _____ of liquor.

10. What is correct regarding intimate partner violence?
    a. Male and females can be victims of domestic abuse.
    b. Substance abuse, obesity, and depression can come from violence.
    c. Intimate partner violence includes controlling behaviors, physical abuse, and sexual abuse.
    d. All of the above

Match the type of elder abuse and neglect with the signs.

11. _____ Leaving the person in a public place

12. _____ Malnutrition, dehydration, lack of proper living conditions, and failing to treat health problems

13. _____ Unexplained sexually transmitted infections, bruising in the genital region, and reports from the older person

14. _____ Stealing from the older person, forging signatures on financial transactions, and any other illegal action that represents a financial loss for the older person

15. _____ Fractures, rope marks, cuts, bruising, dislocations, broken glasses, giving too little or too much medication, bleeding, and sudden changes in the person's personality or behavior

16. _____ Not communicating, withdrawn, agitated, and symptoms that mimic dementia

a. physical abuse
b. sexual abuse
c. emotional abuse
d. neglect
e. abandonment
f. financial abuse

J. Coaching on Diagnostic Tests and Treatment Plans
Match the procedure with the description.

1. _____ Uses x-rays to create pictures of cross-sections of the body. May require IV or oral contrast medium.

2. _____ Uses low-dose x-ray test that measures calcium and other minerals in the bone.

3. _____ An x-ray picture of the breasts used to find tumors.

4. _____ Uses powerful magnets and radio waves to create images of the body.

5. _____ Imaging test that uses an IV radioactive substance (tracer) to identify disease in the organs and tissues.

6. _____ Detects electrical activity in the brain using electrodes that are placed on the scalp.

a. mammography
b. MRI
c. EEG
d. PET
e. CT scan
f. bone density scan

Match the medical laboratory test with the common patient preparations. Answers may be used more than once.

7. _____ No preparation required.

8. _____ May need to fast overnight. May need to refrain from eating meat for a period of time.

9. _____ May require NPO (except for water) prior to the test.

10. _____ Two days prior to the test, refrain from sexual intercourse.

11. _____ Specimen is collected by the patient and returned to a specific medical laboratory for testing.

12. _____ Two days prior to the test, the patient should not douche or use vaginal medications or spermicidal products.

a. creatinine
b. lipid profile
c. Pap test
d. Cologuard stool DNA test

Select the correct answer.

13. When coaching patients on treatments to do at home, a medical assistant may need to discuss
    a. ways to remember to take medications.
    b. safely discarding used needles.
    c. safely discarding expired or unwanted medications.
    d. all of the above.

14. Which of the following should *not* be done when a patient is monitoring their blood pressure at home?
    a. Relax for 5 minutes before taking a blood pressure reading.
    b. Avoid caffeine and exercise for 15 minutes before the reading.
    c. Use the same area for the BP reading.
    d. Avoid smoking for 30 minutes before the reading.

15. Which of the following should be done when a patient is monitoring their blood pressure at home?
    a. Keep legs uncrossed and support the back and feet.
    b. Empty a full bladder and refrain from talking during the procedure.
    c. Use the correct cuff size and place the cuff on a bare arm.
    d. All of the above.

K. Care Coordinator

1. What is an advantage of care coordination?
   a. Greater efficiency in providing patient care
   b. Reduced cost and better patient care
   c. Encourages patients to focus on goals and self-management
   d. All of the above

2. The care coordinator communicates between the _____ and the
   _____ _____.

3. A patient navigator has been described as a type of _____.

4. Which of the following is a role for the medical assistant as a patient navigator/care coordinator?
   a. Provide patients with resources based on their needs and barriers.
   b. Schedule and sequence appointments.
   c. Discuss special needs patients have with their healthcare team.
   d. All of the above.

5. Which of the following is a role for the medical assistant as a patient navigator/care coordinator?
   a. Interview patients to identify their needs and barriers to wellness and healthcare.
   b. Make sure the required information is communicated to and from specialty departments.
   c. Identify community resources for the patient.
   d. All of the above.

CERTIFICATION PREPARATION

Circle the correct answer.

1. Coaching provides patients with
   a. skills.
   b. knowledge.
   c. support and confidence.
   d. all of the above.

2. Providing patients with information on routine screenings and showing patients how to do self-exams is what type of coaching?
   a. Disease prevention
   b. Health maintenance
   c. Diagnostic tests
   d. Specific needs

3. Providing patients with information on respiratory hygiene practices, recommended vaccines, and nicotine cessation is what type of coaching?
   a. Disease prevention
   b. Health maintenance
   c. Diagnostic tests
   d. Specific needs

4. When a patient is experiencing sadness and uncertainty when grieving, what stage of Kübler-Ross' theory is the person in?
   a. Denial
   b. Anger
   c. Bargaining
   d. Depression

5. Language barriers are barriers to learning in the _____ domain.
   a. psychomotor
   b. affective
   c. cognitive
   d. a and c

6. According to Erikson's theory, an adolescent is in which stage?
   a. Identity versus Role Confusion
   b. Intimacy versus Isolation
   c. Industry versus Inferiority
   d. Generativity versus Stagnation

7. What colorectal cancer screening test requires no patient preparation and consists of a computer analysis that checks the stool for cancer and precancerous cells?
   a. gFOBT
   b. FIT
   c. PET
   d. Cologuard stool DNA test

8. Which imaging procedure uses x-rays to create pictures of cross-sections of the patient's body?
   a. X-ray
   b. Computed tomography scan
   c. Magnetic resonance imaging
   d. Mammography

9. What diagnostic test provides an x-ray picture of the breasts and is used to find tumors?
   a. X-ray
   b. Computed tomography scan
   c. Magnetic resonance imaging
   d. Mammography

10. What diagnostic test uses high-frequency sound waves to create an image of the organs and structures?
    a. Ultrasound
    b. Computed tomography scan
    c. Magnetic resonance imaging
    d. Mammography

WORKPLACE APPLICATIONS

1. Working in family medicine, Suzanne works with people of all ages. Describe tips to remember when coaching/working with patients of the following ages.

   a. 1-year-old _____

   _____

   b. 2-year-old _____

   _____

   c. 5-year-old _____

   _____

   d. 8-year-old _____

   _____

   e. 14-year-old _____

   _____

   f. 30-year-old _____

   _____

   g. 72-year-old _____

   _____

   _____

2. Suzanne is coaching a patient about the early warning signs of malignant melanoma. Describe the ABCDE rule.

_____

_____

_____

_____

INTERNET ACTIVITIES

1. Using the FDA website (https://www.fda.gov/), research "disposal of unused medications" in the home environment. Create a poster, PowerPoint, or paper summarizing your research. Focus on these areas:
   a. Using authorized collectors for disposal (e.g., take-back programs)
   b. Disposal in household trash
   c. Disposing of fentanyl patches

2. Using the CDC website (https://www.cdc.gov/), research recommended immunizations for children. Create a poster, PowerPoint, or paper summarizing your research. Focus on five recommended childhood immunizations and address the following for each:
   a. Name of immunization
   b. Why is it recommended or what does it prevent?
   c. Schedule of the vaccine (or the ages when a child should receive the immunization)
   d. Side effects of the vaccine

3. Using the CDC website (https://www.cdc.gov/), research recommended immunizations. Create a poster, PowerPoint, or paper summarizing your research. Focus on immunizations prior to, during, and after pregnancy.
   a. What is recommended? Why is it recommended?
   b. What is not recommended?

Procedure 22.1   Coach a Patient on Disease Prevention

Name _____   **Date** _____   **Score** _____

Tasks: Coach a patient on the recommended vaccinations for their age. Adapt the coaching for any communication barrier and the patient's developmental life stage. Document the coaching in the patient's health record.

Scenario: You are working with Dr. David Kahn. You need to room Charles Johnson (date of birth [DOB] 03/03/19XX), and his record indicates he has not been seen in several years. Charles has significant hearing loss, and he communicates by signing. His wife interprets for him. You look in his health record and see that he is due for influenza, Td, and recombinant zoster (shingles) vaccines. Per the provider's standing order, you need to coach adult patients on potential vaccines they are due for during the initial rooming process.

Directions: Role-play this scenario with two peers, who will play Charles and his wife. You are the medical assistant.

Equipment and Supplies:
- Vaccine Information Statements (VIS) (available at https://www.immunize.org/vis/)
- Patient's health record

Standard: Complete the procedure and all critical steps in _____ minutes with a minimum score of 85% within two attempts (*or as indicated by the instructor*).

Scoring: Divide the points earned by the total possible points. Failure to perform a critical step, indicated by an asterisk (*), results in grade no higher than an 84% (*or as indicated by the instructor*).

Time: Began_____ Ended_____ Total minutes: _____

Steps:	Point Value	Attempt 1	Attempt 2
1. Wash hands or use hand sanitizer.	5		
2. Greet the patient. Identify yourself. Verify the patient's identity with full name and date of birth. Explain what you will be doing.	10		
3. Arrange the chairs so the patient can see both you and the person signing. Speak slowly. Pause as needed to allow person signing to finish with the last statement. Look at the patient when communicating.	15		
4. Use simpler language when talking. Speak clearly and respectfully, while maintaining the patient's dignity. Allow time for the patient to respond. Listen to the patient's concerns. Use active listening skills. Use appropriate eye contact. Focus on the patient and avoid distractions. (*Refer to the Affective Behaviors Checklist – Respect and Active Listening and the Grading Rubric*)	15*		
5. Ask the patient if he has received vaccines somewhere else over the past few years.	5		
Scenario update: Patient has not seen any healthcare providers over the last few years. The only vaccines received were given in this facility. 6. Describe the vaccines that are due. Use the VIS for each vaccine as you coach the patient on the purpose of the vaccine.	15*		

Scenario update: The patient knows the shingles vaccine is not covered and costs more than $200. He refuses the shingles vaccine, and he does not believe in getting the influenza vaccine. He is interested in getting the Td vaccine. 7. Ask the patient which vaccines he is interested in getting. If he refuses, be respectful of his choice. Any reason he gives for the refusal should be communicated to the provider.	**15**		
8. Document the coaching in the patient's health record. Include the provider's name, what was taught, how the patient responded, and any vaccines refused.	**20**		
Total Points	**100**		

Affective Behavior	**Affective Behaviors Checklist** ***Directions:*** *Check behaviors observed during the role-play.*					
Respect	**Negative, Unprofessional Behaviors**	**Attempt**		**Positive, Professional Behaviors**	**Attempt**	
		1	**2**		**1**	**2**
	Rude, unkind, fake/false attitude, disrespectful, impolite, unwelcoming			Courteous, sincere, polite, welcoming		
	Unconcerned with person's dignity; brief, abrupt			Maintained person's dignity; took time with person		
	Unprofessional verbal communication; inappropriate questions			Professional verbal communication		
	Negative nonverbal behaviors, poor eye contact			Positive nonverbal behaviors, proper eye contact		
	Other:			Other:		
Active Listening	Biased, offensive			Remained neutral		
	Interrupted			Refrained from interrupting		
	Did not allow for silence or pauses			Allowed for periods of silence		
	Negative nonverbal behaviors (rolled eyes, yawned, frowned, avoided eye contact)			Positive nonverbal behaviors (smiled, nodded head, appropriate eye contact)		
	Distracted (looked at watch, phone)			Focused on patient, avoided distractions		
	Other:			Other:		

Grading Rubric for the Affective Behaviors Checklist **Directions:** *Based on checklist results, identify the points received for the procedure checklist. Indicate how the behaviors demonstrated met the expectations.*		**Points for Procedure Checklist**	**Attempt 1**	**Attempt 2**
Does not meet Expectation	• Response lacked respect or active listening. • Student demonstrated more than 2 negative, unprofessional behaviors during the interaction.	0		
Needs Improvement	• Response lacked respect or active listening. • Student demonstrated 1 or 2 negative, unprofessional behaviors during the interaction.	0		
Meets Expectation	• Response was respectful. Demonstrated active listening.. No negative, unprofessional behaviors observed. • More practice is needed for behavior to appear natural and for student to appear comfortable and at ease.	15		
Occasionally Exceeds Expectation	• Response was respectful. Demonstrated active listening, professional nonverbal communication. No negative, unprofessional behaviors observed. • At times student appeared comfortable and at ease; but more practice is needed for behavior to become natural and consistent with a professional medical assistant.	15		
Always Exceeds Expectation	• Response was respectful. Demonstrated active listening, professional nonverbal communication. No negative, unprofessional behaviors observed. • Student's behaviors appeared natural and comfortable. Behaviors are consistent with a professional medical assistant.	15		

Documentation

Comments

CAAHEP Competencies	Step(s)
V.P.3.b. Coach patients regarding: medical encounters	Entire procedure
X.P.3. Document patient care accurately in the medical record	8
A.4. Demonstrate active listening.	4
ABHES Competencies	**Step(s)**
5.d. Adapt care to address the developmental stages of life	4
8.h. Teach self-examination, disease management and health promotion	6
8.j. Make adaptations for patients with special needs (psychological or physical limitations)	3, 4
8.k. Make adaptations to care for patients across their lifespan	4

Procedure 22.2   Develop a List of Community Resources and Facilitate Referrals

Name _____ Date _____ Score _____

Tasks: As a patient navigator, develop a current list of community resources that meet the patient's health-care needs. Discuss the resources with the patient and facilitate referrals to the chosen resources.

Scenario 1: Robert Caudill (DOB 10/31/19XX) was just diagnosed with dementia. He currently lives with his daughter, Ruby, who works full time. Ruby is feeling overwhelmed with being his only caregiver and realizes that she needs to find someone to care for her father while she is working.

Scenario 2: Leslie Green (DOB 08/03/20XX) just tested positive for pregnancy. She does not feel that she has a support system to help her make decisions.

Scenario 3: Ella Rainwater's husband of 30 years died suddenly 1 month ago. Ella (DOB 07/11/19XX) stated that she feels alone and has no one to talk to. Her daughter feels that Ella needs the support of others who have gone through the same thing.

Directions: The instructor will assign each student a scenario. For steps 1 and 2, research resources for the scenario. For the remaining steps, role-play the scenario with two peers.

Equipment and Supplies:
* Computer with Internet or a telephone book
* Paper and pen
* Community Resource Referral Form (Work Product 22.1) or referral form
* Patient's health record

Standard: Complete the procedure and all critical steps in _____ minutes with a minimum score of 85% within two attempts (*or as indicated by the instructor*).

Scoring: Divide the points earned by the total possible points. Failure to perform a critical step, indicated by an asterisk (*), results in grade no higher than an 84% (*or as indicated by the instructor*).

Time: Began_____ Ended_____ Total minutes: _____

Steps:	Point Value	Attempt 1	Attempt 2
1. Using the assigned scenario, identify the possible types of community resources that would assist the patient or family. Identify three different types of resources (e.g., medical equipment, support group) that would meet the patient's needs.	5		
2. Using the Internet or the phone book, identify two local resources for each of the three kinds of resources (i.e., find two assisted living resources, two medical equipment suppliers, and so on). Make a list of six resources for the patient and family. Include the following: a. Organization's name b. Address and contact information c. Summary of the services provided d. Cost and other relevant information	30		
Scenario update: Role-play the scenario indicated by the instructor. 3. Provide the patient or family member with the list of six resources. Describe the services offered and any costs.	15*		

4.	Allow the patient or family member time to review the services. Answer any questions.	**10**		
5.	Use professional, tactful verbal and nonverbal communication as you work with the patient or family member.	**10***		
6.	Role-play making the community referrals. Have the patient or family member decide on two or more services they are interested in. Complete the referral document. Have the patient provide any additional information required on the form. Call the community resource agency and provide the referral information to the representative (a peer).	**20***		
7.	Document the patient education and the referrals in the health record.	**10**		
	Total Points	**100**		

Documentation

Comments

CAAHEP Competencies	Step(s)
V.P.7. Use a list of community resources to facilitate referrals.	3-6
X.P.3. Document patient care accurately in the medical record	7
ABHES Competencies	**Step(s)**
5. Human Relations b.3) List organizations and support groups that can assist patients and family members of patients experiencing terminal illnesses	1, 2
8.i. Identify community resources and Complementary and Alternative Medicine practices (CAM)	1, 2

Work Product 22.1   Community Resource Referral Form

To be used with Procedure 22.2.

Name _____   **Date** _____   **Score** _____

Patient's Name:	Date of Birth:

Community Resource Information:

Agency: _____   Contact Name: _____

Address: _____   Phone number: _____

_____   Website: _____

Services
Provided:

Agency: _____   Contact Name: _____

Address: _____   Phone number: _____

_____   Website: _____

Services
Provided:

Agency: _____   Contact Name: _____

Address: _____   Phone number: _____

_____   Website: _____

Services
Provided:

Agency: _____   Contact Name: _____

Address: _____   Phone number: _____

_____   Website: _____

Services
Provided:

Nutrition and Health Promotion

chapter

23

CAAHEP Competencies	Assessment
IV.C.1.a. Identify dietary nutrients including: carbohydrates	Skills and Concepts – B. 1-11, D. 1; Certification Preparation – 1
IV.C.1.b. Identify dietary nutrients including: fat	Skills and Concepts – D. 1-19; Certification Preparation – 3
IV.C.1.c. Identify dietary nutrients including: protein	Skills and Concepts – C. 1-6, D. 1; Certification Preparation – 2
IV.C.1.d. Identify dietary nutrients including: minerals	Skills and Concepts – E. 3-17; Certification Preparation – 4
IV.C.1.e. Identify dietary nutrients including: electrolytes	Skills and Concepts – E. 2, 4-17
IV.C.1.f. Identify dietary nutrients including: vitamins	Skills and Concepts – E. 1, 18-37; Certification Preparation – 6
IV.C.1.g. Identify dietary nutrients including: fiber	Skills and Concepts – B. 8-11
IV.C.1.h. Identify dietary nutrients including: water	Skills and Concepts – E. 41-43
IV.C.2. Identify the function of dietary supplements	Skills and Concepts – E. 38
IV.C.3.a. Identify the special dietary needs for: weight control	Skills and Concepts – I. 2-3
IV.C.3.b. Identify the special dietary needs for: diabetes	Skills and Concepts – I. 5-8; Certification Preparation – 7
IV.C.3.c. Identify the special dietary needs for: cardiovascular disease	Skills and Concepts – I. 10-13
IV.C.3.d. Identify the special dietary needs for: hypertension	Skills and Concepts – I. 9-11; Certification Preparation – 8
IV.C.3.e. Identify the special dietary needs for: cancer	Skills and Concepts – K. 6-8; Workplace Applications – 2
IV.C.3.f. Identify the special dietary needs for: lactose sensitivity	Skills and Concepts – J. 9
IV.C.3.g. Identify the special dietary needs for: gluten-free	Skills and Concepts – J. 7-8; Certification Preparation – 9
IV.C.3.h. Identify the special dietary needs for: food allergies	Skills and Concepts – J. 1-6

CAAHEP Competencies	Assessment
IV.C.3.j. Identify the special dietary needs for: eating disorders	Skills and Concepts – K. 4
IV.C.4. Identify the components of a food label.	Skills and Concepts – G. 1-7
IV.P.1. Instruct a patient regarding a dietary change related to a patient's special dietary needs	Procedure 23.1
A.3. Demonstrate empathy for patients' concern	Procedure 23.1

ABHES Competencies	Assessment
2. Anatomy and Physiology d. Apply a system of diet and nutrition 1) Explain the importance of diet and nutrition	Skills and Concepts – A. 1, 4
2.d.2) Educate patients regarding proper diet and nutrition guidelines	Procedure 23.1
2.d.3) Identify categories of patients that require special diets or diet modifications	Skills and Concepts – H. 2; I. 2, 5, 7-10, 12; J. 6, 8-9; Workplace Applications – 1-2

VOCABULARY REVIEW

Using the word pool on the right, find the correct word to match the definition. Write the word on the line after the definition.

Group A

1. The chemical process that occurs within a living organism to maintain life _____

2. A field of study that examines the substances in food that help us grow and stay healthy _____

3. Special proteins that speed up the chemical reactions in the body _____

4. Chemicals in food that the body uses for energy, growth, and development _____

5. Result when fats are broken down; used by the body for energy and tissue development _____

6. The process of smaller molecules being used to build larger molecules with the use of energy _____

7. The process of breaking down molecules into smaller molecules resulting in energy being released _____

8. Found in protein-containing foods. Released during the digestion of protein foods in the intestines; carried by the blood to cells, where they are used to make proteins _____

9. Results when carbohydrates are broken down; main sugar found in the blood and used as the main source of energy _____

10. A unit that measures how much energy is in a particular food _____

Word Pool
- amino acid
- anabolism
- calorie
- catabolism
- enzymes
- fatty acids
- glucose
- metabolism
- nutrients
- nutrition

Group B

1. The rate the body burns calories while the person is at rest
_____

2. Nutrient used for energy and to regulate protein and fat metabolism
_____

3. Cannot be made by the body and must be in the food eaten
_____

4. Created by the body and do not need to be in food
_____

5. Foods lacking vitamins, minerals, and fiber
_____

6. A hormone produced by the beta cells in the pancreas; moves glucose into the cells so it can be used for energy
_____

7. A nutrient that is broken down into amino acids
_____

8. A hormone produced by the alpha cells in the pancreas; works on the liver to release glycogen and thereby prevent dangerously low blood glucose levels _____

9. Foods that have all the essential amino acids to support the body
_____

10. Nutrients added back into a food after they were lost during food processing _____

Word Pool
- basal metabolic rate
- carbohydrate
- complete proteins
- enriched
- essential nutrients
- glucagon
- insulin
- nonessential nutrients
- non-nutrient–rich
- protein

Group C

1. Synthetic or natural substances found in food and supplements; may prevent or delay some types of cell damage
_____

2. Providing information in a supportive environment that allows people to grow, change, or improve their situation
_____

3. Average daily level of food intake needed to meet the nutrient requirements of most healthy people _____

4. The food and drink a person typically consumes when there are no dietary limitations _____

5. A rapidly progressing, life-threatening allergic reaction; characterized by hives, swelling of the mouth and airway, difficulty breathing, wheezing, and loss of consciousness
_____

6. A credentialed healthcare professional who is trained in nutrition and is able to apply the information to the dietary needs of healthy and ill patients _____

7. Foods that do not contain all the essential amino acids
_____

8. Nutrients are added to a food; these nutrients were never originally in the food _____

Word Pool
- anaphylaxis
- antioxidant
- coaching
- fortified
- incomplete proteins
- recommended dietary allowance
- registered dietitian
- regular diet

ABBREVIATIONS
Write out what each of the following abbreviations stands for.

1. BMR _____

2. GI _____

3. LDL _____

4. HDL _____

5. USDA _____

6. mg _____

7. DV _____

8. GERD _____

9. CDC _____

10. BMI _____

11. LAGB _____

12. FDA _____

13. DASH _____

14. AHA _____

SKILLS AND CONCEPTS
Answer the following questions. Write your answer on the line or in the space provided.

A. Metabolism
Define the following terms by matching the definition with the term.

1. _____ The rate the body burns calories while the person is at rest

2. _____ A unit that measures how much energy is in a particular food

3. _____ Foods lacking vitamins, minerals, and fiber

4. _____ Created by the body and do not need to be in food

5. _____ Also called *nutrient dense*; foods high in nutrients and low in calories

6. _____ Cannot be made by the body and must be in the food eaten

a. essential nutrients
b. basal metabolic rate
c. calorie
d. nonessential nutrients
e. non-nutrient–rich
f. nutrient-rich

Select the correct answer.

7. What factor affects the number of calories a person burns each day?
   a. How much the person exercises
   b. The amount of fat and muscle on the person's body
   c. The person's basal metabolic rate (BMR)
   d. All of the above

8. What factor affects the BMR?
   a. Genetics, sex, and age
   b. Weight and body surface area
   c. Body fact percentage and diet
   d. All of the above

9. Which statement is correct regarding BMR?
   a. A lower body temperature results in an increased BMR.
   b. Starvation and low-calorie diets can reduce BMR.
   c. BMR increases with age.
   d. Thyroxin decreases BMR.

B. Carbohydrates

1. What is correct regarding carbohydrates?
   a. About 45-65% of our daily calories should come from carbohydrates.
   b. Carbohydrates include simple sugars, starches, and fiber.
   c. Carbohydrates are used for energy and to regulate protein and fat metabolism.
   d. All of the above

2. _____ increases the blood glucose level and _____ helps it move out of the bloodstream to the cells to be used for energy.

3. Glucose is also stored in the liver and muscles as _____.

4. When glycogen is released back into the blood, it increases the _____ levels.

5. Which of the following does *not* contain a simple sugar?
   a. Legumes
   b. Candy
   c. Fruit
   d. Honey

6. Which of the following does *not* contain complex carbohydrates?
   a. White bread
   b. Starchy vegetables
   c. Syrups
   d. Whole grain products

7. Which of the following is *not* a carbohydrate?
   a. Legumes
   b. Fruit
   c. Chicken
   d. Bread

8. _____ dissolves in water and forms a gel-like substance, which softens the stool.

9. Soluble fiber lowers the _____ level by slowing sugar absorption and lowers the _____ level by binding to fatty acids.

10. _____ bulks up the stool and helps prevent constipation.

11. _____ are usually taken to reduce constipation and contain natural or synthetic soluble fiber.

C. Protein

1. Proteins are
   a. broken down into amino acids.
   b. used as a source of energy in the absence of carbohydrates.
   c. used to make proteins in the body.
   d. all of the above.

2. _____ cannot be made by the body, and thus must come from protein-containing food eaten throughout the day.

3. _____ can be made by the body from essential amino acids or in the normal breakdown of proteins.

4. Foods that have all of the essential amino acids to support the body are called _____ and foods that do not contain all the essential amino acids are called _____.

5. Which of the following foods are *not* a complete protein?
   a. Eggs
   b. Legumes
   c. Dairy products
   d. Fish

6. Which of the following foods are *not* proteins?
   a. Meat
   b. Poultry
   c. Peanut butter
   d. Prunes

7. Omega-3 fatty acids
   a. are a group of proteins.
   b. are found in fish and some nuts and seeds.
   c. reduce blood cholesterol, heart disease risk, inflammation, and depression.
   d. all of the above
   e. b and c

D. Fat

1. Fats provide _____ calories per gram, whereas carbohydrates and proteins provide only _____ calories per gram.

2. About _____ of our daily calories should come from fats and less than _____ from saturated fatty acids.

3. The body uses fat
   a. as a source of energy if glucose is not available.
   b. for healthy hair, brain development, controlling inflammation, and blood clotting.
   c. for vitamin absorption.
   d. all of the above

4. _____ and _____ are involved with brain development, controlling inflammation, and blood clotting.

Match the following descriptions with the correct type of fats.

5. _____ Liquid at room temperature, two types

6. _____ Increases LDL and decreases HDL levels

7. _____ Solid at room temperature.

8. _____ Also called *hydrogenated fats*

9. _____ Decreases the LDL level

10. _____ Increases the LDL level

11. _____ Found in margarine and hydrogenated oils

12. _____ Found in olive, canola, sunflower, and corn oil

13. _____ Created when hydrogen is added to vegetable oils during food manufacturing

14. _____ Found in butter, cheese, whole milk, coconut oil, and palm oil

a. saturated fats
b. unsaturated fats
c. trans-fatty acid

Select the correct answer or fill in the blank.

15. Triglycerides are
    a. a type of fat in the body.
    b. made by the liver from calories we do not use.
    c. found in foods.
    d. all of the above

16. Lowering the triglyceride level can be done by
    a. cutting back on calories.
    b. avoiding sugary and refined foods.
    c. limiting the amount of alcohol consumed.
    d. all of the above

17. Cholesterol is
    a. a type of lipid found in foods such as egg yolks, meats, shellfish, and cheese.
    b. used to make hormones, vitamin C, bile acids, and cell membranes.
    c. created by the gallbladder.
    d. all of the above

18. _____ is considered "good" cholesterol since it helps move the cholesterol from the tissues to the liver and the liver removes it from the body.

19. _____ is considered "bad" cholesterol since it moves cholesterol to tissues, including arteries.

E. Other Dietary Nutrients

Match the descriptions with the correct term.

1. _____ Organic substances needed by the body in very small amounts for specific roles
2. _____ Naturally occurring inorganic substances (e.g., iron, zinc, and calcium)
3. _____ Found in the body fluid and have an electrical charge
4. _____ Needed in larger amounts in the body; also called *macrominerals*
5. _____ Needed in smaller amounts in the body; also called *microminerals*

a. mineral
b. electrolytes
c. vitamins
d. major minerals
e. trace minerals

Select the correct answer.

6. Which of the following is *not* a major mineral?
   a. Iron
   b. Calcium
   c. Potassium
   d. Sodium

7. Which of the following is *not* a trace mineral?
   a. Fluoride
   b. Copper
   c. Chromium
   d. Magnesium

Match the minerals' role in the body with the correct mineral.

8. _____ Found in thyroid hormone, which is involved with metabolism, growth, and development
9. _____ Used in the metabolism of carbohydrates and fats; also aids in insulin action and glucose metabolism
10. _____ Part of hemoglobin found in the red blood cell, used for energy metabolism
11. _____ For healthy teeth and bones; muscle and nerve function, blood clotting, blood pressure regulation, immune system health
12. _____ Helps form red blood cells; involved with keeping the blood vessels, nerves, immune system, and bones healthy
13. _____ Used for making proteins, taste perception, wound healing, immune system health, production of sperm, normal growth
14. _____ For proper muscle and nerve function, fluid balance
15. _____ Antioxidant; found in seafood and grains
16. _____ Needed to make proteins; for muscle and nerve function and immune system health
17. _____ For proper fluid balance; stomach acid

a. calcium
b. chloride
c. sodium
d. magnesium
e. iron
f. zinc
g. iodine
h. selenium
i. chromium
j. copper

Match the vitamins' role in the body with the correct vitamin.

18. _____ Antioxidant; helps form red blood cells and helps the body use vitamin K

19. _____ Works with vitamin B$_{12}$ to help form blood cells; important in pregnancy to prevent spina bifida

20. _____ Used in bone growth; made by the body after being in the sun

21. _____ Used in digestive process and skin and nerve functions; treats low HDL and high LDL cholesterol and triglyceride levels

22. _____ Used for nervous system, muscle function, and carbohydrate metabolism

23. _____ Antioxidant; helps form and maintain healthy teeth, bones, mucous membranes, soft tissue, and skin

24. _____ Used for fat and carbohydrate metabolism; also used in the production of hormones and cholesterol

25. _____ Antioxidant; promotes healthy gums and teeth; helps absorb iron; maintains healthy tissue and promotes wound healing

26. _____ Blood clotting; made in the intestine

27. _____ Works with other B vitamins; important for growth and red blood cell production

a. vitamin A
b. vitamin D
c. vitamin E
d. vitamin K
e. vitamin c
f. thiamine
g. riboflavin
h. niacin
i. biotin
j. folate

Match the vitamin deficiency with the correct vitamin.

28. _____ Bleeding

29. _____ Beriberi

30. _____ Night blindness

31. _____ Hair loss, cheilitis, glossitis

32. _____ Pellagra

33. _____ Bone pain, muscle weakness

34. _____ Anemia, diarrhea

35. _____ Pernicious anemia, confusion

36. _____ Hemolytic anemia, neurologic deficits

37. _____ Scurvy

a. vitamin A
b. vitamin D
c. vitamin E
d. vitamin K
e. vitamin C
f. thiamine
g. folate
h. niacin
i. biotin
j. cobalamin

Select the correct answer or fill in the blank.

38. Dietary supplements are
    a. oral products that can include a vitamin, mineral, amino acid, herb, or another substance.
    b. used to provide nutrients that are not obtained in the foods we eat and drink.
    c. all of the above.

39. Free radicals are
    a. natural by-products of normal metabolic processes.
    b. produced due to lifestyle and environmental factors.
    c. involved in the inflammation process.
    d. all of the above.

40. Antioxidants
    a. protect cells from free radicals.
    b. limit the damage free radicals can do to the cells.
    c. include vitamins A, C, and E, along with beta-carotene, lycopene, lutein, and selenium.
    d. all of the above

41. _____ makes up more than two-thirds of the body's weight and is the basis for the fluids in the body.

42. Water
    a. keeps the body temperature normal with perspiration.
    b. lubricates organs and cushions joints.
    c. helps prevent and relieve constipation by moving food through the intestines.
    d. all of the above.

43. Our need for water _____ in hot weather, when we are more active, or when we have a fever, diarrhea, or vomiting.

F. Food Guides and Dietary Guidelines

1. The focus of _____ is to make healthy food choices.

2. MyPlate's message includes
    a. fill half of the plate with grains.
    b. eat whole milk and yogurt.
    c. drink and eat less saturated fat, sodium, and added sugars.
    d. all of the above.

3. What are the two focuses of the Dietary Guidelines published by the USDA? _____

    _____

4. The current recommendation for sodium consumption for individuals 14 years and older is fewer than _____ milligrams of sodium a day.

5. The current daily recommendation for alcohol consumption for men is _____ drink(s) and for women _____ drink(s) per day.

G. Food Labels

1. The _____ contains the nutritional information and the ingredient list.

2. Food labels provide information in both the _____ and the _____, which reflects the % Daily Value (DV).

3. The % Daily Value is the percentage of the nutrient in a single serving in terms of the daily recommended amount based on a(n) _____ calorie diet.

4. Food labels provide information on
    a. number of servings per container and the serving size.
    b. the calories per serving.
    c. the %DV for total fat, cholesterol, sodium, and total carbohydrates.
    d. all of the above.

5. Food labels provide information on
   a. saturated and trans-fats.
   b. dietary fiber and total sugars.
   c. protein.
   d. all of the above.

6. Ingredients on food labels are listed in order of weight, starting with the one that weighs the _____ and ending with the one that weighs the _____.

7. _____ or _____ in the ingredient list indicate the presence of trans-fats in the product.

H. Prescribed Diets with Consistency Modifications
Match the description with the correct diet.

1. _____ Foods are soft in texture, low in fiber, and easy for a person to digest and eliminates food that is hard to chew and swallow.

2. _____ Used before and after surgery, difficulty chewing or swallowing, and in preparation for tests or procedures.

3. _____ Foods are prepared for easier chewing and swallowing using household tools.

4. _____ Made up of foods and beverages that are liquid at room temperature.

5. _____ Used for diarrhea, vomiting, nausea, immediately after surgery, and in preparation for intestinal procedures.

6. _____ Made up of foods and beverages that are liquid at room temperature and includes milk products.

7. _____ Used when recovering from surgery or a lengthy illness or with chewing or swallowing problems due to illness or dental problems.

8. _____ Used after head, neck, or mouth surgery; issues with swallowing, poorly fitting dentures, no teeth, or those too ill to chew.

9. _____ The food and drink a person typically consumes when there are no dietary limitations.

10. _____ Used to lower cholesterol levels, control blood glucose levels, and reduce constipation.

11. _____ Include foods that are soft and low in fiber, eliminating spicy, fried, and raw foods.

12. _____ Used when the intestine is narrowed due to a tumor or with a flare-up of intestinal disease.

13. _____ Used to treat gastroesophageal reflux disease, ulcers, and nausea and vomiting.

a. full liquid diet
b. regular diet
c. clear liquid diet
d. full liquid diet
e. soft diet
f. mechanical soft diet
g. low-fiber diet
h. high-fiber diet
i. bland diet

I. Prescribed Diets with Nutrient Modifications

Select the correct answer or fill in the blank.

1. The provider will refer patient to a(n) _____ if the patient needs to make a dietary change, which will be a lifestyle change (e.g., for diabetes or hypertension).

2. For people to lose 1 to 2 pounds per week, they need to reduce their calorie intake by _____ to _____ calories a day or increase their exercise to burn more calories.

3. Tips for people trying to achieve a healthy weight include
   a. eat healthy meals and control portion sizes.
   b. set realistic goals.
   c. track foods and beverages consumed along with physical exercise.
   d. all of the above.

4. _____ is the amount of food we eat and _____ is a standard measurement of food.

5. People with diabetes need to monitor their _____ intake.

Match the following diabetic eating plans with the description.

6. _____ A person keeps track of the amount of carbohydrates eaten each day. Carbohydrates are measured in grams.

7. _____ This diet plan grouped similar foods—carbohydrates, meats, and fats—that had the same amount of carbohydrate, protein, fat, and calories. Each food item had a measurement to indicate how much could be eaten for that exchange.

8. _____ Using a 9-inch dinner plate: half of the plate is filled with non-starchy vegetables, one-quarter is filled with protein, and the last quarter is filled with a grain and starch vegetable. The meal is completed with a serving of fruit, dairy, and a non-sweetened beverage.

a. exchange list system
b. create your plate
c. carbohydrate counting meal plan

Select the correct answer or fill in the blank.

9. When a patient has hypertension, what nutrient must the patient monitor and work to decrease in their diet? _____

10. Excessive sodium in a person's diet can lead to _____, thus increasing the risk for _____ and _____.

11. The DASH eating plan
    a. is recommended for patients with hypertension and/or cardiovascular disease.
    b. is used to prevent hypertension and cardiovascular disease.
    c. has a goal to reduce the blood pressure and decrease the LDL and triglyceride levels.
    d. all of the above.

12. What is encouraged with the Heart Healthy Diet plan?
    a. Limiting sodium
    b. Limiting added sugars and saturated fats
    c. Drinking alcohol in moderation
    d. All of the above

13. The AHA Eating Healthy Recommendations include
    a. eating fish, skinless poultry, lean and extra-lean meat, nuts, seeds, beans, and legumes; limit fatty or processed meats and red meats.
    b. eating whole grains for at least half of the daily servings.
    c. using polyunsaturated and monounsaturated oils; avoid hydrogenated oils and tropical oils.
    d. all of the above.

14. People with _____ and _____ are often prescribed a low-protein diet.

J. Diets for Allergies and Intolerances

1. Which is *not* in the top nine food allergens?
   a. Milk, eggs, and wheat
   b. Fish, crustacean shellfish, and strawberries
   c. Sesame and wheat
   d. Tree nuts, peanuts, and soybeans

2. A person with a(n) _____ needs to eliminate the allergen from their diet.

3. With the _____, people with a suspected food allergy remove the suspicious foods from their diet and slowly add the foods back into their diet, one at a time, to identify the allergen.

4. _____ means that the protein in the allergic food is similar to that in other foods and the person's immune system cannot tell the proteins apart and thus reacts to similar foods.

5. _____, also called *oral allergy syndrome*, is caused by cross-reacting allergens found in pollens, raw foods, and tree nuts.

6. _____ is an allergy to a specific sugar molecule found in mammals, including gelatin, some vaccines and medications, cosmetics, and milk products.

7. People with _____ are put on a gluten-free diet.

8. Gluten is found in
   a. wheat, rye, barley, and malt products.
   b. soybeans.
   c. oats and rice.
   d. all of the above.

9. A lactose intolerance or lactose sensitivity
   a. is not an allergy and occurs because the small intestine does not produce enough lactase.
   b. causes bloating, cramps, diarrhea, nausea, and gas.
   c. is treated by avoiding milk products or using an oral enzyme replacement supplement.

K. Nutritional Needs for Various Populations

1. By _____ months of age, a child started on soft, puréed solid foods.

2. As an adult grows older, the metabolism _____ and the caloric needs _____.

3. What are the dietary recommendations for lactation (breastfeeding)?
    a. Eat a healthy diet.
    b. May need to take a vitamin supplement.
    c. Drink additional water to maintain the milk volume.
    d. All of the above.

4. Treatment for eating disorder includes
    a. psychological, behavioral, and nutritional therapies.
    b. dietary needs focused on correcting nutritional imbalances and restoring weight.
    c. nutritional plans focused on consuming a wide and balanced range of foods.
    d. all of the above.

5. The ketogenic diet
    a. consists of very low-carbohydrate, high-fat, and adequate protein foods.
    b. is used by some people with epilepsy.
    c. is used by some people who want to lose weight.
    d. all of the above.

6. A person who has HIV or AIDS
    a. needs to eat a well-balanced diet.
    b. may struggle with nausea, diarrhea, constipation, and poor appetite.
    c. may need to take a daily vitamin and mineral supplement.
    d. all of the above.

7. A person who has cancer and is undergoing treatment may experience
    a. appetite changes and diarrhea or constipation.
    b. fatigue, dry mouth, and nausea.
    c. weight gain or loss.
    d. all of the above.

8. What should *not* be done by a patient who is experiencing side effects from cancer treatment?
    a. Eat a diet rich in spicy and fatty foods.
    b. Eat six to eight small meals a day.
    c. Eat high-calorie and high-protein foods.
    d. Avoid foods with a strong odor.

9. What should *not* be done by a patient who is experiencing side effects from cancer treatment?
    a. Drink 8 to 10 cups of liquid daily.
    b. Drink a full glass of liquid with each meal.
    c. Limit caffeine and alcohol.
    d. Eat small bites and chew the food well.

CERTIFICATION PREPARATION
Circle the correct answer.

1. What foods or beverages contain carbohydrates?
    a. Cookies, cakes, and other sweets
    b. Regular soda pop and milk products
    c. Breads and cereals
    d. All of the above

2. What foods contain protein?
    a. Fish, meat, and poultry
    b. Fruits and vegetables
    c. Tree nuts and legumes
    d. Both a and c

3. Which foods contain fat?
   a. Fruits and vegetables
   b. Legumes
   c. Butter and cheese
   d. Rice and pasta

4. Which is *not* a mineral?
   a. Potassium
   b. Folate
   c. Calcium
   d. Copper

5. Which protect cells from free radicals and include vitamins A and C, lutein, and selenium?
   a. Antioxidants
   b. Minerals
   c. Vitamins
   d. Electrolytes

6. Which is a water-soluble vitamin?
   a. A
   b. B
   c. D
   d. E

7. What type of foods would be limited on a diabetic eating plan?
   a. Poultry and fish
   b. Breads and pastas
   c. Cakes and cookies
   d. b and c

8. What types of foods would be limited on a low-sodium diet for hypertension?
   a. Frozen dinners and canned foods
   b. Olives and pickles
   c. Soy sauce, ketchup, and mustard
   d. All of the above

9. What types of foods would be limited on a gluten-free diet?
   a. Oatmeal and rice
   b. Potatoes and corn
   c. Barley and wheat
   d. All of the above

10. What factors impact what foods a person purchases?
    a. Cost and convenience
    b. Background and culture
    c. Emotional comfort and routine
    d. All of the above

WORKPLACE APPLICATIONS

1. Working in family medicine, Kayla coaches people of all ages. Describe the nutritional needs for each of the following patients.

   a. 0- to 6-month-old _____

   _____

   b. 2-year-old _____

   _____

   c. 16-year-old female who has her menses _____

   _____

2. Kayla is coaching an older patient who is undergoing chemotherapy for cancer. The patient's mouth is extremely sore, which makes eating difficult. What tips could Kayla give this patient regarding nutrition and oral care?

   _____

   _____

   _____

3. Kayla is coaching a patient with alpha-gal syndrome. Describe the condition and what might cause it.

_____

_____

_____

INTERNET ACTIVITIES

1. Using appropriate online resources, research a diet in this chapter. Create a poster, PowerPoint, or paper summarizing your research. Focus on these areas:
    a. What foods are included in the diet?
    b. Why is the diet typically ordered?

2. Using the tools on MyPlate website (https://www.myplate.gov/), track your food intake for 3 days. At the end of the 3 days, write a brief paper addressing these points:
    a. What are your dietary strengths? What did you do well?
    b. What are your dietary weaknesses? What do you need to work on?
    c. Select one weakness and plan how to improve that dietary issue.
    d. What was your overall impression of the tools you used on MyPlate website?

Procedure 23.1   Instruct a Patient on a Dietary Change

Name _____   **Date** _____   **Score** _____

Tasks: Instruct a patient regarding a dietary change related to a patient's special dietary needs. Show empathy for the patient's concerns regarding the dietary change. Document in the patient's health record.

Equipment and Supplies:
- Patient's health record
- Heart-Healthy Diet brochure

Scenario: You are working with Dr. Angela Perez, a family practice provider. She just finished seeing Al Neviaser (date of birth [DOB] 6/21/19XX). Dr. Perez orders that the patient be given instructions on a heart-healthy diet.

Directions: Role play the scenario with a peer. You are the medical assistant, and the peer is the patient.

Standard: Complete the procedure and all critical steps in _____ minutes with a minimum score of 85% within two attempts (*or as indicated by the instructor*).

Scoring: Divide the points earned by the total possible points. Failure to perform a critical step, indicated by an asterisk (*), results in grade no higher than an 84% (*or as indicated by the instructor*).

Time: Began_____ Ended_____ Total minutes: _____

Steps:	Point Value	Attempt 1	Attempt 2
1. Assemble supplies needed for the provider's order. Ensure that the patient can read and understand the written materials. Verify the order if you have any questions.	5		
2. Greet the patient. Identify yourself. Verify the patient's identity with the full name and date of birth. Explain the order from the provider. Answer any questions the patient may have.	10		
3. Position yourself at the same level as the patient. Angle yourself toward the patient. Have a poised position.	5		
4. Accurately instruct the patient on the new diet. Use the written materials as you discuss the new eating plan.	15*		
5. Use words that the patient can understand. Refrain from jargon and medical terminology. Use professional verbal and nonverbal communication.	10		
Scenario update: After going over the heart-healthy eating plan, Mr. Neviaser states he is not sure this diet is for him. He likes his red meat and does not like to eat fish. He does not have a lot of money to buy expensive fresh fruits and vegetables. 6. Demonstrate empathy by listening to the patient and learning about their experiences and concerns. Use therapeutic communication techniques and positive nonverbal behaviors, including appropriate eye contact. Show your support and respect. *(Refer to the Affective Behaviors Checklist – Respect and Empathy and the Grading Rubric)*	15*		
7. Based on the patient's concerns, provide food alternatives that would meet the eating plan requirements.	15*		

8.	Evaluate the patient's understanding of the teaching by asking the patient to summarize the eating plan or describe a day's worth of meals. Answer any questions the patient may have.	15			
9.	Document the instruction in the patient's health record. Include the order, instruction given, written materials provided, and the patient's feedback.	10			
	Total Points	100			

Affective Behavior	Affective Behaviors Checklist **Directions:** *Check behaviors observed during the role-play.*					
Respect	**Negative, Unprofessional Behaviors**	**Attempt**		**Positive, Professional Behaviors**	**Attempt**	
		1	**2**		**1**	**2**
	Rude, unkind, fake/false attitude, disrespectful, impolite, unwelcoming			Courteous, sincere, polite, welcoming		
	Unconcerned with person's dignity; brief, abrupt			Maintained person's dignity; took time with person		
	Unprofessional verbal communication; inappropriate questions			Professional verbal communication		
	Negative nonverbal behaviors, poor eye contact			Positive nonverbal behaviors, proper eye contact		
	Other:			Other:		
Empathy	Did not listen to patient's responses			Listened to patient; learned about patient		
	Lack of respect and support demonstrated			Showed respect and support		
	Lack of therapeutic communication techniques used			Used therapeutic communication techniques		
	Negative nonverbal behaviors (e.g., positioning, frowning, poor eye contact)			Positive nonverbal behaviors (e.g., at the same level as patient, smiled, good eye contact)		
	Other:			Other:		

Grading Rubric for the Affective Behaviors Checklist Directions: *Based on checklist results, identify the points received for the procedure checklist. Indicate how the behaviors demonstrated met the expectations.*		Point Value	Attempt 1	Attempt 2
Does not meet Expectation	• Response fails to show respect and empathy for patient's concerns. • Student demonstrated more than two negative, unprofessional behaviors during the interaction.	0		
Needs Improvement	• Response fails to show respect and empathy for patient's concerns. • Student demonstrated one or two negative, unprofessional behaviors during the interaction.	0		
Meets Expectation	• Response shows respect and empathy for patient's concerns; no negative, unprofessional behaviors observed. • More practice is needed for behavior to appear natural and for student to appear comfortable and at ease.	15		
Occasionally Exceeds Expectation	• Response shows respect and empathy for patient's concerns; no negative, unprofessional behaviors observed. • At times student appeared comfortable and at ease; but more practice is needed for behavior to become natural and consistent with a professional medical assistant.	15		
Always Exceeds Expectation	• Response shows respect and empathy for patient's concerns; no negative, unprofessional behaviors observed. • Student's behaviors appeared natural and comfortable. Behaviors are consistent with a professional medical assistant.	15		

Documentation

Comments

CAAHEP Competencies	Step(s)
IV.P.1. Instruct a patient regarding a dietary change related to a patient's special dietary needs	Entire procedure
A.3. Demonstrate empathy for patients' concern	6
ABHES Competencies	**Step(s)**
2.d.2) Educate patients regarding proper diet and nutrition guidelines	Entire procedure

Surgical Supplies and Instruments

CAAHEP Competencies	Assessments
III.C.3.b. Identify the following as practiced within an ambulatory care setting: surgical asepsis	Skills and Concepts – D. 1-10
III.P.4. Prepare items for autoclaving	Procedure 24.1
III.P.5. Perform sterilization procedures	Procedure 24.2
ABHES Competencies	Assessments
8. Clinical Procedures a. Practice standard precautions and perform disinfection/sterilization techniques	Procedure 24.2

VOCABULARY REVIEW

Using the word pool on the right, find the correct word to match the definition. Write the word on the line after the definition.

Group A

1. An agent that causes partial or complete loss of sensation _____

2. A thick-walled, dormant form of bacteria that is very resistant to disinfection measures _____

3. To cut or separate tissue with a cutting instrument or scissors _____

4. A disease-causing organism _____

5. Localized collections of pus, which may be under the skin or deep in the body, that cause tissue destruction _____

6. A metal rod with a smooth, rounded tip that is placed in hollow instruments to reduce injury to body tissues during insertion _____

7. A liquid substance that dilutes or lessens the strength of a solution or mixture _____

8. Contraction of the muscles causing the narrowing of the inside tube of the vessel _____

9. A metal probe that is inserted into or passed through a catheter, needle, or tube used for clearing purposes or to facilitate passage into a body orifice _____

10. Not lasting, enduring, or permanent _____

Word Pool
- diluent
- pathogen
- transient
- spore
- anesthetic
- abscess
- vasoconstriction
- dissect
- stylus
- obturator

Group B

1. Capable of burning, corroding, or destroying living tissue
   _____

2. The act of scraping a body cavity with a surgical instrument such as a curette _____

3. Not permitting penetration _____

4. A recess in the upper part of the vagina caused by protrusion of the cervix into the vaginal wall _____

5. Allowing for penetration _____

6. Open condition of a body cavity or canal
   _____

7. The opening or widening of the circumference of a body orifice with a dilating instrument _____

8. Invasion of body tissues by microorganisms, which then multiply and damage tissues _____

9. A rigid tube that surrounds a blunt trocar or a sharp, pointed trocar, which is inserted into the body _____

Word Pool
- cannula
- fornix
- dilation
- curettage
- patency
- infection
- permeable
- impervious
- caustic

SKILLS AND CONCEPTS

Answer the following questions. Write your answer on the line or in the space provided.

A. Preparing for Minor Surgery

1. The minor surgery room, also known as the _____, should be near a workroom with a sink and an autoclave.

2. Which of the following would be stored in the minor surgery room?
   a. Surgical supplies
   b. Wound care equipment
   c. Medications
   d. Biopsy containers
   e. All of the above

3. Before the procedure, the surgical site on the patient must be disinfected with a(n) _____ to reduce the number of _____ on the skin. This process will remove _____ flora and reduce the _____ flora.

4. Topical anesthetics are applied directly to the _____, whereas local anesthetics are _____ at the site of the procedure.

5. What form(s) are topical anesthetics available in? Choose all that apply.
   a. Sprays
   b. Gels and lotions
   c. Swabs and foams
   d. Injectables

6. Many local anesthetics contain _____, which causes vasoconstriction at that site that keeps the anesthetic in the tissues longer and can minimize bleeding.

Match the additional surgical supply with its use.

7. _____ Sterilized gauze squares or strips saturated with petroleum jelly or petrolatum

8. _____ Surgical sponges

9. _____ Syringes and needles

10. _____ Sterile dressing and bandaging materials

a. Used to inject local anesthetics and irrigate wounds
b. Used to pack wounds
c. Used on the surgical site after the procedure is complete
d. Used to absorb blood and protect tissues during surgery

B. Surgical Instruments
Name the instruments pictured in the following figures.

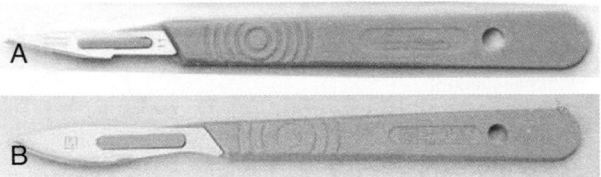

1. _____

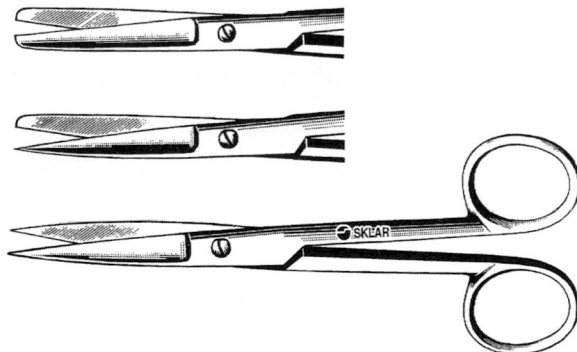

2. _____

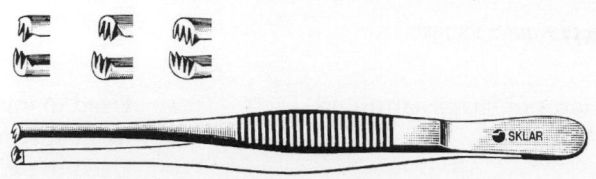

3. _____

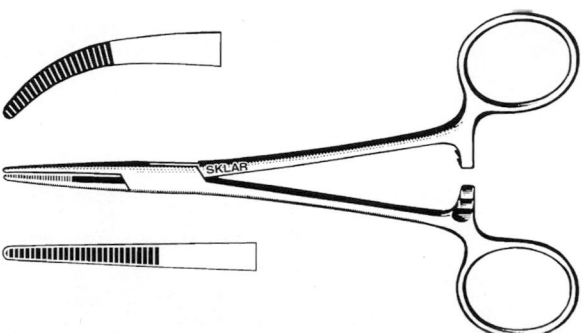

4. _____

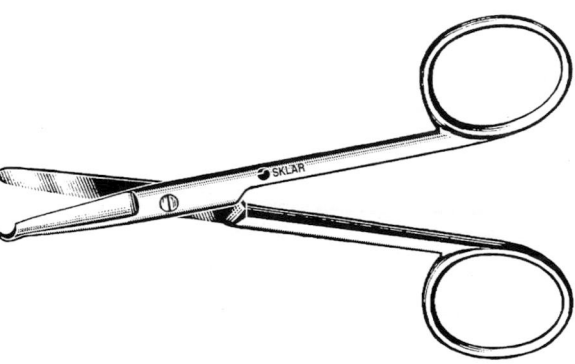

5. _____

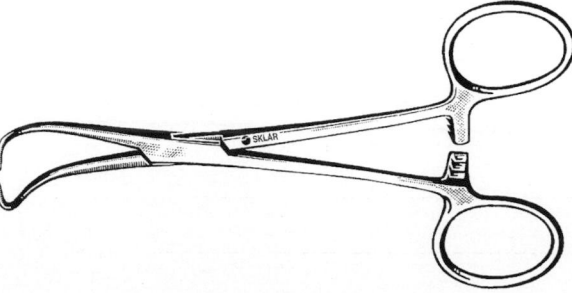

6. _____

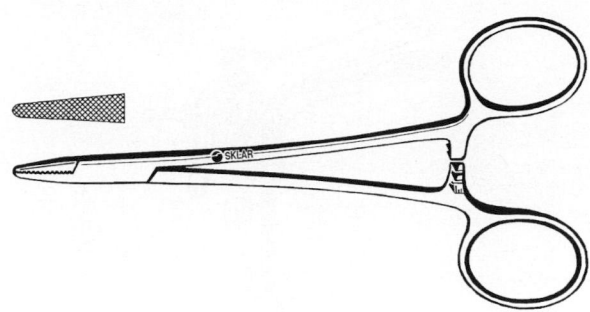

7. _____

8. _____

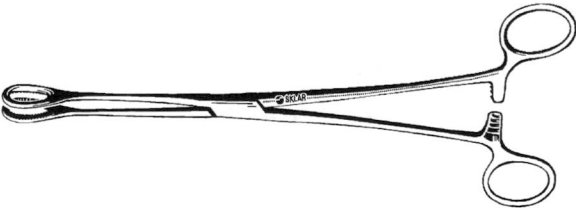

9. _____

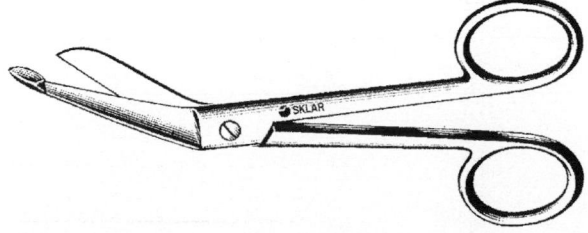

10. _____

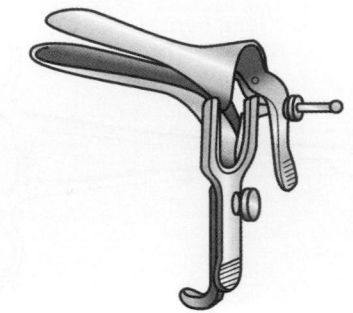

11. _____

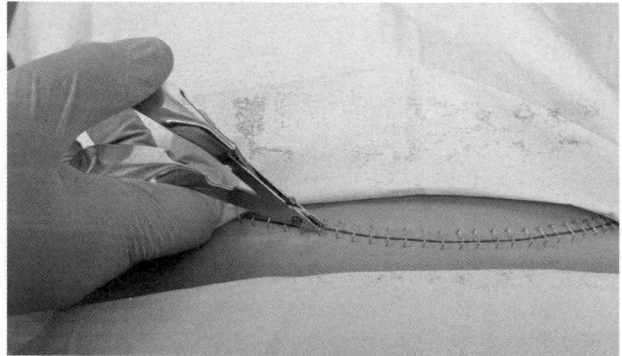

12. _____

13. List four groups of surgical instruments and give an example of each.

a. _____

_____

b. _____

_____

c. _____

_____

d. _____

_____

Name the specialty instruments pictured in the following figures.

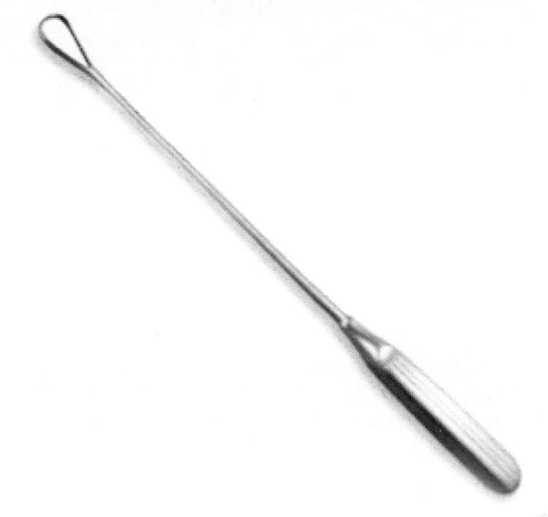

14. _____

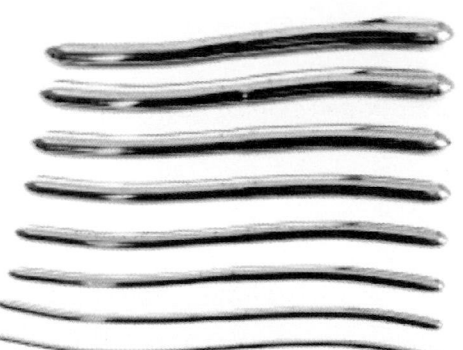

15. _____

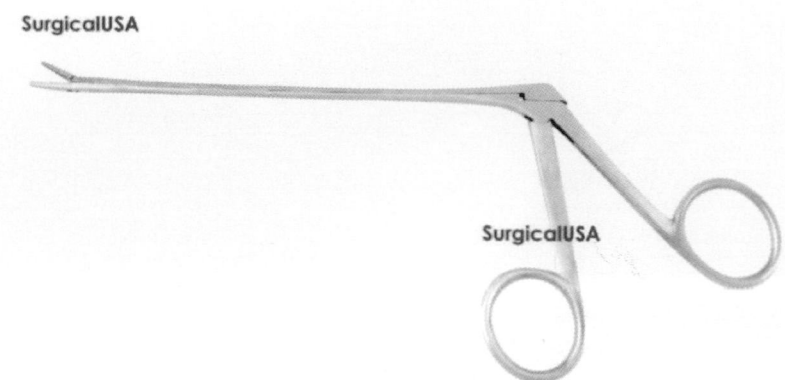

16. _____

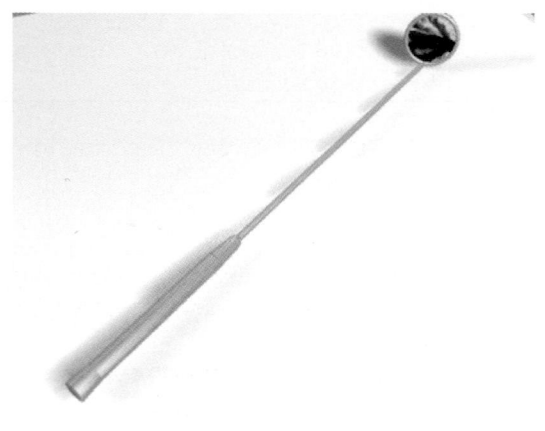

17. _____

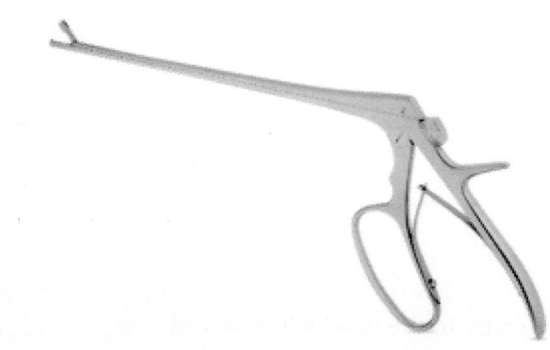

18. _____

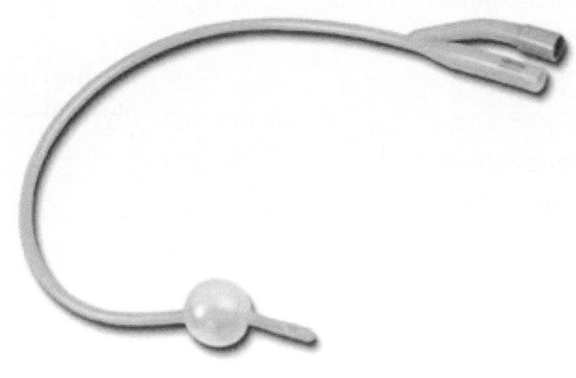

19. _____

C. Drapes, Sutures, and Other Closure Material

1. Advantages of using tissue adhesives include which of the following?
   a. Creates a flexible, water-resistant protective coating for the wound.
   b. Eliminates the need for suture removal.
   c. Results in better cosmetic outcomes because there is no scarring from suture entry.
   d. All of the above
   e. None of the above

2. Absorbable sutures are used to close inner layers of a deep incision or laceration and are dissolved by the body's enzymes. Nonabsorbable suture and also used to close inner layers of a deep incision but must be removed after healing is complete.
   a. The first statement is true, and the second statement is false.
   b. The first statement is false, and the second statement is true.
   c. Both statements are true.
   d. Both statements are false.

Label the suture as either absorbable or nonabsorbable.

3. _____ Dexon
4. _____ Silk
5. _____ Dacron
6. _____ PDS
7. _____ Maxon
8. _____ Prolene

a. absorbable
b. nonabsorbable

9. When the suture is attached directly to the needle it is considered _____.

10. When nonabsorbable suture is use on the face they should be removed in _____ days, on the neck _____ days, on the scalp _____ days, on the trunk and upper extremities _____ days, and on the lower extremities _____ days.

D. Surgical Asepsis and Preparation of Surgical Instruments

Determine if the following procedures require medical or surgical asepsis.

1. _____ Administering oral medication
2. _____ Inserting sutures
3. _____ Measuring an oral temperature
4. _____ Applying a bandage to the forearm
5. _____ Performing a needle biopsy
6. _____ Removing a sebaceous cyst
7. _____ Obtaining a Pap specimen
8. _____ Inserting a urinary catheter
9. _____ Incision and drainage of an abscess
10. _____ Applying a dressing to an open wound

          a. medical asepsis
          b. surgical asepsis

11. A(n) _____ sterilization indicator changes color when exposed to the proper sterilization time, _____, and steam.

12. _____ sterilization indicators should be used _____.

Match the following autoclave problem with the cause.

13. _____ Damp autoclave paper
14. _____ Corroded instruments
15. _____ Spotted or stained instruments
16. _____ Steam leakage
17. _____ Chamber door does not open

a. Caused by mineral deposits on instruments; residual detergents from cleaning; mineral deposits from tap water
b. Caused by worn gasket
c. Caused by vacuum in chamber
d. Caused by clogged chamber drain; goods removed from chamber too soon after cycle; improper loading
e. Caused by poor cleaning; residual soil; exposure to hard chemicals (e.g., iodine, salt, and acids); inferior instruments

18. _____ practices refer to items being considered sterile until something causes contamination, such as the package becoming wet or the packing material is torn.

CERTIFICATION PREPARATION

Circle the correct answer.

1. Choose the smallest diameter of suture strand.
   a. 0
   b. 5-0
   c. 5
   d. 1-0

2. The recommended way to clean sharp instruments is to
   a. use an ultrasonic cleaner.
   b. wear appropriate PPE.
   c. use the proper concentration of disinfectant.
   d. rinse instruments with sterile water before sterilizing.

3. The jaws of which instrument are shorter and stronger than hemostat jaws?
   a. Splinter forceps
   b. Towel forceps
   c. Needleholder
   d. Suture scissors

4. Which is one of the strongest nonabsorbable sutures?
   a. Dacron
   b. Vicryl
   c. Silk
   d. Maxon

5. _____ is the complete destruction of microorganisms and spores. This technique is mandatory for any procedure that invades the body's skin or tissues, such as surgery.
   a. Disinfection
   b. Sterilization
   c. Medical asepsis
   d. Surgical asepsis

6. The recommended temperature for sterilization in an autoclave is
   a. 98.6° F.
   b. 104° F.
   c. 121° C.
   d. 37.6° C.

7. What is the complete destruction of pathogens and spores?
   a. Sanitization
   b. Disinfection
   c. Sterilization
   d. Germicide

8. Which instrument would be damaged by the high temperature and steam under pressure of autoclaves and must be disinfected after each procedure?
   a. Endoscope used in an endoscopy
   b. Microscope used for microsurgery
   c. Electrosurgical tip used for electrosurgery
   d. Laser tip used for laser surgery

9. Which gynecologic instrument is used to remove polyps, secretions, and bits of placental tissue?
   a. Uterine curette
   b. Endocervical curette
   c. Schroeder uterine vulsellum forceps
   d. Both a and b

10. Which ophthalmologic and otolaryngologic instrument is used to remove foreign bodies or polyps?
    a. Krause nasal snare
    b. Hartmann "alligator" ear forceps
    c. "Buck" ear curette
    d. All of the above

WORKPLACE APPLICATIONS

1. Melissa, the medical assistant, is preparing instruments for the autoclave. What rules must she follow when wrapping the instruments?

   _____

   _____

   _____

   _____

2. Tony Carmini, 5 years old, was brought to the clinic today by his mother for treatment of a laceration above his right eyebrow. Rather than suturing the wound, the provider may decide to use either adhesive skin closure strips or skin adhesive. Why are these suturing alternatives a good choice for this patient? Describe both skin closure materials in your answer.

_____

_____

_____

_____

3. Tom is working with a medical assistant student who is at WMFM Clinic for her practicum. What guidelines should Tom explain to the student about unloading the autoclave?

_____

_____

_____

_____

INTERNET ACTIVITIES

1. Using internet resources, research the use of surgical staples. Create a poster presentation, a PowerPoint presentation, or write a paper that summarizes your research. Include the following points in your project:
   a. What types of surgeries use staples to close a wound?
   b. How are they applied?
   c. How are they removed?

2. One of medical assistant's duties is to purchase supplies for minor office procedures. Search the internet for equipment and supplies typically needed to perform such procedures. Print a list of materials and prices. Share the information with your classmates. Did you find anything surprising?

Procedure 24.1   Wrap Instruments and Supplies for Sterilization in an Autoclave

Name _____ Date _____ Score _____

Task: To place dry, inspected, and sanitized supplies and instruments inside appropriate wrapping materials for sterilization and storage without contamination.

Equipment and Supplies:
- Dry, inspected, and sanitized instruments
- Double-ply autoclave paper
- Autoclave tape
- Sterilization strip
- Waterproof, felt-tipped pen
- Gloves (if part of office policy)

Standard: Complete the procedure and all critical steps in _____ minutes with a minimum score of 85% within two attempts (*or as indicated by the instructor*).

Scoring: Divide the points earned by the total possible points. Failure to perform a critical step, indicated by an asterisk (*), results in grade no higher than an 84% (*or as indicated by the instructor*).

Time: Began _____ Ended _____ Total minutes: _____

Steps:	Point Value	Attempt 1	Attempt 2
1. Wash or sanitize your hands. Collect and assemble already inspected, sanitized instruments to be wrapped. Gloves may be worn.	10		
2. Place the double-ply autoclave paper on a clean, flat surface.	10		
3. Place the instruments diagonally at the approximate center of the double-ply autoclave paper. Make sure the size of the square is large enough for the items.	15*		
4. Open any hinged instruments. If the instrument is sharp, its teeth or tip should be shielded with cotton or gauze.	15*		
5. Place a sterilization strip in the center of the pack to check for sterilization standards.	10		
6. Bring up the bottom corner of the wrap and fold back a portion of it.	10		
7. Repeat the previous step with each corner, making sure to turn back a portion each time.	10		
8. Fold the last flap over.	10		
9. Secure with autoclave tape and label the package with the date, including the year, contents, and your initials.	10		
Total Points	100		

Comments

CAAHEP Competencies	Step(s)
III.P.4. Prepare items for autoclaving	Entire procedure
ABHES Competencies	**Step(s)**
4.a. Identify appropriate procedures for sterilization of 1. Instruments 2. Surgical equipment 3. Surgical towels, drapes, or dressings	Entire procedure
4.c. Utilize proper instrument and tray packaging for sterilization	Entire procedure
8.a. Practice standard precautions and perform disinfection/sterilization techniques	Entire procedure

Procedure 24.2   Operate the Autoclave

Name _____ Date _____ Score _____

Task: To sterilize properly prepared supplies and instruments using the autoclave.

Equipment and Supplies:
- Autoclave
- Wrapped items ready to be sterilized
- Heat-resistant gloves

Standard: Complete the procedure and all critical steps in _____ minutes with a minimum score of 85% within two attempts (*or as indicated by the instructor*).

Scoring: Divide the points earned by the total possible points. Failure to perform a critical step, indicated by an asterisk (*), results in grade no higher than an 84% (*or as indicated by the instructor*).

Time: Began_____ Ended_____ Total minutes: _____

Steps:	Point Value	Attempt 1	Attempt 2
NOTE: *The specific instructions for operating an autoclave may vary based on the model number and manufacturer. Refer to the instructions that accompany the autoclave to be sure the appropriate steps are followed.*			
1. Check the water level in the reservoir and add distilled water as necessary.	5		
2. Turn the control to "Fill" to allow water to flow into the chamber. The water flows until you turn the control to its next position. Do not let the water overflow.	5		
3. Load the chamber with wrapped items, spacing them for maximum circulation and penetration.	10*		
4. Close and seal the door.	5		
5. Turn the control setting to "On" or "Autoclave" to start the cycle.	5		
6. Watch the gauges until the temperature gauge reaches at least 121°C (250°F) and the pressure gauge reaches 15 lbs. of pressure.	10*		
7. Set the timer for the desired time.	5		
8. At the end of the timed cycle, turn the control setting to "Vent."	5		
9. Wait for the pressure gauge to reach zero.	5		
10. Standing behind the autoclave door, carefully open the chamber door 1/4".	10		
11. Leave the autoclave control at "Vent" to continue releasing heat.	10		
12. Allow complete drying of all articles.	5		
13. Using heat-resistant gloves, remove the items from the chamber and place the sterilized packages on dry, covered shelves or open the autoclave door and allow the items to cool completely before removal and storage.	10		
14. Turn the control knob to "Off" and keep the door slightly ajar.	10		
Total Points	**100**		

Comments

CAAHEP Competencies	Step(s)
III.P.5. Perform sterilization procedures	Entire procedure
ABHES Competencies	**Step(s)**
4.b. Identify modes of sterilization 1. Autoclave	Entire procedure
1.d. List the general responsibilities and skills of the medical assistant	Entire procedure

Assisting with Surgical Procedures

CAAHEP Competencies	Assessments
III.C.7. Identify the implications for failure to comply with Center for Disease Control (CDC) regulations in healthcare settings	Skills and Concepts – D. 9, 10
I.P.8. Instruct and prepare a patient for a procedure or a treatment	Procedures 25.1, 25.6, 25.7, 25.8
III.P.3 Perform hand washing	Procedure 25.2
III.P.6. Prepare a sterile field	Procedures 25.4, 25.5, 25.6
III.P.7. Perform within a sterile field	Procedures 25.3, 25.4, 25.5, 25.6
III.P.8. Perform wound care	Procedures 25.6, 25.7
III.P.9. Perform dressing change	Procedure 25.7
III.P.10. a. Demonstrate proper disposal of biohazardous material: sharps	Procedures 25.6, 25.8
III.P.10. b. Demonstrate proper disposal of biohazardous material: regulated waste	Procedures 25.6, 25.7, 25.8
X.P.3. Document patient care accurately in the medical record	Procedures 25.6, 25.7, 25.8
ABHES Competencies	**Assessments**
1. General Orientation d. List the general responsibilities and skills of the medical assistant	All procedures
8. Clinical Procedures a. Practice standard precautions and perform disinfection/sterilization techniques	Procedure 25.2
8. Clinical Procedures e. Perform specialty procedures, including but not limited to minor surgery, cardiac, respiratory, OB-GYN, neurological, and gastroenterology	All procedures
9.c Dispose of biohazardous materials	Procedures 25.6, 25.7

VOCABULARY REVIEW

Using the word pool on the right, find the correct word to match the definition. Write the word on the line after the definition.

1. Keen watchfulness to detect danger _____

2. Early scar tissue that appears pale, contracted, and firm

    _____

3. Vapor, smoke, and particle debris produced by laser procedures

    _____

4. The stoppage of bleeding _____

5. Near; close together _____

Word Pool
- plume
- vigilance
- approximated
- hemostasis
- cicatrix

SKILLS AND CONCEPTS

Answer the following questions. Write your answer on the line or in the space provided.

A. Surgical Procedures

Match the following procedures with their description.

1. _____ Electrosurgery

2. _____ Laser

3. _____ Microsurgery

4. _____ Endoscopic procedures

5. _____ Cryosurgery

a. Involves the use of a very low-temperature probe to destroy tissue by freezing it on contact

b. A high-frequency current is used to cut through tissue and coagulate blood vessels

c. A fiberoptic instrument with a miniature camera mounted on a flexible tube is used to examine the inside of an organ or cavity; the procedure's name reflects the organs or areas explored

d. Tiny light beams are used to treat specific tissues while causing minimal damage to surrounding tissues and limited scar formation

e. An operating microscope is used to perform delicate surgical procedures

6. Which of the following are tips about the grounding pad used with electrosurgery?
   a. The pad must be tight against the patient's skin.
   b. Apply the pad over a bony area.
   c. Do not place the pad over body hair.
   d. Both a and c are correct.

7. _____ surgery is often used for the excision of lesions, diseases of the eye, and cosmetic procedures.

8. A medical device that consists of a miniature camera mounted on a flexible tube with an optical system and a light source is used for _____.

9. Joint aspiration is also known as the _____ and involves removing _____ from a joint.

B. Preparation for Surgical Procedures

1. Preoperative preparation may include which of the following?
   a. Blood and urine tests
   b. Completion of a consent form
   c. Gathering of the current history concerning any recent illnesses
   d. Medications and allergies
   e. All of the above

2. Before an informed consent form is signed, the patient should understand which of the following?
   a. What procedure will be performed and why it should be done
   b. Potential risks and benefits of the surgery
   c. Alternative treatments and the possible risks of any alternative treatment
   d. All of the above

3. The goal of skin preparation is to reduce the number of _____ to limit the transference of harmful _____ at the incision site.

4. Place the following steps for skin preparation in the correct order:

   a. _____ Shave the site.

   b. _____ Dry the area using a circular technique, starting in the center of the incision site and moving outward.

   c. _____ Provide sufficient friction for 5 minutes.

   d. _____ Wash the incision site with antiseptic soap on a gauze sponge in a circular motion, starting at the center of the site and moving outward for one rotation.

   e. _____ Place a sterile drape/towel over the area.

   f. _____ Rinse the area with sterile normal saline.

   g. _____ Discard the sponge and begin again with a new one.

5. When preparing the room for a minor surgical procedure, the medical assistant should keep in mind that sterile supplies that have been open longer than _____ are considered nonsterile.

C. Assisting with Surgical Procedures

1. When setting up a sterile field, the Mayo stand must first be _____.

2. The two most common sources of contamination when a sterile field is set up are _____ and _____.

3. When passing instruments to the provider, the medical assistant should use a(n) _____ motion so that the provider does not have to look up. Describe the process of passing instruments to the provider.

4. The medical assistant should hold all instruments by the _____ and pass the handle ends into the provider's palm or fingers.

5. When giving a patient postoperative instructions, what are the warning signs that the patient should report immediately?

   _____

   _____

D. Wound Care

1. A wound from surgery or a knife would be considered a(n) _____ wound, whereas a wound with torn or mangle tissues from a dull or blunt instrument would be considered a(n) _____ wound.

Match the description with the correct phase of wound healing.

2. _____ Encompasses wound health and new growth; tissues repair themselves

3. _____ Blood vessels contract to control hemorrhage and platelets form a network that acts as a glue to plug the wound

4. _____ Collagen is produced to give wounded tissues strength and forms scar tissue

5. _____ Focused on destroying bacteria and removing debris

a. Phase 1
b. Phase 2
c. Phase 3
d. Phase 4

6. What are the reasons for applying a sterile dressing?

    a. _____

    b. _____

    c. _____

    d. _____

7. A(n) _____ is a sterile covering placed over a wound.

8. _____ hold dressings in place and help maintain even pressure, support the affected part, and protect the wound form injury and contamination.

You fail to wear gloves when changing a patient's dressing. During the procedure, you got blood on your hands. Discuss the implication for failing to comply with CDC regulations in healthcare settings. Answer the following questions:

9. How might your actions (of not wearing gloves) impact the patient's health and safety? _____

_____

_____

_____

10. How might your actions (of not wearing gloves) impact your health and safety? _____

_____

_____

_____

_____

CERTIFICATION PREPARATION

Circle the correct answer.

1. For which postoperative condition should the patient call the provider's office?
   a. Redness around the operative site
   b. Fever or swelling
   c. Increasing or severe pain
   d. All of the above

2. The LEEP excisional procedure is considered
   a. endoscopy.
   b. laser surgery
   c. microsurgery.
   d. electrosurgery.

3. Which statement is *not* true about informed consent for surgery?
   a. The patient must provide his or her own witness for the signature.
   b. The patient must understand the potential risks and benefits of the surgery.
   c. The patient must understand the possible risks of any alternative treatment.
   d. The patient cannot give consent if he or she has received preoperative medication.

4. Which endoscope is rigid?
   a. Laparoscope
   b. Colonoscope
   c. Bronchoscope
   d. Gastroscope

5. Which wound passes through to a body organ or cavity?
   a. Incised wound
   b. Lacerated wound
   c. Puncture wound
   d. Penetrating wound

6. In which phase of wound healing is fibrin most involved?
   a. First phase
   b. Second phase
   c. Third phase
   d. Fourth phase

7. Which bandage material is superior for covering round, narrow surfaces such as fingers or toes?
   a. Plain roller gauze
   b. Wrinkled crepe-type roller bandage
   c. Elastic bandage
   d. Seamless tubular gauze bandage

8. Which is a violation of sterile technique?
   a. Holding a sterile article above waist level
   b. Facing a sterile field
   c. Reaching over a sterile field
   d. Placing a sterile item in the center of the a sterile field

9. The purpose of a sterile fenestrated drape is
   a. comfort and warmth for the provider.
   b. to provide a sterile area around the operative site.
   c. to prevent the patient from observing the operative site.
   d. to protect the patient's clothing from blood and other secretions.

10. Cryosurgery involves
    a. freezing temperatures.
    b. sound waves.
    c. x-rays.
    d. chemicals.

WORKPLACE APPLICATIONS

1. Minor surgical procedures such as laser surgery are commonly done in Melissa's office. What is the medical assistant's role in laser surgery?

   _____

   _____

   _____

   _____

2. The provider has ordered open wound healing for a patient with a traumatic injury. What does this mean? How does healing occur? What are some of the advantages of this type of healing process?

_____

_____

_____

_____

INTERNET ACTIVITIES

1. Using internet resources, research a procedure that is commonly performed in a primary care facility. Create a poster presentation, a PowerPoint presentation, or write a paper that summarizes your research. Include the following points in your project:
    a. Describe the procedure and the instruments needed.
    b. What preoperative patient preparation is needed?
    c. What would be the medical assistant's role in this procedure?

2. Using internet resources, research healthcare-associated infections. Create a poster presentation, a PowerPoint presentation, or write a paper that summarizes your research. Include the following points in your project:
    a. Describe a healthcare-associated infection.
    b. How is sterile technique connected to healthcare-associated infections?
    c. What can a medical assistant do to prevent healthcare-associated infections?

Procedure 25.1   Perform Skin Prep for Surgery

Name _____ Date _____ Score _____

Tasks: To prepare the patient's skin and remove hair from the surgical site to reduce the risk of wound contamination.

Equipment and Supplies:
- Disposable skin prep kit, or collect the following:
  - Gauze
  - Cotton-tipped applicators
  - Soap
  - Gloves
  - Electric clippers
  - Two small bowls
  - Antiseptic or antiseptic swabs (e.g., Betadine swabs)
  - Sterile normal saline solution
  - Optional: cotton balls, nail pick, scrub brush
- Sterile drape
- Biohazard waste container
- Biohazard sharps container
- Patient's health record

Standard: Complete the procedure and all critical steps in _____ minutes with a minimum score of 85% within two attempts (*or as indicated by the instructor*).

Scoring: Divide the points earned by the total possible points. Failure to perform a critical step, indicated by an asterisk (*), results in grade no higher than an 84% (*or as indicated by the instructor*).

Time: Began_____ Ended_____ Total minutes: _____

Steps:	Point Value	Attempt 1	Attempt 2
1. Wash hands or use hand sanitizer.	5		
2. Greet the patient. Identify yourself. Verify the patient's identity with full name and date of birth. Explain the procedure to be performed in a manner that is understood by the patient. Answer any questions the patient may have on the procedure.	5		
3. Ask the patient to remove any clothing that might interfere with exposure of the site and provide a gown if needed.	5		
4. Assist the patient into the proper position for site exposure. Provide a drape if necessary to protect the patient's privacy.	5		
5. Expose the site. Use a light if necessary.	5		
6. If hair is present, the area may need to be shaved. Put on gloves and shave the required area with electric clippers.	10		
7. While wearing gloves, open the skin prep pack and add the soap to the two bowls.	5		
8. Start at the incision site and begin washing with the soap on a gauze sponge in a circular motion, moving from the center to the edges of the area to be scrubbed.	10*		

9. After one complete wipe, discard the sponge and begin again with a new sponge soaked in the antiseptic solution.	5		
10. Repeat the process, using sufficient friction for 5 minutes (or follow office policy for the length of time required for a particular prep).	5		
11. Rinse the area with sterile normal saline solution.	5		
12. Dry the area, using the same circular technique with dry sponges. The area may be dried by blotting with a sterile towel.	10*		
13. Paint on the antiseptic with the cotton-tipped applicators or gauze sponges, using the same circular technique and never returning to an area that has already been painted	10		
14. Place a sterile drape and/or towel over the area.	5		
15. Answer all the patient's questions to relieve anxiety about the upcoming surgical procedure.	5		
16. Document completion of the skin prep in the patient's health record.	5		
Total Points	**100**		

Documentation

Comments

CAAHEP Competencies	Step(s)
I.P.8. Instruct and prepare a patient for a procedure or treatment	Entire procedure
ABHES Competencies	**Step(s)**
8.e. Perform specialty procedures, including but not limited to minor surgery, cardiac, respiratory, OB-GYN, neurological, and gastroenterology	Entire procedure
1.d. List the general responsibilities and skills of the medical assistant	Entire procedure

Procedure 25.2   Perform a Surgical Hand Scrub

Name _____ Date _____ Score _____

Task: To scrub the hands with surgical soap using friction, running water, and a disposable sterile brush to sanitize the skin before assisting with any procedure that requires surgical asepsis.

Equipment and Supplies:
- Sink with foot, knee, or arm control for running water
- Surgical soap in a dispenser
- Towels (sterile towels if indicated by office policy)
- Nail file or orange stick
- Sterile disposable brush

Standard: Complete the procedure and all critical steps in _____ minutes with a minimum score of 85% within two attempts (*or as indicated by the instructor*).

Scoring: Divide the points earned by the total possible points. Failure to perform a critical step, indicated by an asterisk (*), results in grade no higher than an 84% (*or as indicated by the instructor*).

Time: Began_____ Ended_____ Total minutes: _____

Steps:	Point Value	Attempt 1	Attempt 2
1. Remove all jewelry.	5		
2. Roll long sleeves above the elbows.	5		
3. Inspect your fingernails for length and your hands for skin breaks.	5		
4. Turn on the faucet and regulate the water to a comfortable temperature, being careful to stand away from the sink to prevent contamination of clothing from contact with the sink or countertop.	5		
5. Keep your hands upright and held at or above waist level.	10*		
6. Clean your fingernails with a file, discard it (in most situations you will drop the file into the sink and discard it later to prevent contamination by lowering your hands and/or touching a waste receptacle), and rinse your hands under the faucet without touching the faucet or the inside of the sink basin.	5		
7. Allow the water to run over your hands from the fingertips to the elbows without moving the arm back and forth under the water.	5		
8. Apply surgical soap from the dispenser to the sterile brush (or use a prepared disposable brush) and start the scrub by scrubbing the palm of the hand in a circular fashion.	5		
9. Continue from the palm to the base of the thumb, then move on to the other fingers, scrubbing from the base, along each side, and across the nail, holding the fingertips upward and remembering to rub between the fingers. After the fingers have been completely scrubbed, clean the posterior surface of the hand in a circular fashion and then proceed to the wrist. The scrub process should take at least 5 minutes for each hand and arm.	10*		
10. Do not return to a clean area after you have moved to the next part of the hand.	5		

11. Wash the wrists and forearms in a circular fashion around the arm while holding your hands above waist level.	5		
12. Rinse the arms and forearms from the fingertips upward, holding the fingers up, without touching the faucet or the inside of the sink basin.	5		
13. Apply more solution without touching any dirty surface and repeat the scrub on the other side, remembering to wash and use friction between each finger with a firm, circular motion.	5		
14. Scrub all surfaces, being careful not to abrade your skin. The second hand and arm should take at least 5 minutes.	5		
15. Rinse thoroughly, keeping your hands up and above waist level. Discard the scrub brush without lowering the arms below the waist.	5		
16. Turn off the faucet with the foot, knee, or forearm lever, if available.	5		
17. Dry your hands with a sterile towel, being careful to keep the fingers pointing upward and your hands above the waist. Do not rub back and forth, dragging contaminants from the dirtier area of the upper arm down toward the hands. Use the opposite end of the towel for the other hand.	5		
18. Using a patting motion, continue to dry the forearms. Discard the towel and keep your hands up and above waist level.	5		
Total Points	100		

Comments

CAAHEP Competencies	Step(s)
III.P.3 Perform hand washing	Entire procedure
ABHES Competencies	**Step(s)**
1.d. List the general responsibilities and skills of the medical assistant	Entire procedure

Procedure 25.3   Put on Sterile Gloves

Name _____   Date _____   Score _____

Task: To put on sterile gloves correctly before performing sterile procedures.

Equipment and Supplies:
- Pair of packaged sterile gloves in your size

Standard: Complete the procedure and all critical steps in _____ minutes with a minimum score of 85% within two attempts (*or as indicated by the instructor*).

Scoring: Divide the points earned by the total possible points. Failure to perform a critical step, indicated by an asterisk (*), results in grade no higher than an 84% (*or as indicated by the instructor*).

Time: Began_____ Ended_____ Total minutes: _____

Steps:	Point Value	Attempt 1	Attempt 2
1. Perform the surgical hand scrub as explained in Procedure 25.2 before putting on sterile gloves.	5		
2. Check that the Mayo stand, or countertop is dust-free and clean. If it is not, disinfect and allow to air dry.	10		
3. Open package and remove the glove pack from the outer package. Place the glove pack on the Mayo stand or countertop. Open the glove pack, being careful not to cross over the open area in the middle of the pack. Remember, a 1-inch area around the perimeter of the glove wrapper is considered nonsterile.	5		
4. Glove your dominant hand first. With your nondominant hand, pick up the glove for your dominant hand with your thumb and forefinger, grabbing the edge of the folded cuff closest to you, which is the inside of the glove, being careful not to cross over the other sterile glove.	10*		
5. Lift the glove up and away from the sterile package.	10		
6. Hold your hands up and away from your body and slide the dominant hand into the glove.	10		
7. Leave the cuff folded.	10		
8. With your gloved dominant hand, pick up the second glove by slipping your gloved fingers into the cuff, extending the thumb up and away from the glove (thumbs up position), so that your gloved fingers touch only the outside of the second glove.	10*		
9. Slide your nondominant hand into the glove without touching the exterior of the glove or any part of the gloved hand.	10		
10. Still holding your hands away from you, unroll the cuff by slipping the fingers into the cuff and gently pulling up and out. Do not touch your bare arm or the internal surface of the glove with any part of the sterile glove.	10		
11. Now, slip your gloved fingers up under the first cuff and unroll it, using the same technique.	10		
Total Points	100		

Comments

CAAHEP Competencies	Step(s)
III.P.7. Perform within a sterile field	Entire procedure
ABHES Competencies	**Step(s)**
1.d. List the general responsibilities and skills of the medical assistant	Entire procedure

Procedure 25.4   Prepare a Sterile Field; Use Transfer Forceps; Pour a Sterile Solution into a Sterile Field

Name _____ Date _____ Score _____

Tasks: To open a sterile instrument pack using correct aseptic technique and create a sterile field; move sterile items on a sterile field or transfer sterile items to a gloved team member; pour a sterile solution into a sterile stainless-steel bowl or container sitting at the edge of a sterile field.

Equipment and Supplies:
- A sterile instrument pack wrapped with autoclave paper that, when opened, will serve as a sterile table drape or field
- Mayo stand or countertop
- Disinfectant and gauze sponges or disinfectant wipes
- Sterile item to move or transfer
- Sterile wrapped transfer forceps
- Bottle of sterile solution
- Sterile bowl or container
- Sink or waste receptacle

Standard: Complete the procedure and all critical steps in _____ minutes with a minimum score of 85% within two attempts (*or as indicated by the instructor*).

Scoring: Divide the points earned by the total possible points. Failure to perform a critical step, indicated by an asterisk (*), results in grade no higher than an 84% (*or as indicated by the instructor*).

Time: Began_____ Ended_____ Total minutes: _____

Steps:	Point Value	Attempt 1	Attempt 2
1. Check that the Mayo stand or countertop is dust-free and clean. If it is not, disinfect and allow to air dry.	5		
2. Wash or sanitize your hands and make sure they are completely dry. If you will be assisting with a surgical procedure immediately after opening the sterile pack, perform the surgical hand scrub as explained in Procedure 25.2.	5		
3. Gather supplies. Check the label of the ordered solution. Check the solution name and the expiration date.	5		
4. If using an autoclaved pack, check the indicator tape for a color change.	5		
5. Open the outside cover. Position the package so that the outer envelope flap is at the top and with the tab facing you.	5		
6. Open the outermost flap. Next, open the first flap away from you. You can cross over the uncovered portion of the Mayo stand as it is not sterile. Do not cross over the pack.	5		
7. Open the second corner, pulling to side.	5		
8. Be careful to lift the flaps by touching only the small, folded-back tab and without touching or crossing over the inner surface of the pack or its contents. Open the remaining two corners of the pack.	10*		
9. You now have a sterile drape as a sterile field from which to work and for the distribution of additional sterile supplies and instruments.	5		

10. Open a package containing sterile transfer forceps. Using sterile technique, handle the sterile forceps by the ring handle only. Always point the forceps tips down.	5*			
11. Grasp an item on the sterile field with the sterile forceps, points down, and move it to its proper position for the procedure, making sure not to cross the sterile field with the hand or contaminated end of the forceps.	5			
12. Set the forceps aside after one-time use.	5			
13. Check the label of the ordered solution when first obtaining the solution.	5			
14. Check the label of the solution for the second time. Place your hand over the label and lift the bottle.	5			
15. Lift the cover of the bottle straight up and then slightly to one side; hold the cover in your nondominant hand facing downward.	5			
16. If the container does not have a double cap, before pouring the solution into the sterile container, pour off a small amount of the solution into a waste receptacle.	10*			
17. Tilt the bottle up to stop the pouring while it is still over the bowl.	5			
18. Check the label of the solution for the third time. Working away from the sterile field, replace the cap (or caps). Be careful not to touch and therefore contaminate the internal surface of the lid.	5			
Total Points	100			

Comments

CAAHEP Competencies	Step(s)
III.P.6. Prepare a sterile field	Entire procedure
III.P.7. Perform within a sterile field	Entire procedure
ABHES Competencies	**Step(s)**
1.d. List the general responsibilities and skills of the medical assistant	Entire procedure

Procedure 25.5   Two-Person Sterile Tray Setup

Name _____ Date _____ Score _____

Task: Perform a sterile tray setup for a cyst removal.

Equipment and Supplies:
- Sterile drape
- Sterile gloves
- In a sealed autoclave pouch; needle holder, operating scissor, tissue forceps, hemostatic forceps
- Suture material with needle
- Sterile 4x4s
- Disposable scalpel

Directions: This procedure involves two people. One person will be act as the nonsterile person and the other will have on sterile gloves and will place the items on the sterile tray.

Standard: Complete the procedure and all critical steps in _____ minutes with a minimum score of 85% within two attempts (*or as indicated by the instructor*).

Scoring: Divide the points earned by the total possible points. Failure to perform a critical step, indicated by an asterisk (*), results in grade no higher than an 84% (*or as indicated by the instructor*).

Time: Began_____ Ended_____ Total minutes: _____

Steps – Nonsterile person	Point Value	Attempt 1	Attempt 2
1. Check that the Mayo stand or countertop is dust-free and clean. If it is not, disinfect and allow to air dry.	5		
2. Wash or sanitize your hands and make sure they are completely dry. If you will be assisting with a surgical procedure immediately after opening the sterile pack, perform the surgical hand scrub as explained in Procedure 25.2.	5		
3. Place the package containing the sterile drape on flat surface near Mayo stand/tray. Check the integrity of the outer package. Open package without touching barrier field.	5		
4. Pick up the sterile drape, by the corner, as you move away from table and allow it to unfold without touching anything else. Drape it over the Mayo stand without crossing over the sterile field.	10		
5. Inspect the sterile 4x4 package for holes and tears; if seen, discard and start over. Slowly pull sides of peel pack of sterile 4x4s away from each other. Maintain control of item inside the package by only opening far enough for sterile person to grab item. Allow the sterile person to take the 4x4s. Inspect and discard wrapper.	10*		
6. Inspect the peel pack of suture for holes and tears; if seen, discard and start over. Slowly pull sides of peel pack of suture away from each other. Maintain control of item inside the package by only opening far enough for sterile person to grab item. Allow the sterile person to take the suture package. Inspect and discard wrapper.	10*		

7.	Inspect the peel pack of scalpel for holes and tears; if seen, discard and start over. Slowly pull sides of peel pack of scalpel away from each other. Maintain control of item inside the package by only opening far enough for sterile person to grab item. Allow the sterile person to take the scalpel. Inspect and discard wrapper.	10*		
8.	Inspect the peel pack of instruments for holes and tears; if seen, discard and start over. Slowly pull sides of peel pack of the instruments away from each other. Maintain control of item inside the package by only opening far enough for sterile person to grab item. Allow the sterile person to take all of the instruments. Inspect and discard wrapper.	10*		
Steps – Sterile person				
9.	Wash or sanitize your hands and make sure they are completely dry. If you will be assisting with a surgical procedure immediately after opening the sterile pack, perform the surgical hand scrub as explained in Procedure 25.2.	5		
10.	Put on sterile gloves.	5		
11.	Remove items from peel pack and maintain sterile technique.	5		
12.	After nonsterile person has indicated that the peel pack has not been compromised, place item on sterile tray. Repeat for all items. Arrange items on sterile tray.	10		
13.	Maintain sterility of sterile field and sterile supplies.	10*		
	Total Points	100		

Comments

CAAHEP Competencies	Step(s)
III.P.6. Prepare a sterile field	Entire procedure
III.P.7. Perform within a sterile field	Entire procedure
ABHES Competencies	**Step(s)**
1.d. List the general responsibilities and skills of the medical assistant	Entire procedure

Procedure 25.6   Assist with Minor Surgery

Name _____ Date _____ Score _____

Tasks: To maintain the sterile field and pass instruments in a prescribed sequence during a surgical procedure that involves the making of a surgical incision and the removal of tissue.

Equipment and Supplies:
- Open patient drape pack on the side counter
- Mayo stand covered with a sterile drape
- Packaged sterile gloves (two pairs)
- Needle and syringe for local anesthetic medication
- Vial of local anesthetic medication
- Alcohol wipes
- Sterile drape
- Disposable scalpel with No. 15 blade
- Tissue forceps
- Skin retractor
- Three hemostats
- Needleholder
- Supply of sterile gauze sponges
- Biohazard waste container
- Sharps container
- Needle with suture material
- Specimen cup
- Laboratory requisitions
- Patient's health record

Standard: Complete the procedure and all critical steps in _____ minutes with a minimum score of 85% within two attempts (*or as indicated by the instructor*).

Scoring: Divide the points earned by the total possible points. Failure to perform a critical step, indicated by an asterisk (*), results in grade no higher than an 84% (*or as indicated by the instructor*).

Time: Began_____ Ended_____ Total minutes: _____

Steps:	Point Value	Attempt 1	Attempt 2
1. Prep the patient's skin with surgical soap and antiseptic solution as explained in Procedure 25.1. Explain the prep procedure to the patient.	3*		
2. Perform the surgical hand scrub as explained in Procedure 25.2.	2		
3. Instruct and prepare the patient for the procedure. Explain the following: what will occur, what the patient should do during the procedure, how long the procedure will take, and what the patient will sense (e.g., feel, smell, etc.).	2*		
4. Position the Mayo stand near the patient and the operative site, making sure the patient understands not to touch the sterile field.	3		
5. Put on sterile gloves using surgical technique as explained in Procedure 25.5.	2		
6. Put on sterile gloves using surgical technique. Grasp the patient drape by holding one edge or corner in each hand.	3		

7.	Drape the surgical site without touching any part of the patient or the operating area with your gloved hands.	5		
8.	If the provider requests medication, such as a local anesthetic, a second circulating assistant holds the vial of local anesthetic so that the provider can read the label and wipes to the top of the vial with the alcohol wipe. The provider withdraws the desired amount using sterile technique.	5		
9.	The provider injects the local anesthetic and waits a few minutes for it to take effect.	2		
10.	Position yourself across from the provider. Arrange the sterile field. Check the placement location on the Mayo stand.	5		
11.	Keep all sharp equipment conspicuously placed on the sterile field.	5		
12.	Pass the scalpel, blade down and handle first, to the provider, or the provider will reach for it. The provider will take the scalpel with the thumb and forefinger in the position ready for use.	5		
13.	Pick up a tissue forceps by the tips and pass it to the provider to grasp a piece of the tissue to be excised.	5		
14.	Dispose of soiled sponges in the biohazard waste container, being careful to keep your hands above your waist and to avoid touching any nonsterile items	5		
15.	Hold clean sponges in your hand to pat or sponge the wound as needed.	3		
16.	Safely position the specimen (if any) where it will not be disturbed in a sterile container on the sterile field.	5		
17.	If there is a bleeding vessel or if a hemostat is requested, pass the hemostat in the manner described in step 13.	5		
18.	Continue to sponge blood from the wound site.	2		
19.	Retract the wound edge, as needed, with a skin retractor.	5		
20.	Continue to monitor the sterile field and assist the provider as needed.	3		
21.	Pass the needle and suture material to close the wound and apply a sterile dressing as requested	5		
22.	Monitor the patient and provide assistance as needed. Provide any patient education required.	5		
23.	Clean up the room. Place sharps in the sharps disposal container and other biohazardous material in the biohazard waste container. Discard other waste in regular waste container. Disinfect the areas used.	5		
24.	Collect the specimen using Standard Precautions, place it in a labeled specimen cup, and send it to the laboratory with the proper requisitions.	5		
25.	Wash hands or use hand sanitizer. Document the procedure, wound condition, and patient education given in the patient's health record.	5		
	Total Points	100		

Documentation

Comments

CAAHEP Competencies	**Step(s)**
I.P.8. Instruct and prepare a patient for a procedure or a treatment.	1, 3
III.P.6. Prepare a sterile field	4
III.P.7. Perform within a sterile field	Entire procedure
III.P.8. Perform wound care	21
III.P.10.a. Demonstrate proper disposal of biohazardous material: sharps	23
III.P.10.b. Demonstrate proper disposal of biohazardous material: regulated wastes	14, 23
X.P.3. Document patient care accurately in the medical record	25
ABHES Competencies	**Step(s)**
1.d. List the general responsibilities and skills of the medical assistant	Entire procedure
9.c. Dispose of biohazardous materials	14, 23

Procedure 25.7   Apply a Sterile Dressing

Name _____ Date _____ Score _____

Tasks: Perform a dressing change; apply a sterile dressing while maintaining aseptic technique; instruct and prepare the patient for the procedure; explain the rationale for the procedure.

Equipment and Supplies:
- Gloves
- Biohazard waste container
- Sterile water or hydrogen peroxide (optional)
- Disposable ruler
- Culture swab
- Lab requisition, label, and plastic specimen bag for transport
- Sterile gloves
- Antiseptic swabs
- Sterile dressing and ABD pad
- Tape
- Mannequin with a wound
- Patient's record

Order: Change dressing and apply a sterile dressing. Culture wound drainage.

Scenario: Dr. Walden ordered a dressing change. You are to apply a sterile dressing after you obtain a culture of the wound drainage. As you are beginning the procedure, the patient asks you questions regarding PPE and the reason for the wound culture. You need to explain the rationale for wearing PPE and why a wound culture is obtained.

Directions: Role-play the scenario with a peer. The peer will be the patient and you are the medical assistant. After the role-play, the rest of the procedure is done on a mannequin.

Standard: Complete the procedure and all critical steps in _____ minutes with a minimum score of 85% within two attempts (*or as indicated by the instructor*).

Scoring: Divide the points earned by the total possible points. Failure to perform a critical step, indicated by an asterisk (*), results in grade no higher than an 84% (*or as indicated by the instructor*).

Time: Began_____ Ended_____ Total minutes: _____

Steps:	Point Value	Attempt 1	Attempt 2
1. Wash hands or use hand sanitizer. Assemble supplies on Mayo stand/tray and place biohazard waste container within easy reach.	2		
2. Greet the patient. Identify yourself. Verify the patient's identity with full name and date of birth. Verify the patient's allergies.	2		
3. Instruct and prepare the patient for the procedure. Explain the procedure to be performed in a manner that is understood by the patient. Explain the following: what will occur, what the patient should do during the procedure, how long the procedure will take, and what the patient will sense (e.g., feel, smell, etc.). Answer any questions the patient may have on the procedure.	3*		

Scenario update: The patient questions why you need to change gloves so much during the procedure. He also asks why the wound culture needs be done. 4. Based on the patient's questions, explain the reason for changing your gloves during the procedure and also for the wound culture. Demonstrate empathy and appropriate nonverbal communication when addressing the patient's questions and concerns.	5*		
Scenario update: The rest of the steps can be done on a mannequin. 5. Put on gloves. Loosen tape on old bandage from edges to the middle, towards the wound. Remove bandage and dressing, one at a time If dressing is stuck, use a small amount of sterile water or hydrogen peroxide to loosen.	3		
6. Check for drainage on the dressing and bandage. Note the color of the drainage. Measure any drainage using a disposable ruler, then discard everything in the biohazard waste container.	5*		
7. Assess the wound. If present, count the sutures or staples. Check if they are intact. Check the wound for signs of infection.	3*		
8. If the wound is open and/or redness or drainage is present: a. Culture the wound using a sterile swab (if ordered). Place in a culture transfer tube. Squeeze the tube to release formalin to preserve the specimen. b. Concisely and accurately report the relevant information (any issues with the wound or wound closures) to the provider. Ask the provider to check the wound before re-dressing.	5*		
9. Remove gloves and place in biohazard waste container.	5		
10. Wash hands or use hand sanitizer.	2		
11. Open and arrange sterile supplies in the order they will be used. Apply the principles of sterile technique.	5*		
12. Put on sterile gloves. State that the nondominant hand will be nonsterile and the dominant hand will be sterile.	5		
13. With the nondominant hand, pick up the antiseptic swab container. With the dominant hand, grasp an antiseptic swab without touching the package. Clean from center of wound to edge, use one roll of the swab and discard in waste container. Start with new swab where you left off with the previous swab. Continue until all the exudate is removed.	10*		
14. With the dominant hand, remove the sterile dressing without touching the package. Place the sterile dressing material over the wound and cover the wound completely.	10*		
15. With the dominant hand, place an ABD pad over the dressing as a bandage.	5		
16. Remove and discard the sterile gloves. Secure the bandage with tape.	5		
17. Provide patient education as needed for wound care.	5		
18. Complete the lab requisition for the culture. Put on gloves. Label the culture tube and place the culture tube in the plastic specimen bag for transport to the lab.	5		
19. Clean up the area. Discard all biohazardous waste in biohazard waste containers. Discard all other waste in the regular waste containers. Disinfect the tables.	3		

20. Remove gloves and dispose of them appropriately. Wash hands or use hand sanitizer.	2			
21. Using the patient's health record, document the following: wound appearance, number of intact sutures or staples (if present), the culture obtained, wound care performed, and the patient education provided.	10*			
Total Points	100			

Documentation

Comments

CAAHEP Competencies	Step(s)
I.P.8. Instruct and prepare a patient for a procedure or a treatment.	3
III.P.8. Perform wound care	Entire procedure
III.P.9. Perform dressing change	Entire procedure
III.P.10.b. Demonstrate proper disposal of biohazardous material: regulated wastes	6, 9, 19
X.P.3. Document patient care accurately in the medical record	21
ABHES Competencies	**Step(s)**
1.d. List the general responsibilities and skills of the medical assistant	Entire procedure
8.e. Perform specialty procedures, including but not limited to minor surgery, cardiac, respiratory, OB-GYN, neurological, and gastroenterology	Entire procedure
9.c. Dispose of biohazardous materials	6, 9, 19

Procedure 25.8 Removal of Sutures and/or Surgical Staples

Name _____ Date _____ Score _____

Task: To remove sutures and/or surgical staples from a healed incision using sterile technique and without injuring the closed wound.

Equipment and Supplies:

Sterile suture removal kit containing the following:
- Suture removal scissors
- Gauze
- Thumb dressing forceps
- Wound closure strips or adhesive bandage strips (e.g., Band-Aids)
- Skin antiseptic swabs (e.g., Betadine swabs)
- Surgical staple remover with 4×4-inch gauze
- Biohazard waste container
- Biohazard sharps container
- Gloves
- Sterile gloves
- Patient's health record

Standard: Complete the procedure and all critical steps in _____ minutes with a minimum score of 85% within two attempts (*or as indicated by the instructor*).

Scoring: Divide the points earned by the total possible points. Failure to perform a critical step, indicated by an asterisk (*), results in grade no higher than an 84% (*or as indicated by the instructor*).

Time: Began_____ Ended_____ Total minutes: _____

Steps:	Point Value	Attempt 1	Attempt 2
1. Wash hands or use hand sanitizer. Assemble the necessary supplies.	5		
2. Greet the patient. Identify yourself. Verify the patient's identity with full name and date of birth. Explain the procedure to be performed in a manner that is understood by the patient. Answer any questions the patient may have on the procedure. Instruct the person to lie or sit still during the procedure.	10*		
3. Position the patient comfortably and support the sutured area.	5		
4. Place dry towels under the site.	5		
5. Check the incision line to make sure the wound edges are approximated and there are no signs of infection such as inflammation, edema, or drainage.	5		
6. Put on gloves. Using antiseptic swabs, cleanse the wound to remove exudate and destroy microorganisms around the sutures or staples. Clean the site from the inside out, starting at the top of the wound and working your way down. Use a new swab if the step must be repeated. Remove gloves and discard.	10*		
7. Open the suture or staple removal pack while maintaining the sterility of the contents.	10*		

8. Place sterile gauze next to the wound site.	5		
9. Put on sterile gloves.	5		
10. Remove the sutures or staples.	5		
11. Remove the gauze holding the sutures or staples. Dispose of sutures in the biohazard waste container. Dispose of staples in the biohazard sharps container.	10*		
12. The provider may apply or may have you apply wound closure strips or an adhesive bandage strip for added support, strength, and protection.	5		
13. Instruct the patient to keep the wound edges clean and dry and not to place excessive strain on the area.	10		
14. Document the procedure, wound condition, number of sutures or staples removed, whether a dressing or bandage was applied, and the instructions on wound care given to the patient.	10		
Total Points	100		

Documentation

Comments

CAAHEP Competencies	Step(s)
I.P.8. Instruct and prepare a patient for a procedure or a treatment	2
III.P.10.a. Demonstrate proper disposal of biohazardous material: sharps	11
III.P.10.b. Demonstrate proper disposal of biohazardous material: regulated medical waste	11
X.P.3. Document patient care accurately in the medical record	14
ABHES Competencies	**Step(s)**
1.d. List the general responsibilities and skills of the medical assistant	Entire procedure

Principles of Electrocardiography

CAAHEP Competencies	Assessments
V.C.8.b. Identify the following related to body systems: abbreviations	Abbreviations – 1-19
I.P.2.a. Perform the following procedures: electrocardiography	Procedure 26.1
I.P.8. Instruct and prepare a patient for a procedure or a treatment	Procedures 26.1, 26.2
X.P.3. Document patient care accurately in the medical record	Procedures 26.1, 26.2
A.1. Demonstrate critical thinking skills	Procedure 26.1
A.3. Demonstrate empathy for patients' concerns	Procedure 26.1
ABHES Competencies	**Assessments**
8. Clinical Procedures d. Assist provider with specialty examination, including cardiac, respiratory, OB-GYN, neurological, and gastroenterology procedures	Procedures 26.1, 26.2
e. Perform specialty procedures, including but not limited to minor surgery, cardiac, respiratory, OB-GYN, neurological, and gastroenterology	Procedures 26.1, 26.2

VOCABULARY REVIEW

Using the word pool on the right, find the correct word to match the definition. Write the word on the line after the definition.

Group A

1. A complete heartbeat _____

2. Electricity is picked up by the electrodes and moves into this machine _____

3. A record or recording of electrical impulses of the heart as produced by an electrocardiograph _____

4. Adhesive patches that conduct electricity from the body to the ECG machine wires _____

5. The use of ultrasonic waves directed through the heart to study the structure and motion of the heart; the visual record produced is called an *echocardiogram* _____

6. During this phase, the heart is at rest and the atria fill with blood _____

7. A myocardial cell forms a strong connection to the next cells through these special junctions _____

8. During this phase, the heart is contracting _____

9. Pacemaker of the heart _____

10. A specialized internodal tract that takes the impulse to the left atria _____

Word Pool
- Bachmann's bundle
- cardiac cycle
- diastole
- echocardiography
- electrocardiogram
- electrocardiograph
- electrodes
- intercalated discs
- sinoatrial node
- systole

Group B

1. An electrically charged atom or the smallest component of an element _____

2. A substance, structure, or event that does not naturally occur in a situation _____

3. Having two poles or electrical charges _____

4. An abnormal heart rate or rhythm _____

5. Having one pole or electrical charge _____

6. A pocket-sized tool used for measuring the height and width of the ECG waves and intervals _____

WORD POOL
- arrhythmia
- artifact
- bipolar
- caliper
- ion
- unipolar

ABBREVIATIONS

Write out what each of the following abbreviations stands for.

1. ECG, EKG_____

2. AV _____

3. SL _____

4. O$_2$ _____

5. CO$_2$ _____

6. SA _____

7. ECHO _____

8. RA _____

9. LA _____

10. LL _____

11. RL _____

12. aV _____

13. UV _____

14. ICS _____

15. PACs _____

16. PVCs _____

17. V-tach _____

18. V-fib _____

19. ICD _____

SKILLS AND CONCEPTS

Answer the following questions.

A. Heart Structures

1. The _____ chambers receive blood from the body and the _____ chambers pump blood out to the body.

2. The _____ divides the right and left sides of the heart.

3. The _____ valve is found between the right atrium and the right ventricle.

4. The _____ valve is between the right ventricle and the pulmonary artery.

5. The _____, or mitral, valve is found between the left atrium and left ventricle.

6. The _____ valve is between the left ventricle and the aorta.

7. The right atrium receives deoxygenated blood from the _____, _____, and _____.

8. Blood empties from the right atrium into the _____.

9. When the ventricles contract, the deoxygenated blood in the right ventricle passes through the opened pulmonary valve and moves into the _____.

10. In the lungs, the blood picks up _____ and gives up _____.

11. The pulmonary vein brings the oxygenated blood back to the _____.

12. When the left atrial chamber contracts, the blood empties into the _____.

13. When the ventricles contract, the blood in the left ventricle moves through the opened aortic valve and into the _____.

14. The _____ bring the oxygenated blood to the heart muscles.

B. Heart's Conduction System

1. The _____ is called the "pacemaker of the heart."

2. The impulse also moves quickly across special bands of tissue called _____.

3. The _____, a specialized intermodal tract, takes the impulse to the left atrium.

4. When the impulse reaches the _____, it moves very slowly through the node.

5. When the impulse leaves the AV node, it moves to the _____.

6. The _____ brings the impulse to the ventricles.

7. The bundle branches split into many _____, which transmit the impulse quickly and efficiently to the ventricular cardiac cells.

Match the stages with the description.

8. _____ When the impulse hits the cell and electrical activity is seen on the ECG

9. _____ Resting state and no electrical activity is seen on the ECG

10. _____ Recovery stage and some electrical activity is seen on the ECG

a. polarization
b. depolarization
c. repolarization

C. ECG Tracing of the Cardiac Cycle
Match the term with the correct description.

1. _____ A period of time between two points or events

2. _____ A deflection from the baseline

3. _____ A form made up of many waves

4. _____ A part of a line between two points

5. _____ Any movement away from the baseline in the tracing

6. _____ A straight line that is also called the *baseline*

a. deflection
b. complex
c. interval
d. isoelectric line
e. segment
f. wave

Match the waves and segments with the correct description. Answers can be used more than once.

7. _____ First isoelectric line after the P wave

8. _____ Follows the last wave in the QRS complex and ends at the start of the T wave

9. _____ Represents ventricular repolarization

10. _____ Created from the electrical impulses moving through the atria

11. _____ Any downward deflection following the R wave and represents the final depolarization of the ventricular walls

12. _____ Follows the T wave but may not be seen

13. _____ Occurs as the impulse moves slowly through the AV node

14. _____ A negative deflection that represents interventricular septal depolarization

15. _____ Represents the repolarization of the Purkinje fibers

16. _____ Represents atrial depolarization

17. _____ Made up of several waves and represents ventricular depolarization and atrial repolarization

18. _____ An isoelectric line and the atrial chambers finish contracting during this time

19. _____ A large, triangular-shaped wave that reflects the depolarization of most of the ventricular walls

20. _____ An isoelectric line on the tracing and the ventricles finish contracting during this time

21. _____ Starts at the beginning of the P wave and ends at the start of the Q wave

22. _____ Time between the end of the atrial depolarization and the start of the ventricular depolarization

23. _____ Starts at the beginning of the Q wave and extends to the end of the T wave

a. P wave
b. PR segment
c. QRS complex
d. Q wave
e. R wave
f. S wave
g. ST segment
h. T wave
i. U wave
j. PR interval
k. QT interval

D. 12-Lead ECG

1. _____ electrodes and lead wires create _____ leads or pictures.

2. _____ or standard leads include leads I, II, and III.

3. The bipolar leads provide pictures of the _____ or _____ plane of the heart.

4. What electrodes and lead wires are used to create the bipolar leads?
   a. Left arm (LA)
   b. Right arm (RA)
   c. Left foot (LL)
   d. All of the above

Select the correct answer.

5. _____ If you see artifact on lead I, which two electrodes and lead wires should you look at?

6. _____ If you see artifact on lead III, which two electrodes and lead wires should you look at?

7. _____ If you see artifact on lead II, which two electrodes and lead wires should you look at?

a. RA and LL
b. RA and LA
c. RA and RL
d. LA and LL

Select the correct answer.

8. _____ If you see artifact on leads I and III, which electrode and lead wire should you look at?

10. _____ What electrodes and lead wire(s) are used to create the augmented leads?

11. _____ If you see artifact on lead aVR, which electrodes and lead wires should you look at?

a. RA
b. LA
c. LL
d. All of the above

Write your answers on the lines.

12. The augmented leads provide pictures of the _____ or _____ plane of the heart.

13. The chest leads provide pictures of the _____ plane of the heart.

14. If you see artifact on lead V_2, which electrode(s) and lead wire(s) should you look at? _____

E. ECG Supplies

1. The small boxes on the ECG paper measure _____ mm.

2. The large boxes on the ECG paper measure _____ mm.

3. When a provider analyzes the ECG tracing, what tool is used to measure the wave forms? _____

4. The vertical lines on an ECG tracing are used to measure the _____ or _____ of the waveform.

5. The horizontal lines measure the _____.

6. When the paper speed (chart speed) is set at 25 mm/second, each small box is _____ seconds and each large box equals _____ seconds.

7. The _____ on electrodes helps pick up the electrical impulses.

F. Electrocardiograph

Match the following settings with the correct descriptions. The answers can be used more than once.

1. _____ Increase this setting for very short waveforms
2. _____ Regulates the speed of the paper during the recording
3. _____ Increase this setting if the heart rate is very fast
4. _____ Default setting is 25 mm/s
5. _____ Default setting is 10 mm/mV
6. _____ Regulates the height (amplitude) of the tracing

a. chart speed
b. gain or sensitivity

Fill in the correct answer.

7. The ECG machine usually prints the _____, a calibration marking, either at the beginning or at the end of the tracing.

8. If the ECG machine is set at 10 mm/mV, the standardization mark will be an upward rectangle that is _____ small boxes tall.

9. If the gain is doubled, then the standardization mark will be _____ in size.

G. ECG Procedure

1. What techniques can be used to prepare the skin for the electrodes?
   a. Wipe the skin with an alcohol pad to remove lotion and sweat.
   b. Use a razor to shave chest hair.
   c. Gently abrade the skin using a gauze sponge or special fine sandpaper tape.
   d. All of the above.

Match the electrode with the correct placement.

2. _____ Placed just above the right wrist or upper arm indicated in the operator's manual.
3. _____ Fourth intercostal space at the left sternal edge.
4. _____ Same horizontal plane as V_4 at the midaxillary line
5. _____ Place on the inner lower right leg, just above the ankle.
6. _____ Midway between V_2 and V_4.
7. _____ Placed just above the left wrist or upper arm indicated in the operator's manual.
8. _____ Same horizontal plane as V_4 at the left anterior axillary line or the midpoint between V_4 and V_6.
9. _____ Place on the inner lower left leg, just above the ankle.
10. _____ Fourth intercostal space at the right sternal edge.
11. _____ Fifth intercostal space on the mid-clavicular line.

a. Right arm (RA)
b. Left arm (LA)
c. Right leg (RL)
d. Left leg (LL)
e. Chest V_1 (V_1)
f. Chest V_2 (V_2)
g. Chest V_3 (V_3)
h. Chest V_4 (V_4)
i. Chest V_5 (V_5)
j. Chest V_6 (V_6)

Match the condition with the placement of electrodes.

12. _____ Place chest electrodes on the right side of the chest using the same intercostal spacing and landmarks. Switch the right and left limb lead wires.

13. _____ Place electrode on the remaining part of the limb. Place the electrode on the opposite limb in the same location.

14. _____ Place the electrode above the covered area. Place the electrode on the opposite limb in the same location.

15. _____ Place the electrodes near the correct area, but not on the area.

a. new surgical incision or wound
b. casted limb
c. dextrocardia
d. amputated limb

H. Troubleshooting Artifact

Match the artifact with the correct description. Answers maybe used more than once.

1. _____ Appears as jagged peaks with irregular heights and spacing

2. _____ Caused by electrical interference

3. _____ Caused by an interruption in the electrical connection

4. _____ Caused by involuntary and voluntary movement

5. _____ The tracing looks normal at the beginning, but then it disappears or goes all over

6. _____ Upward and downward movement of the waveform and the isoelectric lines shift locations

7. _____ Appears as a series of small spikes that creates a thick-looking tracing

8. _____ Caused by breathing, poor skin preparation, old electrodes, and the placement of electrodes

a. wandering baseline artifact
b. somatic tremor artifact
c. AC interference artifact
d. interrupted baseline artifact

Match the artifact with the corrective action to take. Answers maybe used more than once.

9. _____ Clean the skin with alcohol and replace the electrodes with new ones.

10. _____ Make sure the muscle-tremor filter is on, if present.

11. _____ Check that all electrodes and lead wires are attached and replace any broken wires.

12. _____ Ensure cell phones are not near the procedure area.

13. _____ Make sure the baseline filter is turned on.

14. _____ Remind the patient not to talk during the procedure.

15. _____ Unplug the ECG machine or any nearby electrical devices.

a. wandering baseline artifact
b. somatic tremor artifact
c. AC interference artifact
d. interrupted baseline artifact

I. Evaluating an ECG Tracing

1. Using the 6-second method, what is the heart rate if 11 P waves appear in a 6-second strip? _____

Match the rhythm with the description.

2. _____ A flat line appears on the tracing and there is an absence of a heartbeat.

3. _____ Normal finding in well-conditioned athletes.

4. _____ Occurs when the ventricles quiver uncontrollably and they are essentially ineffective at pumping any blood.

5. _____ Occurs when the atria contract faster than the ventricles (up to 300 beats per minute) and they become out of sync with the ventricles.

6. _____ Occurs when the ventricles beat at a rapid rate (up to 250 beats per minute).

7. _____ A normal rhythm.

8. _____ Occur when the ventricles contract sooner than they should. The QRS complex appears before a P wave.

9. _____ Occurs when there is a disruption or slowing of the electrical impulse through the heart; three degrees of this arrhythmia.

10. _____ Occur when the atria contract sooner than they should. The P wave can be abnormally shaped, or an extra P wave can be seen.

a. sinus rhythm
b. sinus bradycardia
c. premature atrial contractions
d. atrial flutter
e. heart block
f. premature ventricular contractions
g. ventricular tachycardia
h. ventricular fibrillation
i. asystole

J. Stress Testing

1. A(n) _____ records the ECG while the patient is exercising.

2. Which of the following is included in the coaching instructions for an exercise stress test?
   a. The patient should wear clothes and shoes for exercising.
   b. The provider will indicate what daily medications should be taken prior to the test.
   c. Stop taking all medications prior to the test.
   d. Only a and b.

3. Which of the following is included in the coaching instructions for an exercise stress test?
   a. The patient should not take a dose of Viagra, Cialis, or Levitra for erectile dysfunction 48 hours before a stress test.
   b. The patient should not smoke or consume caffeine or alcohol 3 hours before the test.
   c. The patient signs a consent form prior to the test.
   d. All of the above.

4. A(n) _____ shows the blood flow into the heart muscle during rest and activity.

K. Remote ECG Monitoring

Match the types of remote ECG monitoring with the correct description.

1. _____ Small device that records the ECG when activated by the patient. The data is sent via phone to the base station.

2. _____ Surgically placed under the skin and catches infrequent arrhythmias missed by other traditional ECG monitoring.

3. _____ Used to monitor the heart over a 24- to 48-hour period while patients go about their normal activities.

4. _____ The recorder is activated by the patient when symptoms occur, and it records the ECG.

a. Holter monitor
b. implantable loop recorder
c. cardiac event recorder
d. transtelephonic monitoring

CERTIFICATION PREPARATION

Circle the correct answer.

1. _____ is a deflection from the baseline.
   a. Interval
   b. Segment
   c. Complex
   d. Wave

2. What ECG wave or segment reflects atrial depolarization?
   a. P wave
   b. Q wave
   c. R and S waves
   d. T wave

3. What ECG wave or segment is a negative deflection and represents interventricular septal depolarization?
   a. P wave
   b. Q wave
   c. R and S waves
   d. T wave

4. What ECG wave or segment represents ventricular repolarization?
   a. P wave
   b. Q wave
   c. R and S waves
   d. T wave

5. _____ is signal distortion or unwanted, erratic movement of the stylus caused by outside interference.
   a. Interval
   b. Deflection
   c. Artifact
   d. Caliper

6. If AC interference artifact appears, what should the medical assistant do?
   a. Check to see if the electrodes and lead wires are attached.
   b. Turn on the muscle-tremor filter.
   c. Help the patient relax.
   d. Separate the lead wires so they do not overlap.

7. _____ is when the ventricles quiver uncontrollably. The patient has no pulse, and is not breathing.
   a. Ventricular fibrillation
   b. Third-degree heart block
   c. Ventricular tachycardia
   d. Atrial flutter

8. _____ results in the absence of a heartbeat.
   a. Ventricular fibrillation
   b. Asystole
   c. Ventricular tachycardia
   d. Premature ventricular contractions

9. Which test involves radioactive substance injected into a vein and a gamma camera used to take images of the blood flow; shows the blood flow into the heart muscle during rest and activity?
   a. Exercise stress test
   b. Implantable loop recorder
   c. Nuclear stress test
   d. Transtelephonic monitor

10. Which device is surgically implanted under the skin in the upper chest and continuously records the ECG for 2-3 years?
    a. Holter monitor
    b. Cardiac event recorder
    c. Transtelephonic monitoring
    d. Implantable loop recorder

WORKPLACE APPLICATIONS

1. Renee is performing an ECG on a patient. How might she prep the patient's skin so the electrodes will adhere?

   _____

   _____

   _____

2. Renee is performing an ECG on a patient. She notices that lead I has upward and downward movement of the waveform. What is occurring and how should she correct the problem?

   _____

   _____

   _____

3. Renee is performing an ECG on a patient. She notices many of the leads have jagged peaks with irregular heights and spacing. What is occurring and how should she correct the problem?

   _____

   _____

   _____

INTERNET ACTIVITIES

1. Using appropriate online resources, research a cardiac test discussed in the "Additional ECG Testing" section. Create a poster, PowerPoint presentation, or a paper and include at least two citations. Discuss the following topics:
   a. Description of the test
   b. Patient education and preparation

2. Using online resources, create an ECG brochure for patients. Include the following in the brochure:
   a. Purpose of the test
   b. Description of the test
   c. Patient instructions

3. Using online resources, research an abnormal rhythm mentioned in the chapter. Identify reasons for the rhythm and possible treatments. In a paper, PowerPoint presentation, or poster, summarize your research and cite your resources.

Procedure 26.1   Perform Electrocardiography

Name _____   Date _____   Score _____

Tasks: Perform electrocardiography. Document the procedure in the patient's health record. Show empathy regarding the patient's concerns and incorporate critical thinking skills when performing patient care.

Equipment and Supplies:
- ECG machine
- Disposable electrodes
- ECG paper
- Alcohol pads
- Razor (optional)
- Gauze pads (optional)
- Patient gown or paper cape
- Tissue
- Disinfecting wipes
- Gloves
- Waste container
- Patient's health record

Standard: Complete the procedure and all critical steps in _____ minutes with a minimum score of 85% within two attempts (*or as indicated by the instructor*).

Scoring: Divide the points earned by the total possible points. Failure to perform a critical step, indicated by an asterisk (*), results in grade no higher than an 84% (*or as indicated by the instructor*).

Time: Began_____ Ended_____ Total minutes: _____

Steps:	Point Value	Attempt 1	Attempt 2
1. Wash hands or use hand sanitizer.	2		
2. Assemble equipment and supplies needed for the ECG procedure. Plug in and turn on the ECG machine. Verify that the standardization and chart/paper speed are correct.	3		
3. Greet the patient. Identify yourself. Verify the patient's identity with full name and date of birth. Make sure the patient's information matches the order and the record. Explain the procedure in a manner that the patient understands. Answer any questions the patient may have about the procedure.	5*		
Scenario update: The patient states that she is really worried that something is wrong with her heart. She states that she is really nervous about having an ECG. 4. Demonstrate empathy by listening to the patient and learning about their experiences and concerns. Use therapeutic communication techniques and positive nonverbal behaviors, including appropriate eye contact. Position yourself at the same level as the patient. Show your support and respect. *(Refer to the Affective Behaviors Checklist – Empathy and the Grading Rubric)*	5*		

5.	Ask the patient to remove all clothing from the waist up, including undergarments, and put on the gown/cape so that the opening is in the front. Ask the patient if assistance is needed. If so, provide help. If not, leave the room and allow the patient time to change. When reentering the room, provide a courtesy knock on the door.	**2**		
6.	Assist the patient into a comfortable supine position on the exam table. Provide support for the legs and arms.	**3**		
7.	Identify the locations for the ECG electrodes on the chest. Prepare the skin. If the patient has a hairy chest, get the person's permission prior to shaving the areas (optional). Wipe each spot with alcohol and allow it to dry. Fold the gauze pad over your index finger and briskly rub the site to abrade the skin (optional).	**5***		
8.	Correctly apply the six chest electrodes. If using tab electrodes, tabs should be pointed towards the waist.	**10**		
9.	Identify the locations for the ECG electrodes on the extremities. Refer to the users' guide for arm electrode position if needed. Wipe each spot with alcohol and allow it to dry. Correctly apply the four limb electrodes to nonbony areas. If using tab electrodes, the lower leg tabs should point toward the waist. The arm/wrist tabs should be pointed toward the fingers.	**10**		
10.	Attach the correct lead wire to each of the electrodes. The wires should follow the natural contour of the body and not overlap.	**10***		
11.	Enter the patient's data into the ECG machine. Identify any changes with the default settings, electrode position, or patient's position.	**3**		
12.	Double-check that the lead wires are in the correct position and attached to the electrodes. Make sure each electrode is attached to the skin. Take any corrective action necessary.	**5***		
13.	Instruct the patient to lie still and not to talk during the tracing. Tell the patient how long the tracing will take.	**5**		
14.	Verify that the filter(s) are on. Check the leads on the screen or monitor. Based on what you observe, use critical thinking skills, and take any corrective action necessary. Run the tracing when the leads look clear and without artifact. *(Refer to the Affective Behaviors Checklist – Critical Thinking and the Grading Rubric)*	**5***		
15.	Check the tracing for clarity, artifact, and abnormal life-threatening rhythms. Based on what you observe, use critical thinking skills, and take any corrective action necessary. *(Refer to the Affective Behaviors Checklist – Critical Thinking and the Grading Rubric)*	**5***		
16.	Disconnect the lead wires and remove the electrodes. Wipe any reside from the patient's skin. Wash your hands or use hand sanitizer. Instruct the patient to get dressed. Ask the patient if assistance is needed. If so, help the patient to dress.	**5**		
17.	Provide the patient with information about following up with the provider. Complete any necessary actions with the ECG (e.g., upload to the electronic health record, mount, and route to the provider).	**2**		
18.	Document accurately in the patient's health record. Indicate the name of the provider ordering the test, what test was performed, how the patient tolerated the test, and what you did with the ECG tracing. You can also add any instructions you provided to the patient regarding follow-up.	**5**		

Scenario update: Perform routine machine maintenance by adding paper to ECG machine or printer. 19. Review the operator's manual on how to change the paper. Gather the new ream of ECG paper (or roll).	5*		
20. Open the machine. Remove the remaining paper and add the new paper per the steps in the manual.	2		
21. Apply gloves and disinfect the lead wires per the operator's manual. Disinfect the exam table. Clean up the work area. Remove the gloves. Wash your hands or use hand sanitizer.	3		
Total Points	100		

Checklist for Affective Behaviors

Affective Behavior	*Directions:* Check behaviors observed during the role-play.					
Critical Thinking	**Negative, Unprofessional Behaviors**	**Attempt**		**Positive, Professional Behaviors**	**Attempt**	
		1	2		1	2
	Coached or told of an issue or problem			Independently identified the problem or issue		
	Failed to ask relevant questions related to the condition			Asked appropriate questions to obtain the information required		
	Failed to consider alternatives; failed to ask questions that demonstrate understanding of principles/concepts			Willing to consider other alternatives; asked appropriate questions that showed understanding of principles/concepts		
	Failed to make an educated, logical judgment/decision			Made an educated, logical judgment/decision based on the protocol		
	Actions or lack of actions demonstrated unsafe practices and/or did not follow the protocol			Took appropriate actions based on observations; actions reflected principles of safe practice		
	Other:			Other:		

Empathy	Did not listen to patient's responses			Listened to patient; learned about patient		
	Lack of respect and support demonstrated			Showed respect and support		
	Lack of therapeutic communication techniques used			Used therapeutic communication techniques		
	Negative nonverbal behaviors (e.g., positioning, frowning, poor eye contact)			Positive nonverbal behaviors (e.g., at the same level as patient, smiled, good eye contact)		
	Other:			Other:		

Grading Rubric for the Affective Behaviors Checklist **Directions:** *Based on checklist results, identify the points received for the procedure checklist. Indicate how the behaviors demonstrated met the expectations.*		**Point Value**	**Attempt 1**	**Attempt 2**
Does not meet Expectation	• Response lacked empathy and/or critical thinking skills. • Student demonstrated more than 2 negative, unprofessional behaviors during the interaction.	0		
Needs Improvement	• Response lacked empathy and/or critical thinking skills. • Student demonstrated 1 or 2 negative, unprofessional behaviors during the interaction.	0		
Meets Expectation	• Response demonstrated empathy or critical thinking; no negative, unprofessional behaviors observed. • More practice is needed for behavior to appear natural and for student to appear comfortable and at ease.	5		
Occasionally Exceeds Expectation	• Response demonstrated empathy or critical thinking; no negative, unprofessional behaviors observed. • At times student appeared comfortable and at ease; but more practice is needed for behavior to become natural and consistent with a professional medical assistant.	5		
Always Exceeds Expectation	• Response demonstrated empathy or critical thinking; no negative, unprofessional behaviors observed. • Student's behaviors appeared natural and comfortable. Behaviors are consistent with a professional medical assistant.	5		

Documentation

Comments

CAAHEP Competencies	Step(s)
I.P.2.a. Perform: the following procedures: electrocardiography	1-18
I.P.8. Instruct and prepare a patient for a procedure or a treatment	3, 13
X.P.3. Document patient care accurately in the medical record	18
A.1. Demonstrate critical thinking skills	14, 15
A.3. Demonstrate empathy for patients' concerns	4
ABHES Competencies	**Step(s)**
8.d. Assist provider with specialty examination, including cardiac, respiratory, OB-GYN, neurological, and gastroenterology procedures	Entire procedure
8.e. Perform specialty procedures, including but not limited to minor surgery, cardiac, respiratory, OB-GYN, neurological, and gastroenterology	Entire procedure

Procedure 26.2   Apply a Holter Monitor

Name _____   Date _____   Score _____

Tasks: Apply a Holter monitor and coach a patient on the procedure. Document the procedure in the patient's health record

Equipment and Supplies:
- Holter monitor, new batteries, flash memory card (if required), carrying case, and operator's manual
- Disposable electrodes
- Razor (optional)
- Sharps container
- Alcohol pads
- Gauze pads (optional)
- Cloth nonallergenic tape (optional)
- Journal
- Waste container
- Patient's health record

Standard: Complete the procedure and all critical steps in _____ minutes with a minimum score of 85% within two attempts (*or as indicated by the instructor*).

Scoring: Divide the points earned by the total possible points. Failure to perform a critical step, indicated by an asterisk (*), results in grade no higher than an 84% (*or as indicated by the instructor*).

Time: Began_____ Ended_____ Total minutes: _____

Steps:	Point Value	Attempt 1	Attempt 2
1. Wash hands or use hand sanitizer.	5		
2. Assemble equipment and supplies needed for the procedure. Insert flash memory card if required. Insert new batteries into the monitor. Consult the operator's manual for the required amount and placement of electrodes.	5		
3. Greet the patient. Identify yourself. Verify the patient's identity with full name and date of birth. Explain the procedure to be performed in a manner that is understood by the patient. Answer any questions the patient may have on the procedure.	10		
4. Ask the patient to remove clothing from the waist up and to sit at the end of the exam table. Ask the patient if assistance is needed. If so, help. If not, leave the room and allow the patient time to change. When reentering the room, provide a courtesy knock on the door.	5		
5. Identify the locations for the electrodes and prepare the skin for the electrodes. Shave the area if the patient has a hairy chest. Wipe the area with the alcohol pad and allow it to dry. Fold the gauze pad over your index finger and briskly rub the site to abrade the skin.	10		
6. Snap the lead wire onto the electrode. Apply the electrodes to the sites as indicated by the manufacturer. Press firmly and make sure the entire electrode adheres completely to the skin.	10		
7. Loop and tape down the wires on the chest.	5		

8.	Attach the patient cable to the monitor if required. Turn on the recorder and set as indicated by the manufacturer. Enter the patient data as indicated.	**10**		
9.	Have the patient get dressed. Assist as needed.	**10**		
10.	Coach the patient regarding making journal entries while wearing the monitor. Provide the required patient education.	**10**		
11.	Assist the patient in scheduling a return appointment in 24 hours. Provide the patient with contact information should a question arise.	**10**		
12.	Document accurately in the patient's health record. Indicate the provider ordering the test, the procedure done, patient education provided, and return appointment.	**10**		
	Total Points	**100**		

Documentation

Comments

CAAHEP Competencies	Step(s)
I.P.8. Instruct and prepare a patient for a procedure or a treatment	3, 10
X.P.3. Document patient care accurately in the medical record	12
ABHES Competencies	**Step(s)**
8.d. Assist provider with specialty examination, including cardiac, respiratory, OB-GYN, neurological, and gastroenterology procedures	Entire procedure
8.e. Perform specialty procedures, including but not limited to minor surgery, cardiac, respiratory, OB-GYN, neurological, and gastroenterology	Entire procedure

Medical Emergencies

CAAHEP Competencies	Assessment
I.C.10.a. Identify the classification of medication, including: indication for use	Skills and Concepts – C. 9-18; Internet Activity – 3
I.C.10.b. Identify the classification of medication, including: desired effect	Skills and Concepts – C. 9-18; Internet Activity – 3
I.C.10.c. Identify the classification of medication, including: side effects	Internet Activity – 3
I.C.10.d. Identify the classification of medication, including: adverse reaction	Internet Activity – 3
I.C.12. Identify basic principles of first aid	Skills and Concepts – D. 2, 7, E. 7, 9-10, F. 8, G. 1-3, H. 6, 12, J. 2
XII.C.2.d. Identify safety techniques that can be used in responding to accidental exposure to: chemicals	Skills and Concepts – E. 10
I.P.13.a. Perform first aid procedures for: bleeding	Procedure 27.5
I.P.13.b. Perform first aid procedures for: diabetic coma or insulin shock	Procedure 27.1
I.P.13.c. Perform first aid procedures for: stroke	Procedure 27.3
I.P.13.d. Perform first aid procedures for: seizures	Procedure 27.3
I.P.13.e. Perform first aid procedures for: environmental emergency	Procedure 27.1
I.P.13.f. Perform first aid procedures for: syncope	Procedure 27.5
X.P.3. Document patient care accurately in the medical record	Procedures 27.1 through 27.6
A.1. Demonstrate critical thinking skills	Procedure 27.2
ABHES Competencies	Assessment
8. Clinical Procedures g. Recognize and respond to medical office emergencies	Procedures 27.1 through 27.7

VOCABULARY REVIEW

Using the word pool on the right, find the correct word to match the definition. Write the word on the line after the definition.

1. A self-refilling bag-valve-mask unit used for artificial respiration that is effective for ventilating and oxygenating intubated patients

   _____

2. Open _____

3. A term used in healthcare settings to indicate an emergency situation and summon the trained team to the scene

   _____

4. Route for delivery of fluids and medications through a needle inserted into the marrow of certain bones

   _____

5. A patient without an appointment _____

6. Tissue death _____

7. Contraction of the muscles causing the narrowing of the inside tube of the vessel _____

8. The application of manual chest compressions and ventilations to patients who are not breathing or do not have a pulse

   _____

9. Itching _____

10. A position on the person's side that helps to keep the airway open and clear _____

Word Pool
- Ambu bag
- cardiopulmonary resuscitation (CPR)
- code
- intraosseous
- necrosis
- patent
- pruritus
- recovery position
- vasoconstriction
- walk-in patient

ABBREVIATIONS

Write out what each of the following abbreviations stands for.

1. CPR _____

2. ET _____

3. LPN _____

4. RN _____

5. IV _____

6. AED _____

7. PPE _____

8. %TBSA _____

9. IM _____

10. RICE _____

11. CVA _____

12. ED _____

13. MI _____

14. EAP _____

15. POTS _____

SKILLS AND CONCEPTS
Answer the following questions.

A. Emergencies In Healthcare Settings
Fill in the blank.

1. The medical assistant must follow the facility's _____ and they cannot assess the patient or give advice.

2. To sort out and classify the injured is called _____.

3. A written flow map to make triage decisions is called a(n) _____.

B. Roles and Documentation in Code Situations
Fill in the blank or select the correct answer.

1. A number of emergency procedures needed to ensure a person's immediate survival is called _____.

2. What procedures are included with basic life support?
   a. Cardiopulmonary resuscitation
   b. Controlling bleeding
   c. Treatment of shock and poisoning
   d. Stabilization of injuries and basic first aid
   e. All of the above

3. Which of the following activities can the medical assistant do in a code situation?
   a. Order treatments and procedures.
   b. Perform CPR and assist with treatments and procedures.
   c. Call 911 when the provider indicates it is needed.
   d. All of the above.
   e. Both b and c.

4. The documentation during a code will provide evidence that the _____ was met in the treatments given to the patient.

C. Emergency Equipment and Supplies
Fill in the blank or select the correct answer.

1. A(n) _____ is a rolling supply cart that contains emergency equipment.

2. The crash cart should be checked _____ by the supervisor or by two qualified employees.

3. Life-saving maneuver to resuscitate a person who has stopped breathing is called _____.

4. A device used to deliver a rescue breath is called a(n) _____.

5. A soft flexible tube that is inserted in the nose and provides a patent airway is called a(n)

    _____.

6. A catheter that is inserted into the trachea through the mouth and provides a patent airway is called a(n)

    _____.

7. What equipment and supplies are needed when a provider performs an endotracheal tube intubation?
    a. Laryngoscope with either a curved (MacIntosh) or straight (Miller) blade
    b. ET tube in the appropriate size and stylet
    c. Ambu-bag
    d. Stethoscope
    e. All of the above

8. A(n) _____ is a device that delivers an electrical shock to the heart muscle in an attempt to restore a normal heartbeat.

Match the desired effect and indication for use with the correct medication.

9. _____ Increases the stimulation of the heart muscle and is used to treat hypotension and heart failure.

10. _____ Blocks or reverses the opioid medication effects and is used for opioid overdose.

11. _____ An antihistamine that reduces the effects of histamine and is used to treat allergic reactions.

12. _____ Hormone that stimulates the liver to release glucose into the blood and is used to treat hypoglycemia.

13. _____ Increases the heart rate and is used to treat bradycardia.

14. _____ Increases the stimulation of the heart muscle and is also a vasoconstrictor and bronchial relaxant; used to treat anaphylaxis, cardiac arrest, severe asthma, and bronchospasms.

15. _____ A vasodilator that is used for congestive heart failure and angina.

16. _____ Slows the heart rate and allows blood to fill the ventricular chambers; treats ventricular tachycardia and ventricular fibrillation.

17. _____ Affects the chemicals in the brain and is used to treat seizures and agitation.

18. _____ Helps restore the regular heart rhythm and is used to treat ventricular arrhythmias.

a. amiodarone
b. atropine
c. diazepam
d. diphenhydramine
e. dopamine
f. epinephrine
g. glucagon
h. lidocaine
i. naloxone
j. nitroglycerin

D. Temperature-Related Emergencies
Fill in the blank or select the correct answer.

1. _____ is caused by exposure to cold temperatures and the person may experience a pins-and-needles sensation followed by numbness in the affected area.

2. What is *not* a first aid procedure for frostbite?
   a. Move the person to a warmer location.
   b. Remove all wet clothing and cover with warm dry clothing.
   c. Observe for signs of hypothermia.
   d. Give the person alcohol to warm them quickly.

3. Which is *not* a sign or symptom of hypothermia?
   a. The core body temperature drops below 96° F
   b. Weak pulse, and slow, shallow breathing
   c. Clumsiness and slurred speech
   d. Drowsiness, confusion, and a loss of consciousness

4. Which of the following is *not* a risk factor for heat injuries?
   a. Dehydration, heart disease, and poor blood circulation
   b. Fever and sunburn
   c. Middle-aged and older adults
   d. Using alcohol and taking antidepressants, anticonvulsants, antipsychotics, and diuretics

5. _____ is a mild heat-related illness that causes muscle pain and spasms in the abdomen, arms, and legs due to electrolyte imbalance.

6. Which is *not* a sign or symptom of heat exhaustion?
   a. Heavy sweating, muscle cramps, nausea, and vomiting
   b. Red, hot, dry skin
   c. Fast, weak pulse and fast, shallow respirations
   d. Tiredness, weakness, dizziness, headache, and fainting

7. Which is *not* a first aid procedure for heat stroke?
   a. Move the person to a shady or air-conditioned area.
   b. Spray or sponge down the person with cool water.
   c. Drink cool sports beverages.
   d. Seek medical attention immediately.

E. Other Environmental Emergencies
Match the description with the type of burn. Answers can be used more than once.

1. _____ Damage to the epidermis and part of the dermis; also called *partial-thickness burn*.

2. _____ Damage to the epidermis, dermis, and subcutaneous tissue; also called *full-thickness burn*.

3. _____ Damage to the epidermis; also called *superficial burn*.

4. _____ Burned area is red and tender; no scar development occurs.

5. _____ Burned area is not painful. Skin appears deep red, pale gray, brown, or black; scar formation is likely.

6. _____ Burned area is red and painful. Blisters may occur and a scar may develop.

a. first-degree burn
b. second-degree burn
c. third-degree burn

Fill in the blank or select the correct answer.

7. For minor burns, seek immediate medical attention and do not remove burned clothing stuck to the skin. For minor burns, soak area in ice water for at least 5 minutes.
   a. Both sentences are correct.
   b. Both sentences are incorrect.
   c. The first sentence is correct, and the second sentence is incorrect.
   d. The first sentence is incorrect, and the second sentence is correct.

8. Which is a sign or symptoms of poisonings?
   a. Bluish lips, cough, and difficulty breathing
   b. Heart palpitations and chest pain
   c. Nausea, vomiting, and abdominal pain
   d. Numbness, tingling, dizziness, weakness, double vision, drowsiness, irritability, and headache
   e. All of the above

9. First aid for poisonings includes checking and monitoring the person's airway, breathing, and pulse. First aid for poisoning also includes ensuring the person vomits the substance.
   a. Both sentences are correct.
   b. Both sentences are incorrect.
   c. The first sentence is correct, and the second sentence is incorrect.
   d. The first sentence is incorrect, and the second sentence is correct.

10. First aid for chemical exposure includes
    a. if the chemical is on the person's clothing, the clothing should be removed.
    b. if the chemical is airborne, bring the person to fresh air.
    c. for chemical exposures of the eye, flush the eye with cool water for 15 minutes while protecting the other eye from an accidental exposure.
    d. all of the above.

11. _____ is a severe allergic reaction that can be life-threatening.

12. Epinephrine administered IM into the _____ absorbs quicker than other sites.

13. A(n) _____ vaccine booster maybe updated after a dirty or deep animal bite or a foreign body in the eye.

14. First aid for a foreign body in the eye is _____.

F. Diabetic Emergencies
Fill in the blank or select the correct answer.

1. _____ is severe hyperglycemia.

2. What causes hyperglycemia?
   a. Took too little insulin
   b. Ate too many carbohydrates
   c. Illness, trauma, or surgery
   d. Using an illegal drug
   e. All of the above

3. Signs and symptoms of hyperglycemia include
    a. very dry mouth, thirst, and frequent urination.
    b. nausea, vomiting, hunger, and stomach pain.
    c. fatigue, rapid pulse, and shortness of breath.
    d. all of the above.

4. IV fluids and insulin are used to treat _____.

5. Severe hypoglycemia is called _____.

6. What causes hypoglycemia?
    a. Took too little of insulin
    b. Ate too few carbohydrates
    c. Drank alcohol
    d. All of the above
    e. Both a and c

7. Signs and symptoms of hypoglycemia include
    a. double or blurry vision.
    b. fast pulse, palpitations.
    c. irritable, aggressive, nervous, headache, and unclear thinking.
    d. shaking, tired, hunger, sweaty, and cold skin.
    e. all of the above.

8. What is used to treat hypoglycemia?
    a. 6 ounces of fruit juice or regular soda
    b. 3 glucose tablets
    c. All of the above

G. Musculoskeletal Emergencies
Fill in the blank or select the correct answer.

1. Which is a first aid step for musculoskeletal emergencies?
    a. Elevate the legs of a person going into shock.
    b. Apply pressure to a bleeding wound with a clean cloth or sterile bandage.
    c. Immobilize the injured area.
    d. All of the above

2. To reduce or limit swelling, apply a(n) _____ to the area.

3. Splint the body part in the position it is in and do not attempt to readjust the area or straighten it. Check the injured area for swelling, paleness, or numbness, which may indicate the ties are too tight.
    a. Both sentences are correct.
    b. Both sentences are incorrect.
    c. The first sentence is correct, and the second sentence is incorrect.
    d. The first sentence is incorrect, and the second sentence is correct.

H. Neurologic Emergencies
Fill in the blank or select the correct answer.

1. _____ is a false sensation that you or your environment is spinning or moving.

2. A(n) _____ is a traumatic brain injury caused by a blow to the head.

3. Signs and symptoms of a concussion include
   a. headache and temporary loss of consciousness right after the incident.
   b. confusion, amnesia, disorientation, irritability, and personality changes.
   c. nausea and vomiting.
   d. listlessness, tiredness, and concentration and memory problems.
   e. all of the above.

4. A(n) _____ is a sudden increase of electrical activity in one or more parts of the brain and _____ is a disorder that causes recurring seizures.

5. It is a medical emergency if the seizure lasts longer than _____ minutes or if a person has multiple seizures without becoming conscious between them.

6. What is the first aid for seizures?
   a. Place the person in the recovery position.
   b. Note the time the seizure began.
   c. Monitor the person's breathing and pulse.
   d. Protect the patient from harm.
   e. All of the above.

Match the description with the correct type of stroke.

7. _____ Occurs when an artery in the brain leaks or ruptures.

8. _____ A blood clot forms in an artery, blocking the blood flow to part of the brain.

9. _____ A blood clot or other debris forms elsewhere in the body and moves into the brain arteries, blocking the blood flow.

10. _____ Occurs when the arterial blood flow to part of the brain is blocked.

a. ischemic stroke
b. thrombotic stroke
c. embolic stroke
d. hemorrhagic stroke

Fill in the blank or select the correct answer.

11. Which are signs or symptoms of a stroke?
    a. Confusion, sudden severe headache, and speech problems
    b. Numbness of the face, arm, or leg
    c. Facial drooping or visual changes
    d. Trouble walking and lack of coordination or balance
    e. All of the above

12. First aid for stroke-type symptoms involves getting help (calling 911) immediately. There is a small window of time during which clot-dissolving medications can be given to help the body break down the clot that is blocking the artery.
    a. Both sentences are correct.
    b. Both sentences are incorrect.
    c. The first sentence is correct, and the second sentence is incorrect.
    d. The first sentence is incorrect, and the second sentence is correct.

I. Respiratory Emergencies
Fill in the blank or select the correct answer.

1. _____, or over-breathing, is rapid and deep breathing.

2. Wheezing, breathlessness, chest tightness, and coughing are signs and symptoms of _____.

3. _____ inhalers, such as albuterol, will lessen an asthma attack within minutes.

4. Which is a sign of a total airway obstruction?
   a. Labored, noisy, or gasping breathing
   b. Stating they are choking
   c. Bluish skin color
   d. All of the above
   e. Both a and c

J. Cardiovascular Emergencies
Fill in the blank or select the correct answer.

1. _____ means fainting, passing out, or having a temporary loss of consciousness.

2. Which is a first aid step for bleeding?
   a. Lower the bleeding extremity below the heart level.
   b. Hold direct pressure over the site and remove the initial gauze every 5 minutes to check the bleeding.
   c. All of the above.
   d. None of the above.

Match the description with the correct type of shock.

3. _____ Caused by a severe allergic reaction; blood pressure drops and the airway narrows.

4. _____ Due to a central nervous system injury and leads to vasodilation (not enough blood can return to the heart) and low blood pressure

5. _____ Due to heart muscle damage caused by a myocardial infarction

6. _____ Due to heavy bleeding or dehydration

7. _____ Caused by a severe infection that affects the functioning of vital organs.

   a. cardiogenic shock
   b. hypovolemic shock
   c. anaphylactic shock
   d. septic shock
   e. neurogenic shock

Select the correct answer.

8. The most common symptom(s) of myocardial infarction include
   a. angina pectoris.
   b. cold sweats.
   c. heartburn.
   d. all of the above.

9. Which medication is used for myocardial infarction?
   a. Epinephrine
   b. Nitroglycerin
   c. Aspirin
   d. All of the above
   e. Both b and c

CERTIFICATION PREPARATION
Circle the correct answer.

1. What is considered a mild heat-related illness that causes muscle pains and spasms due to electrolyte imbalance?
   a. Heat stroke
   b. Heat exhaustion
   c. Heat cramps
   d. Hypothermia

2. What is considered a partial-thickness burn?
   a. First-degree burn
   b. Second-degree burn
   c. Third-degree burn
   d. Fourth-degree burn

3. Which type of burn causes erythema, tenderness, and physical sensitivity, but no scar development occurs?
   a. First-degree burn
   b. Second-degree burn
   c. Third-degree burn
   d. Fourth-degree burn

4. An adult has burns on his back, left arm and hand, and left foot and leg. Using the Rule of Nines, estimate the percentage of total burn surface area.
   a. 18%
   b. 27%
   c. 36%
   d. 45%

5. Which animal is *not* a common carrier of rabies?
   a. Guinea pig
   b. Raccoon
   c. Bat
   d. Fox

6. What is a symptom of a concussion?
   a. Confusion and amnesia
   b. Ringing in the ears
   c. Temporary loss of consciousness right after the incident
   d. All of the above

7. What is a symptom of a cerebrovascular accident?
   a. Confusion and speech difficulty
   b. Numbness of the face, arm, or leg
   c. Problem seeing in one or both eyes
   d. All of the above

8. What is *not* a sign of a partial airway obstruction?
   a. Forceful or weak coughing
   b. Bluish skin color
   c. Labored, noisy, or gasping breathing
   d. Panicked appearance, extreme anxiety, or agitation

9. What is a possible cause of syncope?
   a. Dehydration
   b. Standing up too quickly
   c. Drop in blood glucose
   d. All of the above

10. What is *not* a typical symptom of shock?
    a. Anxiety and agitation
    b. Chest pain
    c. Nausea
    d. Diaphoresis

WORKPLACE APPLICATIONS

1. A medical assistant suspects a patient is starting to have an allergic reaction. What should the medical assistant do? What will the provider order? How should the medication be administered?

   _____

   _____

   _____

2. Gabe was rooming Mr. Smith, who stated, "I think I am having a heart attack." What are the common symptoms of a myocardial infarction (MI)?

   _____

   _____

   _____

3. Dr. Walden ordered nitroglycerin for Mr. Smith. How does nitroglycerin work in the body? _____

   _____

   _____

   _____

INTERNET ACTIVITIES

1. Using online resources, research one of the following conditions: seizures, cerebrovascular accident, asthmatic attack, and MI. Create a poster presentation, a PowerPoint presentation, or write a paper summarizing your research. Include the following points in your project:
   a. Description of the condition
   b. Etiology
   c. Signs and symptoms
   d. Diagnostic procedures
   e. Treatments

2. Using online resources, research a condition listed in #1. Create a patient education flyer based on your research. Include the following points in your flyer:
   a. Description of the condition
   b. Risks factors
   c. Warning signs and symptoms
   d. Actions the individual should take when experiencing the signs and symptoms

3. Research the following medications: diphenhydramine, epinephrine, glucagon, naloxone, and nitroglycerin. Using a reliable online drug resource, identify for each medication:
   a. Indication for use
   b. Desired effects
   c. Side effects
   d. Adverse reactions

   Write a short paper addressing each of these four areas for each medication.

Procedure 27.1 Provide First Aid for a Patient with an Environmental Emergency and Insulin Shock

Name _____ Date _____ Score _____

Task: Provide first aid to an individual who has a dog bite and hypoglycemia.

Background Information: For someone with hypoglycemic symptoms, test the blood glucose level. If the blood glucose is under 70 and the patient is conscious and able to swallow, give 4 ounces of fruit juice or regular soda or 3 glucose tablets. Test the blood glucose in 15 minutes. Continue with these steps until the glucose level is 70 or above.

Scenario: You are working with Dr. Martin, a family practice provider. Maude Crawford (date of birth [DOB} 12/22/19XX) is being seen for a dog bite on her left arm. The wound is still bleeding.

Directions: Role-play the scenario with a peer, who will be the patient, and you are the medical assistant.

Equipment and Supplies:
- Gloves and sterile gauze
- Sugary drink (4 oz. fruit juice or regular soda) or three glucose tablets
- Patient's health record

Standard: Complete the procedure and all critical steps in _____ minutes with a minimum score of 85% within two attempts (*or as indicated by the instructor*).

Scoring: Divide the points earned by the total possible points. Failure to perform a critical step, indicated by an asterisk (*), results in grade no higher than an 84% (*or as indicated by the instructor*).

Time: Began_____ Ended_____ Total minutes: _____

Steps:	Point Value	Attempt 1	Attempt 2
1. Wash hands or use hand sanitizer.	5		
2. Greet the patient. Identify yourself. Verify the patient's identity with full name and date of birth.	15		
3. Apply gloves. Place sterile gauze over the wound and apply direct pressure to control the bleeding.	20*		
4. Identify when the patient had her last tetanus booster.	10		
Scenario update: Mrs. Crawford has diabetes and states that she thinks she has low blood sugar. She has blurry vision, tremors, and a headache. She asks you for something to eat. According to the facility's policy, you check her blood glucose level, and it is 48 mg/dL. 5. Obtain a sugary drink or glucose tablets. Indicate how much to give to the patient.	20*		
Scenario update: After 15 minutes, her blood glucose level is 59 mg/dL. You notify the provider while a coworker stays with the patient. 6. Describe follow-up care for the patient. (See the background information.)	20		

Scenario update: After 15 minutes, her blood glucose level is 82 mg/dL. You notify the provider. 7. Document the situation in the patient's health record. Include the blood glucose levels, your actions, the provider who was notified, and the patient's response.	**10**		
Total Points	**100**		

Documentation

Comments

CAAHEP Competencies	Step(s)
I.P.13.b. Perform first aid procedures for: diabetic coma or insulin shock	5-6
I.P.13.e. Perform first aid procedures for: environmental emergency	3-4
X.P.3. Document patient care accurately in the medical record	7
ABHES Competencies	**Step(s)**
8. g. Recognize and respond to medical office emergencies	Entire procedure

Procedure 27.2 Incorporate Critical Thinking Skills When Performing Patient Assessment

Name _____ Date _____ Score _____

Task: Use critical thinking skills while performing a patient assessment regarding a neurologic emergency.

Scenario: You are working with Dr. Martin, a family practice provider. Maude Crawford's daughter calls concerned about her mother. The daughter stated that Maude Crawford (DOB 12/22/19XX) fell and hit her head.

Directions: Role-play the scenario with a peer. The peer will be the daughter, and you will be the medical assistant. The peer can make up information regarding the scenario. Your instructor will be the provider.

> **WMFM Clinic – Neurologic Emergency Phone Protocol:**
> Obtain the patient's name, date of birth, signs/symptoms, and the history of the situation. After call, document situation, symptoms, and action in the patient's health record.
>
> If a patient reports the following neurologic concerns, send the patient to the emergency department via the ambulance immediately.
> - Seizure or seizure like symptoms lasting 3 or more minutes
> - Passing out or fainting; dizziness or weakness that does not go away
> - Sudden or unusual headache that starts suddenly
> - Unable to see or speak, sudden confusion
> - Neck or spine injury
> - Injuries that cause loss of feeling or inability to move
> - Head injury with passing out, fainting, or confusion
> - Facial drooping or sudden speech difficulties or visual problems
>
> If a patient reports the following concerns, schedule a visit for the same day. If no appointments are available, consult the triage nurse or the provider regarding the situation.
> - Headache/migraine
> - Nonemergent neurologic concern such as muscle stiffness or rigidity that is progressively getting worse, insomnia, or a history of blurry or double vision.

Equipment and Supplies:
- Patient's health record
- Paper and pen
- Emergency Phone Protocol for clinic

Standard: Complete the procedure and all critical steps in _____ minutes with a minimum score of 85% within two attempts (*or as indicated by the instructor*).

Scoring: Divide the points earned by the total possible points. Failure to perform a critical step, indicated by an asterisk (*), results in grade no higher than an 84% (*or as indicated by the instructor*).

Time: Began_____ Ended_____ Total minutes: _____

Steps:	Point Value	Attempt 1	Attempt 2
1. Obtain the patient's name and date of birth.	20*		
2. Using critical thinking skills, ask appropriate questions to obtain information about the patient's condition. Write down the patient's issues or concerns or the situation. *(Refer to the Affective Behaviors Checklist – Critical Thinking and the Grading Rubric)*	20		
Scenario update: The daughter stated that Maude was "knocked out" for about a minute. She has been acting differently since the fall. You need to follow the Neurological Emergency Phone Protocol. 3. Complete the protocol and determine what actions to take using critical thinking skills. *(Refer to the Affective Behaviors Checklist – Critical Thinking and the Grading Rubric)*	20		
4. Instruct the caller on what should be done based on the protocol. Talk with the provider if needed.	20*		
5. Document the call in the patient's health record. Include the caller's name, the patient's condition (e.g., signs, symptoms, and concerns), name of the protocol used, information given to the caller, and the provider who was notified.	20*		
Total Points	100		

Affective Behavior	Affective Behaviors Checklist **Directions:** *Check behaviors observed during the role-play.*					
Critical Thinking	**Negative, Unprofessional Behaviors**	**Attempt**		**Positive, Professional Behaviors**	**Attempt**	
		1	**2**		**1**	**2**
	Coached or told of an issue or problem			Independently identified the problem or issue		
	Failed to ask relevant questions related to the condition			Asked appropriate questions to obtain the information required		
	Failed to consider alternatives; failed to ask questions that demonstrated understanding of principles/concepts			Willing to consider other alternatives; asked appropriate questions that showed understanding of principles/concepts		
	Failed to make an educated, logical judgment/decision; actions or lack of actions demonstrated unsafe practices and/or did not follow the protocol			Made an educated, logical judgment/decision based on the protocol; actions reflected principles of safe practice		
	Other:			Other:		

Grading Rubric for the Affective Behaviors Checklist **Directions:** *Based on checklist results, identify the points received for the procedure checklist. Indicate how the behaviors demonstrated met the expectations.*		Points for Procedure Checklist	Attempt 1	Attempt 2
Does not meet Expectation	• Response fails to show critical thinking. • Student demonstrated more than 2 negative, unprofessional behaviors during the interaction.	0		
Needs Improvement	• Response fails to show critical thinking. • Student demonstrated 1 or 2 negative, unprofessional behaviors during the interaction.	0		
Meets Expectation	• Response demonstrates critical thinking; no negative, unprofessional behaviors observed. • More practice is needed for behavior to appear natural and for student to appear comfortable and at ease.	20		
Occasionally Exceeds Expectation	• Response demonstrates critical thinking; no negative, unprofessional behaviors observed. • At times student appeared comfortable and at ease; but more practice is needed for behavior to become natural and consistent with a professional medical assistant.	20		
Always Exceeds Expectation	• Response demonstrates critical thinking; no negative, unprofessional behaviors observed. • Student's behaviors appeared natural and comfortable. Behaviors are consistent with a professional medical assistant.	20		

Documentation

Comments

CAAHEP Competencies	Step(s)
X.P.3. Document patient care accurately in the medical record	5
A.1. Demonstrate critical thinking skills	3
ABHES Competencies	**Step(s)**
8.g. Recognize and respond to medical office emergencies	Entire procedure

Procedure 27.3 Provide First Aid for a Patient With a Stroke and Seizure Activity

Name _____ Date _____ Score _____

Tasks: Provide first aid to an individual having a stroke and seizure activity. Document care in the health record.

Scenario: You are working with Dr. Martin, a family practice provider. Walter Biller (DOB 1/4/19XX) arrives for his appointment.

Directions: Role-play the scenario with a peer, who will be the patient, and you are the medical assistant.

Equipment and Supplies:
- Watch, stethoscope, and sphygmomanometer
- Folded towel, blanket, or coat
- Patient's health record
- Gloves and other personal protective equipment (as required)

Standard: Complete the procedure and all critical steps in _____ minutes with a minimum score of 85% within two attempts (*or as indicated by the instructor*).

Scoring: Divide the points earned by the total possible points. Failure to perform a critical step, indicated by an asterisk (*), results in grade no higher than an 84% (*or as indicated by the instructor*).

Time: Began_____ Ended_____ Total minutes: _____

Steps:	Point Value	Attempt 1	Attempt 2
1. Wash hands or use hand sanitizer.	5		
2. Greet the patient. Identify yourself. Verify the patient's identity with full name and date of birth.	5		
Scenario update: As you room Mr. Biller, you notice that he seems to be dragging his left leg when walking, the left side of his face is drooping, and he states his left arm is weak. You suspect that he might be having a stroke. He asks for a drink of water when you get to the exam room. 3. You call for help and assist the patient onto the examination table. Place the patient in the recovery position with his head slightly raised.	10*		
4. Monitor the patient's airway. Obtain the patient vital signs.	10		
5. Speak calmly to the patient. Do not give the patient anything to drink.	10		
Scenario update: While you are waiting for the provider, Mr. Biller starts to jerk his arms and he becomes unresponsive. 6. Keep the patient in the recovery position. Note the time when the seizure started. Gently raise the chin to tilt the head back slightly to open the airway. Yell for help if help has not arrived.	15*		
7. Continue to monitor his pulse rate and respiration rate. Put on gloves and other personal protective equipment as needed.	10		
8. Clear any hard or sharp items away from the patient. Place a soft, folded towel, blanket, or coat under the patient's head.	10		

9.	Remove the patient's glasses (if on) and loosen any constrictive clothing around the neck. Stay with the person until they are fully awake and continue to monitor the respiration and pulse rates.	10		
10.	Document the first aid measures you provided in the order that they occurred. In addition, document the seizure activity you witnessed, the length of the episode, and the provider notified.	15		
	Total Points	100		

Documentation

.

Comments

CAAHEP Competencies	Step(s)
I.P.13.c. Perform first aid procedures for: stroke	Entire procedure
I.P.13.d. Perform first aid procedures for: seizures	6-9
X.P.3. Document patient care accurately in the medical record	10
ABHES Competencies	**Step(s)**
8.g. Recognize and respond to medical office emergencies	Entire procedure

Procedure 27.4   Provide First Aid for a Choking Patient

Name _____   Date _____   Score _____

Tasks: Provide first aid to a conscious adult who is choking. Document it in the health record.

Scenario: You are working with Dr. Martin, a family practice provider. As you return from lunch, you notice that an adult visitor is having an issue. It appears that she had been eating fast food and now she is holding her neck with both hands. She appears to be panicking.

Directions: Role-play the scenario with a peer. The peer will be the visitor, and you will be the medical assistant.

Equipment and Supplies:
- Patient's health record
- Gloves
- Mannequin

Standard: Complete the procedure and all critical steps in _____ minutes with a minimum score of 85% within two attempts (*or as indicated by the instructor*).

Scoring: Divide the points earned by the total possible points. Failure to perform a critical step, indicated by an asterisk (*), results in grade no higher than an 84% (*or as indicated by the instructor*).

Time: Began_____ Ended_____ Total minutes: _____

Steps:	Point Value	Attempt 1	Attempt 2
1. Approach the person and ask, "Are you choking?"	10		
Scenario update: She nods her head yes and cannot speak. She is standing. 2. Yell for help. Put on gloves if available. Stand behind the victim with your feet slightly apart. Reach your arms around the person's waist.	15*		
3. Make a fist and place it just above the person's navel. Make sure your thumb side is next to the person. Grasp the fist tightly with your other hand.	15*		
Scenario update: The next steps must be done on a mannequin. 4. With the correct hand position, make quick, upward and inward thrusts with your fist. Do 5 abdominal thrusts before doing back blows.	15*		
5. Stand behind the person and wrap one arm around the person's upper body. Position the person so they are bent forward with the chest parallel to the ground.	15		
6. Use the heel of your other hand to give a firm blow between the shoulder blades. Check to see if the object dislodges. If not, continue by giving another 4 back blows.	10		
7. Continue to give 5 abdominal thrusts followed by 5 back blows until the object is dislodged or the person loses consciousness. Note: If the person faints or loses consciousness, lower the person to the floor. Call 911 (or the local emergency number) or have someone else call. Begin CPR, starting with chest compressions. Check to see if the item is in the airway. Remove it only if it is loose.	10		

Scenario update: After two sets of abdominal thrusts and back blows, the woman coughs out a piece of food. She can now talk. 8. Arrange for the person to be seen by the provider. Document the first aid measures you provided in the order that they occurred.	10		
Total Points	100		

Documentation

Comments

CAAHEP Competencies	Step(s)
X.P.3. Document patient care accurately in the medical record	8
ABHES Competencies	**Step(s)**
8.g. Recognize and respond to medical office emergencies	Entire procedure

Procedure 27.5 Provide First Aid for a Patient With a Bleeding Wound, Fracture, or Syncope

Name _____ Date _____ Score _____

Tasks: Provide first aid to an individual with a suspected fracture, a bleeding wound, and syncope. Document the first aid you provide.

Scenario: You are returning from lunch and see a person fall at the entrance of the healthcare facility. He is an older man and complains of pain in his right lower arm. His arm looks deformed and is bleeding. You call for help. A provider comes, and coworkers bring supplies. The provider tells you to care for the wound and splint the arm before moving the individual. You have a coworker helping you.

Directions: Role-play the situation with two peers. One peer will be the patient and the other peer will be a coworker. You will be the medical assistant.

Equipment and Supplies:
- Gloves
- Sterile gauze
- Bandage
- Splinting material (e.g., SAM splint)
- Coban wrap or gauze roll

Standard: Complete the procedure and all critical steps in _____ minutes with a minimum score of 85% within two attempts (*or as indicated by the instructor*).

Scoring: Divide the points earned by the total possible points. Failure to perform a critical step, indicated by an asterisk (*), results in grade no higher than an 84% (*or as indicated by the instructor*).

Time: Began_____ Ended_____ Total minutes: _____

Steps:	Point Value	Attempt 1	Attempt 2
1. Wash your hands or use hand sanitizer if possible. Identify yourself to the patient. Obtain the patient's name and date of birth as you put on gloves.	10		
2. Using sterile gauze, apply direct pressure over the wound to stop the bleeding. Make sure to immobilize the injured arm as you apply pressure. If possible, elevate the arm to help slow the bleeding. If the blood seeps through the gauze, apply another layer of gauze on the initial one. Continue with the direct pressure until the bleeding stops.	15*		
3. Once the bleeding has stopped, cover the dressing with a bandage. Remember to immobilize the injured arm as you work.	10		
Scenario update: As you apply the bandage to the injured arm, the patient states he does not feel good. He says he feels dizzy and thinks he is going to pass out. Your peer takes over by supporting his arm, and the man faints. He is still breathing and has a pulse. 4. Position the patient on his back. Continue to check his respirations and pulse rates.	15*		
5. Loosen any constrictive clothing around the neck and chest. Raise the legs above the heart level (about 12 inches).	15*		

Scenario update: After a few minutes, he starts to come around. He jokes that blood makes him faint. As he is lying on his back talking with you, you need to splint his injured arm. 6. Use the splint material and shape it to the injured arm. Do not straighten the arm. Apply the splint beyond the joint above and the joint below the injury.	**15***		
7. Use Coban or a gauze roll to secure the splint in place. Encourage the patient to hold the injured arm against his chest as he moves.	**10***		
8. Document the first aid measures you provided in the order they occurred. Note that the provider was at the scene.	**10**		
Total Points	**100**		

Documentation

Comments

CAAHEP Competencies	Step(s)
I.P.13.a. Perform first aid procedures for: bleeding	2, 3
I.P.13.f. Perform first aid procedures for: syncope	4, 5
X.P.3. Document patient care accurately in the medical record	8
ABHES Competencies	**Step(s)**
8.g. Recognize and respond to medical office emergencies	Entire procedure

Procedure 27.6 Provide First Aid for a Patient With Shock

Name _____ Date _____ Score _____

Tasks: Provide first aid to an individual who is in shock. Document the first aid you provide.

Scenarios: You are working with Dr. Julie Walden. The administrative medical assistant at the reception desk notifies you that Robert Caudill (DOB 10/31/19XX) is here and looks very ill. You bring the patient and his wife immediately back to the procedure room because it is the only available room. He asks to move to the exam table, and you assist him as he transfers to the table. You obtain his vital signs, which are P 92, irregular, 1+; R 26, regular, shallow; BP 72/48 RA, lying; and T 103.2° F.

Directions: Role-play the scenario with two peers. One peer will be the patient and the other will be the wife. You will be the medical assistant.

Equipment and Supplies:
- Stethoscope
- Watch
- Pen
- Sphygmomanometer (blood pressure cuff)
- Pillows, blankets, or small stool to help elevate the feet
- Exam table

Standard: Complete the procedure and all critical steps in _____ minutes with a minimum score of 85% within two attempts (*or as indicated by the instructor*).

Scoring: Divide the points earned by the total possible points. Failure to perform a critical step, indicated by an asterisk (*), results in grade no higher than an 84% (*or as indicated by the instructor*).

Time: Began_____ Ended_____ Total minutes: _____

Steps:	Point Value	Attempt 1	Attempt 2
1. Call for help. Monitor the patient's breathing and pulse until the provider arrives.	10		
Scenario update: The provider examines the patient and suspects septic shock. You administer 2 L of oxygen per nasal cannula as the provider ordered. The triage RN inserts an IV and administers IV fluids. The provider directs another medical assistant to call 911. 2. Raise the patient's legs 12 inches.	15*		
3. Make sure the patient's head is flat on the bed.	10*		
4. Loosen the person's clothing. Make sure the clothing does not restrict the neck and chest area.	15*		
5. Obtain a pulse rate, respiration rate, and blood pressure. Continue to monitor the patient's airway, pulse rate, and respiration rate.	15		
6. While monitoring the patient, speak calmly with him. Use a gentle tone of voice. Demonstrate calming body language (e.g., do not appear scared, rushed, or out of control).	15		
7. Talk calmly with the patient's wife and explain what is occurring. Answer any questions the wife may have.	10		

8.	Document the first aid measures you provided in the order they occurred. Indicate which provider examined the patient. In addition, document the administration of oxygen and the vital signs obtained.	**10**		
	Total Points	**100**		

Documentation

Comments

CAAHEP Competencies	Step(s)
X.P.3. Document patient care accurately in the medical record	8
ABHES Competencies	**Step(s)**
8.g. Recognize and respond to medical office emergencies	Entire procedure

Procedure 27.7   Provide Rescue Breathing, Cardiopulmonary Resuscitation (CPR), and Automated External Defibrillator (AED)

Name _____ Date _____ Score _____

Tasks: Perform rescue breathing and CPR. Use the AED machine.

Scenario: You are in the healthcare facility parking lot and find a person on the ground. No one is around.

Directions: Role-play the scenario with a peer. Your peer will be the person on the ground. You will be the medical assistant.

Equipment and Supplies:
- AED machine with adult pads
- Barrier ventilation device
- Mannequin
- Gloves (if available)

Standard: Complete the procedure and all critical steps in _____ minutes with a minimum score of 85% within two attempts (*or as indicated by the instructor*).

Scoring: Divide the points earned by the total possible points. Failure to perform a critical step, indicated by an asterisk (*), results in grade no higher than an 84% (*or as indicated by the instructor*).

Time: Began_____ Ended_____ Total minutes: _____

Steps:	Point Value	Attempt 1	Attempt 2
1. Check the scene for safety. Is it safe to approach and provide help to the victim?	5		
2. Check the person's response. Tap the individual on the shoulder and shout, "Are you all right?" Pause for a few moments for a response.	5		
Scenario update: There is no response from the individual. A bystander comes up and you direct that person to find an AED machine. 3. Call 911 and answer the questions from the dispatcher.	10		
4. Put on gloves if available. Roll the person over if the person is face down. Roll the person as an entire unit, supporting the head, neck, and back. Open the airway and assess the respirations and the pulse for 10 seconds. Note: Occasional gasping is not considered breathing. a. *Person is breathing and has a pulse*: Monitor the person until the emergency responders arrive. If needed and if no head, neck, or spinal injury is suspected, place the patient in the recovery position. b. *Person is not breathing and has a pulse*: Give 1 breath every 5-6 seconds. Check the pulse every 2 minutes. If pulse remains, continue with rescue breathing. If pulse is absent, start CPR. c. *Person is not breathing and has no pulse*: Give CPR, starting with compressions. Give 15 compressions and 2 breaths.	20*		

Scenario update: The individual has a weak pulse and is not breathing. (Use a mannequin for the following steps.) 5. Use a barrier device if available. Pinch the person's nose and give each rescue breath over 1 second. Watch for the chest to rise. Give the appropriate amount of ventilations for the person's age. Continue to monitor the pulse as you give rescue breaths. *Note:* If the person had been choking, look in the mouth before giving a rescue breath. If you see the object, sweep it out with your finger. You can also provide nose ventilation if the mouth is injured. Stoma ventilation must be done if the person has a stoma (in the throat area).	**10***		
Scenario update: When you check the pulse again, there is no pulse. 6. Place your hands at the correct location on the chest. Bring your shoulders directly over the victim's sternum as you compress downward. Keep your elbows locked.	**10**		
7. Give 15 compressions at the appropriate depth. Give two ventilations and watch for the chest to rise. Continue with the cycle. Give approximately 100 compressions per minute to an adult.	**10***		
Scenario update: After two cycles, a bystander brings an AED but does not know how to use it. The bystander also does not know CPR. You need to stop the CPR and use the AED. 8. Turn on the AED and follow the directions. Attach the AED pads to the individual's bare dry chest. Attach the pads to the machine if required. *Note*: Make sure to remove any medication patches and medication residue from the chest before applying the pads.	**10***		
9. Have everyone stand back from the patient by announcing, "Stand clear." Push the analyze button and allow the machine to analyze the heartbeat.	**10***		

10. Follow the prompts on the AED machine.
   a. Shock advised: Announce, "Stand clear" and make sure no one is touching the individual. Press the shock button. After the shock, do CPR for 2 minutes, starting with compressions. Continue following the prompts until the emergency responders arrive.
   b. Shock not advised: Continue doing CPR for 2 minutes, starting with compressions. Continue following the prompts until the emergency responders arrive.
	10*		

Total Points	**100**		

Comments

ABHES Competencies	Step(s)
8.g. Recognize and respond to medical office emergencies	Entire procedure

Principles of Pharmacology

CAAHEP Competencies	Assessment
I.C.10.a. Identify the classifications of medications including: indications for use	Certification Preparation – 9; Workplace Applications – 1; Internet Activities – 3
I.C.10.b. Identify the classifications of medications including: desired effects	Vocabulary Review – A. 1, 3, 4, 6, 8; Certification Preparation – 10; Workplace Applications – 1; Internet Activities – 3
I.C.10.c. Identify the classifications of medications including: side effects	Workplace Applications – 2; Internet Activities – 3
I.C.10.d. Identify the classifications of medications including: adverse reactions	Workplace Applications – 2; Internet Activities – 3

ABHES Competencies	Assessment
1. General Orientation d. List the general responsibilities and skills of the medical assistant	Skills and Concepts – E. 2
1.f. Comply with federal, state, and local health laws and regulations as they relate to healthcare settings	Skills and Concepts – F. 2-5
6. Pharmacology a. Identify drug classification, usual dose, side effects and contraindications of the top most commonly used medications.	Workplace Applications – 1-2; Internet Activities – 3
6.c. 1) Identify parts of prescriptions	Skills and Concepts – K. 2-5
6.c. 2) Identify appropriate abbreviations that are accepted in prescription writing	Abbreviations – 5-9, 16, 18-24, 26-48; Procedure 28.1
6.c. 3) Comply with legal aspects of creating prescriptions, including federal and state laws	Procedure 28.1
6.d. Properly utilize the *Physician's Desk Reference (PDR),* drug handbooks, and other drug references to identify a drug's classification, usual dosage, usual side effects, and contraindications	Internet Activities – 3

VOCABULARY REVIEW

Using the word pool on the right, find the correct word to match the definition. Write the word on the line after the definition.

Group A

1. A medication that prevents or reduces inflammation _____

2. A medication that slows down the cell's activity _____

3. A drug that reduces or eliminates pain _____

4. A drug that destroys or inhibits the growth of bacteria _____

5. By-products of drug metabolism _____

6. A drug that prevents or alleviates heart arrhythmias _____

7. A medication that increases the cell's activity _____

8. A substance (i.e., medication or chemical) that prevent the clotting of blood _____

9. A substance that inhibits the growth of microorganisms on living tissue _____

10. A medication that kills cells or disrupts parts of cells _____

Word Pool
- antiarrhythmic
- anticoagulant
- antiinflammatory
- antiseptic
- antibiotic
- analgesic
- depressing
- destroying
- metabolites
- stimulating

Group B

1. Information that appears on the drug label and addresses serious or life-threatening risks _____

2. Comparing a document with another document to ensure that they are consistent _____

3. A disease that occurs when a person cannot stop or limit the use of a drug, even after negative consequences have been experienced _____

4. Medical doctors who have been specially trained to diagnose and treat patients with mental, emotional, and behavioral conditions _____

5. Directions given by a provider for a specific medication to be administered to a patient _____

6. An identifier assigned by the Centers for Medicare and Medicaid Services (CMS) that classifies the healthcare provider by license and medical specialties _____

7. Indicates the greatest amount of medication a person should have within a 24-hour period _____

8. Physical characteristics of a medication (e.g., tablet and suspension) _____

Word Pool
- addiction
- boxed warning
- form
- maximum dosage
- medication order
- National Provider Identifier
- psychiatrists
- reconciling

ABBREVIATIONS

Write out what each of the following abbreviations stands for.

1. IV _____

2. ID _____

3. NAS _____

4. SUBQ _____

5. PO _____

6. ung _____

7. soln, sol. _____

8. cap _____

9. tinct _____

10. IM _____

11. C _____

12. F _____

13. m _____

14. cm _____

15. mm _____

16. tab(s) _____

17. kg _____

18. g _____

19. mg _____

20. mcg _____

21. gr _____

22. gtt(s) _____

23. L _____

24. mL _____

25. lb _____

26. fl oz _____

27. qt _____

28. pt _____

29. Tbs, tbsp _____

30. tsp _____

31. AM, a.m. _____

32. PM, p.m. _____

33. pc _____

34. ac _____

35. ad lib _____

36. d _____

37. noc, noct _____

38. hr, h _____

39. $\bar{p}$ _____

40. min _____

41. qh _____

42. prn _____

43. q4h _____

44. q6h _____

45. qam _____

46. tid _____

47. bid _____

48. qid _____

49. STAT _____

50. ASA _____

51. K _____

52. Fe _____

53. NS _____

54. MOM _____

55. NSAID _____

56. PPD _____

57. OTC _____

58. aq _____

59. med _____

60. NKA _____

61. NKDA _____

62. NPO _____

63. a̅a̅ _____

64. c̅ _____

65. s̅ _____

66. x _____

67. qs _____

68. Rx _____

69. Sig _____

70. VO _____

SKILLS AND CONCEPTS
Answer the following questions.

A. Introduction
Fill in the blank.

1. _____ is the study of the properties, actions, and uses of drugs.

2. A(n) _____ is a chemical substance used to cure, treat, prevent, or diagnose disease.

3. Unpleasant effects of a drug in addition to the desired or therapeutic effect are called _____.

B. Pharmacology Basics
Match the medication with the correct sources of drug.

1. _____ Synthetic insulin

2. _____ Iron, iodine, and zinc

3. _____ *Penicillium chrysogenum*

4. _____ Heparin and lanolin

5. _____ Digitalis and quinidine

a. natural – animals
b. natural – plants
c. natural – minerals
d. natural – microbiologic substances
e. synthetic

Match the descriptions with the correct uses of drugs.

6. _____ Drugs that do not cure or treat the disease but improve the quality of life

7. _____ Drugs used to diagnose or monitor a condition

8. _____ Drugs that relieve the symptoms while the body fights off the disease

9. _____ Drugs used to prevent pregnancy

10. _____ Drugs used to increase the blood levels of naturally occurring substances in the body

11. _____ Drugs used to prevent diseases

12. _____ Drugs that eliminate the disease

13. _____ Medications used to maintain or enhance health

a. prevention
b. treatment
c. diagnosis
d. cure
e. contraceptive
f. health maintenance
g. palliation
h. replacement

C. Pharmacokinetics
Match the description with the correct term.

1. _____ Placed under the tongue to dissolve

2. _____ Injected into the muscle

3. _____ The study of drug absorption, distribution, metabolism, and excretion in the body

4. _____ Placed between the cheek and the gums to dissolve and absorb quickly

5. _____ The harmful and deadly effect of a medication that can develop due to the buildup of medication or by-products in the body

6. _____ The means by which a drug enters the body

7. _____ Injected just below the skin; moves into the capillaries or the lymphatic vessels and is brought to the bloodstream

8. _____ Where a drug enters the body

9. _____ Injected directly into the bloodstream

10. _____ The movement of drug from the site of administration to the bloodstream

a. pharmacokinetics
b. route
c. site of administration
d. absorption
e. toxicity
f. sublingual
g. buccal
h. intramuscular
i. subcutaneous
j. intravenous

Match the description with the correct term.

11. _____ A series of chemical processes whereby enzymes change drugs in the body

12. _____ Medications that are administered in an inactive form

13. _____ Tissues where drugs accumulate, and the drugs are slowly released into the bloodstream

14. _____ The movement of metabolites out of the body

15. _____ The movement of absorbed drug from the blood to the body tissues

a. distribution
b. reservoirs
c. metabolism
d. prodrugs
e. excretion

Fill in the blank.

16. Most metabolites are excreted through the _____ and _____.

17. Medications are limited when a female is breastfeeding her baby, because drugs can be _____ in the breast milk.

18. Drugs are _____ by the body through stool, urine, breast milk, sweat, exhaled air, and saliva.

19. Young children, older adults, and those with kidney disease are at risk for the _____ of metabolic drug by-products in the body.

D. Drug Action
Fill in the blank or select the correct answer.

1. Which statement is correct regarding drug action?
   a. Infants and older adults have problems metabolizing and excreting medications.
   b. Thinner people require less medication than heavier people.
   c. Women can react differently to some medications compared to men.
   d. Certain foods affect a drug's action.
   e. All of the above.

2. Pharmacogenomics or _____ is the study of how genetic factors influence a person's metabolic response to a specific medication.

3. Medication effects that are seen at the site of administration are _____ effects and medication effects that are seen throughout the body are _____ effects.

4. _____ are also called *desired effects*.

5. The provider may prescribe a higher initial dose, called a(n) _____, which helps to quickly increase the medication level in the blood.

6. The blood concentrations of a medication that are high enough to produce the drug's therapeutic effect is called the _____.

7. A(n) _____ is the amount of medication needed to keep the blood levels within the therapeutic range.

8. An unexpected or life-threatening reaction to a medication is called a(n) _____.

9. _____ is an extreme hypersensitivity to a specific drug that can cause life-threatening symptoms, including swelling of the mouth and airway, dyspnea, wheezing, loss of consciousness, and death.

10. _____ is a peculiar response to a certain drug.

11. _____ is the need for a larger dose to get the same therapeutic or desired effect.

12. _____ is the strong psychological or physical need to take a certain drug.

E. Drug Legislation and the Ambulatory Care Setting
Fill in the blank.

1. _____ means to order a medication as a treatment for a condition, which is done by doctors and advanced-practice professionals.

2. _____ means to give a prescribed dose of medication to a patient, which is done by medical assistants, nurses, and providers.

3. ____ _____ means to give a supply of medication that the patient will take later, which is the role of the pharmacist.

4. The _____ enforces the Food, Drug, and Cosmetic Act and is responsible for the safety, effectiveness, security, and quality of drugs and cosmetics.

5. The _____ enforces the Controlled Substances Act and oversees the manufacturing, importation, possession, use, and distribution of legal controlled substances.

F. Compliance with the Controlled Substance Act
Fill in the blank or select the correct answer.

1. Providers prescribing controlled substances need a DEA registration number, which is good for _____ years.

2. Which is correct regarding the storage of controlled substances?
   a. They need to be kept in a locked cabinet or safe of substantial construction.
   b. Keys should be placed in a locked area accessible only to authorized persons.
   c. They should be stored in a different location than non-narcotic medications.
   d. All of the above

3. Periodic _____ of the log with the actual inventory count is important to identify missing medications.

4. An inventory of all controlled substances must be done at least _____, unless required more often by law.

5. The controlled substance inventory and log records need to be kept for _____ years.

6. _____ of controlled substances means using the medication for personal reasons.

G. Brand and Generic Drugs

1. The _____ name or _____ name is assigned by the manufacturer and no other company can use that name.

2. The _____ name is assigned by the U.S. Adopted Name Council.

3. The _____ name represents the exact formula of the medication.

4. The _____ name is used to list the medication in the U.S. Pharmacopeia and in the National Formulary (USP-NP).

H. Drug Reference Information
Match the description with the correct term.

1. _____ Indicates recommended changes in dosages for special populations
2. _____ Indicates necessary actions or special care that needs to be taken when the patient is on the medication
3. _____ Conditions or diseases for which the drug is used
4. _____ The time during which the drug is present in the blood at great enough levels to produce a response
5. _____ Provides information on how the medication should be given
6. _____ The time it takes for the drug to produce a response
7. _____ How the drug provides therapeutic results in the body, or the use of the drug
8. _____ This section describes known undesirable experiences associated with the medication
9. _____ The time it takes for the drug to reach its greatest effective concentration in the blood
10. _____ Includes medications, foods, and beverages that may either increase or reduce the medication level in the blood
11. _____ Reasons or conditions that make administration of the drug improper or undesirable
12. _____ The time it takes half of the drug to be metabolized or eliminated by normal biologic processes

a. indications
b. dosage considerations
c. administration
d. action
e. adverse reactions
f. duration
g. interactions
h. contraindications
i. precautions
j. biologic half-life
k. onset
l. peak

I. Forms of Medications
Match the description with the correct form of medication.

1. _____ Designed to break down over time
2. _____ Clear sweetened liquid preparation that contains alcohol
3. _____ A sugar and water solution that contains flavoring and medicinal substance
4. _____ Medication in a hard or soft gelatin shell
5. _____ A suspension of medication in a gas, usually used for respiratory or sinus conditions
6. _____ A solid medication containing the active medication and an antacid
7. _____ Semisolid, greasy drug preparations that are applied to the skin, rectum, or nasal mucosa
8. _____ Solid formed by compressed powdered medication; may be coated
9. _____ Coated to pass through the acidic environment of the stomach and break down in the base environment of the intestines
10. _____ A notched tablet, which can be split into half with a pill cutter or splitter

a. tablet
b. capsule
c. scored tablet
d. buffered
e. enteric-coated tablet or capsule
f. extended-release tablet or capsule
g. ointment and paste
h. elixir
i. syrup
j. aerosol

J. Types of Medication Orders

Fill in the blank.

1. A(n) _____ order is given over the phone or in person, whereas a(n) _____ order is given in writing, such as an electronic message.

Match the description with the correct type of order.

2. _____ Medication that is given on an "as needed" basis for specific signs and symptoms.

3. _____ Medication taken at a regular interval until it is canceled or expired.

4. _____ Medication is administered one time right now.

5. _____ Order applies to all patients who meet specific criteria.

6. _____ Medication is administered one time.

a. routine order
b. standing order
c. PRN order
d. single or one-time order
e. stat order

K. Prescriptions

Fill in the blank.

1. A(n) _____ is a written order by a provider to the pharmacist.

Match the description with the correct part of a prescription.

2. _____ Medication name and strength

3. _____ Directions to the pharmacist, how much to dispense, refills, and if generics are permitted

4. _____ The Rx symbol; means take

5. _____ Directions to the patient regarding the dose and timing of the medication

a. superscription
b. inscription
c. signature
d. subscription

CERTIFICATION PREPARATION

Circle the correct answer.

1. The rate of medication absorption is influenced by the
   a. blood flow to the absorption area.
   b. route.
   c. conditions at the site of the absorption.
   d. all of the above.

2. Which statement is true regarding metabolism?
   a. Most drug metabolism occurs in the liver.
   b. Young children, older adults, and those with kidney disease have issues metabolizing medications.
   c. Prodrugs change to inactive forms of drugs during metabolism.
   d. a and c

3. _____ means one drug reduces or blocks the effect of another drug.
   a. Toxicity
   b. Synergism
   c. Antagonism
   d. Potentiation

4. _____ means one drug increases the effect of the second drug.
   a. Toxicity
   b. Synergism
   c. Antagonism
   d. Potentiation

5. _____ means to give a prescribed dose of medication to a patient.
   a. Dispense
   b. Administer
   c. Prescribe
   d. Treatment

6. What is the classification of amoxicillin?
   a. Analgesic
   b. Antianxiety
   c. Antibiotic
   d. Antidepressant

7. What is the classification of atenolol?
   a. Antianxiety
   b. Anticonvulsant
   c. Antidepressant
   d. Antihypertensive

8. What is the classification of albuterol?
   a. Cholesterol-lowering agent
   b. Bronchodilator
   c. Corticosteroid
   d. Antihypertensive

9. Which classification of medication increases urinary output and lowers blood pressure?
   a. Laxative
   b. Corticosteroid
   c. Antihypertensive
   d. Diuretic

10. What is the action of an antiemetic?
    a. Treats depression
    b. Reduces nausea and vomiting
    c. Treats bacterial infections
    d. Reduces blood glucose level

WORKPLACE APPLICATIONS

1. Using Table 28.4, Information on Commonly Prescribed Medications, complete the table. Identify the indications for use and the desired effects for the medication classifications listed.

Medication Classification	Indications for Use	Desired Effects
Analgesics (narcotic)		
Antianxiety		
Antibiotics		
Anticoagulants		
Anticonvulsants		
Antidepressants (SSRIs)		
Antigout		
Antihyperglycemics		
Antihypertensives		
Antiinflammatories		
Antiplatelets		

Medication Classification	Indications for Use	Desired Effects
Bronchodilators		
Cholesterol-lowering agents		
Contraceptive (oral)		
Corticosteroids (oral)		
Diuretics		
Hormone replacement (insulin)		
Muscle relaxants		
Stimulants		

2. Using Table 28.4, Information on Commonly Prescribed Medications, complete the table. Identify the two side effects and two adverse reactions for the following medication classifications.

Class	Generic Name	Side Effects	Adverse Reaction
Analgesics (narcotic)	hydrocodone/acetaminophen		
Antianxiety (benzodiazepines)	alprazolam		
Antibiotics (penicillin)	amoxicillin		
Anticoagulants	warfarin		
Anticonvulsants	gabapentin		
Antidepressant	escitalopram		
Antihyperglycemics	metformin		
Antihypertensive	propranolol		

Class	Generic Name	Side Effects	Adverse Reaction
Bronchodilators	albuterol		
Cholesterol-lowering agents	atorvastatin		
Diuretics	furosemide		
Proton-pump inhibitors	omeprazole		

INTERNET ACTIVITIES

1. Using online resources, identify four reliable websites that can be used for medication information. Cite the websites.

2. Using the internet, research the Prescribers' Digital Reference website (https://www.pdr.net/) or the MedlinePlus website (https://medlineplus.gov/). Summarize the following points in a paper, Power-Point Presentation, or in a poster.
   a. What types of drug information are available?
   b. How can a medical assistant use this website?
   c. What resources are available on this website?

3. Using appropriate online drug reference resources, research one medication from 12 different classifications listed in Table 28.3. The medications should not be listed on Table 28.4. Cite your references. In a paper, PowerPoint presentation, or poster, address the following points for each of the 12 medications:
   a. Generic name
   b. Trade names (in the U.S. only)
   c. Usual adult dose
   d. Classification
   e. Indication for use
   f. Desired effects
   g. Contraindications (list two or more)
   h. Side effects (list five or more)
   i. Adverse reactions (list three or more)

Procedure 28.1   Prepare a Prescription

Name _____   Date _____   Score _____

Tasks: Prepare prescriptions using a prescription refill protocol. Use approved abbreviations.

Scenario: You receive a call from Noemi Rodriguez (DOB 11/04/19XX). She is requesting refills on three of her prescriptions from Jean Burke, NP. She saw Jean Burke 10 months ago. Noemi has no known allergies (NKA). She is doing well with the prescriptions and has no concerns. You determine it is time for refills. Her prescriptions include Coumadin 5 mg, 1 tablet orally daily; Tenormin 50 mg, 1 tablet orally daily; and Plendil 5 mg, 1 tablet orally daily.

Prescription Refill Protocol
Walden-Martin Family Medicine Clinic

Description: A Certified Medical Assistant (CMA) can refill current hypertensive medications that fall within the guidelines of this protocol.

Step 1	Step 2	
For medications to be refilled, the following points need to be addressed.	Qualifying Medications	Prescription Refill
• Has the person seen the provider within the last year? • Is the prescription for a hypertensive, hyperlipidemia, or hyperthyroidism medication, a current prescription? • Is the person free of concerns or complications due to the medication? • Is it time for a refill? (The medical assistant must verify that it is time for a refill.) If the answers to the above questions are all YES, then proceed to Step 2. If any of the answers to the above questions are NO, then schedule the person for an appointment with the provider.	amlodipine amlodipine/benazepril atenolol atenolol/chlorthalidone benazepril captopril diltiazem enalapril felodipine fosinopril irbesartan isradipine lisinopril losartan nifedipine quinapril ramipril	Extend the current prescription for 6 months. Instruct patient that in 6 months: • A visit to the provider will be required • Blood pressure reading will be required • Lab work may be required

Equipment and Supplies:
- SimChart for the Medical Office (SCMO) or paper prescriptions (Work Product 28.1) and pen
- Prescription refill protocol
- Drug reference book or online resource

Standard: Complete the procedure and all critical steps in _____ minutes with a minimum score of 85% within two attempts (or as indicated by the instructor).

Scoring: Divide the points earned by the total possible points. Failure to perform a critical step, indicated by an asterisk (*), results in grade no higher than an 84% (or as indicated by the instructor).

Time: Began_____ Ended_____ Total minutes: _____

Steps:	Point Value	Attempt 1	Attempt 2
1. Using the scenario, look up the generic medication names using the drug reference book or online resource.	10		
2. Read the prescription refill protocol. Compare the generic names to the list of medications given. Identify medication(s) that meet the protocol.	10		
3. Prepare prescription(s) for refill according to the protocol using SCMO or paper prescriptions. • Using SCMO. Search for the patient. Verify the date of birth before selecting the patient. On the INFO PANEL, select Phone Encounter. Complete the fields on the Create New Encounter window and save. Check the box beside the No known allergy statement on the allergy screen and save. Select Order Entry from the Record dropdown list and select Add in the Out-of-office section. • Using paper prescriptions: Add in the patient's complete name, date of birth, and address.	20		
4. Using the information in the scenario, complete the prescription information on either the paper prescription or in the SCMO fields. Use only approved abbreviations.	20		
5. Complete any additional prescription(s) as needed by the prescription refill protocol.	30		
6. Review the prescriptions for any errors. Void the prescription and redo if needed. Note: After the provider signs the prescriptions and depending on the facility's policy, the medical assistant may need to document the refill in the health record. This cannot be done until the provider approves the prescriptions.	10		
Total Points	100		

Comments

ABHES Competencies	Step(s)
6. Pharmacology c.2) Identify appropriate abbreviations that are accepted in prescription writing	4
6.c.3) Comply with legal aspects of creating prescriptions, including federal and state laws	Entire procedure

Work Product 28.1   Prescriptions

To be used with Procedure 28.1.

Walden-Martin Family Medical Clinic
1234 AnyStreet, AnyTown, AnyState, 12345
Phone: 123-123-1234 Fax: 123-123-5678

Jean Burke NP, Family Nurse Practitioner

Patient: _____   DOB: _____

Address: _____   Date: _____

℞   Route:

Sig:

Disp:

Refills:

❑   Generics permitted

_____
Jean Burke, NP
NPI#:1234567891

Walden-Martin Family Medical Clinic
1234 AnyStreet, AnyTown, AnyState, 12345
Phone: 123-123-1234 Fax: 123-123-5678

Jean Burke NP, Family Nurse Practitioner

Patient: _____   DOB: _____

Address: _____   Date: _____

℞   Route:

Sig:

Disp:

Refills:

❑   Generics permitted

_____
Jean Burke, NP
NPI#:1234567891

Walden-Martin Family Medical Clinic
1234 AnyStreet, AnyTown, AnyState, 12345
Phone: 123-123-1234 Fax: 123-123-5678

Jean Burke NP, Family Nurse Practitioner

Patient: _____   DOB: _____

Address: _____   Date: _____

Rx

Route:

Sig:

Disp:

Refills:

❑   Generics permitted

_____
Jean Burke, NP
NPI#:1234567891

Pharmacology Math

CAAHEP Competencies	Assessments
II.C.1.a. Define basic units of measurement: the metric system	Math for Medications – D. 1-13; Certification Preparation – 5
II.C.1.b. Define basic units of measurement: the household system	Math for Medications – C. 1-8; Certification Preparation – 1
II.C.2. Identify abbreviations used in calculating medication dosages	Abbreviations – 1-17
II.P.1. Calculate proper dosages of medication for administration	Procedure 29.1
II.P.4. Apply mathematical computations to solve equations	Math for Medications – C. to K.; Chapter Review – 1-10; Procedure 45.1
I.P.5. Convert among measurement systems	Math for Medications – C. 10, 12, 15, 17, 19, 21-32; Chapter Review – 2-4; Procedure 45.1

ABHES Competencies	Assessments
6. Pharmacology b. Demonstrate accurate occupational math and metric conversions for proper medication administration	Math for Medications – A. to K.

VOCABULARY REVIEW

Using the word pool on the right, find the correct word to match the definition. Write the word on the line after the definition.

1. Holds a specified quantity of medication in a single-use container _____

2. The number obtained by multiplying two or more numbers together _____

3. A grant from the government that gives a creator (or manufacturer) of an invention the sole right to produce, use, and sell the product for a set period of time _____

4. A tablet with a groove on the surface, used for splitting it in half _____

5. The sole right to market an approved medication granted by the FDA _____

6. The quantity of medication to be administered at one time _____

Word Pool
- exclusivity
- dosage
- patient
- product
- scored tablet
- unit-dose packaging
- patent

ABBREVIATIONS

Write out what each of the following abbreviations stands for.

1. C_____

2. F_____

3. m _____

4. cm _____

5. mm _____

6. kg_____

7. g_____

8. mg _____

9. mcg _____

10. gtt(s) _____

11. L_____

12. mL _____

13. fl oz _____

14. qt _____

15. pt _____

16. Tbs, tbsp _____

17. tsp _____

SKILLS AND CONCEPTS

Answer the following questions.

A. Drug Labels

1. The _____ or brand name is the manufacturer's name for the drug, and it is capitalized, and copyright-protected.

2. The _____ name is used by all manufacturers who make that specific medication.

3. _____ is the amount of drug in the unit dose.

4. _____ indicates the batch of drug the medication came from.

5. The _____ is a unique 10-digit number indicating the product and is required by federal law to be on all prescription and nonprescription medication packages and inserts in the U.S.

MATH BASICS
Answer the following questions. Write your answer on the line or in the space provided.

A. Fractions
Convert the improper fractions into whole numbers.

1. $35/5 =$ _____
2. $40/8 =$ _____
3. $20/5 =$ _____
4. $42/6 =$ _____
5. $81/9 =$ _____
6. $63/3 =$ _____

Simplify the improper fractions.

7. $38/5 =$ _____
8. $40/3 =$ _____
9. $24/5 =$ _____
10. $42/8 =$ _____
11. $81/10 =$ _____
12. $61/3 =$ _____

Solve and simplify the answer.

13. $2/3 \times 4/2 =$ _____
14. $1/3 \times 2/4 =$ _____
15. $5/7 \times 2/5 =$ _____
16. $3/5 \times 5/2 =$ _____
17. $4/7 \times 10/5 =$ _____
18. $6/7 \times 4/2 =$ _____
19. $2/3 \div 4/9 =$ _____
20. $1/3 \div 2/6 =$ _____
21. $5/7 \div 2/14 =$ _____
22. $3/5 \div 5/15 =$ _____
23. $4/7 \div 10/21 =$ _____
24. $6/3 \div 4/6 =$ _____

B. Decimals
Convert the fraction to a decimal.

1. $38/10 =$ _____
2. $46/10 =$ _____
3. $26/5 =$ _____
4. $43/5 =$ _____
5. $71/10 =$ _____
6. $61/5 =$ _____

C. Percentages
Convert to a percentage.

1. $28/100 =$ _____
2. $63/100 =$ _____
3. $13/100 =$ _____
4. $3/10 =$ _____
5. $7/10 =$ _____
6. $1/10 =$ _____

MATH FOR MEDICATIONS

Answer the following questions. Write your answer on the line or in the space provided. Follow the healthcare rules for writing numbers when writing your answers.

A. Rounding Numbers

Round the following numbers to the nearest tenth.

1. 2.367 = _____

2. 102.65 = _____

3. 2.634 = _____

4. 1.98 = _____

5. 0.658 = _____

6. 42.212 = _____

7. 3.09 = _____

8. 2.096 = _____

9. 9.98 = _____

10. 37.788 = _____

11. 12.456 = _____

12. 4.22 = _____

B. Roman Numerals

Write the number or Roman numeral on the line.

1. vi = _____

2. iiss = _____

3. x = _____

4. ivss = _____

5. iii = _____

6. ix = _____

7. 7 = _____

8. 3.5 = _____

9. 6.5 = _____

10. 9.5 = _____

11. 5 = _____

12. 3 = _____

C. Household System

Define the basic units of measurement by writing the equivalent on the line.

1. 1 kg – _____ lb

2. 1 Tbs = _____ mL

3. 5 mL = _____ tsp

4. 1 oz = _____ mL

5. 1 oz = _____ tsp

6. 1 lb = _____ oz

7. 3 tsp = _____ Tbs

8. 1 oz = _____ Tbs

Solve the following problems. Round your answers to the nearest tenth.

9. 9 tsp = _____ Tbs

10. 15 Tbs = _____ mL

11. 12 Tbs = _____ tsp

12. 45 mL = _____ Tbs

13. 90 mL = _____ oz

14. 5.5 oz = _____ Tbs

15. 3 oz = _____ mL

16. 21 Tbs = _____ oz

17. 8 tsp = _____ mL

18. 4 oz = _____ tsp

19. 55 mL = _____ tsp

20. 36 tsp = _____ oz

Solve the problems below using the lb and kg equivalents. Round your answer to the nearest tenth.

21. 24 kg = _____ lb

22. 34 kg = _____ lb

23. 52 lb = _____ kg

24. 67.58 lb = _____ kg

25. 58.9 kg = _____ lb

26. 189 kg = _____ lb

27. 310 lb = _____ kg

28. 78.9 lb = _____ kg

29. 108 kg = _____ lb

30. 56.7 kg = _____ lb

31. 123 lb = _____ kg

32. 222 lb = _____ kg

Solve the problems below using the oz and lb equivalents. Round your answer to the nearest tenth.

33. 13 oz = _____ lb

34. 9 oz = _____ lb

35. 15 oz = _____ lb

36. 10 oz = _____ lb

Solve the problems below using the oz and lb equivalents. Round the following to the nearest hundredth.

37. 3 oz = _____ lb

38. 2 oz = _____ lb

39. 7 oz = _____ lb

40. 5 oz = _____ lb

D. Metric System
Write the answer on the line.

1. In the metric system, _____ is measured in liters.

2. In the metric system, _____ is measured in meters.

3. In the metric system, _____ is measured in grams.

Define the basic units of measurement by writing the equivalent on the line.

4. 1 L = _____ mL

5. 1 L = _____ cc

6. 1 mL = _____ cc

7. 1 mg = _____ mcg

8. 1 m = _____ cm

9. 1 m = _____ mm

10. 1 cm = _____ mm

11. 1 g = _____ mg

12. 1 g = _____ mcg

13. 1 kg = _____ g

Solve the problems below using metric equivalents. Do not round your answers.

14. 2 kg = _____ g

15. 2.3 g = _____ mg

16. 5500 g = _____ kg

17. 6758 mg = _____ g

18. 3.1 g = _____ mg

19. 90 mL = _____ cc

20. 230 cm = _____ m

21. 31 cc = _____ mL

22. 5 m = _____ cm

23. 5.7 kg = _____ g

24. 108 mL = _____ L

25. 3456 mm = _____ m

26. 123 L = _____ mL

27. 0.05 m = _____ mm

28. 270 mcg = _____ mg

E. Temperature Conversion

Solve the problems below using the F and C conversions. Round your answer to the nearest tenth.

1. 124° F = _____ ° C

2. 96.3° F = _____ ° C

3. 39.6° C = _____ ° F

4. 123° C = _____ ° F

5. 103.6° F = _____ ° C

6. 48.9° F = _____ ° C

7. 32.9° C = _____ ° F

8. 85.7° C = _____ ° F

9. 98.6° F = _____ ° C

10. 230° F = _____ ° C

11. 66.4° C = _____ ° F

12. 101.2° C = _____ ° F

F. Number of Tablets Needed for Entire Course

For each problem, calculate the number of tablets the patient will need for the entire course. Write your answers on the lines and label your answers.

1. Prescription: XYZ medication 200 mg, 5 tabs bid x 6 days. _____

2. Prescription: XYZ medication 250 mg, 2 tabs qid x 14 days. _____

3. Prescription: XYZ medication 50 mg, 3 tabs bid x 10 days. _____

4. Prescription: XYZ medication 70 mg, 4 tabs tid x 3 days. _____

5. Prescription: XYZ medication 40 mg, 6 tabs bid x 7 days. _____

6. Prescription: XYZ medication 90 mg, 3 tabs qid x 20 days. _____

7. Prescription: XYZ medication 75 mg, 4 tabs bid x 14 days. _____

8. Prescription: XYZ medication 100 mg, 2 tabs tid x 5 days. _____

9. Prescription: XYZ medication 400 mg, 3 tabs bid x 8 days. _____

10. Prescription: XYZ medication 300 mg, 3 tabs qid x 14 days. _____

G. Number of Tablets per Dose

For each problem, calculate the number of tablets that the patient will take per dose. Round your answers to the nearest tenth. Write your answers on the lines and label your answers.

1. **Order:** ABC 175 mg po. **Stock:** ABC 350 mg po scored tablets. _____

2. **Order:** ABC 120 mcg po. **Stock:** ABC 80 mcg po scored tablets. _____

3. **Order:** ABC 185 mg po. **Stock:** ABC 370 mg po scored tablets. _____

4. **Order:** ABC 80 mg po. **Stock:** ABC 32 mg po scored tablets. _____

5. **Order:** ABC 125 mg po. **Stock:** ABC 25 mg po scored tablets. _____

6. **Order:** ABC 2.25 mg po. **Stock:** ABC 4.5 mg po scored tablets. _____

7. **Order:** ABC 195 mg po. **Stock:** ABC 65 mg po scored tablets. _____

8. **Order:** ABC 180 mg po. **Stock:** ABC 45 mg po scored tablets. _____

9. **Order:** ABC 45 mcg po. **Stock:** ABC 90 mcg po scored tablets. _____

10. **Order:** ABC 50 mg po. **Stock:** ABC 12.5 mg po scored tablets. _____

H. Liquid Medication Dose with Matching Labels

For each problem, calculate how many milliliters to give. Round your answers to the nearest tenth. Write your answers on the lines and label your answers.

1. **Order:** ABC 2200 units. **Stock:** ABC 2600 units/mL. _____

2. **Order:** ABC 8 mg. **Stock:** ABC 25 mg/3 mL. _____

3. **Order:** ABC 130 mg. **Stock:** ABC 250 mg/mL. _____

4. **Order:** ABC 75 mcg. **Stock:** ABC 125 mcg/2 mL. _____

5. **Order:** ABC 80 mg. **Stock:** ABC 50 mg/mL. _____

6. **Order:** ABC 60 mg. **Stock:** ABC 100 mg/mL. _____

7. **Order:** ABC 250 units. **Stock:** ABC 180 units/mL. _____

8. **Order:** ABC 85 mg. **Stock:** ABC 130 mg/mL. _____

9. **Order:** ABC 800 mg. **Stock:** ABC 1500 mg/2 mL. _____

10. **Order:** ABC 40 mg. **Stock:** ABC 200 mg/2 mL. _____

11. **Order:** ABC 100 mg. **Stock:** ABC 60 mg/mL. _____

12. **Order:** ABC 70 mg. **Stock:** ABC 40 mg/mL. _____

I. Liquid Medication Dose with Nonmatching Labels

For each problem, calculate how many milliliters to give. Round your answers to the nearest tenth. Write your answers on the lines and label your answers.

1. **Order:** ABC 1700 mg. **Stock:** ABC 2.8 g/3 mL. _____

2. **Order:** ABC 1 g. **Stock:** ABC 2500 mg/2 mL. _____

3. **Order:** ABC 120 mg. **Stock:** ABC 1 g/2 mL. _____

4. **Order:** ABC 750 mg. **Stock:** ABC 1.2 g/2 mL. _____

5. **Order:** ABC 800 mg. **Stock:** ABC 5 g/5 mL. _____

6. **Order:** ABC 2.3 g. **Stock:** ABC 1500 mg/mL. _____

7. **Order:** ABC 800 mg. **Stock:** ABC 2 g/mL. _____

8. **Order:** ABC 450 mg. **Stock:** ABC 1.2 g/3 mL. _____

9. **Order:** ABC 550 mg. **Stock:** ABC 1.2 g/2 mL. _____

10. **Order:** ABC 400 mg. **Stock:** ABC 2 g/4 mL. _____

11. **Order:** ABC 760 mg. **Stock:** ABC 3 g/2 mL. _____

12. **Order:** ABC 1.2 g. **Stock:** ABC 900 mg/mL. _____

J. Solution Dose

For each problem, calculate how many milliliters to give. Round your answers to the nearest tenth. Write your answers on the lines and label your answers.

1. **Order:** ABC 50 mg. **Stock:** ABC 4% solution. _____

2. **Order:** ABC 300 mg. **Stock:** ABC 15% solution. _____

3. **Order:** ABC 80 mg. **Stock:** ABC 6% solution. _____

4. **Order:** ABC 60 mg. **Stock:** ABC 5% solution. _____

5. **Order:** ABC 30 mg. **Stock:** ABC 4% solution. _____

6. **Order:** ABC 48 mg. **Stock:** ABC 3% solution. _____

7. **Order:** ABC 65 mg. **Stock:** ABC 8% solution. _____

8. **Order:** ABC 80 mg. **Stock:** ABC 10% solution. _____

9. **Order:** ABC 67 mg. **Stock:** ABC 4% solution. _____

10. **Order:** ABC 25 mg. **Stock:** ABC 4% solution. _____

11. **Order:** ABC 35 mg. **Stock:** ABC 2% solution. _____

12. **Order:** ABC 230 mg. **Stock:** ABC 15% solution. _____

K. Pediatric Doses

For each problem, calculate how many milliliters to give. Remember to round to the nearest thousandth when working through the problem and round your final answer to the nearest tenth. Write your answers on the lines and label your answers.

1. **Patient's wt:** 60 lb. **Medication order:** 0.5 mg/kg. **Stock medication:** 10 mg/mL.
   _____

2. **Patient's wt:** 122 lb. **Medication order:** 3 mg/kg. **Stock medication:** 180 mg/mL.
   _____

3. **Patient's wt:** 66 lb. **Medication order:** 0.6 mg/kg. **Stock medication:** 50 mg/2 mL.
   _____

4. **Patient's wt:** 82 lb. **Medication order:** 1.2 mg/kg. **Stock medication:** 80 mg/2 mL.
   _____

5. **Patient's wt:** 78 lb. **Medication order:** 0.5 mg/kg. **Stock medication:** 10 mg/mL.
   _____

6. **Patient's wt:** 59 lb. **Medication order:** 1.5 mg/kg. **Stock medication:** 30 mg/mL.
   _____

7. **Patient's wt:** 48 lb. **Medication order:** 0.8 mg/kg. **Stock medication:** 60 mg/2 mL.

   _____

8. **Patient's wt:** 39 lb. **Medication order:** 0.4 mg/kg. **Stock medication:** 6 mg/mL.

   _____

9. **Patient's wt:** 96 lb. **Medication order:** 1.7 mg/kg. **Stock medication:** 90 mg/2 mL.

   _____

10. **Patient's wt:** 66 lb. **Medication order:** 0.8 mg/kg. **Stock medication:** 40 mg/2 mL.

   _____

11. **Patient's wt:** 98 lb. **Medication order:** 0.2 mg/kg. **Stock medication:** 20 mg/mL.

   _____

12. **Patient's wt:** 68 lb. **Medication order:** 0.6 mg/kg. **Stock medication:** 50 mg/mL.

   _____

READING SYRINGES

For each picture, write what each line is equal to in column A. Then indicate the readings for B, C, and D in the columns. Label your answers and follow the healthcare rules when writing numbers (see textbook Chapter 29, Pharmacology Math). Note: All syringes without the word "unit" are calibrated in mL.

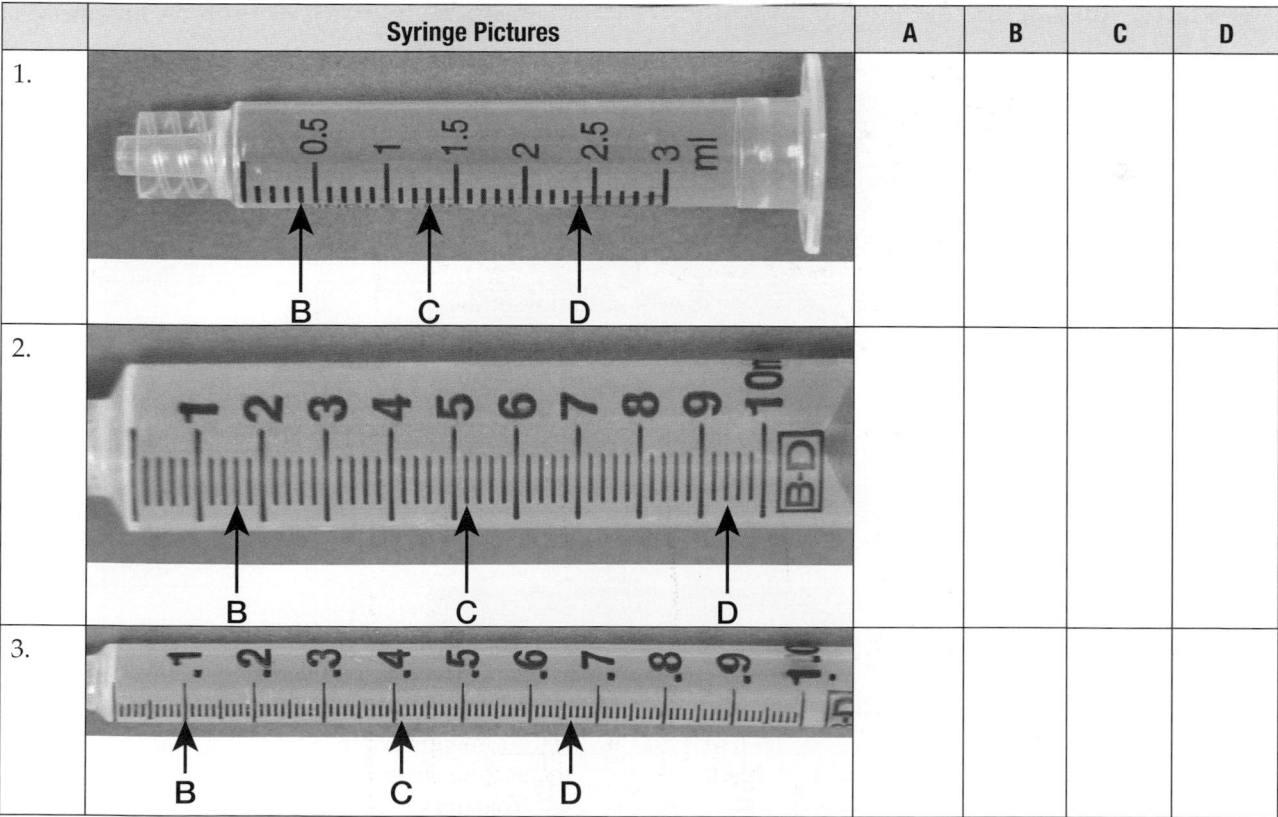

Syringe Pictures	A	B	C	D
1.				
2.				
3.				

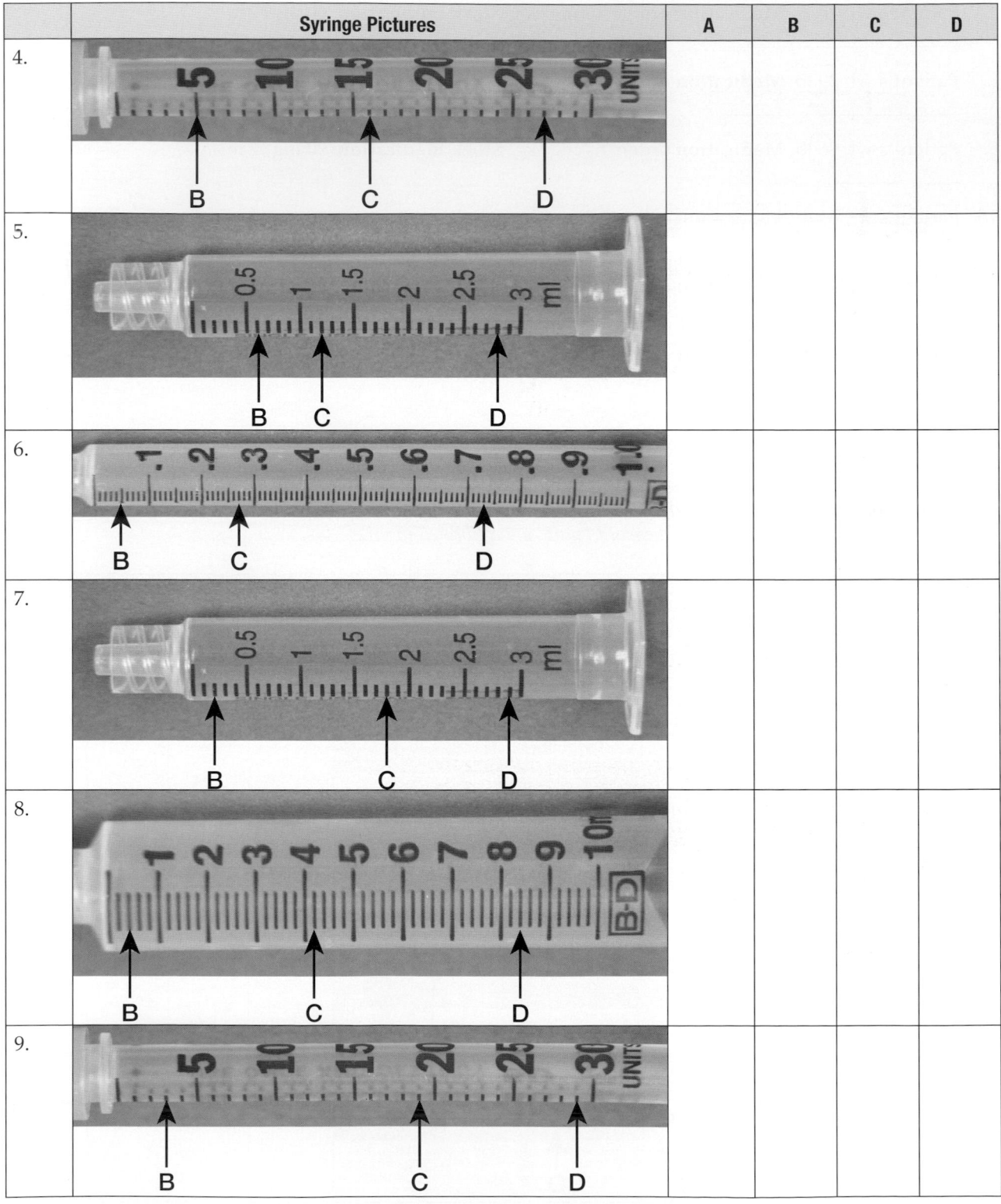

Syringe Pictures	A	B	C	D
4.				
5.				
6.				
7.				
8.				
9.				

Syringe Pictures	A	B	C	D
10. 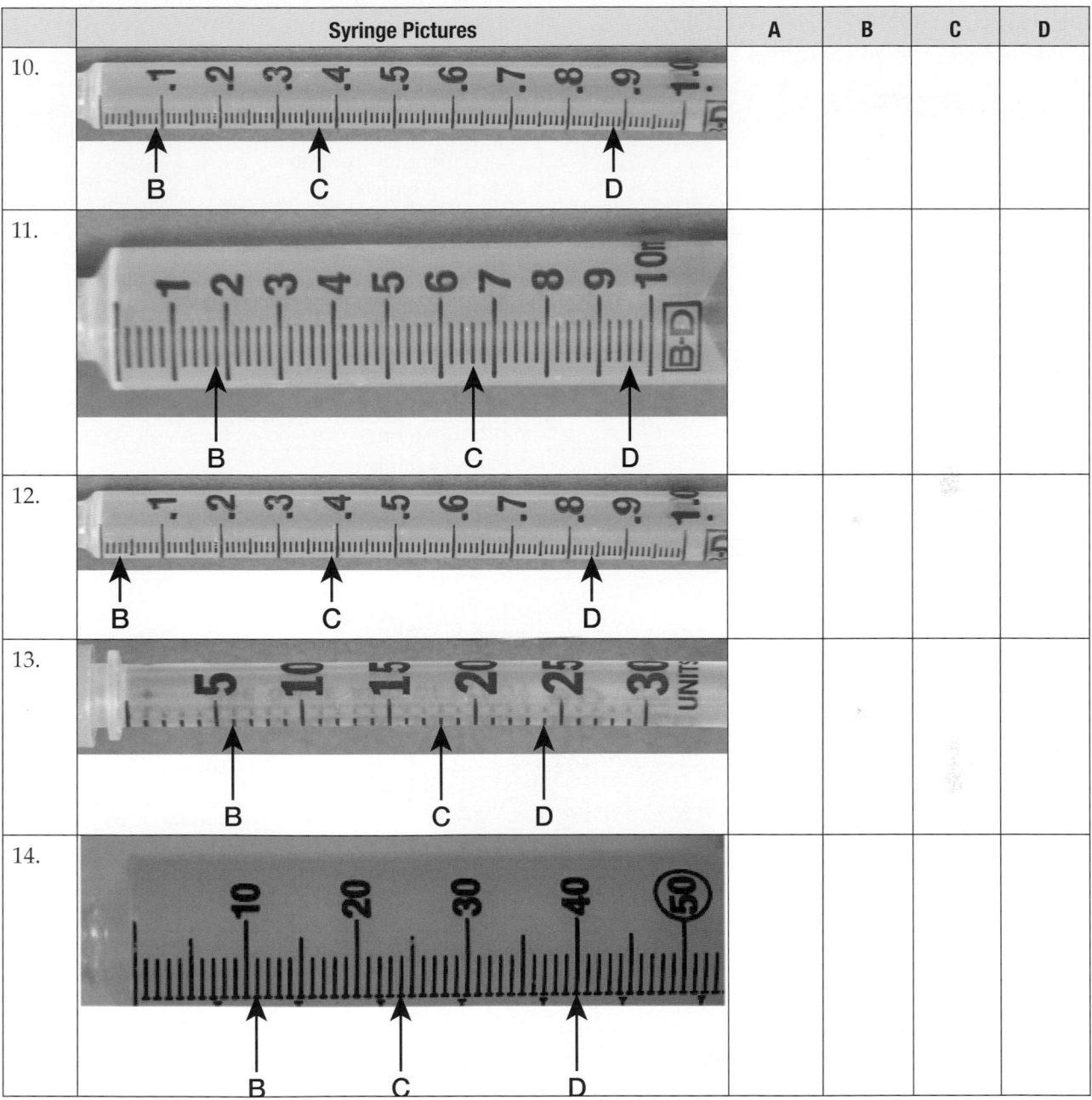				
11.				
12.				
13.				
14.				

CERTIFICATION PREPARATION

Round answers to the nearest tenth. Circle the correct answer.

1. 12 tsp = _____ Tbs
   a. 36
   b. 24
   c. 3
   d. 4

2. 5 oz = ___ mL
   a. 150
   b. 50
   c. 25
   d. 10

3. 63.5 kg = _____ lb
   a. 28.9
   b. 29
   c. 139.7
   d. 140

4. 220.2 lb = _____ kg
   a. 484
   b. 484.4
   c. 100
   d. 100.1

5. 8632 mg = _____ g
   a. 86.32
   b. 8.632
   c. 863.2
   d. 0.8632

6. 23° C = _____° F
   a. 99
   b. 44.8
   c. 73.4
   d. −16.2

7. Order: ABC 240 mcg po. Stock: ABC 160 mcg po scored tablets. How many tablets will the patient take per dose?
   a. 2 tablets
   b. 1.5 tablets
   c. 0.7 tablet
   d. 0.5 tablet

8. Order: ABC 20 mg. Stock: ABC 30 mg/2 mL. How many mL will you give?
   a. 0.7 mL
   b. 1.3 mL
   c. 0.6 mL
   d. 1.5 mL

9. Order: ABC 1.5 g. Stock: ABC 2500 mg/2 mL. How many mL will you give?
   a. 1 mL
   b. 0.1
   c. 0.6 mL
   d. 1.2 mL

10. Patient's wt: 64 lb. Medication order: 0.8 mg/kg. Stock medication: 60 mg/2 mL. How many mL will you give?
    a. 1.7 mL
    b. 0.8 mL
    c. 0.9 mL
    d. 0.4 mL

WORKPLACE APPLICATIONS

1. A child weighs 48 lb and Dr. Walden ordered 0.3 mg/kg. The medication label states 20 mg/mL. How many mL will you give? _____

2. A child weighs 32 lb and Dr. Walden ordered 0.2 mg/kg. The medication label states 4 mg/mL. How many mL will you give? _____

3. A child weighs 23 lb and Dr. Walden ordered 0.3 mg/kg. The medication label states 10 mg/mL. How many mL will you give? _____

INTERNET ACTIVITIES

1. Using appropriate online resources, research medication errors in healthcare facilities. Create a poster, PowerPoint presentation, or a paper and include at least two citations. Discuss the following topics:
   a. Leading causes of medication errors
   b. How a medical assistant can prevent medication errors

Procedure 29.1   Calculate Proper Dosages of Medication for Administration

Name _____   Date _____   Score _____

Tasks: Calculate dosages for oral medication, injectable medication, and dosages for children.

Orders:
- Order 1: Dr. Martin orders ABC medication 135 mg. Stock bottle reads: 45 mg scored tablets
- Order 2: Dr. Martin orders ABC medication 650 mg. Stock bottle reads: 1300 mg scored tablets
- Order 3: Dr. Martin orders XYZ medication 430 mg IM. Stock bottle reads: 1000 mg/2 mL
- Order 4: Dr. Martin orders XYZ medication 680 mg IM. Stock bottle reads: 1200 mg/mL
- Order 5: Dr. Martin orders MNO medication 3 mg/kg IM. Child weighs 53 pounds. Stock bottle reads: 125 mg/mL
- Order 6: Dr. Martin orders MNO medication 5 mg/kg IM. Child weighs 71 pounds. Stock bottle reads: 225 mg/mL

Equipment and Supplies:
- Provider's order
- Paper and pencil
- Calculator (optional per instructor)

Standard: Complete the procedure and all critical steps in _____ minutes with a minimum score of 85% within two attempts (*or as indicated by the instructor*).

Scoring: Divide the points earned by the total possible points. Failure to perform a critical step, indicated by an asterisk (*), results in grade no higher than an 84% (*or as indicated by the instructor*).

Time: Began_____ Ended_____ Total minutes: _____

Steps:	Point Value	Attempt 1	Attempt 2
1. Using Order 1, calculate the number of tablets to give the patient. Label your answer.	10*		
2. Using Order 2, calculate the number of tablets to give the patient. Label your answer.	10*		
3. Using Order 3, calculate the amount in milliliters to give the patient. Round your answer to the nearest tenth. Label your answer.	15*		
4. Using Order 4, calculate the amount in milliliters to give the patient. Round your answer to the nearest tenth. Label your answer.	15*		
5. Using Order 5, calculate the amount in milliliters to give the patient. Round your answer to the nearest tenth. Label your answer.	20*		
6. Using Order 6, calculate the amount in milliliters to give the patient. Round your answer to the nearest tenth. Label your answer.	20*		
7. Double-check your answers to ensure the correct dose will be given.	10		
Total Points	100		

Comments

CAAHEP Competencies	Step(s)
II.P.1. Calculate proper dosages of medication for administration	Entire procedure
II.P.4. Apply mathematical computations to solve equations	Entire procedure
II.P.5. Convert among measurement systems	5-6
ABHES Competencies	**Step(s)**
6.b. Demonstrate accurate occupational math and metric conversions for proper medication administration	Entire procedure

Administering Medications

CAAHEP Competencies	Assessment
I.P.4.a. Verify the rules of medication administration: right patient	Procedures 30.1, 30.7 through 30.10
I.P.4.b. Verify the rules of medication administration: right medication	Procedures 30.1 through 30.10
I.P.4.c. Verify the rules of medication administration: right dose	Procedures 30.1 through 30.10
I.P.4.d. Verify the rules of medication administration: right route	Procedures 30.1 through 30.10
I.P.4.e. Verify the rules of medication administration: right time	Procedures 30.1 through 30.10
I.P.4.f. Verify the rules of medication administration: right documentation	Procedures 30.1, 30.7 through 30.10
I.P.5. Select proper sites for administering parenteral medication	Procedures 30.7 through 30.10
I.P.6. Administer oral medications	Procedure 30.1
I.P.7. Administer parenteral (excluding IV) medications	Procedures 30.7 through 30.10
II.P.1. Calculate proper dosages of medication for administration	Procedure 30.1
III.P.2. Select appropriate barrier/personal protective equipment (PPE)	Procedures 30.7 through 30.10
III.P.10.a. Demonstrate proper disposal of biohazardous material: sharps	Procedures 30.2 through 30.10
X.P.3. Document patient care accurately in the medical record	Procedures 30.1, 30.7 through 30.10
ABHES Competencies	**Assessment**
4. Medical Law and Ethics a. Follow documentation guidelines	Procedures 30.1, 30.7 through 30.10
8. Clinical Procedures a. Practice standard precautions and perform disinfection/sterilization techniques	Procedures 30.7 through 30.10
8.f. Prepare and administer oral and parenteral medications and monitor intravenous (IV) infusions	Procedures 30.1 through 30.10

VOCABULARY REVIEW

Using the word pool on the right, find the correct word to match the definition. Write the word on the line after the definition.

1. Another name for 0.9% sodium chloride _____

2. A dried substance (powder) that has been restored to a fluid form so it can be injected _____

3. Redness _____

4. Resistance to flow _____

5. Affecting the area where applied_____

6. A raised mark on the skin _____

7. Affecting the entire body _____

8. A liquid substance that dilutes or lessens the strength of a solution or mixture _____

9. Solid particles that settle out of a liquid _____

10. To withdraw fluid using suction _____

11. The inner measurement of a hollow space in a needle

    _____

12. The hardening of a normally soft tissue _____

Word Pool
- aspirate
- diluent
- erythema
- gauge
- induration
- local
- normal saline
- precipitate
- reconstituted
- systemic
- viscosity
- wheal

ABBREVIATIONS

Write out what each of the following abbreviations stands for.

1. EHR_____

2. VIS_____

3. Tdap _____

4. po_____

5. SL_____

6. MDI_____

7. IM _____

8. SUBQ_____

9. ID_____

10. IV _____

11. G _____

12. OSHA _____

13. TST _____

14. HIV _____

15. BCG_____

16. PPD _____

17. TB _____

18. NTM _____

19. QFT-Plus_____

20. Td _____

21. MMR_____

22. CDC_____

SKILLS AND CONCEPTS
Answer the following questions.

A. Introduction to the Nine Rights of Medication Administration
Fill in the blank.

1. Physical characteristics of a medication (e.g., tablet, suspension) are considered the

   _____.

2. The means by which a drug enters the body is called the _____.

Match the description with the correct right.

3. _____ Compare the medication amount to the provider's order.

4. _____ Respect patient's wishes, notify the provider of the refusal, and document the refusal and the provider who was notified.

5. _____ Compare the medication name and form to the provider's order.

6. _____ Must document the medication administration after giving the medication.

7. _____ Ask the patient or parent/guardian to state his or her full name and date of birth; information must match the order and the patient's health record.

8. _____ Compare the medication to the provider's order or look at the patient's vaccination history and age to ensure it is the correct time.

9. _____ Must tell the patient the name of the medication, who ordered it, verify the patient's allergies, and explain the action and common side effects of the medication.

10. _____ Compare the way the drug enters the body to the provider's order.

11. _____ Give it the correct way, perform any assessments prior to giving the medication, and give food or water if required.

a. right medication
b. right dose
c. right route
d. right time
e. right patient
f. right education
g. right to refuse
h. right technique
i. right documentation

Match the right to when it is done when administering medication. Answers can be used more than once.

12. _____ Right dose
13. _____ Right time
14. _____ Right patient
15. _____ Right education
16. _____ Right medication
17. _____ Right technique
18. _____ Right route
19. _____ Right to refuse
20. _____ Right documentation

a. completed when preparing medications
b. completed with the patient prior to administration
c. done after giving the medication

Select the correct answer.

21. When is the medication label checked against the provider's order?
    a. First check is done when the medication is taken from the storage area.
    b. Second check is done before measuring the medication.
    c. Third check is done before returning the medication to the storage area.
    d. All of the above.

B. Administering Vaccines
Match the description or vaccines with the correct type of vaccine. Answers can be used more than once.

1. _____ Hib, hepatitis B, HPV, pertussis, pneumococcal, meningococcal, and shingles

2. _____ Hepatitis A, (injectable) influenza, (injectable) polio, and rabies

3. _____ Diphtheria and tetanus

4. _____ MMR, varicella, and yellow fever

5. _____ Use specific pieces of the microorganism, which creates a very strong immune response

6. _____ Use the toxin made by the microorganism

7. _____ The microorganism is dead

8. _____ The microorganism is alive but weakened in the laboratory

a. inactivated vaccine
b. live-attenuated vaccine
c. subunit, recombinant, polysaccharide, and conjugate vaccines
d. toxoid vaccine

Fill in the blank.

9. Patients may not receive a live-virus vaccine if they were vaccinated with another live-virus vaccine less than _____ days earlier.

10. Patients may not receive a live-virus vaccine if they are _____, immunocompromised, or receiving chemotherapy or high-dose steroid therapy.

C. Routes of Medication

Fill in the blank or select the correct answer.

1. If _____ tablets are crushed, chewed, or cut, a person gets the dose faster than they should, resulting in an overdose.

2. If _____ tablets are crushed, chewed, or cut, the protective nature of the coating is lost.

3. _____ medications are placed under the tongue.

4. _____ medications are placed between the cheek and the gums.

5. _____ medications are placed on the skin and absorbed into the bloodstream.

6. What must a medical assistant do when applying a transdermal patch?
   a. Write the date and time on the new patch.
   b. Wear gloves, remove the old patch, and wipe off any residual medication.
   c. Place the new patch in a new location.
   d. All of the above.

7. Applying a drug to a mucous membrane or the skin is considered use of the _____ route.

8. Medications given via the nasal route should be charted as _____.

9. The _____ route means to administer medication to the eye.

10. The _____ route means to administer medication to the ear.

11. _____ means to bathe or flush open wounds or body cavities.

12. The _____ route involves administration by infusion, injection, or implantation.

13. _____ means to administer within a muscle.

14. _____ means to administer beneath the skin.

15. _____ means to administer within the dermis.

D. Needles and Syringes

Match the description to the correct part of the hypodermic needle.

1. _____ Hollow space inside the needle
2. _____ Slanted end of the shaft
3. _____ Where the needle attaches
4. _____ Attaches or screws onto the syringe

a. hub
b. hilt
c. bevel
d. lumen

Fill in the blank.

5. A(n) _____ safety needle is designed so that the needle is automatically covered after the injection.

6. A(n) _____ safety needle requires the healthcare professional to activate the safety device.

E. Working with the Needle and Syringe
Select the correct answer.

1. Never recap a needle that has been used on a patient; cover the needle with the safety device. Needles can be recapped until they are used on a patient.
    a. Both statements are correct.
    b. Both statements are incorrect.
    c. The first statement is correct, and the second statement is incorrect.
    d. The first statement is incorrect, and the second statement is correct.

2. When uncapping a needle, hold the cover with your nondominant hand and the syringe with your dominant hand. Pull your hands apart vertically in a smooth continuous motion.
    a. Both statements are correct.
    b. Both statements are incorrect.
    c. The first statement is correct, and the second statement is incorrect.
    d. The first statement is incorrect, and the second statement is correct.

3. When recapping a needle, use the one-handed scoop technique. If the needle touches the outside surface of the cover or any other surface, it is *not* contaminated.
    a. Both statements are correct.
    b. Both statements are incorrect.
    c. The first statement is correct, and the second statement is incorrect.
    d. The first statement is incorrect, and the second statement is correct.

F. Preparing Parenteral Medication
Select the correct answer or fill in the blank.

1. Which medication(s) should be discarded and *not* used?
    a. Medication that looks abnormal in color or clarity.
    b. Medication that has precipitate at the bottom of the vial.
    c. Expired medications.
    d. Medications that are no longer sterile.
    e. All of the above,

2. Which supplies are used when preparing medication from an ampule?
    a. Filter needle and a safety needle
    b. Syringe
    c. Ampule opener or breaker
    d. All of the above

3. A(n) _____ is a plastic or glass container with a rubber stopper that is covered by a cap.

4. 0.9% sodium chloride is also called _____.

5. When multidose vials are opened, they are only good for _____ days.

Match the description with the correct step when reconstituting powdered medication.

6. _____ Add in air and withdraw the dose needed.

7. _____ Remove air from the powdered medication vial and put air into the diluent vial.

8. _____ Mix the liquid with the powdered medication.

9. _____ Withdraw liquid from the diluent vial and add it to the powdered medication vial.

a. Step 1
b. Step 2
c. Step 3
d. Step 4

Fill in the blank.

10. Insulin is measured in _____.

11. Insulins like NPH are _____ and require _____ before withdrawing the medication.

G. Giving Parenteral Medications

Select the correct answer or fill in the blank.

1. Which is an advantage of parenteral medication administration?
   a. It is useful when the patient has gastrointestinal distress or is unconscious.
   b. It offers good absorption compared with other routes, such as the oral route.
   c. The onset is more rapid than with other routes.
   d. Some types of parenteral medications have a longer duration.
   e. All of the above.

2. Pain with the injection and a risk of infection due to the injection are disadvantages of parenteral medications. The predictable absorption rate for those with poor circulation is also another disadvantage.
   a. Both statements are correct.
   b. Both statements are incorrect.
   c. The first statement is correct, and the second statement is incorrect.
   d. The first statement is incorrect, and the second statement is correct.

3. When selecting an injection site, avoid scar tissue, bones, blood vessels, abrasions, and wounds. Select a site that is large enough to hold the amount of medication injected.
   a. Both statements are correct.
   b. Both statements are incorrect.
   c. The first statement is correct, and the second statement is incorrect.
   d. The first statement is incorrect, and the second statement is correct.

4. If the needle breaks off and it is not visible, mark the spot with a pen and yell for help. If the injection was given in the arm, place a tourniquet below the spot to prevent the needle from moving in the body.
   a. Both statements are correct.
   b. Both statements are incorrect.
   c. The first statement is correct, and the second statement is incorrect.
   d. The first statement is incorrect, and the second statement is correct.

5. With intramuscular injections, if a bone is hit during the procedure, pull the needle out about _____ inch and give the medication.

6. _____ is a severe allergic reaction that can be life-threatening.

7. Which are symptoms of anaphylaxis?
   a. Warm feeling, flushing, throat tightening, difficulty swallowing, and cough
   b. Shortness of breath, dyspnea, and wheezing
   c. Anxiety, loss of consciousness, and shock
   d. Pain or cramping, vomiting, diarrhea, palpitations, and dizziness
   e. All of the above

8. The first-line medication for anaphylaxis is _____.

H. Intradermal Tuberculin Testing
Select the correct answer or fill in the blank.

1. Patients with a history of BCG vaccination may have a(n) _____ reaction to the TST.

2. Which patient should *not* receive a TST?
   a. A patient with a history of a severe reaction to a TST.
   b. A patient with a history of a positive TST result.
   c. A patient who had a live virus vaccine 8 weeks ago.
   d. All of the above.
   e. Both a and b.

3. When performing a TST, tuberculin purified protein derivative _____ is given intradermally in the forearm.

4. After a patient is given the tuberculin purified protein derivative, the wheal must be _____ in diameter, or the test must be repeated.

5. The patient returns within _____ hours to have the test read.

6. When reading a TST, the induration is measured across the forearm using a millimeter ruler. The erythema is also measured in millimeters.
   a. Both statements are correct.
   b. Both statements are incorrect.
   c. The first statement is correct, and the second statement is incorrect.
   d. The first statement is incorrect, and the second statement is correct.

7. A(n) _____ reaction means the person reacted to the test even though no *M. tuberculosis* is present.

8. A(n) _____ reaction means the person may not have reacted to the test, even though the patient is infected with *M. tuberculosis*.

9. Which is a reason for a false-negative result with a TST?
   a. Weakened immune system
   b. Exposure to TB infection within previous 12 to 15 weeks
   c. Patient is younger than 12 months old
   d. All of the above
   e. Both a and b

10. With two-step TST testing, a booster effect can occur, causing the body to "remember" the infection after the second TST. The second TST can be done 1 to 3 weeks after the initial test was read.
    a. Both statements are correct.
    b. Both statements are incorrect.
    c. The first statement is correct, and the second statement is incorrect.
    d. The first statement is incorrect, and the second statement is correct.

I. Subcutaneous Injections
Select the correct answer or fill in the blank.

1. The medication absorbs _____ in the subcutaneous layer compared with medications injected into the muscles.

2. If a 5/8-inch needle is used, then the medical assistant should use a _____-degree angle.

3. If a 1/2-inch needle is used, then a _____-degree angle should be applied.

4. When giving a SUBQ injection in the abdomen, the site is located below the _____ to the iliac crests and stay _____ inches away from the umbilicus.

5. When giving a SUBQ injection in the outer posterior aspect of the upper arm, be at least _____ inches above the elbow.

6. When giving a SUBQ injection in the anterior aspect of the thigh, the _____ of the thigh from the front midline to the outer thigh is used.

J. Intramuscular Injections
Select the correct answer or fill in the blank.

1. Intramuscular injections absorb faster than SUBQ injections because there are more _____ in the muscles.

2. When administering an IM injection, it is important to use a _____-degree angle for entry.

3. Once the needle is in the site, the medical assistant should aspirate by pulling back on the plunger for _____ seconds and check for blood in the syringe.

4. If blood appears in the barrel, change needles, and inject the medication in a new site. Immunizations do not need to be aspirated.
    a. Both statements are correct.
    b. Both statements are incorrect.
    c. The first statement is correct, and the second statement is incorrect.
    d. The first statement is incorrect, and the second statement is correct.

5. When doing the air lock technique for an IM injection, the medical assistant can skip removing the bubbles and just measure the exact amount of medication ordered. The medical assistant needs to add 0.5 mL to 0.7 mL of air into the syringe.
    a. Both statements are correct.
    b. Both statements are incorrect.
    c. The first statement is correct, and the second statement is incorrect.
    d. The first statement is incorrect, and the second statement is correct.

6. When finding the deltoid muscle, place a finger on the _____ and then two fingers below that to find the top of the site and the bottom of the site is at the anterior axillary fold.

7. The vastus lateralis can be used for patients of any age. The vastus lateralis site uses the middle third of the thigh and the site extends from the midline of the thigh to the midline of the outer thigh.
    a. Both statements are correct.
    b. Both statements are incorrect.
    c. The first statement is correct, and the second statement is incorrect.
    d. The first statement is incorrect, and the second statement is correct.

8. When finding the ventrogluteal site, your palm is placed on the patient's greater trochanter, with your fingers pointing toward the person's head and your thumb toward the groin. Your index finger is on or pointing to the anterior superior iliac spine and your middle finger is moved back on the iliac crest toward the buttock.
   a. Both statements are correct.
   b. Both statements are incorrect.
   c. The first statement is correct, and the second statement is incorrect.
   d. The first statement is incorrect, and the second statement is correct.

9. When giving an IM injection, use a _____ to _____ -gauge needle.

10. The maximum volume for a deltoid injection for an adult is _____ mL.

11. When giving two IM injections in the same muscle, separate the injections by _____ inch(es).

CERTIFICATION PREPARATION
Circle the correct answer.

1. When providing the "right education" prior to medication administration, what must the medical assistant do?
   a. Give the name of the medication and who ordered the medication.
   b. Give the desired effect or action and common side effects of the medication.
   c. Verify the patient's allergies.
   d. All of the above.

2. Which type of medication is placed under the tongue?
   a. Transdermal
   b. Inhaled
   c. Sublingual
   d. Buccal

3. What is *not* proper procedure when administering buccal medications?
   a. Always use the same cheek.
   b. Give water immediately after administering the medication.
   c. Allow smoking and eating just prior to administration of the medication.
   d. None of the above are proper procedure.

4. The parenteral route is administered by
   a. implantation.
   b. infusion.
   c. injection.
   d. all of the above.

5. Which syringe and needle would be most appropriate for a TST?
   a. 3 mL syringe; 1/2 inch, 25-gauge needle
   b. 3 mL syringe; 5/8 inch, 21-gauge needle
   c. 1 mL syringe; 3/8 inch, 27-gauge needle
   d. 1 mL syringe; 1/2 inch, 23-gauge needle

6. Which is true regarding TST?
   a. A TST and a live virus vaccine can be given on the same day.
   b. A TST can be given 2-3 weeks after a live virus vaccine.
   c. A live virus vaccine does not impact the TST results.
   d. Options a and b are true.

7. Which syringe and needle would be most appropriate for an adult subcutaneous 90-degree injection?
   a. 3 mL syringe; 1/2 inch, 25-gauge needle
   b. 3 mL syringe; 5/8 inch, 21-gauge needle
   c. 1 mL syringe; 3/8 inch, 27-gauge needle
   d. 1 mL syringe; 5/8 inch, 23-gauge needle

8. When giving an IM vaccine injection to an 8-month-old child, which site is used?
   a. Deltoid
   b. Vastus lateralis
   c. Ventrogluteal
   d. Only a and b

9. Which syringe and needle would be most appropriate to use when giving a deltoid IM injection to an adult male weighing 180 pounds?
    a. 3 mL syringe; 5/8 inch, 25-gauge needle
    b. 3 mL syringe; 1 1/4 inch, 22-gauge needle
    c. 1 mL syringe; 1 inch, 20-gauge needle
    d. 3 mL syringe; 1 inch, 27-gauge needle

10. Which syringe and needle would be most appropriate to use when giving a deltoid IM injection to 5-year-old child?
    a. 3 mL syringe; 5/8 inch, 20-gauge needle
    b. 3 mL syringe; 1 1/4 inch, 22-gauge needle
    c. 3 mL syringe; 5/8 inch, 23-gauge needle
    d. 1 mL syringe; 1 inch, 27-gauge needle

WORKPLACE APPLICATIONS

1. You are giving an analgesic to a patient. You need to obtain the patient's pain level rating before you give the medication. Describe how you would explain a 0 to 10 pain scale to an adult.

_____

_____

_____

_____

2. The patient states, "I am a recovering alcoholic." Explain why it is important for the medical assistant to communicate this information to the provider.

_____

_____

_____

_____

3. A patient needs a two-step TST. The patient asks Gabe why one test is not "good enough." Describe how Gabe would answer the patient.

_____

_____

_____

_____

INTERNET ACTIVITIES

1. Using the CDC website (https://www.cdc.gov/), research two routine Vaccine Information Statements (VIS). In a paper, PowerPoint presentation, or poster, address the following points:
    a. For each VIS:
        i. Name the vaccine.
        ii. Discuss reasons to get the vaccine.
        iii. Indicate who should get the vaccine.
        iv. List the situations when the vaccine should not be given.
        v. Describe the risks from the vaccine, including the common, uncommon, and very rare problems.
    b. Describe severe allergic reactions and what should be done.

2. Using the CDC website (https://www.cdc.gov/), search for "vaccines and immunization." Go to Vaccine and Immunization home page and then click on link for healthcare providers. Review the materials and tools available to healthcare professionals. Create a paper, PowerPoint Presentation, or poster and summarize your findings.

3. Using the CDC website (https://www.cdc.gov/), search for "travelers health." Review the materials and tools available to travelers and healthcare professionals. Create a paper, PowerPoint Presentation, or poster and summarize your findings.

Procedure 30.1   Administering Oral Medications

Name _____ Date _____ Score _____

Tasks: Calculate the dose to give. Prepare a liquid and a solid medication and administer medications to a patient. Document medication administration.

Equipment and Supplies:
- Provider's orders
- Patient's health record
- Drug reference information
- Liquid medication and a solid medication (use drug labels shown)
- Paper cup
- Plastic medication cup
- Marker
- Medication tray
- Glass of water

Orders: Diltiazem 240 mg po and cephalexin suspension 375 mg po.

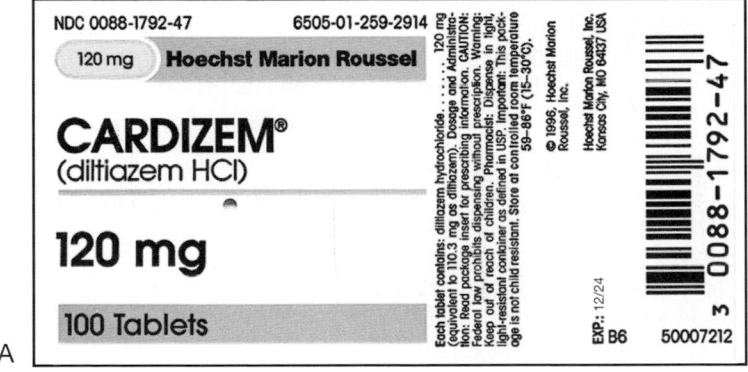

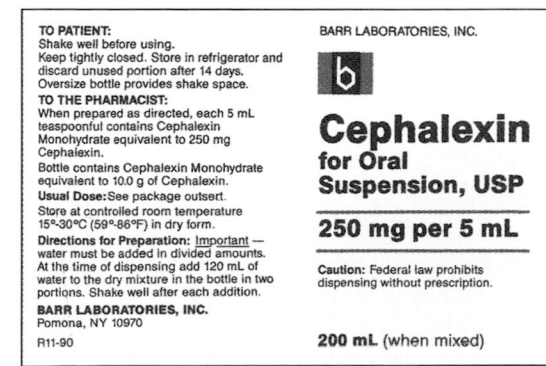

(From Brown M, Mulholland JM: Drug calculations: process and problems for clinical practice, ed 9, St. Louis, 2012.)

Standard: Complete the procedure and all critical steps in _____ minutes with a minimum score of 85% within two attempts (*or as indicated by the instructor*).

Scoring: Divide the points earned by the total possible points. Failure to perform a critical step, indicated by an asterisk (*), results in grade no higher than an 84% (*or as indicated by the instructor*).

Time: Began_____ Ended_____ Total minutes: _____

Steps:	Point Value	Attempt 1	Attempt 2
1. Using the drug reference information and the orders, review the information on the medications.	5		
2. Using the orders and the drug labels shown, calculate the amount of medication you need to give. Verify the right doses with the instructor. Verify if it is the right time for the order if that applies.	10*		
3. Wash your hands or use hand sanitizer. Select the right medications from the storage area. Check each medication label against the order. Check for the right name, form, and route. Check the expiration date to make sure the drug is not expired.	5*		
4. Assemble the supplies required to prepare the medications. Using the marker, write the medication name and dose on the appropriate cups.	5		
5. Perform the second medication check. Check each medication label against the order. Check for the right name, form, and route.	5*		
6. For the solid medication: Remove the cover of the container and hold it so the inside is facing up. Carefully pour the correct number of tablets into the cover. If you pour too many into the cover, pour the extra tablets back into the bottle. When you have the correct number of tablets in the cover, pour them from the cover into the paper cup. Place the cover on the container. Make sure not to contaminate the inside of the container or the cover.	10*		
7. For liquid medication: a. Place the plastic medication cup on a high, even surface. Uncover the bottle and place the cover on the counter, making sure the inside is facing up. Place your palm over the medication label. Position yourself so you are eye level with the medication cup. b. Pour the medication into the cup until the lowest point of the meniscus is at the measurement needed. c. If too much medication is poured into the cup, flush the extra down the sink. Replace the cover on the bottle without contaminating the inside of the cover or bottle.	10*		
8. Place the medication cups on the medication tray. Clean up the area.	5		
9. Perform the third medication check. Check each medication label against the order. Check for the right name, form, and route. Verify that the amount of medication in each cup is correct according to the order.	5*		
10. Prior to entering the exam room, knock on the door and wait a moment. Greet the patient. Identify yourself. Verify the patient's identity with full name and date of birth. Make sure the patient's information matches the order and the record. Explain what you are going to do.	10*		
11. Provide the right education to the patient. Explain the medication ordered, the desired effect, and common side effects, and identify the provider who ordered it. Answer any questions the patient may have. Use language the patient can understand. Ask the patient if they have any allergies. If the patient refuses the medication, notify the provider.	10		
12. Perform the right technique. Do any assessments required prior to giving the medication. If the patient can have water with the medication, have water available.	5		

13. Allow patients to take the medication in their hand or to use the cup. Stay with the patient until the medication has been taken.	5		
14. Document the procedure in the health record. Include assessments done; allergies; teaching or instructions provided; the name of the provider who ordered the medication; the medication's name, dose, and route; and how the patient tolerated the medication. For vaccines and controlled substances, add the lot number, the expiration date, and the manufacturer's number.	10*		
Total Points	100		

Documentation

Comments

CAAHEP Competencies	Step(s)
I.P.4.a. Verify the rules of medication administration: right patient	10
I.P.4.b. Verify the rules of medication administration: right medication	3, 5, 9
I.P.4.c. Verify the rules of medication administration: right dose	2, 6, 7, 9
I.P.4.d. Verify the rules of medication administration: right route	3, 5, 9
I.P.4.e. Verify the rules of medication administration: right time	2
I.P.4.f. Verify the rules of medication administration: right documentation	14
I.P.6. Administer oral medications	Entire procedure
II.P.1. Calculate proper dosages of medication for administration	2
X.P.3. Document patient care accurately in the medical record	14
ABHES Competencies	**Step(s)**
4. Medical Law and Ethics a. Follow documentation guidelines	14
8. Clinical Procedures f. Prepare and administer oral and parenteral medications and monitor intravenous (IV) infusions	Entire procedure

Procedure 30.2 Prepare Medication from an Ampule

Name _____ Date _____ Score _____

Task: Prepare medication from an ampule.

Equipment and Supplies:
- Provider's order
- Ampule of medication
- Gauze or ampule breaker
- Alcohol wipes
- Filter needle and hypodermic safety needle
- 3 mL syringe
- Biohazard sharps container
- Waste container
- Drug reference information
- Marker

Order: 0.9% sodium chloride 0.7 mL IM

Standard: Complete the procedure and all critical steps in _____ minutes with a minimum score of 85% within two attempts (*or as indicated by the instructor*).

Scoring: Divide the points earned by the total possible points. Failure to perform a critical step, indicated by an asterisk (*), results in grade no higher than an 84% (*or as indicated by the instructor*).

Time: Began _____ Ended _____ Total minutes: _____

Steps:	Point Value	Attempt 1	Attempt 2
1. Wash your hands or use hand sanitizer. Using the drug reference information and the order, review the information on the medication if needed. Clarify any questions you have with the provider.	5		
2. Select the right medication from the storage area. Check the medication label against the order. Check for the right name, form, and route. Check the expiration date to make sure the drug is not expired. Verify the right dose and the right time.	5*		
3. Assemble the supplies required for the procedure.	5		
4. Perform the second medication check. Check the medication label against the order. Check for the right name, form, dose, and route.	5*		
5. Attach the filter needle to the syringe without contaminating the unit. Using a marker, label the syringe with the medication name.	5*		
6. Gently tap the medication from the head of the ampule or hold the ampule securely, upright in your hand. Quickly move your hand downward. After all the medication has drained into the body of the ampule, wipe the neck with an alcohol wipe.	5		

7.	Place the ampule breaker over the head of the ampule (following the directions from the manufacturer) or wrap the neck with gauze. Hold the body with your nondominant hand. With your dominant hand, firmly hold the head (or breaker) between your first two fingers and thumb. Quickly snap off the head of the ampule, making sure it breaks away from your body and others.	10*		
8.	Discard the breaker or gauze with the ampule head in a biohazard sharps container.	5		
9	Place the ampule on a flat surface. Uncover the filter needle and insert the needle into the ampule without contaminating the needle. Keeping the bevel in the medication, pull the plunger upward, aspirating the medication into the syringe. Tilt the ampule as you remove all the medication.	10		
10.	Recap the needle using the one-handed scoop technique. Perform the third medication check. Check the medication label against the order. Check for the right name, form, and route. Discard the ampule in the biohazardous sharps container.	5*		
11.	Remove the filter needle and attach a new needle without contaminating the unit. Discard the filter needle in the biohazardous sharps container.	5*		
12.	Hold the syringe in a vertical position with the uncapped needle pointed upward. Tap the barrel carefully with the fingertips or a pen to move the air bubbles up to the top of the barrel. Once all the air bubbles are at the top, push the plunger slowly to the correct calibration marking for the ordered dose. Recap the needle.	10*		
13.	Double-check the dose of medication measured against the order. Make sure no air bubbles are in the syringe.	10*		
14.	Maintain the sterility of the medication and the needle throughout the procedure.	10*		
15.	Clean up the work area. Packaging and other waste should be discarded in the waste container.	5		
	Total Points	100		

Comments

CAAHEP Competencies	Step(s)
I.P.4.b. Verify the rules of medication administration: right medication	2, 4, 10
I.P.4.c. Verify the rules of medication administration: right dose	2, 4, 12, 13
I.P.4.d. Verify the rules of medication administration: right route	2, 4, 10
I.P.4.e. Verify the rules of medication administration: right time	2
III.P.10.a. Demonstrate proper disposal of biohazardous material: sharps	10, 11
ABHES Competencies	**Step(s)**
8. Clinical Procedures f. Prepare and administer oral and parenteral medications and monitor intravenous (IV) infusions	Entire procedure

Procedure 30.3   Prepare Medication Using a Prefilled Sterile Cartridge

Name _____ Date _____ Score _____

Tasks: Prepare medication using a prefilled sterile cartridge. Discard a prefilled sterile cartridge with a reusable holder.

Equipment and Supplies:
- Provider's order
- Prefilled sterile cartridge
- Hypodermic safety needle (if needed)
- Carpuject cartridge holder
- Biohazard sharps container
- Waste container
- Drug reference information

Order: 0.9% sodium chloride 1.6 mL IM

Standard: Complete the procedure and all critical steps in _____ minutes with a minimum score of 85% within two attempts (*or as indicated by the instructor*).

Scoring: Divide the points earned by the total possible points. Failure to perform a critical step, indicated by an asterisk (*), results in grade no higher than an 84% (*or as indicated by the instructor*).

Time: Began_____ Ended_____ Total minutes: _____

Steps:	Point Value	Attempt 1	Attempt 2
1. Wash your hands or use hand sanitizer. Using the drug reference information and the order, review the information on the medication if needed. Clarify any questions you have with the provider.	5		
2. Select the right medication from the storage area. Check the medication label against the order. Check for the right name, form, and route. Check the expiration date to make sure the drug is not expired. Verify the right dose and the right time.	5*		
3. Assemble the supplies required for the procedure.	5		
4. Perform the second medication check. Check the medication label against the order. Check for the right name, form, dose, and route.	5*		
5. Break the seal. With one hand on the needle cover and the other on the barrel of the prefilled cartridge, move your hands together until you hear a pop. If needed, remove the cover on the cartridge and attach a covered safety needle.	5		
6. Hold the Carpuject holder so the opening (for the barrel) is facing up. Pull the plunger rod out until it clicks. Turn the blue lock until it clicks. This should increase the space between the blue lock and the flange.	10		
7. Insert the cartridge into the Carpuject holder. To secure the cartridge, turn the blue lock on the Carpuject holder until it clicks. The space between the blue lock and the flange should decrease. Turn the white plunger rod until it screws onto the rubber stopper.	10*		

8.	Remove the cover. Hold the syringe unit in a vertical position with the uncapped needle or tip pointed upward. Tap the barrel carefully with the fingertips or a pen to move the air bubbles up to the top of the barrel. Once all the air bubbles are at the top, push the plunger slowly to the correct calibration marking for the ordered dose.	10*		
9.	Recap the needle using the one-handed scoop technique. Perform the third medication check. Check the medication label against the order. Check for the right name, form, and route.	10*		
10.	Double-check the dose of medication measured against the order. Make sure no air bubbles are in the syringe.	5*		
11.	Maintain sterility of the medication and the needle throughout the procedure.	10		
12.	After giving the injection, unscrew the plunger rod and pull out until it clicks. Turn the blue lock until it clicks. The space between the blue lock and the flange should increase in size.	5		
13.	Carefully invert the Carpuject holder over a biohazardous sharps container to discard the cartridge. Hold the Carpuject holder firmly so it does not end up in the sharps container.	10*		
14.	Disinfect the Carpuject holder. Clean up the work area. Waste should be put in the waste container.	5		
	Total Points	100		

Comments

CAAHEP Competencies	Step(s)
I.P.4.b. Verify the rules of medication administration: right medication	2, 4, 9
I.P.4.c. Verify the rules of medication administration: right dose	2, 4, 8, 10
I.P.4.d. Verify the rules of medication administration: right route	2, 4, 9
I.P.4.e. Verify the rules of medication administration: right time	2
III.P.10.a. Demonstrate proper disposal of biohazardous material: sharps	13
ABHES Competencies	**Step(s)**
8. Clinical Procedures f. Prepare and administer oral and parenteral medications and monitor intravenous (IV) infusions	Entire procedure

Procedure 30.4 Prepare Medication from a Vial

Name _____ Date _____ Score _____

Task: Prepare medication from a vial.

Equipment and Supplies:
- Provider's order
- Vial of medication
- Alcohol wipes
- Hypodermic safety needle and 3 mL syringe or needle/syringe unit
- Biohazard sharps container
- Waste container
- Drug reference information
- Marker

Order: 0.9% sodium chloride 1.2 mL IM

Standard: Complete the procedure and all critical steps in _____ minutes with a minimum score of 85% within two attempts (*or as indicated by the instructor*).

Scoring: Divide the points earned by the total possible points. Failure to perform a critical step, indicated by an asterisk (*), results in grade no higher than an 84% (*or as indicated by the instructor*).

Time: Began_____ Ended_____ Total minutes: _____

Steps:	Point Value	Attempt 1	Attempt 2
1. Wash your hands or use hand sanitizer. Using the drug reference information and the order, review the information on the medication if needed. Clarify any questions you have with the provider.	5		
2. Select the right medication from the storage area. Check the medication label against the order. Check for the right name, form, and route. Check the expiration date to make sure the drug is not expired. Verify the right dose and the right time.	5*		
3. Assemble the supplies required for the procedure.	5		
4. Perform the second medication check. Check the medication label against the order. Check for the right name, form, dose, and route.	5*		
5. Open the syringe and needle. Tighten the preassembled syringe and needle unit or attach the needle to the syringe. Using a marker, label the syringe with the medication name.	5		
6. Mix the medication by rolling it with your hands if needed. Remove the cap on the vial (if present). Clean the rubber stopper with an alcohol wipe. Let the stopper dry.	5*		
7. With the syringe in a vertical position, pull the syringe plunger down. Draw up an amount of air equal to the amount of medication ordered.	5*		
8. Hold the vial firmly against a flat surface. Insert the needle into the center of the dried rubber stopper. Inject the aspirated air above the fluid in the vial.	5		

9.	With the palm of your nondominant hand facing upward, grasp the vial between your middle and index fingers. Keeping the syringe unit in the vial, pick up and invert them. Use your thumb and the ring and little fingers of your nondominant hand to stabilize the syringe in the vial.	10		
10.	With the syringe at eye level, pull the plunger down using your dominant hand. Fill the syringe with more medication than what was ordered.	10		
11.	Continue to hold the vial/needle/syringe unit in a vertical position (with the needle pointing upward) with your nondominant hand. With your dominant hand, either use your fingers or a pen to tap the bubbles to the top of the barrel.	5		
12.	Once all the air bubbles are at the top, push the plunger slowly to the correct calibration marking for the ordered dose.	10*		
13.	Double-check that no air bubbles are in the syringe and the right dose was measured. If everything is correct, remove the vial from the syringe/needle unit.	5*		
14.	Use the one-hand scoop technique to cover the needle. Perform the third medication check. Check each medication label against the order. Check for the right name, form, and route.	5*		
15.	Maintain sterility of the medication and the needle throughout the procedure.	10*		
16.	Clean up the work area.	5		
	Total Points	100		

Comments

CAAHEP Competencies	Step(s)
I.P.4.b. Verify the rules of medication administration: right medication	2, 4, 14
I.P.4.c. Verify the rules of medication administration: right dose	2, 4, 13
I.P.4.d. Verify the rules of medication administration: right route	2, 4, 14
I.P.4.e. Verify the rules of medication administration: right time	2
ABHES Competencies	**Step(s)**
8. Clinical Procedures f. Prepare and administer oral and parenteral medications and monitor intravenous (IV) infusions	Entire procedure

Procedure 30.5 Reconstituting Powdered Medication

Name _____ Date _____ Score _____

Tasks: Reconstitute powdered medication and prepare the dose of medication.

Equipment and Supplies:
- Provider's order
- Vial of powdered medication
- Vial of diluent
- Alcohol wipes
- Two hypodermic syringes (a 3 mL and a larger syringe)
- Two hypodermic safety needles
- Biohazard sharps container
- Waste container
- Drug reference information
- Marker

Order: (Powdered medication name) 0.5 mL IM or use the order provided by the instructor.

Standard: Complete the procedure and all critical steps in _____ minutes with a minimum score of 85% within two attempts (*or as indicated by the instructor*).

Scoring: Divide the points earned by the total possible points. Failure to perform a critical step, indicated by an asterisk (*), results in grade no higher than an 84% (*or as indicated by the instructor*).

Time: Began_____ Ended_____ Total minutes: _____

Steps:	Point Value	Attempt 1	Attempt 2
1. Wash your hands or use hand sanitizer. Using the drug reference information and the order, review the information on the medication if needed. Clarify any questions you have with the provider.	2		
2. Select the right medication from the storage area. Check the medication label against the order. Check for the right name, form, and route. Check the expiration date to make sure the vials are not expired. Verify the right dose and the right time. Read the medication label to determine the correct diluent. Obtain the diluent and check the name, route, and expiration date.	5*		
3. Assemble the supplies required for the procedure. If needed, calculate the dose of medication required.	3		
4. Perform the second medication check. Check the medication labels against the order and directions for reconstituting the powder. Check for the right name, form, and route.	5*		
5. Open and assemble the syringes and needles. Using a marker, label the 3-mL syringe with the medication name.	2		
6. Remove the caps on the vials. Clean the rubber stoppers with an alcohol wipe. Let the stoppers dry.	3*		
7. With the powdered medication vial on a firm surface, insert the needle of the largest volume syringe unit. Make sure the tip stays out of the powder. Pull back on the plunger and withdraw air equal to the amount of diluent that must be added. Pull the needle/syringe out of the stopper.	5*		

8.	Using the syringe with the aspirated air (equal to the amount of diluent needed), insert the needle into the center of the dried rubber stopper of the diluent vial. Push the air into the vial, but do not force the air into the vial. Make sure the needle is not in the fluid.	**5**		
9.	With the palm of your nondominant hand facing upward, grasp the vial between your middle and index fingers. Keeping the syringe unit in the vial, pick up and invert them. Use your thumb and the ring and little fingers of your nondominant hand to stabilize the syringe in the vial. Pull down on the plunger until you have more diluent than what you need.	**5**		
10.	Continue to hold the vial/needle/syringe unit in a vertical position (with the needle pointing upward) with your nondominant hand. With your dominant hand, either use your fingers or a pen to tap the bubbles to the top of the barrel.	**5**		
11.	Once all the air bubbles are at the top, push the plunger slowly to the correct calibration marking for the ordered dose. Keep the syringe at eye level.	**5***		
12.	Double-check that no air bubbles are in the syringe and the right dose was measured. If everything is correct, remove the vial from the syringe/needle unit.	**5***		
13.	Using an alcohol wipe, clean the rubber stopper of the powdered medication vial. With the vial flat on a hard surface, insert the needle into the dried stopper. Push the diluent into the vial. If resistance is met, take your finger off the plunger and allow air to fill in the syringe. Gradually work all the diluent into the vial. Withdraw the needle from the vial and discard the needle and syringe in the biohazardous sharps container.	**5***		
14.	Gently mix the vial by rolling it in your palms. Mix the medication until all the powder is dissolved.	**2**		
15.	Clean the rubber stopper of the powdered medication vial with an alcohol wipe. Let the stopper dry. With the second syringe in a vertical position, pull the syringe plunger down. Draw up an amount of air equal to the amount of medication ordered.	**3***		
16.	Hold the vial firmly against a flat surface. Insert the needle into the center of the dried rubber stopper. Inject the aspirated air above the fluid in the vial.	**2**		
17.	With the palm of your nondominant hand facing upward, grasp the vial between your middle and index fingers. Keeping the syringe unit in the vial, pick up and invert them. Use your thumb and the ring and little fingers of your nondominant hand to stabilize the syringe in the vial.	**3**		
18.	With the syringe at eye level, pull the plunger down using your dominant hand. Fill the syringe with more medication than what was ordered.	**5**		
19.	Continue to hold the vial/needle/syringe unit in a vertical position (with the needle pointing upward) with your nondominant hand. With your dominant hand, either use your fingers or a pen to tap the bubbles to the top of the barrel.	**5**		
20.	Once all the air bubbles are at the top, push the plunger slowly to the correct calibration marking for the ordered dose.	**5***		
21.	Double-check that no air bubbles are in the syringe and the right dose was measured. If everything is correct, remove the vial from the syringe/needle unit.	**5***		

22. Use the one-hand scoop technique to cover the needle. Perform the third medication check. Check each medication label against the order. Check for the right name, form, and route.	5*		
23. Maintain sterility of the medication and the needle throughout the procedure.	5		
24. If the medication is in a multidose vial, label the vial with the expiration date, diluent added, and your initials. Clean up the work area. Put the packaging and other waste in the waste container. Discard the vial(s) in the biohazardous waste container.	5		
Total Points	100		

Comments

CAAHEP Competencies	**Step(s)**
I.P.4.b. Verify the rules of medication administration: right medication	2, 4, 22
I.P.4.c. Verify the rules of medication administration: right dose	2, 20, 21
I.P.4.d. Verify the rules of medication administration: right route	2, 4, 22
I.P.4.e. Verify the rules of medication administration: right time	2
III.P.10.a. Demonstrate proper disposal of biohazardous material: sharps	13, 24
ABHES Competencies	**Step(s)**
8. Clinical Procedures f. Prepare and administer oral and parenteral medications and monitor intravenous (IV) infusions	Entire procedure

Procedure 30.6   Mixing Two Insulins

Name _____   **Date** _____   **Score** _____

Task: Mix two types of insulin in one syringe.

Equipment and Supplies:
- Provider's order
- Regular insulin vial
- NPH insulin vial
- Alcohol wipes
- U100 insulin needle and syringe unit
- Biohazard sharps container
- Waste container
- Drug reference information
- Marker

Order: Regular insulin 16 units mixed with NPH insulin 30 units SUBQ.

Standard: Complete the procedure and all critical steps in _____ minutes with a minimum score of 85% within two attempts (*or as indicated by the instructor*).

Scoring: Divide the points earned by the total possible points. Failure to perform a critical step, indicated by an asterisk (*), results in grade no higher than an 84% (*or as indicated by the instructor*).

Time: Began_____ Ended_____ Total minutes: _____

Steps:	Point Value	Attempt 1	Attempt 2
1. Wash your hands or use hand sanitizer. Using the drug reference information and the order, review the information on the medication if needed. Clarify any questions you have with the provider.	5		
2. Select the right medications from the storage area. Check the medication labels against the order. Check for the right name, form, and route. Check the expiration date to make sure the vials are not expired. Verify the right dose and the right time.	5*		
3. Assemble the supplies required for the procedure. If the insulin is cold, roll the vials in your hands to warm the medication.	5		
4. Perform the second medication check. Check the medication labels against the order. Check for the right name, form, and route.	5*		
5. Open and assemble the syringe and needle. Using a marker, label the syringe with the medication name. Mix the NPH insulin by rolling the vial in your hands. If present, remove the metal or plastic caps on the vials. Clean the rubber stoppers with an alcohol wipe. Let the stoppers dry.	10*		
6. With the syringe in a vertical position, pull the syringe plunger down. Draw up an amount of air equal to the amount of NPH insulin ordered. With the NPH vial on a firm surface, insert the needle in the rubber stopper. Inject the air into the NPH vial, keeping the needle tip out of the medication. Withdraw the needle from the stopper.	5		
7. With the syringe in a vertical position, pull the syringe plunger down. Draw up an amount of air equal to the amount of Regular insulin ordered. With the Regular vial on a firm surface, insert the needle into the rubber stopper. Inject the air into the Regular vial, keeping the needle tip out of the medication.	5		

8.	With the palm of your nondominant hand facing upward, grasp the vial between your middle and index fingers. Keeping the syringe unit in the vial, pick up and invert them. Use your thumb, ring, and little fingers of your nondominant hand to stabilize the syringe in the vial. Pull down on the plunger until you have more Regular insulin than what you need.	5		
9.	Continue to hold the vial/needle/syringe unit in a vertical position (with the needle pointing upward) with your nondominant hand. With your dominant hand, either use your fingers or a pen to tap the bubbles to the top of the barrel.	5		
10.	Once all the air bubbles are at the top, push the plunger slowly to the correct calibration marking for the ordered dose. Keep the syringe at eye level.	5*		
11.	Double-check that no air bubbles are in the syringe and the right dose was measured. If everything is correct, remove the vial from the syringe/needle unit.	5*		
12.	Using an alcohol wipe, wipe the rubber stopper of the NPH vial. Calculate the total amount of insulin that needs to be given.	5*		
13.	With the NPH vial flat on a hard surface, insert the needle into the dried stopper. With the palm of your nondominant hand facing upward, grasp the vial between your middle and index fingers. Keeping the syringe unit in the vial, pick up and invert them. Use your thumb and the ring and little fingers of your nondominant hand to stabilize the syringe in the vial. Pull down on the plunger until the rubber stopper reaches the calibration mark required. Do not withdraw any extra NPH insulin.	10*		
14.	Double-check that no air bubbles are in the syringe and the right dose was measured. If everything is correct, remove the vial from the syringe/needle unit.	5*		
15.	Use the one-handed scoop technique to cover the needle. Perform the third medication check. Check each medication label against the order. Check for the right name, form, and route.	5*		
16.	Maintain sterility of the medication and the needle throughout the procedure.	10*		
17.	Clean up the work area. Put the packaging and other waste in the waste container. Place the insulin vials back in their storage location.	5		
	Total Points	100		

Comments

CAAHEP Competencies	Step(s)
I.P.4.b. Verify the rules of medication administration: right medication	2, 4, 15
I.P.4.c. Verify the rules of medication administration: right dose	2, 10, 11, 13, 14
I.P.4.d. Verify the rules of medication administration: right route	2, 4, 15
I.P.4.e. Verify the rules of medication administration: right time	2
ABHES Competencies	**Step(s)**
8. Clinical Procedures f. Prepare and administer oral and parenteral medications and monitor intravenous (IV) infusions	Entire procedure

Procedure 30.7 Administer an Intradermal Injection

Name _____ Date _____ Score _____

Tasks: Prepare medication from a vial, administer an intradermal injection, read the tuberculin skin test, and document in the health record.

Equipment and Supplies:
- Provider's order
- Patient's health record
- Vial of medication
- Alcohol wipes
- 1 mL syringe with 1/4 to 1/2-inch, 25- to 27-gauge safety needle
- Bandage (if per facility's policy)
- Medication tray
- Biohazard sharps container
- Waste container
- Drug reference information
- Gloves
- Marker and pen
- Millimeter ruler

Order: Tuberculin purified protein derivative (PPD) (5 tuberculin units) 0.1 mL ID

Standard: Complete the procedure and all critical steps in _____ minutes with a minimum score of 85% within two attempts (*or as indicated by the instructor*).

Scoring: Divide the points earned by the total possible points. Failure to perform a critical step, indicated by an asterisk (*), results in grade no higher than an 84% (*or as indicated by the instructor*).

Time: Began _____ Ended _____ Total minutes: _____

Steps:	Point Value	Attempt 1	Attempt 2
1. Wash your hands or use hand sanitizer. Using the drug reference information and the order, review the information on the medication if needed. Clarify any questions you have with the provider.	2		
2. Select the right medication from the storage area. Check the medication label against the order. Check for the right name, form, and route. Check the expiration date to make sure the drug is not expired. Verify the right dose and the right time.	2*		
3. Assemble the supplies required for the procedure. Perform the second medication check. Check the medication label against the order. Check for the right name, form, dose, and route.	3*		
4. Open the syringe and needle. Tighten the preassembled syringe and needle unit or attach the needle to the syringe. Using a marker, label the syringe with the medication name. Mix the medication by rolling it with your hands if needed. Remove the cap on the vial (if present). Clean the rubber stopper with an alcohol wipe. Let the stopper dry. With the syringe in a vertical position, pull the syringe plunger down. Draw up an amount of air equal to the amount of medication ordered. Hold the vial firmly against a flat surface. Insert the needle into the center of the dried rubber stopper. Inject the aspirated air above the fluid in the vial.	5		

5.	With the palm of your nondominant hand facing upward, grasp the vial between your middle and index fingers. Keeping the syringe unit in the vial, pick up and invert them. Use your thumb and the ring and little fingers of your nondominant hand to stabilize the syringe in the vial.	3		
6.	With the syringe at eye level, pull the plunger down using your dominant hand. Fill the syringe with more medication than what was ordered. Continue to hold the vial/needle/syringe unit in a vertical position (with the needle pointing upward) with your nondominant hand. With your dominant hand, either use your fingers or a pen to tap the bubbles to the top of the barrel. Once all the air bubbles are at the top, push the plunger slowly to the correct calibration marking for the ordered dose.	5*		
7.	Double-check that no air bubbles are in the syringe and the right dose was measured. If everything is correct, remove the vial from the syringe/needle unit. Use the one-hand scoop technique to cover the needle. Perform the third medication check. Check each medication label against the order. Check for the right name, form, and route. Place syringe on a medication tray and clean up the work area.	5*		
8.	Maintain sterility of the medication and the needle throughout the procedure.	5*		
9.	Prior to entering the exam room, knock on the door and wait a moment. Greet the patient. Identify yourself. Verify the patient's identity with full name and date of birth. Make sure the patient's information matches the order and the record. Explain what you are going to do.	5*		
10.	Provide the right education to the patient. Explain the medication ordered, the desired effect, and common side effects; also identify the provider who ordered it. Answer any questions the patient may have. Use language the patient can understand. Ask the patient if they have any allergies. If the patient refuses the medication, notify the provider.	5		
11.	Perform the right technique. Ask the patient: • Can you return in 48 to 72 hours for the reading? • Have you ever had BCG? • Have you ever had a TB skin test? If yes, did you have a reaction to it?	5		
12.	Use hand sanitizer and put on gloves.	2*		
13.	Have the patient extend a forearm. With the palm facing upward, identify an appropriate site for an injection. The site should be 2 to 4 inches below the elbow. Loosen the cap on the needle, but still protect the needle from contamination. Open the alcohol wipes.	3*		
14.	Place your nondominant hand to the side of the site, pulling the skin taut. Option: Place your nondominant hand on the back of the patient's forearm, pulling the skin taut	3		
15.	Cleanse the site with an alcohol wipe using a circular motion. Move from the center outward, using some friction to help clean the site. Create about a 2-inch circle at the site. Let the site dry while continuing to hold the area.	5*		
16.	Pick up the syringe and tip it to remove the cover. Grasp the syringe in your dominant hand, using your thumb and index finger. Make sure to have no fingers under the syringe. Ensure that the bevel is up.	3		
17.	At a 5- to 15-degree angle, slowly insert the needle until the bevel is covered with skin. Carefully lower the syringe to the skin and hold it steady with your dominant hand.	5		

18. Carefully move your nondominant hand to the plunger. Slowly and steadily inject the medication by pressing on the plunger. If a 6- to 10-mm wheal does not appear, repeat the test at least 2 inches from the site.	**5**		
19. Double-check the barrel of the syringe to make sure all the medication was administered. Withdraw the needle. Activate the needle's safety device with one hand.	**5***		
20. Discard the needle/syringe in a biohazardous sharps container. Make sure to put the needle in first.	**3***		
21. Do not massage the area. Per the facility's policy, if the person has a light-colored shirt with long sleeves, offer a bandage. Place the bandage on very loosely to just absorb any blood from the site.	**2**		
22. Observe the patient for any adverse reactions. Clean up the area. Discard the waste in the waste container. Sanitize your hands.	**2**		
23. Document the procedure in the health record. Include assessments done, allergies, teaching or instructions provided; the medication name, dose, and route; the name of the provider who ordered the medication; and how the patient tolerated the medication. Also include the manufacturer, the lot number, and the expiration date of the vial.	**5***		
Scenario update: Patient returns for the reading. 24. Check the health record to identify the location of the test. Greet the patient. Identify yourself. Verify the patient's identity with full name and date of birth. Make sure the patient's information matches the order and the record. Explain what you are going to do.	**2***		
25. Palpate the site for an induration. If an induration is felt, ask patients if you can write on their arm. Using a ballpoint pen, draw a line toward the induration from the outer edge of the arm. Repeat on the other side. Option: Palpate the induration to find the edge and then mark it with a pen. Repeat on the other side. Using a millimeter ruler, accurately measure the distance between the two points.	**5**		
26. Document the reading in the patient's health record. Include the reason for the patient's visit, the test site, the size of the induration in millimeters, and the name of the provider who was notified.	**5***		
Total Points	**100**		

Documentation

Comments

CAAHEP Competencies	Step(s)
I.P.4.a. Verify the rules of medication administration: right patient	9
I.P.4.b. Verify the rules of medication administration: right medication	2, 3, 7
I.P.4.c. Verify the rules of medication administration: right dose	2, 3, 6, 7
I.P.4.d. Verify the rules of medication administration: right route	2, 3, 7
I.P.4.e. Verify the rules of medication administration: right time	2
I.P.4.f. Verify the rules of medication administration: right documentation	23
I.P.5. Select proper sites for administering parenteral medication	13
I.P.7. Administer parenteral (excluding IV) medications	Entire procedure
III.P.2. Select appropriate barrier/personal protective equipment.	12
III.P.10.a. Demonstrate proper disposal of biohazardous material: sharps	20
X.P.3. Document patient care accurately in the medical record	23, 26
ABHES Competencies	**Step(s)**
4. Medical Law and Ethics a. Follow documentation guidelines	23, 26
8. Clinical Procedures a. Practice standard precautions and perform disinfection/sterilization techniques	12
8.f. Prepare and administer oral and parenteral medications and monitor intravenous (IV) infusions	Entire procedure

Procedure 30.8   Administer a Subcutaneous Injection

Name _____ Date _____ Score _____

Tasks: Prepare medication from a vial, administer a subcutaneous injection, and document the medication administration in the health record.

Equipment and Supplies:
- Provider's order
- Patient's health record
- Vial of medication
- Alcohol wipes
- 3 mL syringe with 1/2-inch or 5/8-inch, 23- to 27-gauge safety needle
- Gauze
- Bandage
- Medication tray
- Biohazard sharps container
- Waste container
- Drug reference information
- VIS for polio vaccine (IPV) (optional)
- Gloves
- Marker

Scenario: Dr. Martin ordered polio vaccine (IPV) 0.5 mL SUBQ for Johnny Parker (DOB 06/15/20XX). (Vial information: ABC Manufacturer, Lot 1234, expires 1 year from today.)

Standard: Complete the procedure and all critical steps in _____ minutes with a minimum score of 85% within two attempts (*or as indicated by the instructor*).

Scoring: Divide the points earned by the total possible points. Failure to perform a critical step, indicated by an asterisk (*), results in grade no higher than an 84% (*or as indicated by the instructor*).

Time: Began_____ Ended_____ Total minutes: _____

Steps:	Point Value	Attempt 1	Attempt 2
1. Wash your hands or use hand sanitizer. Using the drug reference information and the order, review the information on the medication if needed. Clarify any questions you have with the provider.	2		
2. Select the right medication from the storage area. Check the medication label against the order. Check for the right name, form, and route. Check the expiration date to make sure the drug is not expired. Verify the right dose and the right time.	2*		
3. Assemble the supplies required for the procedure. Perform the second medication check. Check the medication label against the order. Check for the right name, form, dose, and route.	3*		

4.	Open the syringe and needle. Tighten the preassembled syringe and needle unit or attach the needle to the syringe. Using a marker, label the syringe with the medication name. Mix the medication by rolling it with your hands if needed. Remove the cap on the vial (if present). Clean the rubber stopper with an alcohol wipe. Let the stopper dry. With the syringe in a vertical position, pull the syringe plunger down. Draw up an amount of air equal to the amount of medication ordered. Hold the vial firmly against a flat surface. Insert the needle into the center of the dried rubber stopper. Inject the aspirated air above the fluid in the vial.	5		
5.	With the palm of your nondominant hand facing upward, grasp the vial between your middle and index fingers. Keeping the syringe unit in the vial, pick up and invert them. Use your thumb and the ring and little fingers of your nondominant hand to stabilize the syringe in the vial.	3		
6.	With the syringe at eye level, pull the plunger down using your dominant hand. Fill the syringe with more medication than what was ordered. Continue to hold the vial/needle/syringe unit in a vertical position (with the needle pointing upward) with your nondominant hand. With your dominant hand, either use your fingers or a pen to tap the bubbles to the top of the barrel. Once all the air bubbles are at the top, push the plunger slowly to the correct calibration marking for the ordered dose.	5*		
7.	Double-check that no air bubbles are in the syringe and the right dose was measured. If everything is correct, remove the vial from the syringe/needle unit. Use the one-hand scoop technique to cover the needle. Perform the third medication check. Check each medication label against the order. Check for the right name, form, and route. Place syringe on a medication tray and clean up the work area.	5*		
8.	Maintain sterility of the medication and the needle throughout the procedure.	5*		
9.	(Peer will play the parent.) Prior to entering the exam room, knock on the door and wait a moment. Greet the parent/patient. Identify yourself. Verify the patient's identity with full name and date of birth. Make sure the patient's information matches the order and the record. Explain what you are going to do.	5*		
10.	Provide the right education to the parent/patient. Explain the medication ordered, the desired effect, and common side effects; also identify the provider who ordered it. Answer any questions the parent/patient may have. Use language the parent/patient can understand. Ask if the patient has any allergies. If the parent/patient refuses the medication, notify the provider.	5		
11.	Use hand sanitizer and put on gloves.	5*		
12.	Loosen the cap on the needle, but still protect the needle from contamination. Open the alcohol wipes. Have gauze and a bandage available.	5		
13.	(Peer will play the patient.) Find the injection site.	5*		
14.	Cleanse the site with an alcohol wipe using a circular motion. Move from the center outward, using some friction to help clean the site. Create about a 2-inch circle at the site. Let the site dry. Avoid waving over or blowing on the alcohol, which contaminates the site.	5*		

15. Perform the right technique. Place a gauze between the index and middle fingers of your nondominant hand. With that hand, use your index finger and thumb to pinch up at the cleansed area.	**5**		
16. Pick up the syringe and tip it to remove the cover. Hold the syringe between the thumb and index finger of your dominant hand. Quickly and smoothly insert the needle into the site at a 45- or 90-degree angle, depending on the needle size. Insert the entire needle. Make sure the needle tip is not pointed toward your nondominant hand.	**5**		
17. <u>One-hand option</u>: Continue to pinch the site. Securely grasp the syringe between your fingers of your dominant hand. With your dominant hand, aspirate if required, and then push the plunger to inject the medication. <u>Two-hand option</u>: Release the pinch and with the nondominant hand, aspirate if required, and then push the plunger to inject the medication.	**5**		
18. Inject the medication at a rate of 1 mL over 10 seconds. Ensure that all the medication has been injected before pulling out the needle at the same angle used for entry. Release the pinch if using the one-handed option.	**5**		
19. Activate the needle's safety device with one hand while using the other hand to cover the site with gauze. Gently apply pressure at the site to stop any bleeding. Apply a bandage if the patient requests it.	**5***		
20. Discard the needle/syringe in a biohazardous sharps container. Make sure the needle goes into the sharps container first.	**5***		
21. Observe the patient for any adverse reactions. Clean up the area. Discard the waste in the waste container. Sanitize your hands.	**5**		
22. Document the procedure in the health record. Include assessments done, allergies, teaching or instructions provided; the name of the provider who ordered the medication; the medication's name, dose, and route; and how the patient tolerated the medication. Also include the manufacturer, the lot number, and the expiration date for vaccines and controlled substances.	**5***		
Total Points	**100**		

Documentation

Comments

CAAHEP Competencies	Step(s)
I.P.4.a. Verify the rules of medication administration: right patient	9
I.P.4.b. Verify the rules of medication administration: right medication	2, 3, 7
I.P.4.c. Verify the rules of medication administration: right dose	2, 3, 6, 7
I.P.4.d. Verify the rules of medication administration: right route	2, 3, 7
I.P.4.e. Verify the rules of medication administration: right time	2
I.P.4.f. Verify the rules of medication administration: right documentation	22
I.P.5. Select proper sites for administering parenteral medication	13
I.P.7. Administer parenteral (excluding IV) medications	Entire procedure
III.P.2. Select appropriate barrier/personal protective equipment.	11
III.P.10.a. Demonstrate proper disposal of biohazardous material: sharps	20
X.P.3. Document patient care accurately in the medical record	22
ABHES Competencies	**Step(s)**
4. Medical Law and Ethics a. Follow documentation guidelines	22
8. Clinical Procedures a. Practice standard precautions and perform disinfection/sterilization techniques	11
8.f. Prepare and administer oral and parenteral medications and monitor intravenous (IV) infusions	Entire procedure

Procedure 30.9   Administer an Intramuscular Injection

Name _____ Date _____ Score _____

Tasks: Prepare medication from a vial, administer an intramuscular injection, and document the medication administration in the health record.

Equipment and Supplies:
- Provider's order
- Patient's health record
- Vial of medication
- Alcohol wipes
- 3 mL syringe
- 22- to 25-gauge, 5/8 to 1 1/2-inch safety needle
- Gauze
- Bandage
- Medication tray
- Biohazard sharps container
- Waste container
- Drug reference information
- VIS for influenza vaccine (optional)
- Gloves
- Marker

Scenario: Dr. Martin ordered influenza vaccine (IIV) 0.5 mL IM for Erma Willis (DOB 12/09/19XX). (Vial information: MN Manufacturer, Lot 7845, expires 1 year from today.)

Standard: Complete the procedure and all critical steps in _____ minutes with a minimum score of 85% within two attempts (*or as indicated by the instructor*).

Scoring: Divide the points earned by the total possible points. Failure to perform a critical step, indicated by an asterisk (*), results in grade no higher than an 84% (*or as indicated by the instructor*).

Time: Began_____ Ended_____ Total minutes: _____

Steps:	Point Value	Attempt 1	Attempt 2
1. Wash your hands or use hand sanitizer. Using the drug reference information and the order, review the information on the medication if needed. Clarify any questions you have with the provider.	2		
2. Select the right medication from the storage area. Check the medication label against the order. Check for the right name, form, and route. Check the expiration date to make sure the drug is not expired. Verify the right dose and the right time.	2*		
3. Assemble the supplies required for the procedure.Perform the second medication check. Check the medication label against the order. Check for the right name, form, dose, and route.	3*		

4.	Open the syringe and needle. Tighten the preassembled syringe and needle unit or attach the needle to the syringe. Using a marker, label the syringe with the medication name. Mix the medication by rolling it with your hands if needed. Remove the cap on the vial (if present). Clean the rubber stopper with an alcohol wipe. Let the stopper dry. With the syringe in a vertical position, pull the syringe plunger down. Draw up an amount of air equal to the amount of medication ordered.Hold the vial firmly against a flat surface. Insert the needle into the center of the dried rubber stopper. Inject the aspirated air above the fluid in the vial.	**5**		
5.	With the palm of your nondominant hand facing upward, grasp the vial between your middle and index fingers. Keeping the syringe unit in the vial, pick up and invert them. Use your thumb and the ring and little fingers of your nondominant hand to stabilize the syringe in the vial.	**3**		
6.	With the syringe at eye level, pull the plunger down using your dominant hand. Fill the syringe with more medication than what was ordered. Continue to hold the vial/needle/syringe unit in a vertical position (with the needle pointing upward) with your nondominant hand. With your dominant hand, either use your fingers or a pen to tap the bubbles to the top of the barrel. Once all the air bubbles are at the top, push the plunger slowly to the correct calibration marking for the ordered dose.	**5***		
7.	Double-check that no air bubbles are in the syringe and the right dose was measured. If everything is correct, remove the vial from the syringe/ needle unit. Use the one-hand scoop technique to cover the needle. Perform the third medication check. Check each medication label against the order. Check for the right name, form, and route. Place syringe on a medication tray and clean up the work area.	**5***		
8.	Maintain sterility of the medication and the needle throughout the procedure.	**5***		
9.	Prior to entering the exam room, knock on the door and wait a moment. Greet the patient. Identify yourself. Verify the patient's identity with full name and date of birth. Make sure the patient's information matches the order and the record. Explain what you are going to do.	**5***		
10.	Provide the right education to the patient. Explain the medication ordered, the desired effect, and common side effects; also identify the provider who ordered the medication. Answer any questions the patient may have. Use language the patient can understand. Ask the patient if they have any allergies. If the patient refuses the medication, notify the provider.	**5**		
11.	Use hand sanitizer and put on gloves.	**5***		
12.	Loosen the cap on the needle, but still protect the needle from contamination. Open the alcohol wipes. Have gauze and a bandage available.	**5**		
13.	Find the site using the landmarks.	**5***		
14.	Cleanse the site with an alcohol wipe using a circular motion. Move from the center outward, using some friction to help clean the site. Create about a 2-inch circle at the site. Let the site dry.	**5***		
15.	Perform the right technique. Place a gauze between the index and middle fingers of your nondominant hand. With that hand, stretch or flatten the site. Hold the site.	**5**		

16. Pick up the syringe and tip it to remove the cover. Hold the syringe like a dart with your dominant hand. Quickly and smoothly insert the needle into the site at a 90-degree angle. Insert the entire needle.	5		
17. <u>One-hand option</u>: Continue to hold the site. Securely grasp the syringe between the fingers of your dominant hand. Place your thumb under the plunger edge and push the plunger out farther to aspirate. <u>Two-hand option</u>: Move the nondominant hand to the plunger. Pull the plunger out farther to aspirate.	5		
18. Aspirate for 5 seconds and check the barrel for blood. If blood is seen, pull out the needle and discard. Restart the procedure. If no blood is seen, inject the medication at a rate of about 10 seconds per milliliter. Ensure that all the medication has been injected before pulling out the needle at the same angle used for entry.	5		
19. Activate the needle's safety device with one hand while using the other hand to cover the site with gauze. Gently apply pressure at the site to stop any bleeding. Apply a bandage if the patient requests it.	5*		
20. Discard the needle/syringe in a biohazardous sharps container. Make sure to put the needle in first.	5*		
21. Observe the patient for any adverse reactions. Clean up the area. Discard the waste in the waste container. Sanitize your hands.	5		
22. Document the procedure in the health record. Include assessments done, allergies, teaching or instructions provided; the name of the provider who ordered the medication; the medication's name, dose, and route; and how the patient tolerated the medication. Also include the manufacturer, lot number, and expiration date for vaccines and controlled substances.	5*		
Total Points	100		

Documentation

Comments

CAAHEP Competencies	Step(s)
I.P.4.a. Verify the rules of medication administration: right patient	9
I.P.4.b. Verify the rules of medication administration: right medication	2, 3, 7
I.P.4.c. Verify the rules of medication administration: right dose	2, 3, 6, 7
I.P.4.d. Verify the rules of medication administration: right route	2, 3, 7
I.P.4.e. Verify the rules of medication administration: right time	2
I.P.4.f. Verify the rules of medication administration: right documentation	22
I.P.5. Select proper sites for administering parenteral medication	13
I.P.7. Administer parenteral (excluding IV) medications	Entire procedure
III.P.2. Select appropriate barrier/personal protective equipment.	11
III.P.10.a. Demonstrate proper disposal of biohazardous material: sharps	20
X.P.3. Document patient care accurately in the medical record	22
ABHES Competencies	**Step(s)**
4. Medical Law and Ethics a. Follow documentation guidelines	22
8. Clinical Procedures a. Practice standard precautions and perform disinfection/sterilization techniques	11
8.f. Prepare and administer oral and parenteral medications and monitor intravenous (IV) infusions	Entire procedure

Procedure 30.10 Administer an Intramuscular Injection Using the Z-track Technique

Name _____ Date _____ Score _____

Tasks: Prepare medication from a vial, administer an intramuscular injection, and document the medication administration in the health record.

Equipment and Supplies:
- Provider's order
- Patient's health record
- Vial of medication
- Alcohol wipes
- 3 mL syringe
- 18-21-gauge, 1- to 1½-inch needle
- Gauze
- Bandage
- Medication tray
- Biohazard sharps container
- Waste container
- Drug reference information
- Gloves
- Marker

Scenario: Dr. Martin ordered iron dextran 0.5 mL IM for Erma Willis (DOB 12/09/19XX). (Vial information: FE Manufacturer, Lot 625, expires 1 year from today).

Standard: Complete the procedure and all critical steps in _____ minutes with a minimum score of 85% within two attempts (*or as indicated by the instructor*).

Scoring: Divide the points earned by the total possible points. Failure to perform a critical step, indicated by an asterisk (*), results in grade no higher than an 84% (*or as indicated by the instructor*).

Time: Began_____ Ended_____ Total minutes: _____

Steps:	Point Value	Attempt 1	Attempt 2
1. Wash your hands or use hand sanitizer. Using the drug reference information and the order, review the information on the medication if needed. Clarify any questions you have with the provider.	2		
2. Select the right medication from the storage area. Check the medication label against the order. Check for the right name, form, and route. Check the expiration date to make sure the drug is not expired. Verify the right dose and the right time.	2*		
3. Assemble the supplies required for the procedure.Perform the second medication check. Check the medication label against the order. Check for the right name, form, dose, and route.	3*		

4.	Open the syringe and needle. Tighten the preassembled syringe and needle unit or attach the needle to the syringe. Using a marker, label the syringe with the medication name. Mix the medication by rolling it with your hands if needed. Remove the cap on the vial (if present). Clean the rubber stopper with an alcohol wipe. Let the stopper dry. With the syringe in a vertical position, pull the syringe plunger down. Draw up an amount of air equal to the amount of medication ordered. Hold the vial firmly against a flat surface. Insert the needle into the center of the dried rubber stopper. Inject the aspirated air above the fluid in the vial.	5		
5.	With the palm of your nondominant hand facing upward, grasp the vial between your middle and index fingers. Keeping the syringe unit in the vial, pick up and invert them. Use your thumb and the ring and little fingers of your nondominant hand to stabilize the syringe in the vial.	3		
6.	With the syringe at eye level, pull the plunger down using your dominant hand. Fill the syringe with more medication than what was ordered. Continue to hold the vial/needle/syringe unit in a vertical position (with the needle pointing upward) with your nondominant hand. With your dominant hand, either use your fingers or a pen to tap the bubbles to the top of the barrel. Once all the air bubbles are at the top, push the plunger slowly to the correct calibration marking for the ordered dose.	5*		
7.	Double-check that no air bubbles are in the syringe and the right dose was measured. If everything is correct, remove the vial from the syringe/needle unit. Use the one-hand scoop technique to cover the needle. Perform the third medication check. Check each medication label against the order. Check for the right name, form, and route. Place syringe on a medication tray and clean up the work area.	5*		
8.	Maintain sterility of the medication and the needle throughout the procedure.	5*		
9.	Prior to entering the exam room, knock on the door and wait a moment. Greet the patient. Identify yourself. Verify the patient's identity with full name and date of birth. Make sure the patient's information matches the order and the record. Explain what you are going to do.	5*		
10.	Provide the right education to the patient. Explain the medication ordered, the desired effect, and common side effects; also identify the provider who ordered the medication. Answer any questions the patient may have. Use language the patient can understand. Ask the patient if they have any allergies. If the patient refuses the medication, notify the provider.	5		
11.	Use hand sanitizer and put on gloves.	5*		
12.	Loosen the cap on the needle, but still protect the needle from contamination. Open the alcohol wipes. Have gauze and a bandage available.	5		
13.	Find the site using the landmarks.	5*		
14.	Perform the right technique. Place a gauze between the index and middle fingers of your nondominant hand. With that hand, displace the tissue.	5		
15.	Cleanse the site with an alcohol wipe using a circular motion. Move from the center outward, using some friction to help clean the site. Create about a 2-inch circle at the site. Let the site dry while continuing to hold the area.	5*		

16. Pick up the syringe and tip it to remove the cover. Hold the syringe like a dart with your dominant hand. Quickly and smoothly insert the needle into the site at a 90-degree angle. Insert the entire needle.	**5**		
17. Continue to hold the site. Securely grasp the syringe between the fingers of your dominant hand. Place your thumb under the plunger edge and push the plunger out farther to aspirate.	**5**		
18. Aspirate for 5 seconds and check the barrel for blood. If blood is seen, pull out the needle and discard. Restart the procedure. If no blood is seen, inject the medication at a rate of about 10 seconds per mL. Ensure that all the medication has been injected. Wait 10 seconds before withdrawing the needle and letting go with your nondominant hand.	**5**		
19. Activate the needle's safety device with one hand while using the other hand to cover the site with gauze. Gently apply pressure at the site to stop any bleeding. Apply a bandage if the patient requests it.	**5***		
20. Discard the needle/syringe in a biohazardous sharps container. Make sure to put the needle in first.	**5***		
21. Observe the patient for any adverse reactions. Clean up the area. Discard the waste in the waste container. Sanitize your hands.	**5**		
22. Document the procedure in the health record. Include assessments done, allergies, teaching or instructions provided; the name of the provider who ordered the medication; the medication's name, dose, and route; and how the patient tolerated the medication. Also include the manufacturer, lot number, and expiration date for vaccines and controlled substances.	**5***		
Total Points	**100**		

Documentation

Comments

CAAHEP Competencies	Step(s)
I.P.4.a. Verify the rules of medication administration: right patient	9
I.P.4.b. Verify the rules of medication administration: right medication	2, 3, 7
I.P.4.c. Verify the rules of medication administration: right dose	2, 3, 6, 7
I.P.4.d. Verify the rules of medication administration: right route	2, 3, 7
I.P.4.e. Verify the rules of medication administration: right time	2
I.P.4.f. Verify the rules of medication administration: right documentation	22
I.P.5. Select proper sites for administering parenteral medication	13
I.P.7. Administer parenteral (excluding IV) medications	Entire procedure
III.P.2. Select appropriate barrier/personal protective equipment.	11
III.P.10.a. Demonstrate proper disposal of biohazardous material: sharps	20
X.P.3. Document patient care accurately in the medical record	22
ABHES Competencies	**Step(s)**
4. Medical Law and Ethics a. Follow documentation guidelines	22
8. Clinical Procedures a. Practice standard precautions and perform disinfection/sterilization techniques	11
8.f. Prepare and administer oral and parenteral medications and monitor intravenous (IV) infusions	Entire procedure

Ophthalmology and Otolaryngology

CAAHEP Competencies	Assessment
I.C.4. Identify major organs in each body system	Skills and Concepts – A. 1-7
I.C.5. Identify the anatomical location of major organs in each body system	Skills and Concepts – A. 1-7
I.C.6. Identify structure and function of the human body across the life span	Skills and Concepts – C. 1-4
I.C.7. Identify the normal function of each body system	Skills and Concepts – A. 8-13, C.13
I.C.8.a. Identify common pathology related to each body system including: signs	Skills and Concepts – D. 5, 23-27, E. 12-15
I.C.8.b. Identify common pathology related to each body system including: symptoms	Skills and Concepts – D. 5, 23-27, E. 12-15
I.C.8.c. Identify common pathology related to each body system including: etiology	Skills and Concepts – D. 18-22, E. 8-11
I.C.8.d. Identify common pathology related to each body system including: diagnostic measures	Skills and Concepts – D. 28-32, E. 16-19
I.C.8.e. Identify common pathology related to each body system including: treatment modalities	Skills and Concepts – D. 28-32, E. 16-19
V.C.8.a. Identify the following related to body systems: medical terms	Vocabulary Review
V.8.b. Identify the following related to body systems: abbreviations	Abbreviations
I.P.3. Perform patient screening following established protocols	Procedures 31.1, 31.2, 31.5
I.P.4.a. Verify the rules of medication administration: right patient	Procedures 31.3, 31.4, 31.6, 31.7
I.P.4.b. Verify the rules of medication administration: right medication	Procedures 31.3, 31.4, 31.6, 31.7
I.P.4.c. Verify the rules of medication administration: right dose	Procedures 31.3, 31.4, 31.6, 31.7
I.P.4.d. Verify the rules of medication administration: right route	Procedures 31.3, 31.4, 31.6, 31.7
I.P.4.e. Verify the rules of medication administration: right time	Procedures 31.3, 31.4, 31.6, 31.7

CAAHEP Competencies	Assessment
I.P.4.f. Verify the rules of medication administration: right documentation	Procedures 31.3, 31.4, 31.6, 31.7
I.P.8. Instruct and prepare a patient for a procedure or a treatment	Procedures 31.1 through 31.7
I.P.9. Assist provider with a patient exam	Procedures 31.1, 31.2, 31.5
III.P.2. Select appropriate barrier/personal protective equipment.	Procedure 31.3, 31.4, 31.6, 31.7
X.P.3. Document patient care accurately in the medical record	Procedures 31.1-31.4, 31.6, 31.7

ABHES Competencies	Assessment
2. Anatomy and Physiology a. List all body systems and their structures and functions	Skills and Concepts – A. 8-13, C. 13
b. Describe common diseases, symptoms, and etiologies as they apply to each system	Skills and Concepts – D. 18-22, E. 8-11
c. Identify diagnostic and treatment modalities as they relate to each body system	Skills and Concepts – D. 28-32, E. 16-19
3. Medical Terminology c. Apply medical terminology for each specialty	Vocabulary Review
d. Define and use medical abbreviations when appropriate and acceptable	Abbreviations
4. Medical Law and Ethics a. Follow documentation guidelines	Procedures 31.1 through 31.4, 31.6, 31.7
8. Clinical Procedures a. Practice standard precautions and perform disinfection/sterilization techniques	Procedures 31.1 through 31.7
c. Assist provider with general/physical examination	Procedures 31.1, 31.2, 31.5

VOCABULARY REVIEW

Using the word pool on the right, find the correct word to match the definition. Write the word on the line after the definition.

Group A

1. A state of rest or balance due to the equal action of opposing forces _____

2. The lowest part of the brain, continuous with the top of the spinal cord _____

3. Having (blood) vessels that conduct or circulate liquids (blood) _____

4. The region of the cerebral cortex that receives auditory data _____

5. Relating to balance when moving at an angle or rotating _____

6. Involving the sensory nerves, especially as they affect hearing _____

7. Involving, relating, or seeing with both eyes _____

8. Relating to balance when moving in a straight line _____

9. The middle part of the brain through which sensory impulses pass to reach the cerebral cortex _____

10. Having two outward curving surfaces on a lens _____

Word Pool
- binocular
- vascular
- biconvex
- sensorineural
- equilibrium
- dynamic equilibrium
- static equilibrium
- medulla oblongata
- thalamus
- auditory cortex

Group B

1. An instrument used to measure intraocular pressure _____

2. A medicine or substance capable of damaging cranial nerve VIII or the organs of hearing and balance _____

3. A sound in one or both ears such as buzzing, ringing, or whistling, occurring without an external stimulus _____

4. Used to diagnose glaucoma and inspect ocular movement _____

5. Farsightedness due to ciliary weakness and loss of elasticity in the lens _____

6. Capable of being heard _____

7. Extreme sensitivity to light _____

8. Any substance or medication that causes constriction of the pupil _____

9. A condition where the ossicles of the middle ear become fused and act as a single unit instead of individual bones, which restricts their movement and results in conductive hearing loss _____

10. Dull or dim vision, with no apparent organic defect _____

Word Pool
- audible
- presbyopia
- amblyopia
- photophobia
- tonometer
- gonioscopy
- miotic
- otosclerosis
- ototoxic
- tinnitus

Group C

1. Dizziness; abnormal sensations of movement when there is none
   _____

2. The unit of measurement used in hearing examinations; a wave frequency equal to 1 cycle per second _____

3. An excessive discharge of sebum from the sebaceous glands, forming greasy scales or crusty areas on the body
   _____

4. Characterized by the formation and/or discharge of pus
   _____

5. To turn the eyelid inside out; this typically is done by the provider to inspect the area for foreign bodies _____

6. Allied healthcare professional who specializes in evaluation of hearing function, detection of hearing impairment, and determination of the anatomic site of impairment
   _____

7. A usually chronic, recurrent skin disease marked by bright red patches covered with silvery scales _____

8. A thin, watery, serum-like drainage _____

9. The lens of the eye flattens to adjust to something seen at a distance or thickens for close vision; process where the lens flattens or thickens its shape _____

Word Pool
- seborrhea
- psoriasis
- suppurative
- vertigo
- accommodation
- Hertz
- audiologist
- serous
- evert

ABBREVIATIONS

Write out what each of the following abbreviations stands for.

1. OD _____

2. ENT _____

3. CNS _____

4. UNHS _____

5. ARMD _____

6. PRK _____

7. LASIK _____

8. LASEK _____

9. CK _____

10. IOL _____

11. IOP _____

12. OME _____

13. L&A _____

14. Hz _____

15. ADA _____

16. ADAA_____

SKILLS AND CONCEPTS

Answer the following questions.

A. Anatomy and Physiology of the Eye

Match the layer of the eyeball with the correct description.

1. _____ Outer layer
2. _____ Middle layer
3. _____ Inner layer

   a.   the choroid, the iris, and the ciliary body
   b.   the retina in the posterior portion and the lens in the anterior portion
   c.   white, opaque sclera and the transparent cornea

4. The retina contains two light-sensitive neurons; _____ function in bright light and detect color while _____ are highly sensitive to light and can function in dim light.

5. There is a natural blind spot in our vision where the _____ is located.

6. _____ maintains the shape of the posterior eyeball and holds the choroid membrane against the retina to ensure an adequate blood supply.

7. _____ helps maintain normal pressure within the eye and provides nutrients to the lens and the cornea.

8. A visual impulse begins with the passage of light through the _____, where light is _____.

9. The _____ adjusts the curvature of the _____ to again refract light rays so that they pass onto the _____.

10. Focused light triggers the photoreceptor cells called _____ and _____.

11. Light energy is converted into a(n) _____.

12. The electrical impulse is sent through the _____ to the _____ of the brain.

13. The brain interprets the light impulses and a picture is created that we perceive as _____.

B. Anatomy and Physiology of the Ear

1. The structures of the outer ear include which of the following?
   a. Auricle or pinna
   b. External auditory canal
   c. Tympanic membrane or eardrum
   d. All of the above
   e. None of the above

2. The three bones of the middle ear are called the _____.

Match the scientific name to the common name of the three bones of the middle ear.

3. _____ Malleus
4. _____ Incus
5. _____ Stapes

a. anvil
b. hammer
c. stirrup

6. The structures of the inner ear include which of the following?
   a. Vestibule
   b. Cochlea
   c. Semicircular canal
   d. All of the above

7. Earwax or cerumen is secreted by modified sweat glands in the _____.

8. The _____ helps equalize the pressure between the middle ear and the throat.

9. The ossicles transmit bone-conducted sound waves through the middle ear to the _____.

10. Sound waves travel through the fluid of the inner ear as _____.

11. Located within the cochlea, the _____ contains receptors for sound.

12. Semicircular canals detect _____ equilibrium, and the vestibule detects _____ equilibrium.

Place the following items in the order in which hearing occurs.

13. Arrange the following items in the order in which hearing occurs.

_____ The sensorineural impulses reach the cochlea.

_____ The brain then interprets the auditory impulse into audible sound and speech patterns.

_____ Sound waves cause the tympanic membrane to vibrate.

_____ Auditory impulse is initiated; it travels through the cochlear nerve to the eighth cranial nerve.

_____ Sound impulses cause the hairlike sensory cells of the cochlea to bend and rub against the nerve fibers.

_____ The sound waves reach the tympanic membrane.

_____ The auditory impulse travels to the thalamus and to the auditory cortex of the temporal lobe of the brain.

_____ The ossicles are vibrated and transmit the waves to the oval window.

_____ The auditory impulse is transmitted to medulla oblongata.

C. Life Span Changes

1. By _____ of age, a baby will be able to follow moving objects and by the age of _____, eye-hand coordination and depth perception are well developed.

2. Young children develop more ear infections that adults because the eustachian tube is _____ and more _____ than in adults.

3. The two most common causes of blindness in older adults are _____ and _____.

4. Hearing loss as we age is referred to as _____.

D. Eye Diseases and Disorders

Match the refractive disorder with the correct description.

1. _____ Hyperopia
2. _____ Myopia
3. _____ Astigmatism
4. _____ Presbyopia

   a. As people age, the lens of the eye becomes less flexible, and the ciliary muscles weaken. When this happens, changing the point of focus from distance to near becomes difficult.
   b. Light enters the eye, and focuses behind the retina. This disorder occurs when the eyeball is too short from the anterior to the posterior wall. An individual has difficulty seeing objects that are close.
   c. Occurs when light rays entering the eye are focused irregularly. This usually occurs because the cornea or the lens is not smooth but has an irregular shape. It is like attempting to focus on objects seen through a wavy piece of window glass.
   d. Occurs when light rays entering the eye focus in front of the retina. This causes objects at a distance to appear blurry and dull. This disorder occurs when the eyeball is too long from front to back. An individual has difficulty seeing objects that are far away.

5. Signs and symptoms of refractive errors include which of the following?
   a. Squinting
   b. Frequent rubbing of the eyes
   c. Headaches
   d. All of the above

6. Traditional treatments for refractive errors are _____ and _____.

Match the term with the correct definition.

7. _____ Strabismus
8. _____ Nystagmus
9. _____ Hordeolum
10. _____ Keratitis
11. _____ Conjunctivitis
12. _____ Nyctalopia

   a. a failure of the eyes to track together
   b. also known as a *stye*; infection of one of the sebaceous glands of an eyelash
   c. inability to see well in dim light
   d. inflammation of the conjunctiva caused by irritation, allergy, or bacterial infection
   e. a constant involuntary movement of one or both eyes
   f. inflammation of the cornea

Match the description with the correct disorder.

13. _____ Progressive deterioration of the macula lutea, which causes loss of central vision

14. _____ Increased intraocular pressure, which damages the optic nerve

15. _____ Abrasion of the outer covering of the eye

16. _____ The blood vessels of the retina become damaged from hyperglycemia, causing blockages in the small blood vessels

17. _____ A cloudy or opaque area in the normally clear lens of the eye that blocks the passage of light into the retina

a. corneal abrasion
b. cataract
c. glaucoma
d. diabetic retinopathy
e. macular degeneration

Match the etiology with the correct disease.

18. _____ Cause is unknown, but hereditary tendency toward development of the most common forms has been noted

19. _____ Diabetes mellitus

20. _____ Foreign body in the eye or direct trauma

21. _____ Breakdown of light-sensitive cells in the region of the macula; new blood vessels form behind the retina and leak blood and fluid

22. _____ Injury to the eye, exposure to extreme heat or radiation, or inherited factors

a. corneal abrasion
b. cataract
c. glaucoma
d. diabetic retinopathy
e. macular degeneration

Match the signs and symptoms with the correct disease.

23. _____ Need to change prescriptions frequently, loss of peripheral vision, impaired dark adaptation; severe pain, headaches, inflammation, photophobia, seeing halos around lights

24. _____ Loss of central vision

25. _____ Pain, inflammation, tearing, photophobia

26. _____ Development of spots or dark strings floating in vision, blurred or fluctuating vision, dark or empty areas in vision, vision loss

27. _____ Diplopia, difficulty with night vision, halo images around lights, increased sensitivity to glare

a. corneal abrasion
b. cataract
c. glaucoma
d. diabetic retinopathy
e. macular degeneration

Match the diagnostic measures and treatments with the correct disease.

28. _____ Comprehensive eye examination, fluorescein angiography, optical coherence tomography; photocoagulation, panretinal photocoagulation, vitrectomy vascular endothelial growth factor inhibitor

29. _____ Based on patient's signs and symptoms, confirmed with the instillation of fluorescein stain; remove foreign body, antibiotic ophthalmic ointment, nonsteroidal antiinflammatory ophthalmic drops, oral analgesics

30. _____ Tonometer with a slit lamp, gonioscopy; miotic and beta-blocker eyedrops, laser surgery

31. _____ Beta carotene, vitamins C and E with zinc and copper

32. _____ Surgical removal of the lens

a. corneal abrasion
b. cataract
c. glaucoma
d. diabetic retinopathy
e. macular degeneration

E. Ear Diseases and Disorders

1. Hearing loss that originates in the external or middle ear that prevents sound vibrations from passing through the external auditory canal, limits the vibration of the tympanic membrane, or interferes with the passage of bone-conducted sound in the middle ear is _____.

2. Hearing loss from an abnormality of the organ of Corti or auditory nerve is _____.

3. Progressive sensorineural deafness associated with aging is _____.

Match the description with the correct disorder.

4. _____ Ear wax that has been pushed up tightly against the eardrum

5. _____ Inflammation of the outer ear

6. _____ Disorder of the inner ear

7. _____ Inflammation of the middle ear

a. otitis externa
b. otitis media
c. impacted cerumen
d. Meniere's disease

Match the etiology with the correct disease.

8. _____ Upper respiratory infection, allergic reaction

9. _____ Psoriasis, abnormally narrow ear canals, excessive amount of hair growing in the ear canals

10. _____ Dermatologic conditions, trauma, continuous use of earplugs or earphones

11. _____ Inner ear seems to have an abnormal amount of fluid

a. otitis externa
b. otitis media
c. impacted cerumen
d. Meniere's disease

Match the signs and symptoms with the correct disease.

12. _____ Vertigo, tinnitus, progressive hearing loss

13. _____ Full feeling, some hearing loss

14. _____ Hearing loss, tinnitus, feeling of fullness, otalgia

15. _____ Severe pain, inflammation and swelling, hearing loss

a. otitis externa
b. otitis media
c. impacted cerumen
d. Meniere's disease

Match the diagnostic measures and treatments with the correct disease.

16. _____ Otoscopic examination; removal, softening of the wax, irrigation of the ear

17. _____ Antibiotic or steroid eardrops

18. _____ Otoscopic examination, tympanogram; "watch and wait," antibiotics, acetaminophen or ibuprofen, myringotomy

19. _____ Medications for nausea and vomiting, salt-restricted diet, diuretics and antihistamines, surgical destruction of the labyrinth

a. otitis externa
b. otitis media
c. impacted cerumen
d. Meniere's disease

F. The Medical Assistant's Role in Examination, Diagnostic Procedures, and Treatments

1. What does each letter of the acronym PERRLA stand for?

    a. P _____

    b. E _____

    c. R _____

    d. R _____

    e. L _____

    f. A _____

Match the description with the correct term.

2. _____ A chart commonly used to test visual acuity

3. _____ A tuning fork test used if the patient reports that hearing is better in one ear than the other

4. _____ Drooping of the upper eyelid

5. _____ A simple procedure that detects color blindness

6. _____ A tuning fork test used to compare air conduction sound with bone conduction sound

7. _____ An abnormal protrusion of the eye

a. blepharoptosis
b. exophthalmia
c. Snellen alphabetical chart
d. Ishihara color vision test
e. Weber hearing test
f. Rinne hearing test

8. _____ measures the lowest intensity of sound an individual can hear.

9. In ophthalmology a medical assistant might help with treatments such as _____ and _____.

10. In otolaryngology a medical assistant might help with treatments such as _____ and _____.

CERTIFICATION PREPARATION
Circle the correct answer.

1. What is buzzing, ringing, or whistling in the ear(s), occurring without an external stimulus?
    a. Vertigo
    b. Presbycusis
    c. Tinnitus
    d. Astigmatism

2. Which is part of the anterior surface of the eye?
    a. Retina
    b. Lens
    c. Optic disc
    d. Macula lutea

3. The colored portion of the eye is called the
    a. iris.
    b. pupil.
    c. retina.
    d. none of the above.

4. What is the term used for a drooping upper eyelid?
    a. Hordeolum
    b. Blepharedema
    c. Keratitis
    d. Blepharoptosis

5. Which structures are located in the middle ear?
    a. Pinna, external auditory canal, tympanic membrane
    b. Semicircular canals, vestibule, cochlea
    c. Malleus, incus, stapes
    d. Oval window, eustachian tube, vestibule

6. The organ of Corti is located in the
    a. middle ear.
    b. semicircular canal.
    c. cochlea.
    d. vestibule.

7. Which could be a sign or symptom of glaucoma?
    a. Mild headaches
    b. Impaired adaptation to the dark
    c. Loss of peripheral vision, often called *tunnel vision*
    d. All of the above

8. Macular degeneration is most commonly diagnosed after age
    a. 45.
    b. 55.
    c. 65.
    d. 75.

9. What is the term for age-related hearing loss?
    a. Presbycusis
    b. Otosclerosis
    c. Otitis media
    d. Paracusis

10. Which condition could be diagnosed in an older adult patient?
    a. Macular degeneration
    b. Glaucoma
    c. Presbycusis
    d. All of the above

WORKPLACE APPLICATIONS

1. Rosie greets her patient, Harry, age 10, and his mother. Harry loves to swim in the pond on the family farm, but recently he has been having pain in his right ear and some discharge of clear fluid. It has been hard for Harry to sleep the last few days because he normally sleeps on his right side. Given this very limited information, what possible condition(s) could cause these signs and symptoms?

_____

_____

2. Rosie is reviewing eye and ear diseases and disorders as part of a continuing education course. Briefly describe the following diagnostic procedures:

    a. Visual acuity test _____

    _____

    b. Tonometry _____

    _____

    c. Audiometry _____

    _____

    d. Speech audiometry _____

    _____

3. Patrick Kachajian has been diagnosed with color blindness.

    a. Describe color blindness. _____

    _____

    b. Briefly describe the signs and symptoms of color blindness. _____

    _____

    c. What test is used to diagnose color blindness? _____

    _____

INTERNET ACTIVITIES

1. Using online resources, research a test used for diagnosing an eye or ear disease. Create a poster presentation, a PowerPoint presentation, or a written paper summarizing your research. Include the following points in your project:
    a. Description of the test
    b. Any contraindications for the test
    c. Patient preparation for the test
    d. What occurs during the test

2. Using online resources, research an eye or ear disease or disorder. Create a poster presentation, a PowerPoint presentation, or a written paper summarizing your research. Include the following points in your project:
    a. Description of the disease
    b. Etiology
    c. Signs and symptoms
    d. Diagnostic procedures
    e. Treatments
    f. Prognosis
    g. Prevention

3. Using online resources, research the effect that diet can have on the management of Meniere's disease. In a one-page paper, summarize the information that you found.

Procedure 31.1   Measuring Distance Visual Acuity

Name _____ Date _____ Score _____

Task: To determine the patient's degree of visual clarity at a measured distance of 20 feet using the Snellen chart.

Equipment and Supplies:
- Patient's health record
- Provider's order
- Snellen eye chart
- Disposable eye occluder or an alcohol wipe to clean the occluder before use
- Pen or pencil and paper

Standard: Complete the procedure and all critical steps in _____ minutes with a minimum score of 85% within two attempts (*or as indicated by the instructor*).

Scoring: Divide the points earned by the total possible points. Failure to perform a critical step, indicated by an asterisk (*), results in grade no higher than an 84% (*or as indicated by the instructor*).

Time: Began_____ Ended_____ Total minutes: _____

Steps:	Point Value	Attempt 1	Attempt 2
1. Wash hands or use hand sanitizer.	5		
2. Prepare the area. Make sure the room is well lit and that a distance marker is 20 feet from the chart.	5		
3. Greet the patient. Identify yourself. Verify the patient's identity with full name and date of birth. Explain the procedure to be performed in a manner that is understood by the patient. Answer any questions the patient may have on the procedure. Instruct the patient not to squint during the test because this temporarily improves vision. The patient should not have an opportunity to study the chart before the test is given. If the patient wears corrective lenses, they should be worn during the test.	5		
4. Position the patient in a standing or sitting position at the 20-foot marker.	10		
5. Check that the Snellen chart is positioned at the patient's eye level.	5		
6. If the occluder is not disposable, disinfect it before the procedure starts. Then instruct the patient to cover the left eye with the occluder and to keep both eyes open throughout the test to prevent squinting.	5		
7. Stand beside the chart and point to each row as the patient reads it aloud, starting with the 20/70 row.	5*		
8. Proceed down the rows of the chart until the smallest row the patient can read with a maximum of two errors is reached. If one or two letters are missed, the outcome is recorded with a minus sign and the number of errors (e.g., 20/40–2). If more than two errors are made, the previous line should be documented.	10*		
9. Record any of the patient's reactions while reading the chart.	10		
10. Repeat the procedure with the left eye, covering the right eye.	10		
11. Repeat the procedure with both eyes uncovered.	10		

12. Disinfect the occluder, if it is not disposable, and wash hands or use hand sanitizer.	**10**		
13. Document the procedure in the patient's record, including the date and time, visual acuity results, and any reactions by the patient. Also record whether corrective lenses were worn.	**10**		
Total Points	**100**		

Documentation

Comments

CAAHEP Competencies	**Step(s)**
I.P.3. Perform patient screening following established protocols	Entire procedure
I.P.8. Instruct and prepare a patient for a procedure or a treatment	3
I.P.9. Assist provider with a patient exam	Entire procedure
X.P.3. Document patient care accurately in the medical record	13
ABHES Competencies	**Step(s)**
4. Medical Law and Ethics a. Follow documentation guidelines	13
8. Clinical Procedures a. Practice standard precautions and perform disinfection/sterilization techniques	1, 6
8. Clinical Procedures c. Assist provider with general/physical examination	Entire procedure

Procedure 31.2 Assess Color Acuity Using the Ishihara Test

Name _____ Date _____ Score _____

Task: To assess a patient's color acuity correctly and record the results.

Equipment and Supplies:
- Patient's health record
- Provider's order
- Room with natural light if possible
- Ishihara color plate book
- Pen, pencil, and paper
- Watch with a second hand

Standard: Complete the procedure and all critical steps in _____ minutes with a minimum score of 85% within two attempts (*or as indicated by the instructor*).

Scoring: Divide the points earned by the total possible points. Failure to perform a critical step, indicated by an asterisk (*), results in grade no higher than an 84% (*or as indicated by the instructor*).

Time: Began_____ Ended_____ Total minutes: _____

Steps:	Point Value	Attempt 1	Attempt 2
1. Assemble the equipment and prepare the room for testing. The room should be quiet and illuminated with natural light.	10		
2. Greet the patient. Identify yourself. Verify the patient's identity with full name and date of birth. Explain the procedure to be performed in a manner that is understood by the patient. Answer any questions the patient may have on the procedure. Use a practice card during the explanation and make sure the patient understands that they have 3 seconds to identify each plate.	10		
3. Hold up the first plate at a right angle to the patient's line of vision and 30 inches from the patient. Be sure both of the patient's eyes are kept open during the test.	15*		
4. Ask the patient to tell you the number on the plate. Record the plate number and the patient's answer.	15		
5. Continue this sequence until all 11 plates have been read. If the patient cannot identify the number on the plate, place an X in the record for that plate number.	15		
6. Include any unusual symptoms such as eye rubbing, squinting, or excessive blinking in your record.	15		
7. Place the book back in its cardboard sleeve and return it to its storage space.	10		
8. Document the procedure in the patient's health record, including the date and time, the testing results, and any patient symptoms shown during the test.	10		
Total Points	100		

Documentation

Comments

CAAHEP Competencies	Step(s)
I.P.3. Perform patient screening following established protocols	Entire procedure
I.P.8. Instruct and prepare a patient for a procedure or a treatment	2
I.P.9. Assist provider with a patient exam	Entire procedure
X.P.3. Document patient care accurately in the medical record	8
ABHES Competencies	**Step(s)**
4. Medical Law and Ethics a. Follow documentation guidelines	8
8. Clinical Procedures c. Assist provider with general/physical examination	Entire procedure

Procedure 31.3 Irrigate a Patient's Eye

Name _____ Date _____ Score _____

Tasks: Irrigate a patient's eye and document patient care.

Equipment and Supplies:
- Provider's order
- Patient health record
- Drug reference information
- Sterile ophthalmic irrigation solution and supplies
- Disposable waterproof pad and towels
- Basin
- Sterile gauze
- Gloves

Standard: Complete the procedure and all critical steps in _____ minutes with a minimum score of 85% within two attempts (*or as indicated by the instructor*).

Scoring: Divide the points earned by the total possible points. Failure to perform a critical step, indicated by an asterisk (*), results in grade no higher than an 84% (*or as indicated by the instructor*).

Time: Began_____ Ended_____ Total minutes: _____

Steps:	Point Value	Attempt 1	Attempt 2
1. Wash hands or use hand sanitizer.	5		
2. Select the right medication (fluid) from the storage area. Check the medication label against the order. Check for the right name, form, and route. Check the expiration date to make sure the fluid is not expired. Verify the right dose and the right time.	5*		
3. Using the drug reference information and the order, review the information on the medication.	5		
4. Perform the second medication check. Check the medication label against the order. Check for the right name, form, dose, and route.	5*		
5. Assemble the supplies required for the procedure.	5		
6. Perform the third medication check. Check the medication label against the order. Check for the right name, form, dose, and route.	5*		
7. Prior to entering the exam room, knock on the door and give it a moment. Greet the patient. Identify yourself. Verify the patient's identity with full name and date of birth. Make sure the patient's information matches the order and the record.	10*		
8. Provide the right education to the patient. Explain the procedure ordered, provider ordering the procedure, the desired effect, and common side effects. Answer any questions the patient may have. Use language the patient can understand. Ask the patient if they have any allergies. If the patient refuses the procedure, notify the provider.	10		

9. Using room-temperature fluid, set up the equipment. If using an IV bag, prime or run fluid through the tubing. If using a prepackaged solution, remove the cover. If using a bulb syringe, pour the required fluid into a basin. Remember to palm the label. Draw the solution into the bulb syringe.	**5**		
10. Assist the patient into a sitting or supine position. Have the patient remove glasses or contact lens. Ask the patient to turn the head towards the side of the affected eye. Place the disposable waterproof pad over the patient's neck and shoulder. Place or have the patient hold the drainage basin next to the affected eye.	**5**		
11. Put on gloves. Moisten a gauze pad with the irrigation fluid. Using the gauze, clean the eyelid from the inner to outer canthus. Discard the gauze after each wipe.	**5**		
12. Perform the right technique. With your nondominant hand, separate and hold the eyelids using the index finger and thumb. With the dominant hand, hold the irrigation equipment on or near the bridge of the nose.	**5***		
13. Direct the solution towards the lower conjunctiva of the inner canthus. Allow a steady flow of solution to slowly flush the eye from the inner to the outer canthus. Do not touch the tip of the irrigation equipment to the eye.	**10***		
14. Continue until the ordered amount of fluid has flushed the eye. Dry the eyelid with sterile gauze, moving from the inner to outer canthus.	**5**		
15. Help the patient into a comfortable position. Clean up the area. Remove gloves and wash hands or use hand sanitizer.	**5**		
16. Document the procedure in the health record. Include allergies, teaching or instructions provided, the provider ordering the irrigation, the fluid used for the irrigation, the amount used, the site, and how the patient tolerated the procedure.	**10***		
Total Points	**100**		

Documentation

Comments

CAAHEP Competencies	Step(s)
I.P.4.a. Verify the rules of medication administration: right patient	7
I.P.4.b. Verify the rules of medication administration: right medication	2, 4, 6
I.P.4.c. Verify the rules of medication administration: right dose	2, 4, 6
I.P.4.d. Verify the rules of medication administration: right route	2, 4, 6
I.P.4.e. Verify the rules of medication administration: right time	2
I.P.4.f. Verify the rules of medication administration: right documentation	16
I.P.8. Instruct and prepare a patient for a procedure or a treatment	8
III.P.2. Select appropriate barrier/personal protective equipment.	11
X.P.3. Document patient care accurately in the medical record	16
ABHES Competencies	**Step(s)**
4. Medical Law and Ethics a. Follow documentation guidelines	16
8. Clinical Procedures a. Practice standard precautions and perform disinfection/ sterilization techniques	11

Procedure 31.4   Instill an Eye Medication

Name _____   Date _____   Score _____

Tasks: Instill an eye drop or ointment and document medication administration.

Equipment and Supplies:
- Provider's order
- Patient health record
- Drug reference information
- Sterile ophthalmic eye drops or ointment
- Sterile gauze
- Gloves

Standard: Complete the procedure and all critical steps in _____ minutes with a minimum score of 85% within two attempts (*or as indicated by the instructor*).

Scoring: Divide the points earned by the total possible points. Failure to perform a critical step, indicated by an asterisk (*), results in grade no higher than an 84% (*or as indicated by the instructor*).

Time: Began_____ Ended_____ Total minutes: _____

Steps:	Point Value	Attempt 1	Attempt 2
1. Wash hands or use hand sanitizer.	5		
2. Select the right medication from the storage area. Check the medication label against the order. Check for the right name, form, and route. Check the expiration date to make sure the drug is not expired. Verify the right dose and the right time.	5*		
3. Using the drug reference information and the order, review the information on the medication.	5		
4. Perform the second medication check. Check the medication label against the order. Check for the right name, form, dose, and route.	5*		
5. Assemble the supplies required for the procedure.	10		
6. Perform the third medication check. Check the medication label against the order. Check for the right name, form, dose, and route.	10*		
7. Prior to entering the exam room, knock on the door and give it a moment. Greet the patient. Identify yourself. Verify the patient's identity with full name and date of birth. Make sure the patient's information matches the order and the record.	10*		
8. Provide the right education to the patient. Explain the medication ordered, provider ordering the medication, the desired effect, and common side effects. Answer any questions the patient may have. Use language the patient can understand. Ask the patient if they have any allergies. If the patient refuses the medication, notify the provider.	10		
9. Assist the patient into a sitting or supine position. Ask the patient to tilt the head backward and look up.	5		
10. Put on gloves. If crusting or draining is present on the eyelid, gently wash the area from the inner to outer canthus. Discard the gauze after each wipe. Dry the area.	10		

11. Perform the right technique. With your nondominant hand holding a sterile gauze, pull the lower conjunctival sac downward creating a pocket for the medication. Instruct the patient to look up.
   a. For the eye drops: with your dominant hand, hold the bottle or the dropper ¾ inch away from the conjunctival sac. Drop the required number of drops into the eye. If the drop misses the eye or the patient blinks, wipe the liquid on the skin and repeat the drop. Have the person gently press against the inner corner of the eye and the nose bone for 1 minute. Have the person keep the eye closed for 2-3 minutes after the administration of the drop.
   b. For eye ointment: with the dominant hand, hold the ointment container above the lower lid. Working from inner to outer canthus, apply a small layer of ointment along the inner lower lid margin. Have the patient close the eye and rub the eyelid in a circular motion. Wipe up any extra ointment.
	10*		

12. Help the patient into a comfortable position. Clean up the area. Remove gloves and wash hands or use hand sanitizer.	5		
13. Document the procedure in the health record. Include allergies; teaching or instructions provided; the provider ordering the medication; the medication name, dose, route; and how the patient tolerated the medication.	10*		
Total Points	100		

Documentation

Comments

CAAHEP Competencies	Step(s)
I.P.4.a. Verify the rules of medication administration: right patient	7
I.P.4.b. Verify the rules of medication administration: right medication	2, 4, 6
I.P.4.c. Verify the rules of medication administration: right dose	2, 4, 6
I.P.4.d. Verify the rules of medication administration: right route	2, 4, 6
I.P.4.e. Verify the rules of medication administration: right time	2
I.P.4.f. Verify the rules of medication administration: right documentation	13
I.P.8. Instruct and prepare a patient for a procedure or a treatment	8
III.P.2. Select appropriate barrier/personal protective equipment.	10
X.P.3. Document patient care accurately in the medical record	13
ABHES Competencies	**Step(s)**
4. Medical Law and Ethics a. Follow documentation guidelines	13
8. Clinical Procedure a. Practice standard precautions and perform disinfection/ sterilization techniques	10

Procedure 31.5 Measuring Hearing Acuity with an Audiometer

Name _____ Date _____ Score _____

Task: To perform audiometric testing of hearing acuity.

Equipment and Supplies:
- Patient's health record
- Provider's order
- Audiometer with adjustable headphones and graph paper
- Quiet area

Standard: Complete the procedure and all critical steps in _____ minutes with a minimum score of 85% within two attempts (*or as indicated by the instructor*).

Scoring: Divide the points earned by the total possible points. Failure to perform a critical step, indicated by an asterisk (*), results in grade no higher than an 84% (*or as indicated by the instructor*).

Time: Began_____ Ended_____ Total minutes: _____

Steps:	Point Value	Attempt 1	Attempt 2
1. Wash hands or use hand sanitizer, assemble the equipment, and bring the patient into a quiet area.	10		
2. Greet the patient. Identify yourself. Verify the patient's identity with full name and date of birth. Explain the procedure to be performed in a manner that is understood by the patient. Answer any questions the patient may have on the procedure.	10		
3. Explain that the audiometer measures whether the patient can hear various sound wave frequencies through the headphones. Each ear is tested separately. When the patient hears a frequency, they should raise a hand or push the button to signal the medical assistant.	10		
4. Place the headphones over the patient's ears, making sure they are adjusted for comfort.	10		
5. The audiometer tests each ear separately, starting at a low frequency. If the results are not automatically recorded by the machine, the medical assistant documents the patient's response to the frequencies on a graph or audiogram. Results for the left ear are marked with an X, and those for the right ear are marked with an O.	10*		
6. Frequencies are increased gradually to test the patient's ability to hear. Each response by the patient is documented.	10		
7. After one ear has been tested, the other ear is then tested, and the results are documented.	10		
8. The results are given to the provider for interpretation or downloaded into the patient's electronic health record for the provider to review.	10		
9. The equipment is sanitized and disinfected according to the manufacturer's guidelines.	10		
10. Wash hands or use hand sanitizer.	10		
Total Points	100		

Comments

CAAHEP Competencies	Step(s)
I.P.3. Perform patient screening following established protocols	Entire procedure
I.P.8. Instruct and prepare a patient for a procedure or a treatment	2, 3
I.P.9. Assist provider with a patient exam	Entire procedure
ABHES Competencies	**Step(s)**
8. Clinical Procedures c. Assist provider with general/physical examination	Entire procedure

Procedure 31.6   Irrigate a Patient's Ear

Name _____ Date _____ Score _____

Tasks: Irrigate a patient's ear and document patient care.

Equipment and Supplies:
- Provider's order
- Patient health record
- Ear wash basin
- Elephant ear wash system (or other ear wash system)
- Disposable waterproof pad and towels
- Thermometer (optional)
- Otoscope and disposable speculum (optional)
- Gauze
- Gloves
- Sterile water or saline
- Waste container

Order: Irrigate left ear with warm sterile water.

Standard: Complete the procedure and all critical steps in _____ minutes with a minimum score of 85% within two attempts (*or as indicated by the instructor*).

Scoring: Divide the points earned by the total possible points. Failure to perform a critical step, indicated by an asterisk (*), results in grade no higher than an 84% (*or as indicated by the instructor*).

Time: Began_____ Ended_____ Total minutes: _____

Steps:	Point Value	Attempt 1	Attempt 2
1. Wash hands or use hand sanitizer.	5		
2. Select the right medication (fluid) from the storage area. Check the medication label against the order. Check for the right name and route; check the expiration date.	5*		
3. Assemble the equipment and supplies needed. Perform the second medication check. Check the medication (fluid) name and route against the order.	5*		
4. Clean up the work area and perform the third medication check. Check the medication (fluid) name and route against the order.	5*		
5. Prior to entering the exam room, knock on the door and give it a moment. Greet the patient. Identify yourself. Verify the patient's identity with full name and date of birth. Make sure the patient's information matches the order and the record.	5*		
6. Provide the right education to the patient. Explain the procedure ordered, provider ordering the procedure, the desired effect, and common side effects of ear irrigations. Answer any questions the patient may have. Use language the patient can understand. If the patient refuses the procedure, notify the provider.	5		

7.	Prepare the equipment. Warm the irrigating solution to body temperature (98.6° F [check with a thermometer]) or until it is lukewarm. Lukewarm is neither hot nor cold. Fill the spray bottle with the fluid. Attach the disposal tip to the nozzle on the hose. If another type of ear wash system is being used, prepare the equipment and the fluid.	5		
8.	Assist the patient into a sitting position. Wrap a waterproof pad around the person's shoulder, protecting the clothing. Have a towel available for the patient if needed. Have the patient tilt his or her head towards the affected ear. Have the patient hold the ear wash basin under the affected ear.	10		
9.	Put on gloves. Using gauze, wipe any debris from the outer ear.	10		
10.	Insert the disposable tip gently into the ear. Do not insert too far since it could injure the canal. If possible, gently pull the pinna up and back if the patient is older than age 3. For patients younger than 3, pull the pinna down and back.	5*		
11.	Keeping the tubing straight, spray the fluid in the ear canal. Aim the fluid towards the top of the ear canal.	5		
12.	Continue irrigating until the solution is used, the maximum time has been reached, the desired result is achieved, or the patient has problems with the procedure. Empty the ear wash basin when it fills. Observe the fluid for any substances (i.e., cerumen).	5		
13.	Dry the outside of the ear with gauze. If facility procedure indicates, use otoscope to observe canal. Attach the speculum to the otoscope. Straighten the ear canal by pulling the appropriate direction on the pinna. Gently insert the otoscope. Observe the canal.	5		
14.	Place a clean, absorbent towel on the examination table. Have the patient rest quietly with the head turned to the irrigated side while you wait for the provider to return to check the affected ear.	10*		
15.	Clean up the work area. Remove your gloves and dispose in the waste container. Sanitize your hands.	5		
16.	Document the procedure in the health record. Include teaching or instructions provided, the provider ordering the irrigation, the fluid used for the irrigation, the amount used, the site, and how the patient tolerated the procedure.	10*		
	Total Points	100		

Documentation

Comments

CAAHEP Competencies	Step(s)
I.P.4.a. Verify the rules of medication administration: right patient	5
I.P.4.b. Verify the rules of medication administration: right medication	2, 3, 4
I.P.4.d. Verify the rules of medication administration: right route	2, 3, 4
I.P.4.f. Verify the rules of medication administration: right documentation	16
I.P.8. Instruct and prepare a patient for a procedure or a treatment	6
III.P.2. Select appropriate barrier/personal protective equipment.	9
X.P.3. Document patient care accurately in the medical record	16
ABHES Competencies	**Step(s)**
4. Medical Law and Ethics a. Follow documentation guidelines	16
8. Clinical Procedures a. Practice standard precautions and perform disinfection/ sterilization techniques	9

Procedure 31.7 Instill Ear Drops

Name _____ Date _____ Score _____

Tasks: Instill ear drops and document medication administration.

Equipment and Supplies:
- Provider's order
- Patient health record
- Drug reference information
- Otic drops
- Gauze
- Gloves

Standard: Complete the procedure and all critical steps in _____ minutes with a minimum score of 85% within two attempts (*or as indicated by the instructor*).

Scoring: Divide the points earned by the total possible points. Failure to perform a critical step, indicated by an asterisk (*), results in grade no higher than an 84% (*or as indicated by the instructor*).

Time: Began_____ Ended_____ Total minutes: _____

Steps:	Point Value	Attempt 1	Attempt 2
1. Wash hands or use hand sanitizer.	5		
2. Select the right medication from the storage area. Check the medication label against the order. Check for the right name, form, and route. Check the expiration date to make sure the drug is not expired. Verify the right dose and the right time.	5*		
3. Using the drug reference information and the order, review the information on the medication.	5		
4. Perform the second medication check. Check the medication label against the order. Check for the right name, form, dose, and route.	5*		
5. Assemble the supplies required for the procedure.	5		
6. Perform the third medication check. Check the medication label against the order. Check for the right name, form, dose, and route.	5*		
7. Prior to entering the exam room, knock on the door and give it a moment. Greet the patient. Identify yourself. Verify the patient's identity with full name and date of birth. Make sure the patient's information matches the order and the record.	10*		
8. Provide the right education to the patient. Explain the medication ordered, provider ordering the medication, the desired effect, and common side effects. Answer any questions the patient may have. Use language the patient can understand. Ask the patient if they have any allergies. If the patient refuses the medication, notify the provider.	10		
9. Assist the patient into a sitting position or in a side-lying position on the unaffected side.	5		
10. Warm the medication bottle with your hands if needed. The drops should be at room temperature. Shake the medication if needed. Put on gloves.	5		

11. Perform the right technique. Have the patient tilt his/her head so the affected ear is upward. If cerumen or drainage is blocking the canal, gently remove it with a cotton-tipped application.	**5**			
12. Remove the cover of the bottle. With your nondominant hand, gently pull the pinna up and back if the patient is older than age 3. This straightens the external auditory canal. For patients younger than 3, pull the pinna down and back.	**5**			
13. Hold the dropper firmly in your dominant hand. Place the tip of the dropper about ½ inch above the ear canal. Be sure not to contaminate the dropper by touching it to the patient. Carefully drop the required number of drops in the patient's ear. Replace the cover.	**10***			
14. Have the patient keep the ear facing up for 3-5 minutes, depending on the medication.	**5**			
15. Help the patient into a comfortable position. Clean up the area. Remove gloves and wash hands or use hand sanitizer.	**5**			
16. Document the procedure in the health record. Include allergies; teaching or instructions provided; the provider ordering the medication; the medication name, dose, route; and how the patient tolerated the medication.	**10***			
Total Points	**100**			

Documentation

Comments

CAAHEP Competencies	Step(s)
I.P.4.a. Verify the rules of medication administration: right patient	7
I.P.4.b. Verify the rules of medication administration: right medication	2, 4, 6
I.P.4.c. Verify the rules of medication administration: right dose	2, 4, 6
I.P.4.d. Verify the rules of medication administration: right route	2, 4, 6
I.P.4.e. Verify the rules of medication administration: right time	2
I.P.4.f. Verify the rules of medication administration: right documentation	16
I.P.8. Instruct and prepare a patient for a procedure or a treatment	8
III.P.2. Select appropriate barrier/personal protective equipment.	10
X.P.3. Document patient care accurately in the medical record	16
ABHES Competencies	**Step(s)**
4. Medical Law and Ethics a. Follow documentation guidelines	16
8. Clinical Procedures a. Practice standard precautions and perform disinfection/ sterilization techniques	10

Dermatology

CAAHEP Competencies	Assessment
I.C.4. Identify major organs in each body system	Skills and Concepts – A. 1-5
I.C.5. Identify the anatomical location of major organs in each body system	Skills and Concepts – A. 1-5
I.C.6. Identify the structure and function of the human body across the life span	Skills and Concepts – C. 1-4
I.C.7. Identify the normal function of each body system	Skills and Concepts – A. 1-9, B. 1-7
I.C.8.a. Identify common pathology related to each body system including: signs	Skills and Concepts – D. 11-20, 35-39
I.C.8.b. Identify common pathology related to each body system including: symptoms	Skills and Concepts – D. 11-20, 35-39
I.C.8.c. Identify common pathology related to each body system including: etiology	Skills and Concepts – D. 1-10, 30-34
I.C.8.d. Identify common pathology related to each body system including: diagnostic measures	Skills and Concepts – D. 21-29, 40-44
I.C.8.e. Identify common pathology related to each body system including: treatment modalities	Skills and Concepts – D. 21-29, 40-44
V.C.8.a. Identify the following related to body systems: medical terms	Vocabulary Review – A. 1-10, B. 1-11
V.C.8.b. Identify the following related to body systems: abbreviations	Abbreviations – 1-10
ABHES Competencies	**Assessment**
2. Anatomy and Physiology a. List all body systems and their structures and functions	Skills and Concepts – A. 1-5
b. Describe common diseases, symptoms, and etiologies as they apply to each system	Skills and Concepts – D. 1-20, 30-39
c. Identify diagnostic and treatment modalities as they relate to each body system	Skills and Concepts – D. 21-29, 40-44
3. Medical Terminology c. Apply medical terminology for each specialty	Vocabulary Review – A. 1-10, B. 1-11
d. Define and use medical abbreviations when appropriate and acceptable	Abbreviations – 1-10

VOCABULARY REVIEW

Using the word pool on the right, find the correct word to match the definition. Write the word on the line after the definition.

Group A

1. To strip off or remove the skin from an area

   _____

2. Naturally or artificially formed layers of material, usually multiple layers _____

3. The most abundant structural protein found in skin and other connective tissues; provides strength and cushioning to many parts of the body _____

4. Kidney disease affecting the capillaries of the nephron (glomeruli); characterized by albuminuria, edema, and hypertension

   _____

5. Form cellular sheets that cover surfaces, both inside and outside the body; cells are closely packed, take on different shapes, and strongly stick to each other _____

6. A highly elastic protein in connective tissue that allows tissues to resume their shape after stretching or contracting; found abundantly in the dermis of the skin _____

7. Cells of the stratum germinativum that produce a brownish pigment called *melanin*; melanin gives skin its color

   _____

8. A disease-causing organism _____

9. Bottom layer _____

10. Formation of a chemical compound from simpler compounds or elements _____

Word Pool
- pathogen
- synthesis
- epithelial cells
- strata
- basal
- melanocytes
- collagen
- elastin
- excoriated
- glomerulonephritis

Group B

1. A reddish pigment that results from the breakdown of red blood cells in the liver _____

2. Discoloration of the skin caused by the escape of blood into the tissues from ruptured blood vessels; typically caused by bruising

   _____

3. Lack of skin pigmentation, especially in patches

   _____

4. The technique of exposing tissue to extreme cold to produce a well-defined area of cell destruction _____

5. A descriptive term for things or conditions that threaten life or well-being; the opposite of benign _____

6. Tiny openings in the surface of the skin that allow gases, liquids, or microscopic particles to pass _____

7. A yellow discoloration of the skin and mucous membranes caused by deposits of bile _____

Word Pool
- hyperplasia
- opaque
- benign
- malignant
- leukoderma
- jaundice
- bilirubin
- petechiae
- ecchymosis
- cryosurgery
- pores

8. Enlargement due to an abnormal multiplication of cells
   _____

9. Very small, round hemorrhage in the skin or mucous membrane
   _____

10. Not transparent; cloudy or murky _____

11. A noncancerous condition, not malignant, harmless
    _____

ABBREVIATIONS
Write out what each of the following abbreviations stands for.

1. UV _____

2. HPV _____

3. HSV-1 _____

4. OTC _____

5. TIM _____

6. DLE _____

7. PDT _____

8. KS _____

9. SLE _____

10. PUVA _____

SKILLS AND CONCEPTS
Answer the following questions. Write your answer on the line or in the space provided.

A. Anatomy of the Integumentary System

1. The upper layer of the skin is the _____, and the lower layer of the skin is the
   _____.

2. Where are new skin cells formed in the epidermis?_____

3. New skin cells are produced in the stratum germinativum and move upward towards the top layer or stratum corneum. During the transition from the basal layer to the upper layer, the cell's cytoplasm is replaced with keratin.
   a. The first statement is true, and the second statement is false.
   b. The first statement is false, and second statement is true.
   c. Both statements are true.
   d. Both statements are false.

4. Which of the following is true about keratin?
   a. It is a hard protein.
   b. It makes the skin waterproof.
   c. It makes the skin abrasion-resistant.
   d. It enables the body to retain moisture.
   e. All of the above.

5. "Peg-like projections that help fasten the dermis and epidermis together" is describing _____.

6. If the dermal-epidermal junction is damaged by a burn, irritation, abrasion, or friction, a(n) _____ may develop at the site of the damage.

Match the term to the correct description. Answers may be used more than once.

7. _____ Located in the axillae, scalp, face, and pigmented skin around the genitals

8. _____ Releases sweat through the pores in the skin

9. _____ Dispersed throughout the body

10. _____ Release a fatty sweat in response to stress

a. Eccrine sweat gland
b. Apocrine sweat gland

11. Subcutaneous tissue is made up of _____ tissue and _____ tissue.

B. Physiology of the Integumentary System

1. The skin _____ the body by providing a flexible, waterproof barrier to the outside environment.

2. The skin acts as a(n) _____ organ by using receptors that can feel pain, pressure, heat, and cold.

3. When we are hot, the skin produces _____ that evaporates and cools us off. When we are cold, the skin _____ blood vessels close to the surface to preserve body heat.

4. The synthesis of _____ starts with the skin. When the skin is exposed to the sun's ultraviolet rays, it manufactures a(n) _____ molecule that is carried to the liver and kidneys where it is converted to the _____ form that can be used by the body.

5. Sensory receptors located throughout the skin include which of the following?
   a. Pain, pressure
   b. Heat, cold
   c. Light, dark
   d. Both a and b

6. The skin is also involved in excretion. Which of the following is excreted by the skin?
   a. Water
   b. Electrolytes
   c. Small amounts of other waste products
   d. All of the above
   e. None of the above

C. Life Span Changes

1. The creamy biofilm that forms in utero to protect the baby's skin from the amniotic fluid is _____.

2. The two highly contagious skin disorders that are often seen in children are _____ and _____.

3. In older adults, masses or thickening of the skin in response to constant friction are called _____ and _____.

4. Bedridden patients may develop _____, also called _____ or _____.

D. Diseases and Disorders of the Integumentary System

Match the etiology with the correct condition.

1. _____ Cold sores or fever blisters caused by HSV-1	a. impetigo
2. _____ Caused by lice that populate the head, body, or pubis	b. acne vulgaris
3. _____ A common superficial infection caused by Streptococcus sp. or *Staphylococcus aureus*	c. rosacea
4. _____ A localized staphylococcal infection that begins as inflammation of a hair follicle or skin gland	d. furuncle
	e. cellulitis
5. _____ Caused by the human papillomavirus	f. fungal infections
6. _____ A hair follicle becomes plugged with oil and dead skins cells	g. herpes simplex
7. _____ An acute infection of the skin and subcutaneous tissue	h. warts
8. _____ Caused by the itch mite *Sarcoptes scabiei*	i. scabies
9. _____ Chronic disease most frequently seen in women between the ages of 30 and 60	j. pediculosis
10. _____ Pathogens infect hair follicles or the nails, causing almost no inflammation in the underlying skin	

Match the signs and symptoms with the correct disease.

11. _____ Begins as a small cut, skin injury, or at the site of a furuncle or ulcer. The site becomes inflamed, edematous, and painful with red streaks along the lymph vessels that lead from the infection	a. impetigo
	b. acne vulgaris
12. _____ Small vesicles on the face that quickly enlarge and rupture, excreting a honey-colored exudate. This forms crusty lesions with an inflamed and moist are underneath	c. rosacea
	d. furuncle
13. _____ Small red bumps on the skin and nits on the body, facial, or pubic hair	e. cellulitis
	f. fungal infections
14. _____ Whiteheads; blackheads; papules and pustules; large, solid, painful nodules; painful, pus-filled lumps beneath the skin's surface	g. herpes simplex
	h. warts
15. _____ Painful ulcers along the gumlines of the mouth or on the lips	i. scabies
16. _____ Little burrows or tunnels can be seen under the skin	j. pediculosis
17. _____ Lesions are pruritic and have a distinct border with scaling areas that have a clear center	
18. _____ Begins as frequent flushing across the nose, forehead, cheeks, and chin. Capillaries dilate and are visible across affected areas as small, red, edematous lines; eye inflammation and photosensitivity	
19. _____ Hyperplasia of the epidermis and a raised, cauliflower-like appearance	
20. _____ A raised, inflamed, and painful area that may produce purulent drainage	

Match the diagnostic measures and treatments with the correct disease.

21. _____ Resolve over time, can be treated with topical chemicals, excised surgically, vaporized with lasers, removed with cryosurgery

22. _____ OTC lotions, topical prescription-strength benzoyl peroxide, antibiotics, retinoids, and oral contraceptives. Light therapy, chemical peels, dietary changes, dermabrasion, laser resurfacing

23. _____ Prescription shampoo, body wash, and lotion

24. _____ Clotrimazole, ketoconazole, nystatin, keep the site clean and dry, wear loose clothing

25. _____ Topical antibiotics, oral antibiotics such as doxycycline

26. _____ Topical antiviral drugs or oral antiviral drugs

27. _____ Oral antibiotics, frequent cleansing of the area, antibiotic ointment, surgical incision and drainage of the purulent material

28. _____ Antibiotic ointment or oral antibiotics, consistent handwashing

29. _____ Oral antibiotics, warm compresses applied locally, analgesics to relieve discomfort

a. impetigo
b. acne vulgaris
c. rosacea
d. furuncle
e. cellulitis
f. fungal infections
g. herpes simplex
h. warts
i. pediculosis

Match the etiology with the correct condition.

30. _____ It alters the amount and quality of the sebum

31. _____ Inherited tendency, often seen in combination with asthma or hay fever

32. _____ Chronic autoimmune disease affecting the face, ears, and scalp

33. _____ An inflammatory response to a skin irritant or from exposure to a substance that causes an allergic reaction

34. _____ An autoimmune disease that affects the life cycle of skin cells; caused by a malfunction in the T lymphocytes that attack healthy skin cells

a. seborrheic dermatitis
b. contact dermatitis
c. eczema (atopic dermatitis)
d. psoriasis
e. discoid lupus erythematosus

Match the signs and symptoms with the correct disease.

35. _____ Redness, edema, pruritus, and vesicles

36. _____ Red patches of skin covered in silvery scales; dry, cracked skin that may bleed and small patches of scaly spots; itching, burning, and pain in round plaques; thick, pitted, or ridged fingernails and toenails; swollen, stiff joints

37. _____ Dry or moist, greasy-appearing scales and yellowish crusts on the scalp, eyebrows, eyelids, and the sides of the nose

38. _____ Sores with inflammation and scarring on the face, ears, scalp; coin-shaped red lesions with inflamed patches with a scaly or crusty appearance

39. _____ Itchy skin; rash on the face, back of the knees, hands, wrists, or feet; a dry, thickened, or scaly appearance of the skin that starts out pink or red but can turn brownish with time

a. seborrheic dermatitis
b. contact dermatitis
c. eczema (atopic dermatitis)
d. psoriasis
e. discoid lupus erythematosus

Match the diagnostic measures and treatments with the correct disease.

40. _____ Observation and patient history; provider-recommended lotion or cream, cold compresses, and 1% hydrocortisone cream

41. _____ Physical examination with complete history and laboratory evaluation, skin biopsy; use of sunscreen and avoidance of sun exposure, corticosteroid creams or ointment used in conjunction with injections

42. _____ Wash affected area, corticosteroid cream, oral corticosteroid medications

43. _____ Observation; creams and ointments, light therapy, oral or injected medications

44. _____ Tar- or sulfur-based shampoos; topical corticosteroids

a. seborrheic dermatitis
b. contact dermatitis
c. eczema (atopic dermatitis)
d. psoriasis
e. discoid lupus erythematosus

45. Using the rule of nines, indicate the percentages for each section of the body for the adult and infant.

A. _____
B. _____
C. _____
D. _____
E. _____
F. _____
G. _____
H. _____
I. _____
J. _____
K. _____
L. _____
M. _____
N. _____
O. _____
P. _____

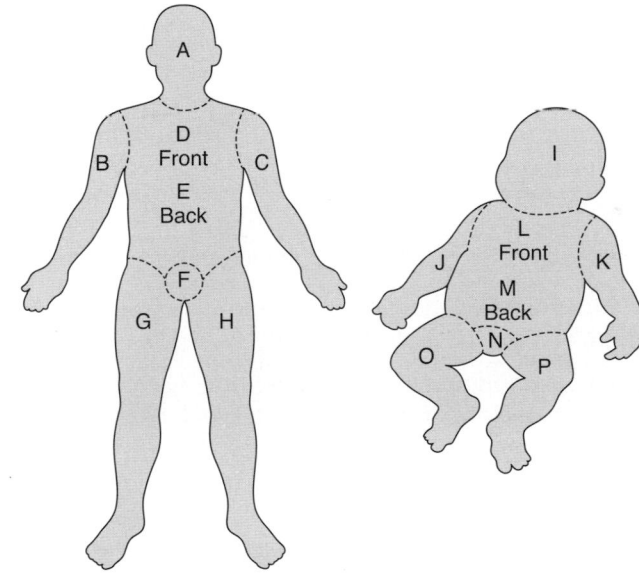

Figure modified from *Bolick et al: Pediatric Acute Care: A Guide to Interprofessional Practice*, ed 2, St. Louis, 2021, Elsevier.

Match the category of burn with the correct description.

46. _____ A burn that damages the epidermis, dermis, and subcutaneous tissue. Pain is not present as the nerve endings have been destroyed.

47. _____ A burn in which only the epidermis is damaged.

48. _____ Rare burn that extends beyond the subcutaneous tissue into the muscle and bone.

49. _____ A burn in which only the first and second layers of the skin are affected.

a. first-degree burn
b. second-degree burn
c. third-degree burn
d. fourth-degree burn

E. Carcinomas of the Skin

Match the type of skin cancer with the correct description.

1. _____ A large brownish spot with darker speckles; a mole that changes in color, size, or feel or that bleeds; a small lesion with an irregular border and portions that appear red, white, blue, or blue-black

2. _____ A firm red nodule; flat lesion with a scaly, crusted surface

3. _____ A pearly or waxy bump; a flat, flesh-colored or brown scar-like lesion

a. basal cell carcinoma
b. squamous cell carcinoma
c. melanoma

F. The Medical Assistant's Role with Examinations, Diagnostic Procedures, and Treatments

1. A glass plate that is held firmly against the skin to permit observation of changes produced in underlying areas when pressure applied is a(n) _____.

2. When an entire lesion is removed for analysis, it is called a(n) _____.

3. When a small section, usually the center, is removed from a designated location in the lesion, it is called _____.

4. When a scalpel or razor is used to remove a growth or lesion for a thin specimen of combined epidermis and upper dermis cells, it is called _____.

Match the treatment to the correct burn.

5. _____ Rinse with cold water until the pain stops, and then cold compresses as needed, elevate the limb.

6. _____ Needs immediate and ongoing medical attention. Cover with a sterile gauze or clean cloth until medical intervention is obtained.

7. _____ Immerse affected area in cool to cold water, analgesics for pain, topical OTC burn cream or aloe vera gel.

a. first-degree burn
b. second-degree burn
c. third-degree burn

8. Mohs surgery is done only for basal cell carcinoma. The procedure involves repeated removal and microscopic examination of the layer of a lesion until no cancerous cells are seen.
   a. The first statement is true, and the second statement is false.
   b. The first statement is false, and the second statement is true.
   c. Both statements are true.
   d. Both statements are false.

9. Which of the following are appearance modification procedures?
   a. Chemical peel, chemoexfoliation
   b. Dermabrasion
   c. Laser resurfacing, photothermolysis
   d. Botox injections
   e. All of the above

CERTIFICATION PREPARATION

Circle the correct answer.

1. Which is an accessory structure of the integumentary system?
   a. Hair
   b. Nails
   c. Sweat glands
   d. All of the above

2. What is the main function of the integumentary system?
   a. Body movement
   b. pH balance
   c. Protection
   d. All of the above

3. _____ is a hard protein material that enhances the skin by making it waterproof, abrasion-resistant, and able to retain moisture.
   a. Keratin
   b. Sebum
   c. Melanin
   d. Collagen

4. Peg-like projections that help fasten the dermis and epidermis together are called
   a. elastin.
   b. pores.
   c. dermal papillae.
   d. stratified epithelium.

5. Which is a sign of melanoma?
   a. A mole that changes in color, size, feel, or that bleeds
   b. A firm, red nodule on the skin
   c. A flat, flesh-colored or brown scar-like lesion
   d. A flat lesion with a scaly or crusted surface

6. What vitamin is synthesized in the skin?
   a. A
   b. B_3
   c. C
   d. D

7. Which disease is a common fungal infection?
   a. Decubitus ulcer
   b. Eczema
   c. Psoriasis
   d. Dermatophytosis

8. Which condition would *not* be found on a child's skin?
   a. Eczema
   b. Birth marks
   c. Melanoma
   d. Freckles

9. Atopic dermatitis is also known as
   a. vitiligo.
   b. seborrheic dermatitis.
   c. psoriasis.
   d. eczema.

10. What is a burn in which only the first and second layers of the skin (epidermis and part of the dermis) are affected?
    a. Fourth-degree burn
    b. Vitiligo
    c. Second-degree burn
    d. Psoriasis

WORKPLACE APPLICATIONS

1. A young mother calls in and says that she is concerned about her school-age son. She got a note from school saying that another student in his class has head lice. She has checked her son's hair and skin, following directions from the school note. The mother found what she thinks are a few nits in his hair.

   a. Which laboratory test will confirm a diagnosis of head lice (pediculosis)? _____

   _____

   b. What organisms can cause pediculosis? _____

   _____

c.   What type of preventive measure can be taken to guard against acquiring a lice infestation?_____

_____

_____

2.   Mai is going over a patient chart in preparation for a follow-up visit with the provider. The patient had a cold injury recently: frostbite on her fingers. Mai was reviewing the signs and symptoms of frostbite. List the signs and symptoms of superficial and deep frostbite.

_____

_____

_____

3.   Helen Rodney is a 42-year-old woman in good health. She had suffered with acne vulgaris when she was in her late teens into her early 30s. Helen has acne scars that she has decided to treat at the dermatologist. She is going to have dermabrasion today. Describe in your own words what a dermabrasion procedure is like. Describe the usual precautions that must be taken by providers and medical assistants during this procedure.

_____

_____

_____

_____

INTERNET ACTIVITIES

1.   Using online resources, research a test used to diagnose an integumentary system disease. Create a poster presentation, a PowerPoint presentation, or a written paper summarizing your research. Include the following points in your project:
   a.   Description of the test
   b.   Any contraindications for the test
   c.   Patient preparation for the test
   d.   What occurs during the test

2.   Using online resources, research a skin disease or condition. Create a poster presentation, a PowerPoint presentation, or a written paper summarizing your research. Include the following points in your project:
   a.   Description of the disease
   b.   Etiology
   c.   Signs and symptoms
   d.   Diagnostic procedures
   e.   Treatments
   f.   Prognosis
   g.   Prevention

3.   Using online resources, research the effect of diet on the management of psoriasis. In a one-page paper, summarize the information you found.

Allergy and Infectious Disease

CAAHEP Competencies	Assessment
I.C.4. Identify major organs in each body system	Skills and Concepts – A. 2-9
I.C.5. Identify the anatomical location of major organs in each body system	Vocabulary Review – A. 6, 8; Skills and Concepts – A. 2-4; Certification Preparation – 2, 9
I.C.6. Identify structure and function of the human body across the life span	Skills and Concepts – C. 1-5; Certification Preparation – 10
I.C.7. Identify the normal function of each body system	Skills and Concepts – A. 1, B. 1-25
I.C.8.a. Identify common pathology related to each body system including: signs	Skills and Concepts – D. 5-8, 19-22, 26, E. 5-8; Certification Preparation – 7, 8; Workplace Applications – 3; Internet Activities – 2
I.C.8.b. Identify common pathology related to each body system including: symptoms	Skills and Concepts – D. 5-8, 19-22, 26, E. 5-8; Certification Preparation – 7, 8; Workplace Applications – 3; Internet Activities – 2
I.C.8.c. Identify common pathology related to each body system including: etiology	Skills and Concepts – D. 1-4, 13-18, E. 1-4; Certification Preparation – 6, 8; Internet Activities – 2
I.C.8.d. Identify common pathology related to each body system including: diagnostic measures	Skills and Concepts – D. 9-12, E. 9-12; Internet Activities – 1, 2
I.C.8.e. Identify common pathology related to each body system including: treatment modalities	Skills and Concepts – D. 9-12, E. 9-12; Internet Activities – 1, 2
I.C.9. Identify Clinical Laboratory Improvement Amendments (CLIA) waived tests associated with common diseases	Certification Preparation – 4
V.C.8.a. Identify the following related to body systems: medical terms	Vocabulary Review – A. 1-10, B. 1-13
V.C.8.b. Identify the following related to body systems: abbreviations	Abbreviations – 1-38
ABHES Competencies	**Assessment**
2. Anatomy and Physiology a. List all body systems and their structures and functions	Vocabulary Review – A. 6, 8; Skills and Concepts – A. 2-4; Certification Preparation – 2, 9

ABHES Competencies	Assessment
b. Describe common diseases, symptoms, and etiologies as they apply to each system	Skills and Concepts – D. 1-4, 5-8, 13-18, 19-22, E. 1-8; Certification Preparation – 6, 8; Internet Activities – 2
c. Identify diagnostic and treatment modalities as they relate to each body system	Skills and Concepts – D. 9-12, E. 9-12; Internet Activities – 1, 2
3. Medical Terminology c. Apply medical terminology for each specialty	Vocabulary Review – A. 1-10, B. 1-13
d. Define and use medical abbreviations when appropriate and acceptable	Abbreviations – 1-38

VOCABULARY REVIEW

Using the word pool on the right, find the correct word to match the definition. Write the word on the line after the definition.

Group A

1. A type of white blood cell that has a large, round nucleus that is surrounded by a thin layer of agranular cytoplasm

    _____

2. The cellular material that fills the area between the nucleus and the cell membrane; contains the organelles of the cell

    _____

3. Disease-causing organisms _____

4. Any living organisms of microscopic size; examples include bacteria, protozoa, fungi, parasites, and helminths; some definitions include viruses, which are not alive

    _____

5. The remains of anything broken down or destroyed; ruins, rubble

    _____

6. A clear, yellowish fluid containing white blood cells in a liquid similar to plasma; comes from the tissues of the body and is moved through the lymphatic vessels and the bloodstream

    _____

7. Large white blood cells that live in the tissues; they engulf foreign particles, microorganisms, and cell debris

    _____

8. Small masses of lymphatic tissue found mostly in the ileum of the small intestine; they are an important part of the immune system because they monitor intestinal bacteria populations and prevent growth of pathogenic bacteria in the intestines

    _____

9. An agranulocyte that engulfs foreign particles, microorganisms, and cell debris in the blood _____

10. The internal environment of the body that is compatible with life; a steady state that is created by all body systems working together to provide a consistent, unvarying internal environment

    _____

Word Pool
- homeostasis
- pathogens
- lymph
- Peyer patches
- monocyte
- lymphocyte
- macrophage
- debris
- microorganism
- cytoplasm

Group B

1. Special proteins that speed up a chemical reaction in the body
   _____

2. A substance that stimulates the production of an antibody when introduced into the body; includes toxins, bacteria, viruses, and other foreign substances _____

3. The production of exact copies of a complex molecule, such as DNA _____

4. The total collection of microorganisms and their genetic material present on or in the human body or a specific site in the human body _____

5. Protein substances produced in the blood or tissues in response to a specific antigen that destroys or weakens the antigen; part of the immune system _____

6. Undifferentiated cells that can become specialized cells in the body _____

7. The ability to live _____

8. A contraction of muscles that causes narrowing of the inside tube of a vessel _____

9. Movements or processes caused by an automatic response that doesn't require thought _____

10. To distinguish one thing from another; to make a distinction between items _____

11. Complete or whole; not altered; unbroken
    _____

12. A substance or structure that can be passed through, especially by liquids or gases _____

13. A pathology characterized by redness, swelling, pain, tenderness, heat, and disturbed function of an area of the body; especially a reaction of tissues to injury _____

14. A disease that is prevalent throughout an entire country, continent, or the whole world _____

Word Pool
- inflammation
- permeable
- differentiate
- intact
- reflexes
- enzymes
- vasoconstriction
- viability
- replication
- stem cells
- antigen
- antibody
- microbiome
- pandemic

ABBREVIATIONS

Write out what each of the following abbreviations stands for.

1. WBC _____

2. RBC _____

3. Igs _____

4. NK _____

5. T_h _____

6. T_c _____

7. T_{reg} _____

8. SLE _____

9. TB _____

10. HDN _____

11. VIS _____

12. AML _____

13. IBD _____

14. MS _____

15. ANA _____

16. CBC _____

17. CMP _____

18. CRP _____

19. ESR _____

20. MRI _____

21. NSAIDs _____

22. AIDS _____

23. HIV _____

24. ELISA _____

25. HAV _____

26. HBV _____

27. HCV _____

28. HDV _____

29. HDE _____

30. EBV _____

31. CT _____

32. PET _____

33. MGUS _____

34. HPI _____

35. PMH _____

36. OTC _____

37. PPD _____

38. RAST _____

SKILLS AND CONCEPTS

Answer the following questions. Write your answer on the line or in the space provided.

A. Anatomy of the Immune and Lymphatic Systems

1. Which of the following is a function of the lymphatic system?
   a. Cleansing the cellular environment, returning proteins and tissue fluids to the blood.
   b. Providing a pathway for the absorption of fats into the bloodstream.
   c. Defending the body against disease.
   d. All of the above

2. Lymph is a cloudy, white fluid containing white blood cells in a liquid similar to plasma. The fluid comes from the tissues of the body and is moved through the lymphatic vessels and the bloodstream.
   a. The first statement is true, the second statement is false.
   b. The first statement is false, the second statement is true.
   c. Both statements are true.
   d. Both statements are false.

3. Which of the following is *not* part of the lymphatic system?
   a. Adenoids
   b. Spleen
   c. Kidneys
   d. Vermiform appendix
   e. All of the above

4. Interstitial flows through which of the following structures?
   a. Lymph vessels
   b. Lymph nodes
   c. Lymph glands
   d. Lymphoid tissue
   e. All of the above

5. _____ are large white blood cells that are called _____ when they enter tissues.

6. The chemical messengers of the immune system are _____.

7. List the granular white blood cells. _____

   _____

8. List the agranular white blood cells. _____

   _____

9. Name the two types of lymphocytes that are part of specific immunity. _____

   _____

B. Physiology of the Immune and Lymphatic Systems

1. The primary function of the immune system is to _____ what is "self" from what is _____, and then destroy anything that is _____.

Match the component of nonspecific immunity with the correct line of defense. Each answer may be used more than once.

2. _____ Phagocytosis

3. _____ Vasoconstriction

4. _____ Intact skin

5. _____ Coughing and sneezing

6. _____ Pyrexia

7. _____ Tears, saliva, and perspiration

8. _____ Interferon

9. _____ Stomach acids and enzymes

10. _____ Cells derived from stem cells in the bone marrow, concentrated in the liver and lungs

a. first line of defense
b. second line of defense

11. Briefly describe the five ways nonspecific immunity and specific immunity differ. _____

_____

_____

_____

_____

12. There are _____ classes of immunoglobulins. Each class responds to different types of _____.

13. Antibody mediated is also known as _____ and involves _____.

Match the type of immunity to correct characteristic.

14. _____ Antibody mediated

15. _____ Cytotoxic T cells

16. _____ B cells

17. _____ Well suited to destroying viruses

18. _____ B cells are the most important cell

19. _____ Recognizes and destroys cancer cells

20. _____ Cells are formed in the bone marrow and migrate to the lymph organs

a. humoral immunity
b. cell mediated immunity

21. Antibodies are _____ that specifically attach to _____. They can _____ toxins or _____ directly.

Match the type of T cell to the correct description.

22. _____ Destroy virus infected cells and tumor cells

23. _____ Assist B cell activation and activation of cytotoxic T cells

24. _____ Help shut down the immune response when antigen is destroyed

25. _____ Rapidly proliferate if an antigen is re-exposed to the body

a. T helper cells
b. cytotoxic T cells
c. memory T cells
d. regulatory T cells

26. _____ is an immune response that causes tissue damage in the host. It is an excessive response to a stimulus or foreign agent.

27. _____ immunity requires the body to respond to an antigen and produce _____ for protection. In _____ immunity, pre-made _____ are given to a person.

C. Life Span Changes

1. When babies are born, some _____ are passed from mother to baby to provide protection for a short time.

2. Babies produce their own antibodies when they are exposed to a pathogen whether by having the _____ or getting a(n) _____.

3. Childhood disorders of the lymphatic and immune systems include which of the following?
   a. Hypersensitivities or allergies to foods, pollen, or pet dander
   b. Childhood leukemias or lymphomas
   c. The development of autoimmune disease in late adolescence
   d. All of the above

4. At what age is multiple myeloma most frequently diagnosed?
   a. 40 years
   b. 50 years
   c. 60 years
   d. 70 years

5. The reduction of _____ and _____ as we age contributes to a lesser response from the immune system to challenges presented.

D. Diseases and Disorders of the Immune System

Match the etiology with the correct condition.

1. _____ Caused by human immunodeficiency virus that attacks the immune system of its host and damages the CD4+ lymphocytes, impairs the immune system's ability to fight infectious agents that can cause disease

2. _____ Can attack many different body systems including joints, skin, kidneys, blood cells, brain, heart, and lungs; cause is unknown, environmental factors such as sunlight, infections, and certain medications seem to provide a trigger

3. _____ Most commonly caused by the Epstein-Barr virus

4. _____ Affects the glands that make tears and saliva, but can also cause damage to other parts of the body; cause is unknown, a triggering mechanism such an infection with a particular virus or bacteria

a. Sjögren's syndrome
b. systemic lupus erythematosus
c. HIV / AIDS
d. infectious mononucleosis

Match the signs and symptoms with the correct condition.

5. _____ Fatigue, fever, swollen lymph nodes, sore throat, swollen tonsils, headache, soft-swollen spleen

6. _____ Swollen joints, low-grade fever, skin changes such as discoloration or rash, weight loss, fatigue, joint pain

7. _____ Flu-like symptoms, swollen lymph nodes, diarrhea, and weight loss

8. _____ Fatigue, fever, skin lesions that appear or worsen with sun exposure, butterfly-shaped rash on the face that covers the cheeks and bridge of the nose, and dry eyes

a. Sjögren's syndrome
b. systemic lupus erythematosus
c. HIV / AIDS
d. infectious mononucleosis

Match the diagnostic measures and treatments with the correct condition.

9. _____ Difficult to diagnose, CBC, erythrocyte sedimentation rate, kidney and liver assessments, and ANA blood tests are done, urinalysis; treatment includes NSAIDs, antimalarial drugs, corticosteroids, immunosuppressants, and biologics

10. _____ History and physical exam, blood tests, including a test to detect antibodies to EBV, CBC; lots of rest, fluids, OTC pain- or fever-reducing medications, and a healthy diet

11. _____ Positive test for the virus; cannot be cured, a regimen of antiviral medications using three drugs from at least two different drug classes

12. _____ Difficult to diagnose, blood tests to look for the presence of antibodies common to this disease, eye tests will be done to measure dryness of the eyes, biopsy of the lip to detect clusters of inflammatory cells; treatment is focused on managing the signs and symptoms, OTC eyedrops and sipping water more frequently, sugarless gum or citrus-flavored hard candies to stimulate saliva flow

a. Sjögren's syndrome
b. systemic lupus erythematosus
c. HIV / AIDS
d. infectious mononucleosis

Match the etiology with the correct hepatitis virus.

13. _____ Sex with an infected partner

14. _____ Person-to-person through fecal-oral contamination

15. _____ Ingesting contaminated food or water

16. _____ Person-to-person transmission through activities that involve percutaneous contact with infected blood or body fluids

17. _____ Sharing needles

18. _____ Ingesting undercooked foods that are contaminated

a. hepatitis A and E
b. hepatitis B, C, D

Match the signs and symptoms with the correct hepatitis virus.

19. _____ Children younger than 6 are frequently asymptomatic

20. _____ Children younger than 5 and newly infected immunosuppressed adults are frequently symptomatic

21. _____ Fever, fatigue, loss of appetite, nausea, vomiting, abdominal pain

22. _____ 30-50% of children older than 5 years are symptomatic

a. hepatitis A and E
b. hepatitis B, C, D

23. Hepatitis _____ is treated aggressively with antiviral medications to minimize the possibility of developing chronic hepatitis.

24. Hepatitis _____ is only possible as a co-infection with hepatitis _____.

25. COVID-19 is caused by the _____ virus and most often causes _____ symptoms.

26. Common signs and symptoms of COVID-19 include which of the following?
    a. Cough
    b. Headache
    c. Shortness of breath
    d. New loss of taste or smell
    e. All of the above

27. At the time that the textbook was written, there are _____ vaccines approved for COVID-19 and _____ antiviral drug(s) to treat COVID-19.

E. Diseases and Disorders of the Lymphatic System
Match the etiology with the correct condition.

1. _____ Idiopathic, but for most people, starts out as MGUS

2. _____ Inflammation of the tonsils caused by common viruses or bacteria

3. _____ Idiopathic; risk factors include family history, age, having had an EBV infection

4. _____ Accumulation of protein-rich fluid that accumulates in the tissue, caused by compromised lymph vessels

a. lymphoma
b. multiple myeloma
c. lymphedema
d. tonsillitis

Match the signs and symptoms with the correct disease.

5. _____ Swelling of all or part of the arm or leg, a feeling of heaviness or tightness, restricted range of motion, recurring infections, fibrosis

6. _____ Sore throat, difficult or painful swallowing, fever, bad breath, stomachache, neck pain or stiff neck

7. _____ Painless swelling of lymph nodes, fatigue, fever, chills, night sweats, and unexplained weight loss

8. _____ None or subtle at first, bone pain, anemia, loss of kidney function, excessive thirst, nausea, loss of appetite, weight loss, constipation, fatigue, frequent infections, weakness or numbness in the legs, and mental confusion

a. lymphoma
b. multiple myeloma
c. lymphedema
d. tonsillitis

Match the diagnostic measures and treatments with the correct disease.

9. _____ Examination of the throat, nose, and ears, palpating the neck for swollen lymph glands, checking for enlargement of the spleen, throat swab, CBC; minimize the symptoms, fluids, comforting foods to sooth the sore throat, OTC medications for pain and fever

10. _____ Test for the presence of M protein, CMP, urinalysis, bone marrow biopsy, MRI, CT, PET; asymptotic-none, targeted cancer therapy, biologic therapy, chemotherapy, radiation therapy, stem cell transplant

11. _____ Presenting signs and symptoms, MRI, CT or ultrasound; reducing the swelling, compression bandages or garments, surgical procedures

12. _____ Physical examination looking for enlarged and nontender lymph nodes, liver, and spleen, CBC, CMP, urinalysis, CT, MRI, PET, lymph node tissue, and/or bone marrow biopsy; chemotherapy, radiation therapy, stem cell transplant, targeted cancer therapy, biologic therapy

a. lymphoma
b. multiple myeloma
c. lymphedema
d. tonsillitis

F. The Medical Assistant's Role with Examination, Diagnostic Procedures, and Treatments

1. What PPE could a patient be asked to put on when presenting with a cough or respiratory issue?
   a. Gloves
   b. Gown
   c. Mask
   d. All of the above

2. A(n) _____ is an important part of any examination. For a patient who has a potential infectious disease, the medical assistant should gather the _____ and review the _____.

3. With a true allergy, the immune response can cause difficulty breathing or hives. With a sensitivity, the immune response is less severe.
   a. The first statement is true, the second statement is false.
   b. The first statement if false, the second statement is true.
   c. Both statements are true.
   d. Both statements are false.

4. Which of the following is true regarding a percutaneous allergy test?
   a. The skin surface is labeled in rows 1.5-2 inches apart.
   b. A small amount of allergen is placed on the skin.
   c. A patch is placed on the skin for 48 hours.
   d. Both a and b are true.

5. Which of the following allergy tests measures the level of antibodies created when a sample of patient's blood is mixed with allergens in the laboratory?
   a. Patch test
   b. Intradermal test
   c. Radioallergosorbent test
   d. All of the above

CERTIFICATION PREPARATION

Circle the correct answer.

1. Which is a granulocyte in the blood?
   a. Neutrophil
   b. Eosinophil
   c. Lymphocyte
   d. Both a and b

2. A monocyte lives in the bloodstream. Where does a macrophage live?
   a. In the bloodstream
   b. In the tissues
   c. Only in the intestines
   d. None of the above

3. What is the main function of the immune system in the body?
   a. To recognize self and destroy anything foreign
   b. To recognize self and recognize foreign
   c. To recognize foreign and preserve foreign
   d. None of the above

4. Which is a CLIA-waived test?
   a. ESR
   b. CRP
   c. CMP
   d. All of the above

5. _____ is/are a collection of WBCs, dead WBCs, bacteria, and tissue cells.
   a. Inflammation
   b. Pyrexia
   c. Pus
   d. Peyer patches

6. EBV causes what condition?
   a. Influenza
   b. Infectious mononucleosis
   c. Strep throat
   d. RSV infections

7. Which could be a sign or symptom of an auto-immune disease?
   a. Skin changes, rashes, or lesions
   b. Low-grade fever and fatigue
   c. Joint pain
   d. All of the above

8. AIDS is caused by which virus?
   a. HIV
   b. Hepatitis B virus
   c. Herpes simplex-1
   d. Epstein-Barr virus

9. Where are Peyer patches located in the body?
   a. Intestines
   b. Brain
   c. Liver
   d. All internal organs

10. Which conditions could be seen in a young child?
    a. Multiple myeloma
    b. Leukemia
    c. Allergies to food
    d. Both b and c

WORKPLACE APPLICATIONS

1. Julia rooms a new patient, Robert, and his mother. Robert is 8 years old and was having an adventure in the woods near his house. About a day later, Robert developed a rash and itching on his legs. His mother suspects poison ivy. A reaction to poison ivy would be what type of hypersensitivity reaction?

   _____

2. Julia is reviewing STIs as part of a continuing education course. Briefly describe the following STIs' common signs and symptoms for males and females.

   a. Syphilis _____

   _____

   b. Chlamydia _____

   _____

3. Monica Green was recently diagnosed with influenza.

   a. What is the cause of influenza? _____

   _____

   b. Briefly describe the signs and symptoms of influenza. _____

   _____

INTERNET ACTIVITIES

1. Using online resources, research a test used for diagnosing a lymphatic or immune system disease. Create a poster presentation, a PowerPoint presentation, or a written paper summarizing your research. Include the following points in your project:
   a. Description of the test
   b. Any contraindications for the test
   c. Patient preparation for the test
   d. What occurs during the test

2. Using online resources, research a lymphatic or immune system disease or condition. Create a poster presentation, a PowerPoint presentation, or a written paper summarizing your research. Include the following points in your project:
   a. Description of the disease
   b. Etiology
   c. Signs and symptoms
   d. Diagnostic procedures
   e. Treatments
   f. Prognosis
   g. Prevention

3. Using online resources, research the effect that diet can have on the management of autoimmune disorders. In a one-page paper, summarize the information you found.

Gastroenterology

CAAHEP Competencies	Assessment
I.C.4. Identify major organs in each body system	Skills and Concepts – B. 2; Certification Preparation – 1
I.C.5. Identify the anatomical location of major organs in each body system	Skills and Concepts – B. 4-10, 16-19, 22, 24-25, 28-29; C. 4, 6; Certification Preparation – 2
I.C.6. Identify structure and function of the human body across the life span	Skills and Concepts – E. 1-3; Certification Preparation – 10
I.C.7. Identify the normal function of each body system	Skills and Concepts – B. 13-15, 20-21, 23, 26-27, 30; C. 2, 3, 5, 7, D. 1-11; Certification Preparation – 3, 5, 6
I.C.8.a. Identify common pathology related to each body system including: signs	Skills and Concepts – G. 11-14, H. 12-16, I. 7-9, J. 1-4; Certification Preparation – 7; Workplace Application – 1; Internet Activities – 2
I.C.8.b. Identify common pathology related to each body system including: symptoms	Skills and Concepts – G. 11-14, H. 12-16, I. 7-9, J. 1-4; Workplace Application – 1; Internet Activities – 2
I.C.8.c. Identify common pathology related to each body system including: etiology	Skills and Concepts – G. 7-10, H. 7-11, I. 4-6; Certification Preparation – 8-9; Internet Activities – 2
I.C.8.d. Identify common pathology related to each body system including: diagnostic measures	Skills and Concepts – G. 15-18, H. 17-21, I. 10-12, J. 5-8, K. 1-11; Workplace Application – 1; Internet Activities – 1-3
I.C.8.e. Identify common pathology related to each body system including: treatment modalities	Skills and Concepts – G. 15-18, H. 17-21, I. 10-12, J. 5-8, K. 12-21; Internet Activities – 2, 3
I.C.9. Identify Clinical Laboratory Improvement Amendments (CLIA) waived tests associated with common diseases	Skills and Concepts – K. 9-11; Certification Preparation – 4
I.C.10.a. Identify the classifications of medications, including indications for use	Skills and Concepts – K. 17-21; Internet Activities – 4
I.C.10.b. Identify the classifications of medications, including desired effects	Skills and Concepts – K. 17-21; Internet Activities – 4
I.C.10.c. Identify the classifications of medications, including side effects	Skills and Concepts – K. 22-26; Internet Activities – 4
I.C.10.d. Identify the classifications of medications, including adverse reactions	Skills and Concepts – K. 22-26; Internet Activities – 4

CAAHEP Competencies	Assessment
V.C.8.a. Identify the following related to body systems: medical terms	Skills and Concepts – K. 12-16; Certification Preparation – 9
V.C.8.b. Identify the following related to body systems: abbreviations	Abbreviations – 1-30
V.P.3.b. Coach patients regarding medical encounters	Procedure 34.2
X.P.3. Document patient care accurately in the medical record	Procedures 34.1, 34.2
I.A. Demonstrate critical thinking skills	Procedure 34.1

ABHES Competencies	Assessment
2. Anatomy and Physiology a. List all body systems and their structures and functions	Skills and Concepts – B. 2, 4-10, 13-30; C. 2-7, D. 1-11
2.b. Describe common diseases, symptoms, and etiologies as they apply to each system	Skills and Concepts – F. 1-6, G. 1-14, H. 1-16, I. 1-9, J. 1-4; Workplace Application – 2, 3; Internet Activities – 2
2.c. Identify diagnostic and treatment modalities as they relate to each body system	Skills and Concepts – G. 15-18, H. 17-21, I. 10-12; J. 5-8, K. 12-21; Workplace Application – 1-3
3. Medical Terminology c. Apply medical terminology for each specialty	Skills and Concepts – K. 12-16; Certification Preparation – 9
3. d. Define and use medical abbreviations when appropriate and acceptable	Abbreviations – 1-30
8. e. Perform specialty procedures, including but not limited to minor surgery, cardiac, respiratory, OB-GYN, neurological, and gastroenterology	Procedure 34.2

VOCABULARY REVIEW

Using the word pool on the right, find the correct word to match the definition. Write the word on the line after the definition.

Group A

1. Folds in the wall of the organ; when the organ (e.g., stomach, bladder, uterus) fills or needs to expand, the ability to unfold is due to _____

2. Secreted by the parietal cells of the stomach; necessary for the absorption of vitamin B_{12} to prevent pernicious anemia _____

3. Wave-like movement from alternating contraction and relaxation of a tubular structure (e.g., intestine), which propels the contents forward _____

4. A mucus-producing membrane that lines tracts and structures of the body (e.g., GI tract, respiratory tract); also called *mucosa* _____

5. A glandular secretion released through a duct _____

6. The cavity, channel, or open space within a tube or tubular organ _____

7. Lid-like structure over the glottis that prevents food and liquids from entering the trachea when swallowing occurs _____

8. A circular muscle that either constricts and closes the opening or relaxes and allows substances to pass through the opening _____

9. A glandular secretion that is released into the blood or lymph directly (does not go through a duct) _____

10. When a substance suspends tiny droplets of one liquid into a second liquid; this allows mixing two liquids that usually do not mix well such as oil and water _____

Word Pool
- emulsifies
- endocrine
- epiglottis
- exocrine
- intrinsic factor
- lumen
- mucous membrane
- peristalsis
- rugae
- sphincter

Group B

1. Surgical removal of all or part of an organ

   _____

2. A surgical procedure where the large intestine is brought though the abdominal wall, creating either a temporary or permanent opening (stoma) to allow stool to pass out of the body

   _____

3. Pain is felt when the pressure on the abdomen is released

   _____

4. Hidden or unseen _____

5. Confined or trapped _____

6. Kidney disorder that can occur after a digestive infection with *E. coli*, Shigella, or Salmonella; red blood cells are destroyed and block the kidneys' filtering system causing acute kidney failure

   _____

7. A crack, cleft, or narrow opening _____

8. Sticky substance made of mucus, food particles, and bacteria that builds up on the exposed part of the tooth

   _____

9. Constriction of a tubular structure, such as an intestine or vessel, leading to a lack of blood supply to the tissues

   _____

10. The surgical connection of separate or severed tubular hollow organs to form a continuous channel _____

11. Pain that is felt at a site in the body at a distance from the cause

    _____

12. A growth or mass protruding from a mucous membrane

    _____

Word Pool
- anastomosis
- colostomy
- fissure
- hemolytic uremic syndrome
- incarcerated
- occult
- plaque
- polyp
- rebound pain
- referred pain
- resection
- strangulation

ABBREVIATIONS

Write out what each of the following abbreviations stands for.

1. GI _____

2. UES _____

3. LES _____

4. CCK _____

5. GER _____

6. GERD _____

7. EGD _____

8. HAV _____

9. PPI _____

10. CVS _____

11. CBC _____

12. HCV _____

13. IPAA _____

14. IBS _____

15. SIBO _____

16. HIDA scan _____

17. ERCP _____

18. NSAID _____

19. HBV _____

20. IBD _____

21. HDV _____

22. iFOBT _____

23. IVIg _____

24. NAFLD _____

25. DRE _____

26. MT-sDNA_____

27. HEV _____

28. gFOBT _____

29. FIT _____

30. UGI _____

SKILLS AND CONCEPTS
Answer the following questions.

A. Introduction
Match the description with the correct term.

1. _____ A subspecialist who treats disorders of the rectum and anus

2. _____ A specialist who focuses only on the liver

3. _____ The healthcare specialty that deals with most digestive diseases and disorders

4. _____ A subspecialty that deals with liver disorders

5. _____ A specialist involved in the diagnosis, treatment, and prevention of disorders of the digestive organs and liver

a. gastroenterology
b. hepatology
c. gastroenterologist
d. proctologist
e. hepatologist

B. Anatomy of the Gastrointestinal Tract

Fill in the blank or select the correct answer.

1. _____ is also called the *digestive tract* and the *alimentary canal*.

2. The GI tract includes the
   a. mouth and pharynx.
   b. esophagus and stomach.
   c. small and large intestines.
   d. all of the above.

3. The cheeks, lips, tongue, hard palate, and soft palate form the _____ , also called the *mouth* or *buccal cavity*.

Match the structures with the correct description.

4. _____ Connects the pharynx to the stomach

5. _____ Fleshy structure that hangs above the throat, at the back of the soft palate

6. _____ Throat

7. _____ Create the roof of the mouth

8. _____ Part of the pharynx located between the epiglottis and the esophagus

9. _____ Part of the pharynx located behind the nasal cavity

10. _____ Part of the pharynx located behind the mouth

    a. pharynx
    b. anterior hard palate and posterior soft palate
    c. esophagus
    d. uvula
    e. laryngopharynx
    f. nasopharynx
    g. oropharynx

Fill in the blank or select the correct answer.

11. The esophagus is lined with a(n) _____ that secretes mucus, helping the mass of food, or bolus, pass into the stomach.

12. A(n) _____ is located at the top and bottom of the esophagus.

13. Tiny glands in the stomach produce
    a. digestive enzymes.
    b. intrinsic factor.
    c. hydrochloric acid and mucus.
    d. bicarbonate.
    e. all of the above.

14. The stomach
    a. produces gastrin and ghrelin.
    b. protects the body by killing bacteria in food.
    c. absorbs alcohol, some water, certain drugs, and some fatty acids.
    d. all of the above.

15. The _____ is located between the pylorus and the small intestine and regulates the passage of food into the small intestine.

Match the description with the correct section of the intestine. Answers can be used more than once.

16. _____ Smallest part of the small intestine; connected to the stomach by the pyloric sphincter

17. _____ A tubelike structure in the lower-right abdomen that is considered the first section of the large intestine

18. _____ Second largest part of the small intestine; connected to the duodenum and the ileum

19. _____ Extends horizontally from the ascending colon to the descending colon

20. _____ Sugars, fatty acids, and amino acids are absorbed in this section.

21. _____ Receives chyme from the small intestine and absorbs fluids and salts

22. _____ Extends vertically on the left side of the abdomen from the transverse colon to the sigmoid colon

23. _____ Receives chyme from the stomach, which mixes with pancreatic enzymes, bile, and bicarbonate

24. _____ Forms an S-shaped curve; attaches to the descending colon and the rectum

25. _____ The vermiform appendix attaches to this section

26. _____ Limited absorption occurs in this section; bile acids and vitamin B_{12} are most often absorbed for reuse in the body

27. _____ Stores the stool until a bowel movement occurs

28. _____ Largest part of the small intestine; connects to the jejunum and the large intestine

29. _____ The second part of the large intestine

a. ileum
b. duodenum
c. jejunum
d. cecum
e. transverse colon
f. ascending colon
g. rectum
h. descending colon
i. sigmoid colon

Select the correct answer.

30. Which of the following is *not* a function of the large intestine?
    a. Reabsorption of water
    b. Reabsorption of electrolytes
    c. Making vitamin C
    d. Eliminating waste products

C. Anatomy of the Accessory Organs
Fill in the blank or select the correct answer.

1. _____ include the salivary glands, liver, gallbladder, and the pancreas.

2. The salivary glands produce and secrete saliva, which contains _____, an enzyme.

3. The liver
   a. produces plasma proteins and bile.
   b. breaks down old or damaged blood cells.
   c. breaks down proteins and fats and produces energy.
   d. removes extra minerals, vitamins, and glucose from the blood.
   e. all of the above

4. The _____ is found in a small area on the underside of the liver.

5. The gallbladder stores and concentrates _____.

6. The _____ is found behind the stomach and in front of the spine and has exocrine and endocrine functions.

7. The pancreas creates
    a. trypsin.
    b. chymotrypsin.
    c. amylase.
    d. lipase.
    e. all of the above

D. Physiology of the Gastrointestinal System
Match the substance with the correct chemical digestive role.

1. _____ Found in pancreatic juices and breaks down proteins into amino acids.

2. _____ Starts to break down complex carbohydrates.

3. _____ Released from the gallbladder and emulsifies fat.

4. _____ Softens and breaks down proteins and other foods.

5. _____ An enzyme in gastric juices that breaks down proteins into amino acids.

6. _____ Found in pancreatic juices and breaks down fats into fatty acids and glycerol.

7. _____ Helps neutralize the acidity of the chyme in the duodenum.

8. _____ Found in pancreatic juices and breaks down carbohydrates into sugars.

9. _____ An enzyme that breaks down lactose into galactose and glucose.

10. _____ An enzyme that breaks down sucrose into glucose and fructose.

11. _____ An enzyme that breaks down maltose into glucose.

a. trypsin and chymotrypsin
b. amylase
c. lipase
d. sodium bicarbonate
e. hydrochloric acid
f. bile
g. salivary amylase
h. pepsin
i. sucrase
j. lactase
k. maltase

E. Life Span Changes of the Gastrointestinal System
Select the correct answer.

1. Which of the following is *incorrect*?
    a. Salivary secretions are insufficient until about 10 months of age.
    b. Pancreatic amylase levels may not be sufficient until 12 to 18 months of age.
    c. Bile salts levels are not sufficient until 6 to 9 months of age.
    d. Lipase levels are not sufficient until 6 to 9 months of age.

2. What change occurs with pregnancy?
   a. Progesterone causes less peristalsis in the digestive system, thus slowing digestion.
   b. Gallbladder emptying may be delayed, leading to gallstone formation.
   c. Morning sickness, constipation, and heartburn can result from digestive system changes.
   d. All of the above

3. What change occurs with age?
   a. The stomach empties slower.
   b. Lactase levels decrease with age, leading to lactose intolerance.
   c. Bacterial overgrowth leads to bloating, weight loss, and pain.
   d. All of the above

F. Mouth Diseases and Disorders
Match the description with the correct disease.

1. _____ An inflammatory disease of the gums that causes redness, swelling, and bleeding.

2. _____ Inflammation of the mouth caused by the herpes simplex virus.

3. _____ A yeast infection of the mouth and tongue.

4. _____ An opening in the upper lip caused by the lip tissues not completely joining before birth.

5. _____ A condition of white patches on the lips and buccal mucosa often associated with tobacco use.

6. _____ The tissue that makes up the roof of the mouth does not completely join before birth.

   a. cleft lip
   b. cleft palate
   c. gingivitis
   d. herpetic stomatitis
   e. leukoplakia
   f. thrush

G. Esophageal and Stomach Diseases and Disorders
Match the description with the correct disease.

1. _____ Occurs when a section of the upper stomach pushes through an opening of the diaphragm into the chest

2. _____ Inflammation of the stomach lining

3. _____ A sore or breakdown in the lining of the stomach or duodenum

4. _____ Stomach motility is slowed, causing delayed gastric emptying

5. _____ The narrowing of the pylorus, the muscular opening between the stomach and the small intestine

6. _____ Rapid gastric emptying

   a. pyloric stenosis
   b. dumping syndrome
   c. hiatal hernia
   d. peptic ulcer
   e. gastritis
   f. gastroparesis

Match the etiology with the correct disease.

7. _____ Caused by a *Helicobacter pylori* (*H. pylori*) bacterial infection
8. _____ Caused by a weakened or an abnormal lower esophageal sphincter
9. _____ Caused by GERD
10. _____ The cause is unknown

a. gastroesophageal reflux disease (GERD)
b. hiatal hernia
c. peptic ulcer
d. Barrett esophagus

Match the signs and symptoms with the correct disease.

11. _____ Chest pain, heartburn, and difficulty swallowing
12. _____ Heartburn, bad breath, nausea, vomiting, chest pain, upper abdominal pain, respiratory problems, and erosion of the teeth
13. _____ Upper abdominal pain at night or when the stomach is empty, nausea, melena, chest pain, fatigue, vomiting and hematemesis, and weight loss
14. _____ Projectile vomiting, weight loss, constant hunger, dehydration, a wavelike motion of the abdomen just before vomiting, and an olive-sized mass in the upper abdomen

a. gastroesophageal reflux disease (GERD)
b. hiatal hernia
c. peptic ulcer
d. pyloric stenosis

Match the diagnostic measures and treatments with the correct disease.

15. _____ Abdominal ultrasound and blood tests to detect electrolyte imbalances; treatment consist of pyloromyotomy or medications
16. _____ Barium swallow and EGD; treatment includes medications for acid reflux and herniorrhaphy
17. _____ Upper GI endoscopy or UGI series, biopsy of the stomach lining, and stool occult blood test; treatment may include antibiotics, H_2 blocker, and a proton-pump inhibitor
18. _____ An upper endoscopy, esophageal manometry, ambulatory acid probe test, and an upper digestive system x-ray; treatment includes lifestyle changes, medications, or surgery

a. gastroesophageal reflux disease (GERD)
b. hiatal hernia
c. peptic ulcer
d. pyloric stenosis

H. Intestinal Diseases and Disorders
Match the description with the correct disease.

1. _____ Occurs when the diverticula become inflamed or infected
2. _____ Also called *gluten-sensitive enteropathy* or *celiac sprue*, is a digestive and an autoimmune disorder
3. _____ A type of inflammatory bowel disease; usually starts in the rectum and spreads into the large intestine
4. _____ A type of inflammatory bowel disease; often affects the ileum
5. _____ A common disorder of the large intestine, though it does not cause harm to the colon
6. _____ An inflammation of the appendix

a. acute appendicitis
b. celiac disease
c. diverticulitis
d. Crohn disease
e. ulcerative colitis
f. irritable bowel syndrome

Match the etiology with the correct disease.

7. _____ Unknown, but it is the result of a defective immune system

8. _____ A blockage in the appendix, which can increase pressure, affect blood flow, and cause inflammation

9. _____ When a diverticulum tears, inflammation and infection can occur

10. _____ A genetic autoimmune disorder

11. _____ No known cause; factors leading to it include severe infection and changes in the intestinal microbes

a. acute appendicitis
b. celiac disease
c. diverticulitis
d. inflammatory bowel disease
e. irritable bowel syndrome

Match the signs and symptoms with the correct disease.

12. _____ Constant lower-left abdomen pain and tenderness, nausea, vomiting, diarrhea, constipation, and fever

13. _____ The pain usually begins near the umbilicus and then moves to the lower right side of the abdomen, low fever, abdominal bloating, anorexia, nausea, and vomiting

14. _____ Persistent diarrhea, abdominal pain, blood in the stool, weight loss, and fatigue

15. _____ Diarrhea, constipation, fatigue, bone or joint pain, depression, anxiety, irritability, missed menstrual periods, anemia, and osteoporosis

16. _____ Abdominal cramping, bloating, constipation, and diarrhea

a. acute appendicitis
b. celiac disease
c. diverticulitis
d. inflammatory bowel disease
e. irritable bowel syndrome

Match the diagnostic measures and treatments with the correct disease.

17. _____ Blood tests and an intestinal biopsy; treated with a gluten-free diet

18. _____ CBC and imaging tests; treated with antibiotics and an appendectomy

19. _____ A colonoscopy, an upper endoscopy, x-ray, and/or CT scan to rule out other diseases; treated with dietary changes, stress management, medications, and probiotics

20. _____ Blood and urine tests and a CT scan; treatment may include antibiotics, analgesics, a liquid diet, and surgery for severe cases

21. _____ Imaging tests, endoscopy exams, and stool samples; treated with corticosteroids, immunomodulators, biologics, and surgery (e.g., colectomy, proctocolectomy) for severe cases

a. acute appendicitis
b. celiac disease
c. diverticulitis
d. inflammatory bowel disease
e. irritable bowel syndrome

I. Diseases and Disorders of the Accessory Organs
Match the description with the correct disease.

1. _____ A condition caused by high levels of bilirubin in the blood
2. _____ An inflammation of the liver
3. _____ Occurs when substances in the bile harden and form stones

a. cholelithiasis
b. jaundice in the newborn
c. hepatitis

Match the etiology with the correct disease.

4. _____ Different types and different causes including viruses, alcohol use, toxins, and certain medications
5. _____ May occur if the bile contains too much cholesterol or bilirubin
6. _____ Can be caused by hyperbilirubinemia, hemorrhage, infection, incompatibility between the mother's blood and the baby's blood, liver malfunction, red blood cell abnormality, and an enzyme deficiency

a. cholelithiasis
b. jaundice in the newborn
c. hepatitis

Match the signs and symptoms with the correct disease.

7. _____ Yellowish coloring to the skin and sclera, listlessness, poor feeding, and high-pitched cries
8. _____ Nausea, vomiting, and referred pain
9. _____ Fatigue, nausea, vomiting, anorexia, abdominal pain, clay-colored stools, dark urine, low-grade fever, joint pain, jaundice, and intense itching

a. cholelithiasis
b. jaundice in the newborn
c. hepatitis

Match the diagnostic measures and treatments with the correct disease.

10. _____ Bilirubin blood levels; treatment may include phototherapy, intravenous immunoglobulin, and exchange transfusion of blood
11. _____ Blood tests and imaging tests; treatment depends on the type and may include liver transplant, bedrest, or medications
12. _____ A gallbladder radionuclide scan, MRI, or endoscopic retrograde cholangiopancreatography (ERCP); treatment may consist of a cholecystectomy or gallstones can be removed during the ERCP

a. cholelithiasis
b. jaundice in the newborn
c. hepatitis

J. Gastrointestinal System Cancers
Match the signs and symptoms with the correct disease.

1. _____ Symptoms are vague and may go unnoticed
2. _____ Jaundice, right abdominal pain, and a lump in the right abdomen
3. _____ Diarrhea, constipation, bloody stools, cramps, bloating, flatus (gas), nausea, vomiting, fatigue, or weight loss
4. _____ White or red patches, bleeding, or a continuous sore in the mouth, loose teeth, pain with swallowing, earache, and lump in the neck

a. oral cancer
b. liver cancer
c. colorectal cancer
d. pancreatic cancer

Match the diagnostic measures and treatments with the correct disease.

5. _____ Blood tests, imaging tests, and biopsy; treatment consists of surgical removal of the tumor or liver transplant, localized treatment, radiation therapy, chemotherapy, immunotherapy, and targeted drug therapies

6. _____ Colonoscopy, biopsy, and a carcinoembryonic antigen (CEA) blood test; treatment consists of a surgical removal of the tumor, polypectomy, colectomy, radiation therapy, chemotherapy, targeted drug therapies, and immunotherapy

7. _____ An endoscopic ultrasound, imaging tests, positron emission tomography, blood test, and biopsies; treatment consist of a surgical removal of the tumor, partial or total pancreatectomy, radiation therapy, and chemotherapy

8. _____ Biopsy of the mouth lesion; treatment consists of surgical removal of the tumor, radiation therapy, chemotherapy, and targeted therapy

a. oral cancer
b. liver cancer
c. colorectal cancer
d. pancreatic cancer

K. The Medical Assistant's Role with Examinations, Diagnostic Measures, and Treatments
Select the correct answer or fill in the blank.

1. During a(n) _____, an endoscope is inserted in the anus and is used to visualize the large intestine.

2. During a(n) _____, an endoscope is inserted into the rectum, sigmoid colon, and descending colon.

3. During a(n) _____, an endoscope is inserted into the mouth and passed through the stomach and duodenum before it is inserted into the bile ducts.

4. During a(n) _____, a proctoscope is used to inspect the rectum.

5. During a computed tomography (CT) colonography, also called a(n) _____, a small tube is inserted into the rectum, the lower colon is inflated with gas, and CT images are taken of the colon and rectum.

6. A(n) _____ is a nuclear scan of the liver, gallbladder, and bile ducts.

7. A(n) _____ is an x-ray evaluation of large intestine after instillation of a barium sulfate enema.

8. A(n) _____, also called an *upper gastrointestinal (UGI) series,* is an x-ray evaluation of the esophagus, stomach, and duodenum after the patient drinks barium sulfate.

9. The _____ includes glucose, electrolytes, liver function, and kidney function tests and some are CLIA-waived tests.

10. The _____ is a CLIA-waived test that detects occult blood in a stool smear.

11. _____, also called a *hepatic function panel* and *liver panel,* measures protein, enzymes, and other substances, and some CLIA-waived tests are available.

12. A(n) _____ is the surgical removal of the appendix.

13. A(n) _____ is the surgical removal of the gallbladder.

14. A(n) _____ is the surgical removal of the colon.

15. A(n) _____ is the surgical redirection of the bowel to a stoma.

16. A total _____ is the surgical removal of all of the stomach.

Match the indication for use and desired effect with the correct medication classification.

17. _____ Treats gastroesophageal reflux disease (GERD) and ulcers by decreasing the amount of acid produced in the stomach.

18. _____ Treats gastric hyperacidity by neutralizing stomach acid.

19. _____ Increases and hastens bowel evacuation by increasing the activating in the large intestine.

20. _____ Controls diarrhea by decreasing the amount of fluids and electrolytes in the bowel and slows peristalsis.

21. _____ Prevents and relieves nausea and vomiting by acting on hypothalamic center in the brain.

a. antacid
b. antidiarrheal
c. antiemetic
d. laxative
e. proton-pump inhibitor

Match the side effects and adverse reactions with the correct medication classification.

22. _____ Dry mouth, sedation, drowsiness, diarrhea, blurred vision

23. _____ Constipation, fatigue, bloody stools, stomach pain or swelling, rash

24. _____ Confusion, drowsiness, arrhythmias, sweating, flushing

25. _____ GI distress, increased urination, metallic taste

26. _____ Nausea, bloating, flatulence, cramping

a. antacid
b. antidiarrheal
c. antiemetic
d. laxative
e. proton-pump inhibitor

CERTIFICATION PREPARATION

Circle the correct answer.

1. Which is/are an accessory structure(s) of the digestive system?
   a. Liver
   b. Pancreas
   c. Large intestine
   d. Both a and b

2. What is the proper order of the sections of the pharynx from top down?
   a. Nasopharynx, laryngopharynx, oropharynx
   b. Oropharynx, laryngopharynx, nasopharynx
   c. Nasopharynx, oropharynx, laryngopharynx
   d. Laryngopharynx, nasopharynx, oropharynx

3. What is/are the main function(s) of the gastrointestinal system?
   a. Digest and absorb nutrients
   b. Ingestion of food
   c. Elimination of waste products
   d. All of the above

4. Which is a CLIA-waived test?
   a. Fecal occult blood test
   b. CT scan
   c. Tissue biopsy
   d. Ova and parasite testing

5. _____ are ring-like muscles that appear throughout the digestive system to keep chyme moving in one direction through the organs.
   a. Sphincter
   b. Arrector pili
   c. Pylorus
   d. Cecum

6. Which is the enzyme secreted by the pancreas to digest carbohydrates and starches?
   a. Lipase
   b. Protease
   c. Amylase
   d. Pepsin

7. Which is a sign of Crohn disease?
   a. Abdominal pain
   b. Diarrhea and blood in the stool
   c. Nausea
   d. Fatigue and lethargy

8. Peptic ulcers can be caused by which bacteria?
   a. *Staphylococcus aureus*
   b. *Helicobacter pylori*
   c. Herpesvirus
   d. All of the above

9. Which is an inflammation of the liver?
   a. Cholelithiasis
   b. Pancreatitis
   c. Diverticulitis
   d. Hepatitis

10. Which condition could be seen in infants?
    a. GERD
    b. Pyloric stenosis
    c. Jaundice
    d. All of the above

WORKPLACE APPLICATION

1. Martha calls into Walden-Martin Family Medical (WMFM) Clinic and speaks to Samuel. She is wondering if she should come in and see a provider because she has been having recurring pain in the upper-right quadrant of her abdomen. The pain can be intense, but then subsides. Sometimes she feels nauseous.

   a. With this limited information, what three conditions could cause these types of symptoms?

      _____

      _____

      _____

   b. What diagnostic tests may be useful in determining the cause of the pain? _____

      _____

      _____

2. Samuel is going over a pamphlet with a patient who has hemorrhoids. The patient asks Samuel to answer a few questions. What is a hemorrhoid? Also, describe the difference between an external and internal hemorrhoid.

   _____

   _____

   _____

   _____

3. Emily Stark is planning a trip to Mexico to get away from the cold upper-Midwest winter. Her provider has recommended that she get a hepatitis A vaccine before her trip.

   a. How is hepatitis A acquired?_____

   _____

   _____

   b. Briefly describe the signs and symptoms of hepatitis._____

   _____

   _____

   _____

   _____

   _____

   _____

INTERNET ACTIVITIES

1. Using online resources, research a test used for diagnosing a gastrointestinal system disease. Create a poster presentation, a PowerPoint presentation, or a written paper summarizing your research. Include the following points in your project:
   a. Description of the test
   b. Any contraindications for the test
   c. Patient preparation for the test
   d. What occurs during the test

2. Using online resources, research a gastrointestinal system disease or condition. Create a poster presentation, a PowerPoint presentation, or a written paper summarizing your research. Include the following points in your project:
   a. Description of the disease
   b. Etiology
   c. Signs and symptoms
   d. Diagnostic measures
   e. Treatments

3. Using online resources, research the effect that diet can have on the diagnostic measures and treatment management of Crohn disease. In a one-page paper, summarize the information that you found.

4. Using Table 34.5, Medication Classifications, select one generic medication from each of the following classifications: antacid, antidiarrheal, antiemetic, laxative, and proton-pump inhibitor. Using a reliable online drug resource, identify for each medication:
   a. Indication for use
   b. Desired effects
   c. Side effects
   d. Adverse reactions

   Write a short paper addressing each of these four areas for each medication.

Procedure 34.1   Use Critical Thinking when Performing Patient Screening

Name _____ Date _____ Score _____

Tasks: Incorporate critical thinking skills when performing patient assessment. Document the patient's history and chief complaint.

Scenario 1: You work at Walden-Martin Family Medical (WMFM) Clinic. A patient calls and states that they have had nausea, vomiting, diarrhea, and abdominal pain for 3 days. You need to gather the patient's information before talking with the provider per the facility's policy.

Scenario 2: You work at WMFM clinic. A patient calls and states that they have had vomiting and constipation for 4 days. You need to gather the patient's information before talking with the provider, per the facility's policy.

Directions: Role-play the scenario with a peer, who is the patient. Your instructor is the provider.

Equipment and Supplies:
- Phone log and pen
- Patient's health record
- Phone

Standard: Complete the procedure and all critical steps in _____ minutes with a minimum score of 85% within two attempts (*or as indicated by the instructor*).

Scoring: Divide the points earned by the total possible points. Failure to perform a critical step, indicated by an asterisk (*), results in grade no higher than an 84% (*or as indicated by the instructor*).

Time: Began_____ Ended_____ Total minutes: _____

Steps:	Point Value	Attempt 1	Attempt 2
1. Answer the telephone by the third ring, speaking directly into the mouthpiece or headset. Speak distinctly, using a pleasant tone and expression, at a moderate rate, and with sufficient volume.	10		
2. Greet the caller, identify the facility and yourself, and offer to help the caller.	10		
3. Verify the identity of the caller and their date of birth; access the patient's record. Note the patient's phone number in case you are disconnected.	5		
4. Determine the caller's needs using therapeutic communication skills.	10		
5. Upon learning the patient's complaint, use critical thinking skills and ask appropriate questions to obtain information about the patient's condition for the provider. Identify the onset, frequency, and duration of the complaint. If related to pain, identify the exact location, quality (e.g., sharp, dull, stabbing), and rating (using a 0–10 pain scale). Identify significant history and factors that increase or decrease the complaint. (*Refer to the Affective Behaviors Checklist – Critical Thinking and the Grading Rubric*)	30*		

Scenario update: You know the provider is available and the patient is willing to be put on hold as you talk with the provider. 6. Discuss the patient's information with the provider. Present the information accurately and logically.	**20**		
7. Upon returning to the phone, give the patient the information from the provider. Conclude the phone call.	**5**		
8. Document the patient interaction, including the patient's medical history, the provider notified, and the information relayed to the patient.	**10**		
Total Points	**100**		

Affective Behavior	Affective Behaviors Checklist **Directions:** *Check behaviors observed during the role-play.*					
	Negative, Unprofessional Behaviors	**Attempt**		**Positive, Professional Behaviors**	**Attempt**	
Critical Thinking		**1**	**2**		**1**	**2**
	Coached or told of an issue or problem			Independently identified the problem or issue		
	Failed to ask relevant questions related to the condition			Asked appropriate questions to obtain the information required		
	Failed to consider alternatives; failed to ask questions that demonstrated understanding of principles/concepts			Willing to consider other alternatives; asked appropriate questions that showed understanding of principles/concepts		
	Failed to make an educated, logical judgment/decision; actions or lack of actions demonstrated unsafe practices and/or did not follow the protocol			Made an educated, logical judgment/decision based on the protocol; actions reflected principles of safe practice		
	Other:			Other:		

Grading Rubric for the Affective Behaviors Checklist **Directions:** *Based on checklist results, identify the points received for the procedure checklist. Indicate how the behaviors demonstrated met the expectations.*		Points for Procedure Checklist	Attempt 1	Attempt 2
Does not meet Expectation	• Response fails to show critical thinking. • Student demonstrated more than 2 negative, unprofessional behaviors during the interaction.	0		
Needs Improvement	• Response fails to show critical thinking. • Student demonstrated 1 or 2 negative, unprofessional behaviors during the interaction.	0		
Meets Expectation	• Response demonstrates critical thinking; no negative, unprofessional behaviors observed. • More practice is needed for behavior to appear natural and for student to appear comfortable and at ease.	30		
Occasionally Exceeds Expectation	• Response demonstrates critical thinking; no negative, unprofessional behaviors observed. • At times student appeared comfortable and at ease; but more practice is needed for behavior to become natural and consistent with a professional medical assistant.	30		
Always Exceeds Expectation	• Response demonstrates critical thinking; no negative, unprofessional behaviors observed. • Student's behaviors appeared natural and comfortable. Behaviors are consistent with a professional medical assistant.	30		

Phone Log

Date: _____ Time: _____ Caller: _____

Documentation

Comments

CAAHEP Competencies	Step(s)
X.P.3. Document patient care accurately in the medical record	8
I.A. Demonstrate critical thinking skills	5

Procedure 34.2   Coach Patient on Preparing for a Colonoscopy

Name _____   Date _____   Score _____

Tasks: Coach a patient on colonoscopy preparation. Document the coaching in the health record.

Scenario: You work at WMFM Clinic. You are working with Dr. David Kahn, who has asked you to coach Charles Johnson (DOB 03/03/19XX) on the colonoscopy patient instructions. Dr. Kahn wants Charles to take his antihypertensive medication the morning of the procedure, 1 hour after finishing the preparation solution.

The ambulatory surgical center requires that Charles not eat or drink anything starting at midnight on the day of the procedure. He needs to arrive 90 minutes before the procedure, which is scheduled at 11 AM. He will be receiving IV sedation during the procedure and will need a driver to take him home.

Directions: Role-play the scenario with a peer, who is the patient. Your instructor is the provider. Make up the location, date, and time of the procedure. Use the following as the patient instructions:

Purpose of the colonoscopy:
- To detect abnormal changes in the large intestine and rectum.

Dietary preparations:
- Two days before the procedure: Do not take fiber supplements or eat foods high in fiber (e.g., nuts, seeds, whole grains, and raw or cooked fruits and vegetables).
- One day before the procedure: Do not eat solid foods, just drink clear liquids (e.g., broth, gelatin, coffee, tea, clear juice, popsicles, and sport drinks). Do not drink red liquids or eat red gelatin. Do not drink or eat dairy products or alcohol.

Colon cleansing:
- Split the preparation solution (e.g., GoLYTELY, Colyte) and take half the evening before the procedure. Take the rest of the solution in the morning. The solution must be completed at least 2 hours before the procedure.
- Usually within 1 hour of starting the preparation solution, liquid stools can occur and continue until 2 hours after completing the solution. Chills, headache, cramping, weakness, nausea, vomiting, and bloating can occur when taking the solution. Drinking the preparation more slowly can help reduce the severe vomiting and cramping.

During the test:
- Sedation is usually given. You will be lying on your side on the exam table.
- The colonoscope will be inserted into your rectum. Air or carbon dioxide is pumped into the intestine to help the provider see the lining of the colon. This can cause some cramping.
- The procedure takes about 30 to 60 minutes.

After the test:
- You will need to recover for about an hour after the test.
- Do not drive. Plan to have someone bring you home.

Equipment and Supplies:
- Patient instructions
- Patient's health record

Standard: Complete the procedure and all critical steps in _____ minutes with a minimum score of 85% within two attempts (*or as indicated by the instructor*).

Scoring: Divide the points earned by the total possible points. Failure to perform a critical step, indicated by an asterisk (*), results in grade no higher than an 84% (*or as indicated by the instructor*).

Time: Began_____ Ended_____ Total minutes: _____

Steps:	Point Value	Attempt 1	Attempt 2
1. Wash hands or use hand sanitizer.	10		
2. Greet the patient. Identify yourself. Verify the patient's identity with full name and date of birth. Explain what you will be doing in a manner that the patient understands. Answer any questions the patient may have.	10		
3. Use simpler language when talking. Speak clearly. Communicate with dignity and respect. Allow time for the patient to respond. Listen to the patient's concerns.	10		
4. Ask the patient if they have ever had a colonoscopy. If so, ask them what they remember about it.	10		
5. Discuss the purpose of the colonoscopy and the preparation involved. Refer to the written instructions that the patient will be taking home.	15		
6. Explain what the patient should expect during and after the procedure.	15		
7. Ask the patient to teach back the preparation to you. Clarify any misconceptions or inaccuracies. Answer any questions the patient may have. Give the patient a phone number to call if they have questions.	10		
8. Let the patient know when to anticipate the results. Also, give the patient the appointment information for the procedure, including the location, date, and time.	10		
9. Document the coaching in the patient's health record. Include the provider's name, what was taught, how the patient responded, and any written directions (including appointment information) sent home with the patient.	10		
Total Points	**100**		

Documentation

Comments

CAAHEP Competencies	Step(s)
V.P.3.b. Coach patients regarding medical encounters	Entire procedure
X.P.3. Document patient care accurately in the medical record	9
ABHES Competencies	**Step(s)**
8.e. Perform specialty procedures, including but not limited to minor surgery, cardiac, respiratory, OB-GYN, neurological, and gastroenterology	Entire procedure

Orthopedics and Rheumatology

CAAHEP Competencies	Assessment
I.C.4. Identify major organs in each body system	Skills and Concepts – A. 8, D. 1-8
I.C.5. Identify the anatomical location of major organs in each body system	Skills and Concepts – B. 1-26, D. 10-14; Certification Preparation – 1, 4
I.C.6. Identify structure and function of the human body across the life span	Skills and Concepts – F. 1-4
I.C.7. Identify the normal function of each body system	Skills and Concepts – A. 9, C. 1-2, E. 1-7; Certification Preparation – 2
I.C.8.a. Identify common pathology related to each body system including: signs	Skills and Concepts – G. 14-21, J. 7-12; Internet Activities – 2, 3
I.C.8.b. Identify common pathology related to each body system including: symptoms	Skills and Concepts – G. 14-21, J. 7-12; Internet Activities – 2, 3
I.C.8.c. Identify common pathology related to each body system including: etiology	Skills and Concepts – G. 7-13, J. 1-6; Certification Preparation – 5, 6; Workplace Application – 1; Internet Activities – 2, 3
I.C.8.d. Identify common pathology related to each body system including: diagnostic measures	Skills and Concepts – G. 22-29, J. 13-18, K. 1-4; Workplace Application – 1, 2; Internet Activities – 1, 2, 3
I.C.8.e. Identify common pathology related to each body system including: treatment modalities	Skills and Concepts – G. 22-29, J. 13-18, K. 5-20; Certification Preparation – 7; Workplace Application – 2-4
I.C.9. Identify Clinical Laboratory Improvement Amendments (CLIA) waived tests associated with common diseases	Skills and Concepts – K. 1-4; Certification Preparation – 3
I.C.10.a. Identify the classifications of medications, including indications for use	Skills and Concepts – K. 11-18; Certification Preparation – 5; Internet Activities – 4
I.C.10.b. Identify the classifications of medications, including desired effects	Skills and Concepts – K. 11-18; Internet Activities – 4
I.C.10.c. Identify the classifications of medications, including side effects	Skills and Concepts – K. 19-26; Internet Activities – 4
I.C.10.d. Identify the classifications of medications, including adverse reactions	Skills and Concepts – K. 19-26; Internet Activities – 4
V.C.8.a. Identify the following related to body systems: medical terms	Skills and Concepts – A. 1-7, K. 5-10
V.C.8.b. Identify the following related to body systems: abbreviations	Abbreviations – 1-17

ABHES Competencies	Assessment
2. Anatomy and Physiology a. List all body systems and their structures and functions	Skills and Concepts – A. 8-9, C. 1-2, D. 1-8, E. 1-7; Certification Preparation – 2
2.b. Describe common diseases, symptoms, and etiologies as they apply to each system	Skills and Concepts – G. 1-21, H. 1-4, I. 1-8, J. 1-12, K. 1-20; Certification Preparation – 5, 6; Workplace Application – 1; Internet Activities – 2, 3
2.c. Identify diagnostic and treatment modalities as they relate to each body system	Skills and Concepts – G. 22-29, J. 13-18; Certification Preparation – 7; Workplace Application – 1, 2, 3; Internet Activities – 2, 3, 4
3. Medical Terminology c. Apply medical terminology for each specialty	Vocabulary Review – A. 1-12, B. 1-12
3.d. Define and use medical abbreviations when appropriate and acceptable	Abbreviations – 1-17

VOCABULARY REVIEW

Using the word pool on the right, find the correct word to match the definition. Write the word on the line after the definition.

Group A

1. Supportive connective tissue that connects bones at a joint
   _____

2. Flexible connective tissue that covers the ends of many bones at the joint _____

3. An immune response against a person's own tissues, cells, or cell parts, as in autoimmune disease, leading to the deterioration of tissue _____

4. Connective tissue that attaches muscles to bone
   _____

5. Soft, gelatinous tissue that consists of blood stem cells that can become white or red blood cells or platelets
   _____

6. A prominence or projection on a bone _____

7. Consists of tightly packed osteons; denser and heavier compared to spongy bone _____

8. Lighter and less dense than compact bone; also called *cancellous bone* _____

9. Hard bony tissue that forms at the ends of fractured bones during the healing process _____

10. Chemicals that help a nerve cell communicate with another nerve cell or muscle _____

11. The formation of the blood cells and platelets
    _____

12. A tough, fibrous connective tissue that attaches muscles to muscles _____

Word Pool
- aponeurosis
- autoimmune
- callus
- cartilage
- compact bone
- hematopoiesis
- ligament
- neurotransmitters
- process
- red bone marrow
- spongy bone
- tendon

Group B

1. A point of communication between two cells

   _____

2. A high-energy molecule, found in every cell, that supplies large amounts of energy for various biochemical processes

   _____

3. An enzyme that destroys acetylcholine and counteracts its action

   _____

4. Occurring in the presence of oxygen _____

5. Occurring without the presence of oxygen

   _____

6. The internal environment of the body that is compatible with life

   _____

7. Involuntary muscle tremors and fine movements

   _____

8. A drug that reduces or eliminates pain _____

9. A drug used to prevent or treat seizures _____

10. Removal of tissue or cells for examination by a pathologist

    _____

11. The partial or complete disappearance of the clinical and subjective characteristics of a chronic or malignant disease

    _____

12. A drug used to suppress the immune system

    _____

Word Pool
- acetylcholinesterase
- adenosine triphosphate
- aerobic
- anaerobic
- analgesic
- anticonvulsant
- biopsy
- fasciculations
- homeostasis
- immunosuppressant
- remission
- synapse

ABBREVIATIONS

Write out what each of the following abbreviations stands for.

1. ATP _____

2. EMG _____

3. ROM _____

4. NMJ _____

5. ACh _____

6. ORIF _____

7. WPI _____

8. SS _____

9. RA _____

10. JA _____

11. DJD _____

12. MD _____

13. CK _____

14. RICE _____

15. DMARDs _____

16. CRP _____

17. RF _____

SKILLS AND CONCEPTS
Answer the following questions.

A. Introduction
Match the following description with the term.

1. _____ A specially trained physician who medically, surgically, and physically treats musculoskeletal disorders

2. _____ A physician who specializes in treating the foot and ankle

3. _____ The healthcare specialty that deals with most skeletal disorders and associated muscle, joint, and ligament conditions

4. _____ A physician who specializes in internal medicine and rheumatology

5. _____ A specialty that deals with disorders of connective tissue, including bone and cartilage

6. _____ The branch of medicine that deals with the diagnosis, treatment, and prevention of foot disorders

7. _____ A physician who is specially trained to diagnose and treat skeletal system disorders

a. orthopedist
b. orthopedic surgeon
c. podiatrist
d. rheumatologist
e. orthopedics
f. podiatry
g. rheumatology

Select the correct answer.

8. The musculoskeletal system consists of
   a. bones and joints.
   b. cartilage, tendons, and ligaments.
   c. muscles.
   d. all of the above.

9. The function of the musculoskeletal system includes
   a. body movement.
   b. support, protection, and framework for the organ systems of the body.
   c. storage of minerals.
   d. the formation of new blood cells.
   e. all of the above.

B. Anatomy of the Skeletal System
Select the correct answer or fill in the blank.

1. Which bone is *not* part of the cranium?
   a. Temporal
   b. Parietal
   c. Zygomatic
   d. Sphenoid
   e. Ethmoid

2. Which bone is also called the *maxilla* or *upper jawbone*?
   a. Lacrimal
   b. Parietal
   c. Zygomatic
   d. Sphenoid
   e. Maxillary

3. Which bone is *not* a facial bone?
   a. Lacrimal
   b. Frontal
   c. Zygomatic
   d. Palatine
   e. Maxillary

4. Which bone is *not* an ossicle?
   a. Malleus
   b. Conchae
   c. Incus
   d. Stapes

5. Which is *not* a region of the vertebral column?
   a. Lumbar
   b. Cervical
   c. Hyoid
   d. Thoracic
   e. Coccygeal

6. There are _____ pairs of true ribs and _____ pairs of false ribs.

Match the following descriptions with the correct bone.

7. _____ Lateral tip of the scapula
8. _____ Wrist bones
9. _____ Protrusion near the neck of the femur
10. _____ Upper arm bone
11. _____ Smaller lower leg bone
12. _____ Kneecap
13. _____ Thigh bone
14. _____ Part of the tibia and located on the inner side of the ankle
15. _____ Breastbone
16. _____ Lower arm bone on the little finger side
17. _____ Heel bone
18. _____ Collarbone
19. _____ Bones in the palm of the hand
20. _____ Shin bone
21. _____ Lower arm bone on the thumb side
22. _____ Finger and toe bones
23. _____ Made up of the ilium, ischium, and pubis
24. _____ Forms the heel and the posterior side of the foot
25. _____ Foot bones
26. _____ Shoulder blade

a. sternum
b. clavicle
c. scapula
d. humerus
e. radius
f. carpals
g. metacarpals
h. phalanges
i. coxal bone
j. femur
k. patella
l. tibia
m. fibula
n. tarsals
o. calcaneus
p. metatarsals
q. acromion process
r. ulna
s. greater trochanter
t. medial malleolus

Match the description with the correct term.

27. _____ Growth plate
28. _____ Bone cells
29. _____ Hollow space inside the diaphysis and contains yellow bone marrow
30. _____ Structural units of compact bone
31. _____ The long shaft of a long bone and made of compact bone
32. _____ The end of a long bone and made of spongy bone
33. _____ Narrow strip between the diaphysis and epiphysis; contains the growth plate

a. diaphysis
b. medullary cavity
c. epiphysis
d. epiphyseal plate
e. ostocytes
f. osteons
g. metaphysis

Match the description with the correct type of joint. Answers can be used more than once.

34. _____ Full range of motion (ROM) joints
35. _____ Limited ROM joints, which are joined together by cartilage that is slightly movable
36. _____ Immovable joints held together by fibrous cartilaginous tissue
37. _____ Also called *synovial joints*
38. _____ Examples of this type of joint include the knee and the hip joint
39. _____ Examples of this type of joint include the vertebrae and the pubic bone
40. _____ An example of this type of joint is a suture line of the skull

a. synarthroses
b. amphiarthroses
c. diarthroses

Fill in the blank.

41. _____ are sacs of synovial fluid located between the bones of the joint and the tendons that hold the muscles in place.

42. The synovial membrane secretes _____ that lubricates the joint.

43. The _____ consists of crescent-shaped cartilage in the knee joint that also cushions the joint.

44. _____ are strong bands of white, fibrous connective tissue that connect one bone to another bone at the joints.

Match the description with the correct type of joint.

45. _____ Allows free movement; an example is the shoulder joint

46. _____ Permits rotation; an example is the joint between the ulna and radius

47. _____ Allows a bone to slide over another bone; found in the wrist

48. _____ Allows for flexion, extension, and other movement; an example is the thumb crossing over the palm of the hand

49. _____ Permits flexion and extension; an example is the elbow

50. _____ Permits flexion, extension, and circular motion; an example is the atlas

a. hinge joint
b. pivot joint
c. saddle joint
d. condyloid joint
e. ball-and-socket joint
f. gliding joint

C. Physiology of the Skeletal System
Select the correct answer.

1. Which of the following is a function of the skeletal system?
   a. Protects, supports, and provides a framework for the organ systems of the body
   b. Develops new bone
   c. Regulates blood calcium levels
   d. Hematopoiesis
   e. All of the above

2. Which of the following statements is *incorrect*?
   a. Osteoclasts and osteoblasts continuously remodel bones.
   b. Osteoblasts break down bone and osteoclasts form bone.
   c. Parathyroid hormone increases the activity of the osteoclasts when the blood calcium level is decreased.
   d. Calcitonin promotes bone formation by the osteoblasts and inhibits bone breakdown by the osteoclasts.

D. Anatomy of the Muscular System

Match the description with the correct type of muscle. Answers can be used more than once.

1. _____ Found in hollow organ walls
2. _____ Found in the walls of the heart
3. _____ Helps with swallowing and eye movements
4. _____ Involuntary, striated muscles
5. _____ Involuntary, nonstriated muscle cells that have a single nucleus
6. _____ Found in the walls of the blood vessels
7. _____ Have multiple nuclei and striations
8. _____ Sphincter muscles
9. _____ Found in the eye and change the size of the iris and the shape of the lens.

a. skeletal muscles
b. smooth muscles
c. cardiac muscles

Select the correct answer.

10. Which muscle is *not* found in the head and neck?
    a. Orbicularis oculi
    b. Zygomaticus
    c. Pectoralis major
    d. Buccinator
    e. Sternocleidomastoid

11. Which muscle is *not* found in the upper extremities?
    a. Deltoid
    b. Latissimus dorsi
    c. Biceps brachii
    d. External oblique

12. Which muscle is *not* found in the abdomen?
    a. Iliopsoas
    b. Rectus abdominis
    c. Diaphragm
    d. Internal oblique
    e. Transversus abdominis

13. Which muscle is *not* found in the lower extremities?
    a. Sartorius
    b. Gluteus maximus
    c. Tibialis anterior
    d. Gastrocnemius
    e. Triceps brachii

14. Which muscle is *not* part of the quadriceps group?
    a. Rectus femoris
    b. Tibialis anterior
    c. Vastus lateralis
    d. Vastus intermedius
    e. Vastus medialis

E. Physiology of the Muscular System
Select the correct answer.

1. Which of the following activities is a primary function of the muscular system?
   a. Maintains body temperature
   b. Muscle contractions provide muscle tone and posture
   c. Provides joint stability
   d. Controls passageways in the body
   e. All of the above

2. Which statement is correct?
   a. For skeletal muscle contraction to occur, it must be stimulated by an impulse.
   b. The neuromuscular junction is the point of contact between the nerve ending and the muscle fiber.
   c. Neurotransmitters are released by the motor neuron in response to a nerve impulse.
   d. All of the above

3. Muscle fatigue
   a. causes muscles to feel weaker, the strength decreases, and the ability to contract may be lost.
   b. is the result of lactic acid buildup from anaerobic respirations.
   c. is corrected by extra oxygen that oxidizes the lactic acid.
   d. all of the above.

Match the descriptions with the correct type of muscle contractions.

4. _____ Sustained and steady contraction response to a stimulus.

5. _____ Muscle contraction usually does not produce movement.

6. _____ A quick, fine movement of a small area of muscles in response to a stimulus.

7. _____ Muscle contraction that usually produces movement at a joint.

a. twitch
b. tetanic
c. isotonic
d. isometric

F. Life Span Changes
Select the correct answer.

1. Which of the following is *incorrect*?
   a. The initial cartilage and fibrous skeletal structures are replaced with bone matrix as a person grows.
   b. The prime time to build bone mass is in middle adulthood.
   c. Bone density increases through calcium-rich diet and regular weight-bearing exercises.
   d. Poor nutrition, smoking, inactivity, and excessive alcohol intake reduce bone density.

2. Which of the following is a common skeletal system change that occurs with age?
   a. Bones lose calcium and other minerals, which reduces the bone mass.
   b. The disks between the vertebrae wear and tear with age.
   c. Loss of height from the compression and curving of the spinal column occurs.
   d. Joints become stiffer and less flexible.
   e. All of the above.

3. Which of the following is a common muscular system change that occurs with age?
   a. Muscle tissue is replaced more slowly.
   b. Muscle tissue may be replaced with tough, fibrous tissue.
   c. Muscles have less ability to contract.
   d. Lean body mass decreases.
   e. All of the above.

4. With the muscle changes, older people experience
    a. loss of strength.
    b. loss of endurance.
    c. fatigue.
    d. reduced activity tolerance.
    e. all of the above.

G. Skeletal System Diseases and Disorders

Match the description with the correct type of fracture.

1. _____ The bone breaks on one side and is bent but still intact on the other side; commonly seen in children.
2. _____ The fracture line does not go across the entire cross section of the bone.
3. _____ The bone fragments are not in alignment.
4. _____ The fracture line resembles a spiral; caused by the bone being twisted.
5. _____ The fracture line goes across the entire cross section of the bone.
6. _____ The bone fragments are driven into each other.

a. incomplete
b. complete
c. displaced
d. greenstick
e. impacted
f. spiral

Match the etiology with the disease.

7. _____ Caused by a lack of vitamin D.
8. _____ Bone mass is lost faster than it can be produced.
9. _____ Occurs from trauma, overuse, or disease.
10. _____ Caused by an overgrowth of bone, herniated disks, tumors, spinal injury, and thickening of ligaments.
11. _____ Unknown etiology but may be related to genetic factors or to a viral infection.
12. _____ Occurs with strenuous activities or lifting heavy objects.
13. _____ Caused by genetic and congenital conditions, such as muscular dystrophy.

a. fractures
b. lordosis
c. osteomalacia and rickets
d. herniated disk
e. Paget disease
f. spinal stenosis
g. osteoporosis

Match the signs and symptoms with the correct disease.

14. _____ Back pain, height loss, stooped posture, and fractures
15. _____ Bone fractures without related injuries, muscle weakness, and widespread bone pain, usually in the hips
16. _____ Numbness, tingling, weakness in the extremities, neck pain, difficulty walking, and bowel and bladder incontinence
17. _____ Pain, swelling, bruising, numbness or tingling, deformity, and difficulty using or inability to use the affected area
18. _____ Foot pain immediately in the morning, after standing, sitting, or intense exercise, and when climbing stairs
19. _____ Uneven shoulders and waist, one shoulder blade may be more prominent, and one hip may be higher than the other
20. _____ Bone pain, joint stiffness, pain, fractures, an enlarged skull, and bowing of the legs
21. _____ Sciatica, back pain, and weakness

a. fractures
b. scoliosis
c. osteomalacia and rickets
d. herniated disk
e. Paget disease
f. cervical spinal stenosis
g. osteoporosis
h. plantar fasciitis

Match the diagnostic measures and treatments with the correct disease.

22. _____ Myelogram, electromyograph, and imaging tests; treated with medications to reduce the pain and inflammation, rest and physical therapy

23. _____ Spinal x-ray, MRI, and CT scan; physical therapy, medications, spinal fusion surgery, treated with back brace, and surgical placement of metal stabilizing rods

24. _____ X-rays, MRI, CT myelogram; treated with surgery, analgesics, physical therapy, and steroid injection

25. _____ Blood tests (e.g., vitamin D, creatinine, electrolytes), bone x-rays, a bone density test, and a bone biopsy; treated with vitamin D, calcium, and phosphorus

26. _____ Bone density test; treated with weight-bearing exercises, calcium and vitamin D, and medications such as bisphosphonates

27. _____ Bone scan, x-rays, and laboratory tests (e.g., alkaline phosphatase and serum calcium); treated with percutaneous image-guided lumbar decompression and bisphosphonates

28. _____ X-ray; treated with casting, splinting, or bracing to immobilize the area

29. _____ Foot x-ray; treated with analgesics, heel and foot stretches, and good arch supports

a. fractures
b. scoliosis
c. osteomalacia and rickets
d. herniated disk
e. Paget disease
f. spinal stenosis
g. osteoporosis
h. plantar fasciitis

H. Arthritic Joint Diseases and Disorders
Fill in the blank.

1. _____ is a term that refers to any inflammatory joint condition.

2. _____, also called *degenerative joint disease* (DJD), can occur in any joint but most often affects the hands, hips, spine, and knees.

3. _____ is an autoimmune and inflammatory disease that often starts in middle age and is common in older adults.

4. _____ is caused by a buildup of uric acid in the body and leads to swollen, red, warm, and stiff joints.

I. Nonarthritic Joint Diseases and Disorders

Match the description with the disease.

1. _____ A partial or incomplete dislocation of the joint
2. _____ The inflammation of the bursa, usually affects the hip, buttock, knee, calf, and shoulder
3. _____ An abnormality of the hip joint in which the femoral head does not fit in the acetabulum as it should
4. _____ Also called *bunion*; an abnormal enlargement of the first metatarsophalangeal (MTP) joint of the great toe, caused by inflammation of the synovial bursa
5. _____ Carpal tunnel syndrome results when the median nerve becomes compressed at the wrist
6. _____ Occurs when a bone has been completely displaced from the joint
7. _____ Also called *runner's knee*; causes pain at the front of the knee around the patella
8. _____ A stretched or torn ligament

a. bursitis
b. carpal tunnel syndrome
c. dislocation
d. subluxation
e. hallux valgus
f. hip dysplasia
g. sprain
h. patellofemoral syndrome

J. Muscular System Diseases and Disorders

Match the etiology with the disease.

1. _____ Congenital or caused by a genetic mutation that disrupts the body's ability to make muscle-protecting proteins
2. _____ Occurs after repeated injury to a joint
3. _____ Caused by falling, jumping, lifting heavy objects, and repetitive muscle movements
4. _____ Caused by a fracture, bruised muscle, severe sprain, or a crushing injury
5. _____ Unknown
6. _____ An autoimmune neuromuscular disease

a. compartment syndrome
b. fibromyalgia
c. muscular dystrophy
d. myasthenia gravis
e. strain
f. tendinitis

Match the signs and symptoms with the disease.

7. _____ Causes pain, swelling, difficulty moving the affected muscle, and muscle spasms
8. _____ Causes muscle weakness, drooping eyelids, facial paralysis, fatigue, hoarseness, and double vision
9. _____ Causes widespread muscle pain, burning, aching, stiffness, soreness, fatigue, sleep disturbances, mood and concentration problems, anxiety, headache, abdominal pain, bloating, constipation, diarrhea, and bladder spasms
10. _____ Causes pain, tenderness, inflammation in the joint area, and a limited range of motion
11. _____ Causes pale skin, swelling, severe pain, and inability to move the extremity
12. _____ Causes frequent falls, trouble running and moving from lying to sitting position, muscle pain and stiffness, and learning disabilities

a. compartment syndrome
b. fibromyalgia
c. Duchenne muscular dystrophy
d. myasthenia gravis
e. strain
f. tendinitis

Match the diagnostic measures and treatments with the correct disease.

13. _____ Usually just an examination; treatment consists of rest, splinting, heat and cold therapy, medications (e.g., analgesics and corticosteroid injections), and physical therapy

14. _____ Measure the compartment's pressure; treated with a fasciotomy

15. _____ No diagnostic tests; treated with medications to minimize pain, exercise, biofeedback, and acupuncture

16. _____ Range of motion and imaging tests to rule out other injuries; treated with rest, ice, compression, and elevation of the area and analgesics

17. _____ Imaging tests (CT or MRI), pulmonary function tests, electromyography (EMG), and an acetylcholine receptor antibody blood test; treatments include resting, using eye patches, avoiding stress and heat exposure, and medications (e.g., neostigmine, immunosuppressants)

18. _____ Creatine kinase (CK) blood test; treatments include corticosteroids, heart medication, range of motion and stretching exercises, braces, and assistive devices

a. compartment syndrome
b. fibromyalgia
c. muscular dystrophy
d. myasthenia gravis
e. strain
f. tendinitis

K. The Medical Assistant's Role with the Examination, Diagnostic Measures, and Treatments

Select the correct answer or fill in the blank.

1. C-reactive protein (CRP)
   a. can be measured by a blood test and some are CLIA-waived tests.
   b. is produced by the liver.
   c. increases with inflammation.
   d. is a nonspecific indicator of inflammation.
   e. all of the above.

2. _____ test, a CLIA-waived blood test, measures how quickly the red blood cells (RBCs) in a blood sample settle to the bottom of the test tube. The quicker they settle, the more it indicates inflammation in the body.

3. _____ test, a CLIA-waived test, looks for antibodies to Borrelia.

4. _____ test, a CLIA-waived blood test, looks for the presence of rheumatoid factor in the blood.

5. _____ is the surgical procedure that involves a puncture of the joint and removal (aspiration) of fluid.

6. _____ is the surgical removal of a bunion.

7. _____ is the surgical procedure that involves opening the muscle compartment to reduce the pressure and restore blood flow.

8. _____ is the surgical removal of a meniscus.

9. _____ is the surgical suturing of a muscle.

10. _____ is the surgical procedure to repair a tendon and muscle.

Match the indication for use and desired effects with the correct medication classification.

11. _____ Used to prevent seizures by reducing excessive stimulation of the brain

12. _____ Treats chronic inflammatory diseases and acute conditions (e.g., poison ivy, asthma) by reducing the inflammation

13. _____ Treats autoimmune disorders by blocking the action of tumor-necrosis factor and preventing inflammation

14. _____ Relieves pain by blocking the pain receptors.

15. _____ Treats arthritis and other inflammatory disorders by reducing inflammation

16. _____ Promotes bone mineral density and reverse the progression of osteoporosis by inhibiting bone reabsorption and/or promotes the use of calcium

17. _____ Treats gout by reducing the uric acid in the body

18. _____ Treats painful musculoskeletal conditions by working on the central nervous system to relax muscles, which decreases the pain

a. analgesic
b. tumor necrosis factor (TNF) inhibitor
c. anticonvulsant and mood stabilizer
d. antigout medication
e. antiinflammatory
f. corticosteroid
g. osteoporosis agent
h. muscle relaxant

Match the side effects and adverse reactions with the correct medication classification.

19. _____ Headache, mood changes, difficulty falling asleep or staying asleep, increased sweating, vision problems, depression, and weight gain

20. _____ Sedation, vertigo, visual disturbances, GI disturbances, and liver complications

21. _____ GI distress, GI bleeding, hepatitis, drowsiness, tinnitus, irregular heart rate, and kidney disorders

22. _____ GI distress, liver and kidney disorders, and tinnitus

23. _____ GI disorders and esophageal irritation

24. _____ GI distress, eye irritation, itching, rash, and blood in urine

25. _____ Drowsiness, clumsiness, tachycardia, GI intolerance, difficulty breathing, fever, weakness, burning in the eyes, and seizures

26. _____ GI distress, weakness, seizures, and bleeding

a. analgesic
b. tumor necrosis factor (TNF) inhibitor
c. anticonvulsant and mood stabilizer
d. antigout
e. antiinflammatory
f. corticosteroid
g. osteoporosis agent
h. muscle relaxant

CERTIFICATION PREPARATION

Circle the correct answer.

1. Which is *not* part of the sternum?
   a. Body
   b. Xiphoid process
   c. Clavicle
   d. Manubrium

2. What is the main function of the musculoskeletal system?
   a. Body movement
   b. pH balance
   c. Waste removal
   d. All of the above

3. Which is a CLIA-waived test?
   a. Erythrocyte sedimentation rate
   b. Rheumatoid factor
   c. Lyme disease blood antibodies
   d. All of the above

4. A ligament connects which two structures?
   a. Muscles to bone
   b. Muscles to muscles
   c. Bones to bones
   d. Muscles to tendons

5. RA is caused by
   a. a bacterial infection that destroys the joints.
   b. a fracture within a joint.
   c. a genetic condition that cannot be prevented.
   d. an autoimmune reaction that attacks the lining of the joints.

6. Which disease is caused by a buildup of uric acid in the blood?
   a. Gout
   b. Osteoporosis
   c. Degenerative joint disease
   d. Lyme disease

7. Which medication classification is used to treat seizures?
   a. Antigout
   b. Corticosteroids
   c. Anticonvulsants
   d. Antiinflammatories

8. Which term means to increase the angle or distance between two bones or parts of the body?
   a. Flexion
   b. Extension
   c. Abduction
   d. Hyperextension

9. Which term means to move the body part toward the midline of the body?
   a. Rotation
   b. Adduction
   c. Abduction
   d. Circumduction

10. Which term means to turn the sole of the foot medially, or inward?
   a. Eversion
   b. Plantar flexion
   c. Dorsiflexion
   d. Inversion

WORKPLACE APPLICATIONS

1. A young woman calls in and says that she is concerned about a rash she has on her leg. She is an avid hiker and spends most of her weekends hiking and camping. She frequently finds ticks on her clothing and is careful about using preventive measures to limit her exposure to tick bites. She has noticed a red rash on her leg today and for the last day or two has been feeling very tired and achy. She is afraid she might have Lyme disease.

   a. What type of testing can be done to help diagnose her condition? _____

   _____

   b. What organism causes Lyme disease? _____

   c. What type of preventive measure can be taken to guard against a tick bite? _____

   _____

   _____

2. Walter Biller is in to see Dr. James Martin at Walden-Martin Family Medical (WMFM) Clinic to go over some tests results. Walter's rheumatoid factor (RF) test is negative, and his C-reactive protein (CRP) and erythrocyte sedimentation rate (ESR) are elevated. What do these results mean?

   _____

   _____

3. Marcie Nguyen was playing softball last night and slid into second base, and in the process, she twisted her ankle. She is afraid she may have a sprained ankle. What is the difference between and strain and a sprain?

    _____

    _____

    How would the injury be treated if the diagnosis is a Grade I ankle sprain? _____

    _____

    _____

INTERNET ACTIVITIES

1. Using online resources, research a test used for diagnosing musculoskeletal disease. Create a poster presentation, a PowerPoint presentation, or a written paper summarizing your research. Include the following points in your project:
    a. Description of the test
    b. Any contraindications for the test
    c. Patient preparation for the test
    d. What occurs during the test

2. Using online resources, research a musculoskeletal disease. Create a poster presentation, a PowerPoint presentation, or an infographic summarizing your research. Include the following points in your project:
    a. Description of the disease
    b. Etiology
    c. Signs and symptoms
    d. Diagnostic measures
    e. Treatments

3. Using online resources, research the three abnormal curvatures of the spine presented in this chapter: lordosis, kyphosis, and scoliosis. In a one-page paper, describe each abnormal curve, the etiologies, signs and symptoms, and describe how it is treated.

4. Using Table 35.4, Medication Classifications, select a generic medication from each of the following classifications: antigout, antiinflammatory, muscle relaxant, osteoporosis agent, and tumor-necrosis factor inhibitor. Using a reliable online drug resource, for each medication identify:
    a. Indications for use
    b. Desired effects
    c. Side effects
    d. Adverse reactions

    Write a short paper addressing each of these four areas for each medication.

Physical Medicine and Rehabilitation

CAAHEP Competencies	Assessment
V.C.8.b. Identify the following related to body system: abbreviations	Abbreviations – 1-12
I.P.8. Instruct and prepare a patient for a procedure or a treatment	Procedures 36.4 through 36.9
V.P.3.b. Coach patients regarding: medical encounters	Procedures 36.1 through 36.9
X.P.3. Document patient care accurately in the medical record	Procedures 36.1 through 36.9

ABHES Competencies	Assessment
4. Medical Law and Ethics a. Follow documentation guidelines	Procedures 36.1 through 36.9
5. Human Relations d. Adapt care to address the developmental stages of life	Procedure 36.7
8. Clinical Procedures h. Teach self-examination, disease management and health promotion	Procedures 36.3 through 36.9
8.i. Identify community resources and complementary and alternative medicine (CAM) practices	Review of Concepts – H. 1-4
8.j. Make adaptations for patients with special needs (psychological or physical limitations)	Procedures 36.8, 36.9
8.k. Make adaptations to care for patients across their lifespan	Procedures 36.7, 36.8

VOCABULARY REVIEW

Using the word pool on the right, find the correct word to match the definition. Write the word on the line after the definition.

1. The normal movement allowed by the joint
   _____

2. A calibrated device designed to measure the arc, angle, or range of motion of a joint _____

3. Connective tissue that attaches muscles to bone
   _____

4. A dry, crackling sound or sensation _____

5. Supportive connective tissue that connects bones at a joint
   _____

6. An instrument used for measuring the degree of muscle power or force _____

7. A physician who specializes in physical medicine and rehabilitation _____

8. Flexible connective tissue that covers the ends of many bones at the joint _____

9. A substance that prevents clotting of blood
   _____

10. A drug that reduces or eliminates pain _____

11. A serious condition that involves increased pressure, usually in the muscles, which leads to compromised blood flow and muscle and nerve damage _____

12. Therapeutic treatments for a disorder _____

13. Contraction of the muscles that causes a narrowing of the inside tube of the blood vessel _____

14. Adhesive patches that conduct electricity from the body to the machine wires _____

15. The standing position when using crutches; crutch tips are 4 to 6 inches to the side and front of each foot _____

Word Pool
- analgesic
- anticoagulant
- cartilage
- compartment syndrome
- crepitation
- dynamometer
- electrodes
- goniometer
- ligaments
- modalities
- physiatrist
- range of motion
- tendons
- tripod position
- vasoconstriction

ABBREVIATIONS

Write out what each of the following abbreviations stands for.

1. PM&R _____

2. PT _____

3. OT _____

4. ADLs _____

5. ROM _____

6. CT _____

7. DEXA _____

8. EMG _____

9. NCV _____

10. CMST _____

11. RICE _____

12. TENS _____

SKILLS AND CONCEPTS

Answer the following questions.

A. Introduction

1. Physical medicine and rehabilitation
   a. are also called *physiatry* or *rehabilitation medicine*.
   b. use therapies and physical agents to diagnose, prevent, and treat disorders.
   c. focus on improving and restoring a patient's ability and quality of life.
   d. all of the above.

2. A(n) _____ is a physician who specializes in physical medicine and rehabilitation.

3. _____ focuses on improving a person's movement, strength, and mobility.

4. _____ focuses on improving a person's ability to perform activities of daily living.

5. List the therapy involved with helping the patient with the following activities:

   a. Bathing and grooming _____

   b. Swallowing and communication _____

   c. Eating _____

   d. Using a walker _____

B. Assisting with the Examination

1. When gathering information on the symptoms for the medical history, what additional information should be obtained?
   a. Details about the onset
   b. What reduces the symptoms
   c. What increases the symptoms
   d. All of the above

2. When describing the 0 to 10 pain scale to a patient, 0 is _____ and 10 is the _____.

C. Assisting with Diagnostic Procedures

Match the following descriptions with the diagnostic procedures.

1. _____ Used with an EMG to test the speed of electrical signals through a nerve
2. _____ A bone density test used to measure the calcium and other minerals in the bone
3. _____ A camera slowly scans the body and takes pictures of the radiotracer that collects in the bones
4. _____ Uses fluoroscopy and contrast medium to evaluate the spinal cord and related structures
5. _____ A series of x-rays taken of a joint after a contrast medium (e.g., dye) is injected into the joint
6. _____ Thin needle electrodes are inserted through the skin into the muscle to pick up the electrical activity in the muscle
7. _____ Imaging test that takes cross-sectional pictures of the body

a. arthrogram
b. bone scan
c. CT
d. DEXA scan
e. EMG
f. myelogram
g. NCV

Fill in the blank.

8. With _____ of a joint, the patient is asked to move the joint as far as possible.

9. With _____ of a joint, the provider moves the joint as far as possible.

10. Muscle strength is _____ in normal conditions.

11. Hand-grip strength can be measured with a(n) _____ or a blood pressure cuff.

D. Assisting with Immobilization Treatments

1. Indicate the size of elastic bandage used for older teens and adults.

   a. For the hand _____

   b. For the forearm, arm, and lower leg _____

   c. For the thigh _____

Match the following descriptions with the immobilization treatment.

2. _____ Used as a bandage over wounds and also limits swelling in the injured or operative extremity; also called a *compression wrap*
3. _____ Consists of a strip of rigid material that immobilizes an extremity
4. _____ Provides stability and protection to the joint while allowing the joint to still function
5. _____ Used to protect and stabilize the ankle and lower leg after an injury or surgery; used for partial, full, or non–weight-bearing extremities
6. _____ A device used to support and immobilize an injured part of the body such as the arm, wrist, or shoulder
7. _____ Applied to immobilize a joint and bones after injury or surgery and provide additional protection; made from fiberglass or plaster

a. brace
b. ankle boot
c. elastic bandage
d. cast
e. sling
f. splint

For each description, match the CMST category addressed and then determine if it is normal or abnormal. Match the descriptions with the answers.

8. _____ The patient is unable to move her fingers on the side of the casted arm.

9. _____ The patient's fingers are warm on the casted extremity and match the warmth on the opposite extremity.

10. _____ The fingers on the casted arm are bluish and pale.

11. _____ The patient's fingers are cooler on the casted extremity compared to the other extremity.

12. _____ The patient can feel light touch on his toes on the casted extremity.

13. _____ The patient is able to move the toes on his casted leg and no swelling is present.

14. _____ The patient states she has a stinging sensation in her fingers on the casted arm. She also indicates the fingers feel like they are sleeping.

15. _____ The toes are pink and match the opposite extremity.

a. color—normal
b. color—abnormal
c. motion—normal
d. motion—abnormal
e. sensation—normal
f. sensation—abnormal
g. temperature—normal
h. temperature—abnormal

E. Assisting with Cold and Heat Therapies

1. Heat and cold therapy should be applied for _____ minutes.

2. _____ is typically used for sprains, strains, fractures, joint injuries, shin splints, and other injuries.

3. A cold application causes vasoconstriction, which results in tissue metabolism _____, _____ oxygen is used, and _____ swelling occurs.

4. _____ is typically used for acute and chronic pain, sinus congestion, and infection.

5. A hot application produces local _____, which increases the blood supply to a local area and helps absorb the extra fluid.

6. A paraffin bath uses melted paraffin and mineral oil warmed to about _____°F.

7. _____ light therapy is used to treat skin conditions and _____ light therapy penetrates deeper, killing pathogens, healing tissue, improving circulation, and relieving pain.

F. Physical Therapy Treatments

1. For orthopedic injuries, RICE is commonly ordered as a treatment for usually the first _____ to _____ hours.

Match the description with the RICE component.

2. _____ Use elastic bandage (e.g., ACE Wrap) or splints to reduce swelling.

3. _____ Reduce activities for a period of time.

4. _____ Raise the injured extremity higher than the level of the heart to help reduce swelling.

5. _____ Apply a cold pack to the injured area for 15 to 20 minutes, 4 to 8 times daily.

a. rest
b. ice
c. compression
d. elevation

Fill in the blank.

6. _____ contractions do not change the muscle length, but they do increase the muscle tension and help maintain a person's strength.

7. _____ contractions cause muscles to shorten and thicken, and movement at a joint.

8. _____ exercises help restore movement after an injury and relieve stiffness and pain.

G. Assisting with Assistive Devices

1. _____ crutches are the most common type and are used when recovering from a foot, ankle, or leg injury or surgery.

2. With _____, the axillary nerves can be temporarily or permanently damaged from poorly fitted crutches or if the patient rests on the top of the crutches while walking.

3. Crutches should be _____ inches below the armpit, _____ inches to the side and front of each foot, and the elbows should be bent _____ degrees when on the handgrips.

4. _____ walkers are also called one-hand walkers.

5. When fitting a walker, the top of the walker grip should be near the _____ and even with the top of the hip line. With the shoulders relaxed and the hands on the grips, the elbows should be bent _____ degrees.

6. When fitting a cane, the top of the cane should be near the _____ and the elbow should be bent _____ degrees when the hand is on the top of the cane.

H. Complementary Therapies

1. With _____, pressure is applied to a person's skin and muscles, and it has been shown to reduce stress, pain, and muscle tension.

2. _____ focuses on the relationship between the spine and the function of the body.

3. _____ involves applying firm pressure on specific points on the body.

4. _____ involves inserting fine needles into specific points on the body.

CERTIFICATION PREPARATION

Circle the correct answer.

1. Which is used to measure a handgrip strength?
   a. Active ROM
   b. Passive ROM
   c. Goniometer
   d. Dynamometer

2. Which provides stability and protection, while allowing the joint to function?
   a. Splint
   b. Immobilizer
   c. Brace
   d. Sling

3. Which should be used to help support a casted arm?
   a. Splint
   b. Immobilizer
   c. Brace
   d. Sling

4. Which of the following are characteristics of fiberglass casts?
   a. Colorful and lightweight
   b. Durable and porous
   c. Can be penetrated by x-rays
   d. All of the above

5. _____ is a serious condition that involves increased pressure, usually in the muscles; it leads to compromised blood flow and muscle and nerve damage.
   a. Crepitation
   b. Compartment syndrome
   c. Stoma
   d. Strain

6. _____ is a dry, crackling sound or sensation.
   a. Crepitation
   b. Compartment syndrome
   c. Stoma
   d. Strain

7. A walker used by patients who can only grasp the walker with one hand.
   a. Hemi-walker
   b. Standard walker
   c. Two-wheel walker
   d. Knee walker

8. Which is *not* a dry cold application?
   a. Chemical cold pack
   b. Ice bag
   c. Cold compress
   d. Bead pack

9. Fit axillary crutches so they are _____ below the armpit.
   a. ½ to 1 inch
   b. 1 to 1 ½ inches
   c. Two fingerwidths
   d. b and c

10. When fitting a cane, what statement is correct?
    a. The cane should be held on the weak side.
    b. The top of the cane should be near the crease in the wrist.
    c. The elbow should be bent 30 degrees.
    d. All of the above

WORKPLACE APPLICATIONS

1. You need to teach a patient how to use the two-point crutch gait. Describe the sequence for this gait.

   _____

   _____

   _____

   _____

2. You need to teach a patient how to use the four-point crutch gait. Describe the sequence for this gait.

_____

_____

_____

_____

3. You need to teach a patient how to use the three-point crutch gait. Describe the sequence for this gait.

_____

_____

_____

4. You need to teach a patient how to sit down and stand up when using a walker. Describe both of these sequences.

_____

_____

_____

INTERNET ACTIVITIES

1. Using a .gov website, research safety tips when using a walker. Your research should also include stepping up or down from a step or curb. Create a poster, PowerPoint, or paper summarizing your research.

2. Using the National Center for Complementary and Integrative Health (https://www.nccih.nih.gov/), research the chiropractic profession, including the following points:
   - Services provided by chiropractic practitioners.
   - Describe the education and licensure of chiropractic practitioners.

   Create a poster, PowerPoint, or paper summarizing your research.

3. Using the National Center for Complementary and Integrative Health (https://www.nccih.nih.gov/), research massage therapy, including the following points:
   - Uses of massage therapy.
   - Requirements to become a massage therapist.

   Create a poster, PowerPoint, or paper summarizing your research.

Procedure 36.1 Apply Elastic Bandages

Name _____ Date _____ Score _____

Tasks: Apply elastic bandages to the forearm using the spiral technique and to the ankle using a figure-eight technique. Document the procedure.

Equipment and Supplies:
- Patient's health record
- Two 3-inch elastic bandages with clip or Velcro closures
- Provider's order

Provider's order: Apply an elastic bandage to the right arm and right ankle.

Standard: Complete the procedure and all critical steps in _____ minutes with a minimum score of 85% within two attempts (*or as indicated by the instructor*).

Scoring: Divide the points earned by the total possible points. Failure to perform a critical step, indicated by an asterisk (*), results in grade no higher than an 84% (*or as indicated by the instructor*).

Time: Began_____ Ended_____ Total minutes: _____

Steps	Possible Points	Attempt 1	Attempt 2
1. Wash hands or use hand sanitizer. Read the provider's order. Assemble the necessary supplies.	5		
2. Greet the patient. Identify yourself. Verify the patient's identity with full name and date of birth. Explain the procedure to be performed in a manner that is understood by the patient. Answer any questions the patient may have on the procedure.	10		
3. Hold the roll so the bandage can be rolled away from you. Using the patient's arm, perform an anchor or circular technique at the distal end.	10		
4. Keep the roll close to the patient and keep it facing upward. With each successive turn, overlap the previous bandage turn by 1/3. Maintain even tension and spacing as you continue to apply the bandage up the forearm. The bandage should be smooth. Finish with the circular technique and then secure the bandage with clips, tape, or Velcro.	15		
5. Hold the roll so the bandage can be rolled away from you. Using the patient's ankle, perform a circular or anchor technique at the starting point near the most distal part of the foot (near the toes). *Note:* The patient's ankle should be at a 90-degree angle. Make sure the end of the bandage is not on the bottom of the foot, which would cause discomfort.	15		
6. Keep the roll close to the patient and keep it facing upward. Slowly circle the bandage around the arch of the foot and then around the ankle. With each successive turn, overlap 2/3 of the previous bandage layer. Maintain even tension and spacing as you continue to apply the bandage on the foot and up the ankle. The bandage should be smooth.	15		
7. Continue until the joint is wrapped and complete the procedure with a circular technique before securing the bandage with clips, Velcro, or tape.	10		

8.	Check the nailbeds for cyanosis; ask the patient whether the bandages are comfortable or feel too tight. Check the pulse on the wrapped extremities, if possible. Have the patient move the fingers and toes on the wrapped extremities.	10		
9.	Document the procedure in the patient's health record. Include the name of the provider ordering the bandage, the procedure done, how the patient tolerated the procedure, and instructions given to the patient.	10		
	Total Score	100		

Documentation

Comments

CAAHEP Competencies	Step(s)
V.P.3.b. Coach patients regarding: medical encounters	2
X.P.3. Document patient care accurately in the medical record	9
ABHES Competencies	**Step(s)**
4. Medical Law and Ethics a. Follow documentation guidelines	9

Procedure 36.2 Apply a Sling

Name _____ Date _____ Score _____

Tasks: Apply a sling to a patient's arm. Document the procedure in the patient's health record.

Scenario: Dr. Kahn orders a commercial sling to be applied to a patient's left arm.

Equipment and Supplies:
- Adult-sized sling
- Provider's order
- Patient's health record

Standard: Complete the procedure and all critical steps in _____ minutes with a minimum score of 85% within two attempts (*or as indicated by the instructor*).

Scoring: Divide the points earned by the total possible points. Failure to perform a critical step, indicated by an asterisk (*), results in grade no higher than an 84% (*or as indicated by the instructor*).

Time: Began_____ Ended_____ Total minutes: _____

Steps	Possible Points	Attempt 1	Attempt 2
1. Wash hands or use hand sanitizer.	10		
2. Read the provider's order. Assemble the equipment. Make sure to have the correct-sized sling for the patient.	10		
3. Greet the patient. Identify yourself. Verify the patient's identity with full name and date of birth. Explain the procedure to be performed in a manner that the patient understands. Answer any questions the patient may have about the procedure.	10		
4. Gently place the arm and elbow in the sling. Support the arm on both sides of the injury. Make sure the sling fits comfortably around the elbow. The patient's hand should come to the end of the sling.	10		
5. Position the strap behind the elbow and pull the strap around the back of the neck. Make sure the strap does not rub against or cut into the skin on the neck. Secure the strap to the loops on the sling near the hand.	20		
6. Adjust the straps so the hand and forearm are elevated about the level of the elbow.	10		
7. Check the CMST of the fingers. Ask the patient if the fingers feel numb or asleep.	20		
8. Document the procedure in the patient's health record. Include the provider's name, the order, what was taught, and how the patient responded.	10		
Total Score	100		

Documentation

Comments

CAAHEP Competencies	Step(s)
V.P.3.b. Coach patients regarding: medical encounters	3
X.P.3. Document patient care accurately in the medical record	8
ABHES Competencies	**Step(s)**
4. Medical Law and Ethics a. Follow documentation guidelines	8

Procedure 36.3   Assist with the Application of a Cast

Name _____   Date _____   Score _____

Tasks: To assist the provider in applying a fiberglass cast. Document the procedure in the patient's health record.

Scenario: You are working with Dr. David Kahn, and he needs to apply a fiberglass cast on the left lower leg of Johnny Parker (DOB 06/15/20XX). You will assist the provider.

Equipment and Supplies:
- Patient's health record
- Rolls of fiberglass
- Basin for casting material
- Bandage
- Stockinette
- Gloves
- Sheet wadding and/or spongy padding
- Stand to support foot (lower extremity)
- Tape
- Scissors
- 2-3 towels
- Water
- Cast care instructions (optional)

Standard: Complete the procedure and all critical steps in _____ minutes with a minimum score of 85% within two attempts (*or as indicated by the instructor*).

Scoring: Divide the points earned by the total possible points. Failure to perform a critical step, indicated by an asterisk (*), results in grade no higher than an 84% (*or as indicated by the instructor*).

Time: Began_____ Ended_____ Total minutes: _____

Steps	Possible Points	Attempt 1	Attempt 2
1. Wash hands or use hand sanitizer. Assemble the necessary equipment.	5*		
2. Greet the patient. Identify yourself. Verify the patient's identity with full name and date of birth. Explain the procedure to be performed in a manner that the patient understands. Answer any questions the patient may have about the procedure.	10*		
3. Seat the patient comfortably, as directed by the provider. If the cast is being applied to the lower extremity, the toes must be supported by a stand.	5		
4. Clean the area that the cast will cover. Note any objective signs and ask about subjective symptoms (chart them at the end of the procedure).	10		
5. Cut the stockinette to fit the area the cast will cover. Apply the stockinette smoothly to the area the cast will cover. Leave 1 or 2 inches of excess stockinette above and below the cast area to finish the cast. Excess stockinette may be cut away where wrinkles form, such as at the front of the ankle.	5		

6.	Apply sheet wadding along the length of the cast using a spiral bandage turn. Extra padding may be used over bony prominences, such as the bones of the elbow or ankle.	**10**		
7.	Put on gloves. With lukewarm water in the basin, wet the fiberglass tape as directed by the provider.	**10**		
8.	Assist as directed as the provider applies the inner layer of fiberglass tape. A length of 1 to 2 inches of stockinette is rolled over the inner layer of the cast to form a smooth edge when the outer layer is applied.	**10**		
9.	As directed by the provider, help open and apply an outer layer of fiberglass tape.	**10**		
10.	Help shape the cast as directed. All contours must be smooth.	**5**		
11.	Discard the water and excess materials. Remove your gloves. Wash hands or use hand sanitizer.	**5***		
12.	Reassure the patient, review cast care verbally, and provide written instructions (optional).	**5***		
13.	Document the procedure in the patient's health record. Include the provider's name, the procedure, what was taught, and how the patient responded.	**10***		
	Total Score	**100**		

Documentation

Comments

CAAHEP Competencies	Step(s)
V.P.3.b. Coach patients regarding: medical encounters	2
X.P.3. Document patient care accurately in the medical record	13
ABHES Competencies	**Step(s)**
4. Medical Law and Ethics a. Follow documentation guidelines	13
8. Clinical Procedures h. Teach self-examination, disease management and health promotion	12

Procedure 36.4 Assist with Cast Removal

Name _____ Date _____ Score _____

Tasks: To remove a cast. Document the procedure in the patient's health record.

Scenario: You are working with Dr. David Kahn, and he orders removal of the lower left leg cast on Johnny Parker (DOB 06/15/20XX).

Equipment and Supplies:
- Patient's health record
- Cast cutter
- Cast spreader
- Large bandage scissors
- Basin of warm water
- Mild soap
- Towel
- Skin lotion

Standard: Complete the procedure and all critical steps in _____ minutes with a minimum score of 85% within two attempts (*or as indicated by the instructor*).

Scoring: Divide the points earned by the total possible points. Failure to perform a critical step, indicated by an asterisk (*), results in grade no higher than an 84% (*or as indicated by the instructor*).

Time: Began_____ Ended_____ Total minutes: _____

Steps	Possible Points	Attempt 1	Attempt 2
1. Wash hands or use hand sanitizer. Assemble the necessary equipment.	15*		
2. Greet the patient. Identify yourself. Verify the patient's identity with full name and date of birth. Explain the procedure to be performed in a manner that the patient understands. Answer any questions the patient may have about the procedure.	15*		
3. Provide adequate support for the limb throughout the procedure. Using the cast cutter, make a cut on the medial and lateral sides of the long axis of the cast.	15		
4. Use the cast spreader to pry apart the two halves. Carefully remove the two parts of the cast. Use the large bandage scissors to cut away the stockinette and padding remaining.	15		
5. Gently wash the area that was covered by the cast with mild soap and warm water. Dry the area and apply a gentle skin lotion.	10		
6. Give the patient appropriate instructions about exercising and using the limb, as directed by the provider.	15		
7. Clean up the area. Wash hands or use hand sanitizer.	5		
8. Document the procedure in the patient's health record. Include the provider's name, the procedure, what was taught, and how the patient responded.	10		
Total Score	**100**		

Documentation

Comments

CAAHEP Competencies	Step(s)
I.P.8. Instruct and prepare a patient for a procedure or a treatment	2
V.P.3.b. Coach patients regarding: medical encounters	6
X.P.3. Document patient care accurately in the medical record	8
ABHES Competencies	**Step(s)**
4. Medical Law and Ethics a. Follow documentation guidelines	8
8. Clinical Procedures h. Teach self-examination, disease management and health promotion	6

Procedure 36.5   Apply a Cold Pack

Name _____   Date _____   Score _____

Tasks: Apply a cold pack (chemical, gel, or bead) to a body area to reduce pain and prevent further swelling per treatment plan. Document the procedure in the patient's health record.

Scenario: You are working with Dr. David Kahn. Johnny Parker (DOB 06/15/20XX) arrives holding his arm and crying. Another medical assistant brings the patient and parent to the exam room. The medical assistant comes out and updates you on Johnny. His parent states that Johnny fell off his bike an hour ago and has since been complaining of pain in his right wrist. The providers in the department have a standing order to apply a cold pack to orthopedic injuries if the patient does not arrive with one in place. The medical assistant asks you to apply the cold pack as he completes the vital signs and medical history on Johnny.

Equipment and Supplies:
- Cold pack (chemical, gel, or bead)
- Towel or another type of protective covering for the cold pack
- Provider's order or standing order for orthopedic injuries
- Patient's health record

Standard: Complete the procedure and all critical steps in _____ minutes with a minimum score of 85% within two attempts (*or as indicated by the instructor*).

Scoring: Divide the points earned by the total possible points. Failure to perform a critical step, indicated by an asterisk (*), results in grade no higher than an 84% (*or as indicated by the instructor*).

Time: Began_____ Ended_____ Total minutes: _____

Steps	Possible Points	Attempt 1	Attempt 2
1. Wash hands or use hand sanitizer.	15*		
2. Read the standing order or the provider's order. Assemble the equipment. If using a chemical cold pack, activate the pack by squeezing it.	15		
3. Greet the patient. Identify yourself. Verify the patient's identity with full name and date of birth. Explain the procedure to be performed in a manner that the patient understands. Answer any questions the patient may have about the procedure.	15*		
4. Cover the cold pack with a towel or protective covering.	15		
5. Position the cold pack over the injured area.	10		
6. Coach the patient on the use of a cold pack. Advise the patient to leave the cold pack in place for 15 to 20 minutes or until the area feels numb, whichever comes first.	15		
7. Document the procedure in the patient's health record. Include the provider's name, the order, what was taught, and how the patient responded.	15*		
Total Score	**100**		

Documentation

| |
| |
| |
| |
| |
| |
| |
| |
| |

Comments

CAAHEP Competencies	Step(s)
I.P.8. Instruct and prepare a patient for a procedure or a treatment	3
V.P.3.b. Coach patients regarding: medical encounters	6
X.P.3. Document patient care accurately in the medical record	7
ABHES Competencies	**Step(s)**
4. Medical Law and Ethics a. Follow documentation guidelines	7
8. Clinical Procedures h. Teach self-examination, disease management and health promotion	6

Procedure 36.6   Apply a Hot Pack

Name _____ Date _____ Score _____

Tasks: Apply a hot pack (chemical, gel, or bead) to an infected wound. Document the procedure in the patient's health record.

Scenario: Dr. Kahn orders a hot pack to be applied to an infected wound for 15 minutes. He also orders coaching for the patient to continue the treatment at home four times a day for the next 3 days.

Equipment and Supplies:
- Hot pack (chemical, gel, or bead)
- Towel or another type of protective covering for the hot pack
- Provider's order
- Patient's health record

Standard: Complete the procedure and all critical steps in _____ minutes with a minimum score of 85% within two attempts (*or as indicated by the instructor*).

Scoring: Divide the points earned by the total possible points. Failure to perform a critical step, indicated by an asterisk (*), results in grade no higher than an 84% (*or as indicated by the instructor*).

Time: Began_____ Ended_____ Total minutes: _____

Steps	Possible Points	Attempt 1	Attempt 2
1. Wash hands or use hand sanitizer.	5		
2. Read the provider's order. Assemble the equipment. If using a chemical hot pack, activate the pack by squeezing it. If the pack needs to be warmed, follow the manufacturer's directions.	15		
3. Greet the patient. Identify yourself. Verify the patient's identity with full name and date of birth. Explain the procedure to be performed in a manner that the patient understands. Answer any questions the patient may have about the procedure.	15*		
4. Cover the hot pack with a towel or protective covering.	15		
5. Position the hot pack over the covered wound.	10		
6. Coach the patient on the use of a hot pack. Advise the patient to leave the hot pack in place for 15 to 20 minutes per the provider's order or until the area feels warm, whichever comes first.	20*		
7. Wash hands or use hand sanitizer.	5		
8. Document the procedure in the patient's health record. Include the provider's name, the order, what was taught, and how the patient responded.	15*		
Total Score	100		

Documentation

Comments

CAAHEP Competencies	Step(s)
I.P.8. Instruct and prepare a patient for a procedure or a treatment	3
V.P.3.b. Coach patients regarding: medical encounters	6
X.P.3. Document patient care accurately in the medical record	8
ABHES Competencies	**Step(s)**
4. Medical Law and Ethics a. Follow documentation guidelines	8
8. Clinical Procedures h. Teach self-examination, disease management and health promotion	6

Procedure 36.7   Coach a Patient in the Use of Axillary Crutches

Name _____ **Date** _____ **Score** _____

Tasks: Fit crutches to the patient. Coach the patient to use crutches. Document your teaching in the patient's health record.

Scenario: You are working with Dr. David Kahn. He has ordered you to teach Daniel Miller (DOB 3/21/20XX) how to use axillary crutches. Daniel broke his left leg, and his treatment plan requires that he not bear weight on the left leg for 6 weeks. Daniel's bedroom is on the second floor, so he has to learn how to use crutches on the stairs also.

Equipment and Supplies:
*   Axillary crutches
*   Handout on crutch walking (optional)
*   Provider's order
*   Patient's health record

Standard: Complete the procedure and all critical steps in _____ minutes with a minimum score of 85% within two attempts (*or as indicated by the instructor*).

Scoring: Divide the points earned by the total possible points. Failure to perform a critical step, indicated by an asterisk (*), results in grade no higher than an 84% (*or as indicated by the instructor*).

Time: Began_____ Ended_____ Total minutes: _____

Steps	Possible Points	Attempt 1	Attempt 2
1. Wash hands or use hand sanitizer.	10*		
2. Read the provider's order. Assemble the equipment.	5		
3. Greet the patient. Identify yourself. Verify the patient's identity with full name and date of birth. Explain the procedure to be performed in a manner that the patient understands. Answer any questions the patient may have about the procedure.	10*		
4. Ensure the patient is wearing shoes and ask the patient to stand up straight. Assist as needed. Fit the crutches to the patient so they are 1 to 1 1/2 inches (about 2 finger widths) below the armpit. The crutch should be about 4 to 6 inches to the side and front of each foot.	5		
5. Adjust the handgrips so they are near the patient's wrist and even with the top of the hip line. This should allow for a 15- to 30-degree bend in the elbow when the patient's hands are on the handgrip.	5		
6. Instruct the patient to keep the injured leg as relaxed as possible. The knee should be slightly bent, and the patient should look forward when walking. Instruct the patient not to bear weight on the axilla.	10		
7. Have the patient start in the tripod position and then move the crutches about 12 inches in front of their body (or less for a child).	5		
8. Have the patient put their weight on the crutches and move the body forward. Finish the step by having the patient swing the "good" or unaffected leg forward. Do not place weight on the "bad" or affected leg. Continue with these steps.	10		

9.	To sit down: Instruct the patient to do the following: Back up to the chair, toilet, or bed until the seat touches the back of the legs. Move the "bad" or affected leg forward, balancing on the "good" or unaffected leg. Hold both crutches on the side with the "bad" or affected leg. Use the free hand to grab the seat or armrest. Slowly sit down.	**5**		
10.	To stand up: Instruct the patient to do the following: Move toward the front of the seat and move the "bad" or affected leg forward. Hold both crutches on the side with the "bad" or affected leg. Use the free hand to push up from the seat to stand up. Balance on the "good" or unaffected leg while placing a crutch in each hand. Balance is needed before moving.	**5**		
11.	To go up the stairs: Instruct the patient to do the following: Step up with the "good" or unaffected leg first. Then bring the crutches up, one in each arm. Finally place weight on the "good" or unaffected leg and bring the "bad" or affected leg up.	**5**		
12.	To go down stairs: Instruct the patient to do the following: With a crutch in each hand, place the crutches on the first step. Then move the "bad" or affected leg forward and down. Lastly, follow with the "good" or unaffected leg.	**5**		
13.	Instruct the patient and family on ways to prevent falls. Wash hands or use hand sanitizer.	**10***		
14.	Document the patient education in the patient's health record. Include the provider's name, the order, what was taught, how the patient responded, how the patient did the demonstration, and any handouts provided.	**10***		
	Total Score	**100**		

Documentation

Comments

CAAHEP Competencies	Step(s)
I.P.8. Instruct and prepare a patient for a procedure or a treatment	3
V.P.3.b. Coach patients regarding: medical encounters	7-13
X.P.3. Document patient care accurately in the medical record	14
ABHES Competencies	**Step(s)**
4. Medical Law and Ethics a. Follow documentation guidelines	14
8. Clinical Procedures h. Teach self-examination, disease management and health promotion	7-13

Procedure 36.8   Coach a Patient in the Use of a Walker

Name _____ **Date** _____ **Score** _____

Tasks: Fit a standard walker to a patient. Coach the patient to use a standard walker. Document teaching in the patient's health record.

Scenario: You are working with Dr. David Kahn. He has ordered you to teach Jana Green (DOB 5/1/19XX) how to use a standard walker. Jana needs the walker for extra stability.

Equipment and Supplies:
- Standard walker
- Walker handout (optional)
- Provider's order
- Patient's health record

Standard: Complete the procedure and all critical steps in _____ minutes with a minimum score of 85% within two attempts (*or as indicated by the instructor*).

Scoring: Divide the points earned by the total possible points. Failure to perform a critical step, indicated by an asterisk (*), results in grade no higher than an 84% (*or as indicated by the instructor*).

Time: Began_____ Ended_____ Total minutes: _____

Steps	Possible Points	Attempt 1	Attempt 2
1. Wash hands or use hand sanitizer.	10*		
2. Read the provider's order. Assemble the equipment.	10		
3. Greet the patient. Identify yourself. Verify the patient's identity with full name and date of birth. Explain the procedure to be performed in a manner that the patient understands. Answer any questions the patient may have about the procedure.	10*		
4. Ensure the patient is wearing shoes and ask the patient to step into the walker. The top of the walker grip should be even with the top of the hip line and near the crease in the wrist when the arms are at the side of the body. Adjust as needed. Keeping the shoulders relaxed and the hands on the grips will ensure the elbows are bent at a 15-degree angle.	15		
5. Have the patient place the walker one step ahead of their body. Instruct the patient to use the "bad" or affected leg to step into the walker. The patient should not touch the front bar with the leg. Have the patient step forward with the other leg to complete the step. The patient will continue with this pattern while holding up the head and looking forward.	15		
6. To sit down: Instruct the patient to back up to the chair, toilet, or bed until the seat touches the back of the legs. The patient can then use one hand to grab the seat or armrest and slowly sit down.	10		
7. To stand up: Instruct the patient to move toward the front of the seat. Have the walker in front of the person. Have the patient use one hand to push up from the seat to stand up and then place hands on the walker. Remind patients to make sure they have their balance before moving.	10		

8.	Instruct the patient on ways to prevent falls. The walker should never be used on stairs or an escalator. If the patient will be using a bag on the front of the walker, instruct them to make sure not to overload it. Make sure to place all four legs of the walker on the ground before moving into the walker. Wash hands or use hand sanitizer.	**10***		
9.	Document the patient education in the patient's health record. Include the provider's name, the order, what was taught, how the patient responded, how the patient did the demonstration, and any handouts provided.	**10***		
	Total Score	**100**		

Documentation

Comments

CAAHEP Competencies	Step(s)
I.P.8. Instruct and prepare a patient for a procedure or a treatment	3
V.P.3.b. Coach patients regarding: medical encounters	3-8
X.P.3. Document patient care accurately in the medical record	9
ABHES Competencies	**Step(s)**
4. Medical Law and Ethics a. Follow documentation guidelines	9
8. Clinical Procedures h. Teach self-examination, disease management and health promotion	3-8

Procedure 36.9   Coach a Patient in the Use of a Cane

Name _____ Date _____ Score _____

Tasks: Fit a cane to a patient. Coach the patient to use a cane. Document teaching in the patient's health record.

Scenario: You are working with Dr. David Kahn. He has ordered you to teach Ella Rainwater (DOB 7/11/19XX) how to use a cane. Ella has left-side weakness.

Equipment and Supplies:
- Cane
- Handout on cane walking (optional)
- Provider's order
- Patient's health record

Standard: Complete the procedure and all critical steps in _____ minutes with a minimum score of 85% within two attempts (*or as indicated by the instructor*).

Scoring: Divide the points earned by the total possible points. Failure to perform a critical step, indicated by an asterisk (*), results in grade no higher than an 84% (*or as indicated by the instructor*).

Time: Began_____ Ended_____ Total minutes: _____

Steps	Possible Points	Attempt 1	Attempt 2
1. Wash hands or use hand sanitizer.	15*		
2. Read the provider's order. Assemble the equipment.	10		
3. Greet the patient. Identify yourself. Verify the patient's identity with full name and date of birth. Explain the procedure to be performed in a manner that the patient understands. Answer any questions the patient may have about the procedure.	10*		
4. Ensure the patient is wearing shoes. The top of the cane should be near the crease in the wrist when the arms are at the side of the body. Adjust as needed. With the patient's shoulders relaxed and hand on the cane, ensure the elbows are bent at a 15-degree angle.	10		
5. Instruct the patient to hold the cane on the "good" or unaffected side. The patient should take a step moving the "bad" or affected leg and the cane forward at the same time and then step forward with the "good" leg. Instruct the patient to lean on the cane as needed.	10		
6. To sit down: Instruct the patient to back up to the chair, toilet, or bed until the seat touches the back of the legs. The patient can then use a hand to grab the seat or armrest and slowly sit down.	5		
7. To stand up: Instruct the patient to move toward the front of the seat and move the "bad" or affected leg forward. The patient can then use a hand to push up from the seat to stand up. Remind patients to make sure to get their balance before moving.	5		

8. To go up the stairs: Instruct the patient to step up with the "good" or unaffected leg first while holding onto the rail. Then the patient should bring up the "bad" or affected leg to the same step. If there is no handrail, the cane and the "bad" leg should be placed on the stair at the same time.	5		
9. To go down stairs: Instruct the patient to hold onto the rail and move the "bad" or affected leg down first. Then the patient should place the "good" or unaffected leg on the same step as the "bad" leg. When there is no handrail, instruct the patient to place the cane on the lower step, then place the "bad" or affected leg, and lastly place the "good" or unaffected leg next to the "bad" or affected leg.	5		
10. Instruct the patient on ways to prevent falls. Wash hands or use hand sanitizer.	10*		
11. Document the patient education in the patient's health record. Include the provider's name, the order, what was taught, how the patient responded, how the patient did the demonstration, and any handouts provided.	15*		
Total Score	100		

Documentation

Comments

CAAHEP Competencies	**Step(s)**
I.P.8. Instruct and prepare a patient for a procedure or a treatment	3
V.P.3.b. Coach patients regarding: medical encounters	5-9
X.P.3. Document patient care accurately in the medical record	11
ABHES Competencies	**Step(s)**
4. Medical Law and Ethics a. Follow documentation guidelines	11
8. Clinical Procedures h. Teach self-examination, disease management and health promotion	5-9
8.j. Make adaptations for patients with special needs (psychological or physical limitations)	4, 5

Neurology

CAAHEP Competencies	Assessment
I.C.4. Identify major organs in each body system	Skills and Concepts – A. 4-8, B. 11-27; Certification Preparation – 1
I.C.5. Identify the anatomical location of major organs in each body system	Skills and Concepts – B. 11-28; Certification Preparation – 6
I.C.6. Identify structure and function of the human body across the life span	Skills and Concepts – E. 15-16
I.C.7. Identify the normal function of each body system	Skills and Concepts – B. 11-21, 23-27, E. 1-14; Certification Preparation – 1, 5
I.C.8.a. Identify common pathology related to each body system including: signs	Skills and Concepts – F. 1-5, 16-20, H. 7-9, J. 6, K. 3, 6, 8, L. 4; Certification Preparation – 7; Workplace Application – 2-3; Internet Activities – 2
I.C.8.b. Identify common pathology related to each body system including: symptoms	Skills and Concepts – F. 1-5, 16-20, H. 7-9, J. 6, K. 3, 6, 8, L.4; Certification Preparation – 7; Workplace Application – 2-3; Internet Activities – 2
I.C.8.c. Identify common pathology related to each body system including: etiology	Skills and Concepts – F. 11-15, G. 1, H. 4-6, J. 1, 5; Internet Activities – 2
I.C.8.d. Identify common pathology related to each body system including: diagnostic measures	Skills and Concepts – F. 21-25, H. 10-12, M. 2-4; Internet Activities – 1-3
I.C.8.e. Identify common pathology related to each body system including: treatment modalities	Skills and Concepts – F. 21-25, H. 10-12, M. 5-21; Internet Activities – 2-4
I.C.10.a. Identify the classifications of medications, including indications for use	Skills and Concepts – M. 10-15
I.C.10.b. Identify the classifications of medications, including desired effects	Skills and Concepts – M. 10-15
I.C.10.c. Identify the classifications of medications, including side effects	Skills and Concepts – M. 16-21
I.C.10.d. Identify the classifications of medications, including adverse reactions	Skills and Concepts – M. 16-21
V.C.8.a. Identify the following related to body systems: medical terms	Skills and Concepts – A. 1-3, H. 1-2, M. 5-9
V.C.8.b. Identify the following related to body systems: abbreviations	Abbreviations – 1-23

CAAHEP Competencies	Assessment
I.P.8. Instruct and prepare a patient for a procedure or a treatment	Procedures 37.3, 37.4
I.P.9 Assist provider with a patient exam	Procedures 37.1, 37.2
X.P.3. Document patient care accurately in the medical record	Procedures 37.1. 37.3, 37.4

ABHES Competencies	Assessment
2. Anatomy and Physiology a. List all body systems and their structures and functions	Skills and Concepts – A. 4-8, B. 11-28, E. 1-14; Certification Preparation – 1, 5, 6
2.b. Describe common diseases, symptoms, and etiologies as they apply to each system	Skills and Concepts – F. 1-20, G. 1-11, H. 1-9, I. 1-4, J. 1-6, J. 1-4, K. 1-12, L. 1-6; Certification Preparation – 7, 10; Workplace Application – 1-3; Internet Activities – 2
2.c. Identify diagnostic and treatment modalities as they relate to each body system	Skills and Concepts – F. 21-25, H. 10-12; Internet Activities – 1-4
3. Medical Terminology c. Apply medical terminology for each specialty	Skills and Concepts – A. 1-3, H. 1-2, M. 5-9
3.d. Define and use medical abbreviations when appropriate and acceptable	Abbreviations – 1-23
4. Medical Law and Ethics a. Follow documentation guidelines	Procedures 37.1. 37.3, 37.4
8. Clinical Procedures	Procedures 37.2, 37.3
e. Perform specialty procedures, including but not limited to minor surgery, cardiac, respiratory, OB-GYN, neurological, and gastroenterology	

VOCABULARY REVIEW

Using the word pool on the right, find the correct word to match the definition. Write the word on the line after the definition.

Group A

1. Consists of several structures including the amygdala, hippocampus, and hypothalamus; plays an important role with behavior, memories, and emotions _____

2. Nerve tissue that lacks the insulation that causes a white appearance to other nerves; looks gray _____

3. Grooves or depressions on the surface of the brain between the gyri _____

4. A ridge in the floor of the lateral ventricle; composed of gray matter; involved with the limbic system and with creating and filing new memories _____

5. Folds or convolutions on the surface of the cerebral hemisphere, which increase the gray matter surface area
_____

Word Pool
- amygdala
- aphasia
- fissure
- gray matter
- gyri
- hippocampus
- limbic system
- pineal gland
- sulci
- tract

6. A system of tissues and/or organs that function together
   _____

7. Partial or complete loss of the ability to articulate ideas or understand written or spoken language _____

8. A small organ in the brain that secretes melatonin, a hormone that regulates the sleep/wake cycle _____

9. A groove that divides an organ into lobes or parts
   _____

10. A small mass of gray matter found in each temporal lobe of the cerebrum that is involved with memories, emotions, and activating the fight-or-flight response; part of the limbic system
    _____

Group B

1. Pertaining to carrying away from a structure
   _____

2. A protective insulation that covers the axons and helps with the transmission of nerve impulses _____

3. Detectable cellular indicators used as a marker for a substance or disease process _____

4. The internal environment of the body that is compatible with life; a steady state that is created by all the body systems working together to provide a consistent and unvarying internal environment _____

5. A chemical that helps a nerve cell communicate with another nerve cell or muscle _____

6. An immune response against a person's own tissues, cells, or cell parts, leading to the deterioration of tissue
   _____

7. A long extension of a nerve fiber that conducts the impulse away from the nerve cell body _____

8. Pertaining to carrying toward a structure
   _____

9. The destination or intended tissue in the nervous impulse (e.g., a muscle) _____

10. A large opening in the base of the skull; forms a passageway for the spinal cord _____

Word Pool
- afferent
- autoimmune
- axons
- biomarkers
- efferent
- foramen magnum
- homeostasis
- myelin sheath
- neurotransmitters
- target tissue

Group C

1. A type of traumatic brain injury resulting from a hit to the head or body that causes the brain to move rapidly back and forth
_____

2. Condition resulting from internal head injuries that occur when a baby or young child is violently shaken _____

3. An abnormal accumulation of cerebrospinal fluid that causes enlargement of the skull and compression of the brain
_____

4. A scale used to measure the level of consciousness and severity of a head injury _____

5. An abnormal blood-filled sac formed from a localized dilation of the wall of a vein, artery, or heart _____

6. Sharp, spasm-like pain in a nerve or along the course of one or more nerves _____

7. A nerve response test that uses electrodes placed on the scalp to measure brain reaction to a stimulus _____

8. A soft membranous gap between the incompletely formed cranial bones of an infant; also called a _soft spot_ _____

9. A drug that reduces or eliminates pain _____

Word Pool
- evoked potential test
- analgesics
- shaken baby syndrome
- fontanel
- concussion
- Glasgow coma scale
- neuralgia
- hydrocephalus
- aneurysm

ABBREVIATIONS

Write out what each of the following abbreviations stands for.

1. CNS _____

2. PNS _____

3. ANS _____

4. CSF _____

5. BBB _____

6. ALS _____

7. AD _____

8. PET _____

9. HD _____

10. MS _____

11. PD _____

12. DHE _____

13. SPECT _____

14. TBI _____

15. NCV _____

16. EMG _____

17. CVA_____

18. TIA _____

19. LP _____

20. EEG_____

21. SBS_____

22. ICP_____

23. DBS _____

SKILLS AND CONCEPTS

Answer the following questions.

A. Introduction

Match the description with the term.

1. _____ A specialist involved in the diagnosis, treatment, and prevention of nervous system diseases and disorders

2. _____ The healthcare specialty that deals with the diseases and disorders of the nervous system

3. _____ A surgeon who operates on the nervous system as treatment for a neurologic disorder

a. neurology
b. neurologist
c. neurosurgeon

Fill in the blank or select the correct answer.

4. Which structure(s) is part of the nervous system?
    a. Brain
    b. Spinal cord
    c. Nerves
    d. Neurons
    e. All of the above

5. The _____ is composed of the brain and the spinal cord.

6. The _____ is made up of the cranial nerves and spinal nerves.

7. The _____ is voluntary and collects information from and returns instructions to the skin, voluntary muscles, and joints.

8. The _____ is involuntary and collects information from and returns instructions to involuntary structures.

B. Central Nervous System

Match the description to the correct term.

1. _____ A bundle of nerve tissue that facilitates communication between the hemispheres

2. _____ Nerve tissue that lacks the insulation that causes the white appearance of other nerves

3. _____ Covers the surface of the hemispheres; also called *gray matter*

4. _____ The largest portion of the brain; divided into two hemispheres

5. _____ Folds or convolutions on the surface of the cerebral hemisphere

6. _____ A groove that divides an organ into lobes or parts

7. _____ Make up the cerebral hemispheres

8. _____ A small mass of gray matter found in each temporal lobe of the cerebrum and involved with memories, emotions, and activating the fight-or-flight response

9. _____ Consists of several structures including the amygdala, hippocampus, and hypothalamus

10. _____ Grooves or depressions on the surface of the brain between the gyri

a. fissure
b. cerebrum
c. corpus callosum
d. gray matter
e. amygdala
f. cerebral cortex
g. limbic system
h. lobes
i. gyri
j. sulci

Match the description with the correct part of the brain.

11. _____ Involved with reading and interpreting visual, auditory, motor, sensory, and memory signals, along with spatial and visual perceptions

12. _____ Found at the back of the brain and handle images from the eyes and connect the information with stored image memories

13. _____ Lie directly behind the forehead and are responsible for personality, intelligence, concentration, self-awareness, problem solving, short-term memory, planning, and judgment

14. _____ Found in the left temporal lobe and is important for language comprehension and speech

15. _____ Found near the motor area of the frontal lobe and receive information from the body regarding touch, pain, and temperature

16. _____ Found in the left frontal lobe and is involved with speech

17. _____ Found in the back of the frontal lobe and controls the voluntary movements on the opposite side of the body

18. _____ A small mass of gray matter found in each temporal lobe of the cerebrum and involved with memories, emotions, and activating the fight-or-flight response

19. _____ Part of the brainstem; connects the hemispheres of the cerebrum with the pons and contains centers to regulate pupillary reflexes and eye movements

20. _____ Found in front of the occipital lobes and processes memories and sensations of taste, touch, sight, and sounds

21. _____ Located below the occipital lobe of the cerebrum and coordinates the equilibrium, or balance, posture, and muscle coordination

a. frontal lobes
b. parietal lobes
c. occipital lobes
d. temporal lobes
e. motor area
f. Broca area
g. sensory areas
h. Wernicke area
i. amygdala
j. thalamus
k. diencephalon
l. cerebellum
m. hypothalamus
n. pineal gland
o. midbrain
p. pons
q. medulla oblongata

22. _____ Is located just above the brainstem and is almost surrounded by the cerebral hemispheres

23. _____ Part of the diencephalon, which processes information going to and from the body and the cerebrum

24. _____ Part of the diencephalon, which controls body temperature, hunger, and thirst

25. _____ A small organ in the brain that secretes melatonin

26. _____ Lowest part of the brainstem; contains vital centers of life

27. _____ Part of the brainstem; serves as a bridge between the medulla oblongata and the cerebrum and helps to regulate respirations

Fill in the blank.

28. The spinal cord passes through the _____ in the skull and is protected by the vertebrae.

29. The spinal cord and brain are covered by _____.

30. The spinal cord is composed of the cell bodies of motor neurons and the myelin-covered _____.

31. There are _____ pairs of spinal nerves that extend from the spinal cord.

Match the description with the correct structure or term.

32. _____ A network of capillaries found in the lateral ventricles and the third and fourth ventricles that secrete cerebrospinal fluid

33. _____ The space below the arachnoid, which is filled with cerebrospinal fluid and blood vessels

34. _____ The space below the dura mater, which contains tiny blood vessels

35. _____ Innermost layer of meninges

36. _____ Middle layer of meninges

37. _____ Outer layer of meninges

a. pia mater
b. dura mater
c. arachnoid matter
d. subarachnoid space
e. subdural space
f. choroid plexus

C. Peripheral Nervous System
Fill in the blank or select the correct answer.

1. The peripheral nerves exiting the brain directly through the skull are called _____.

2. The _____ nerves exit the spinal canal through spaces between the vertebrae.

3. A(n) _____ is created when nerve fibers from several spinal nerves form a network.

4. Spinal nerves
    a. are named by their vertebrae location.
    b. are named by number.
    c. carry information to and from the brain through the spinal cord.
    d. all of the above.

5. _____ are skin surface areas supplied by a single afferent spinal nerve.

D. Cells of the Nervous System
Fill in the blank or select the correct answer.

1. Neurons are
    a. called *parenchymal cells.*
    b. composed of a cell body, dendrites, and an axon.
    c. all of the above.

2. A neuroglia is called a *stromal cell* or _____.

3. Which statement is *incorrect* regarding neuroglial cells?
    a. Schwann cells form the myelin sheath that covers the axons of peripheral nerves.
    b. Microglia help form the blood-brain barrier.
    c. Oligodendrocytes are found in the central nervous system (CNS).
    d. Microglia engulf and destroy microorganisms or debris.

E. Physiology of the Nervous System
Fill in the blank or select the correct answer.

1. The nervous system works in partnership with the _____ system to help the body respond to its internal and external environments.

2. Which of the following is a main function of the nervous system?
    a. Collecting information about the external and internal environments
    b. Processing this information and making decisions about action
    c. Directing the body to put into action the decisions made
    d. All of the above

3. The basic flow of information in the nervous system includes:

    a. _____ or sensory neurons, which collect stimuli received from receptors.

    b. The brain and spinal cord process the information and direct the necessary response. The central nervous system contains _____, nerve cells, that connect sensory and motor neurons.

    c. The response from the CNS is sent via the _____ or motor neurons.

4. The _____ nervous system is the part of the peripheral nervous system that sends motor impulses to the skeletal muscles.

5. A(n) _____ is an involuntary, almost instantaneous movement in response to a specific stimulus.

6. A(n) _____ arc consists of sensory neurons, interneurons, and motor neurons.

7. The patellar reflex is an example of a(n) _____ arc.

8. The _____ nervous system consists of nerves that conduct impulses from the brainstem or spinal cord to cardiac and smooth muscle tissue and glands.

9. The autonomic nervous system
   a. controls the muscles in the blood vessel walls, organs, and glands.
   b. regulates breathing, the heart rate, sweating, circulation, and digestion.
   c. controls skeletal muscles.
   d. all of the above.
   e. both a and b.

10. The _____ nervous system can produce a "fight-or-flight" response.

11. Which of the following is caused by the "fight-or-flight" response?
    a. Increased heart rate and blood pressure
    b. Increased digestive system processes
    c. Decreased blood glucose levels
    d. All of the above

12. Which of the following is caused by the parasympathetic nervous system response?
    a. Slows the heart rate
    b. Lowers the blood pressure
    c. Decreases the digestive functions
    d. Reduces adrenal and sweat gland activity
    e. All of the above

13. A(n) _____ is a self-propagating wave of electrical impulse that travels along the surface of a neuron membrane.

14. Which of the following are neurotransmitters?
    a. Epinephrine and norepinephrine
    b. Dopamine and enkephalins
    c. Serotonins and endorphins
    d. All of the above

15. Which change occurs as a child grows?
    a. The process of myelination occurs, increasing the child's brain size.
    b. With age, learning and thinking processes become more complex.
    c. All of the above

16. Which change occurs with age?
    a. Nerve cells are lost from the brain and spinal cord.
    b. Plaques and neurofibrillary tangles form in the brain.
    c. Nerve impulses become slower, thus increasing the reaction time.
    d. All of the above.
    e. Only b and c.

F. Neurodegenerative Diseases and Disorders

Match the description with the correct sign or symptom.

1. _____ Involuntary muscle contractions

2. _____ Rhythmic, purposeless muscle movements

3. _____ Sharp, spasm-like pain in a nerve or along the course of one or more nerves

4. _____ Memory loss

5. _____ Feelings of prickling, burning, or numbness

a. neuralgia
b. paresthesia
c. spasms
d. tremors
e. amnesia

Match the description with the correct disease.

6. _____ A progressive neurodegenerative disorder that affects movement and the dopamine-producing neurons in the brain gradually die

7. _____ A progressive neurodegenerative disorder, also known as *Huntington chorea*

8. _____ A degenerative disease of the brain; characterized by disorientation, memory failure, speech disturbance, and a loss of mental capacity, and is the most common cause of dementia

9. _____ An autoimmune neurodegenerative disorder that causes the myelin sheath to be damaged, affecting the brain and spinal cord

10. _____ Also called *Lou Gehrig disease*; a progressive neurologic disorder that attacks the motor neurons in the brain and spinal cord

a. amyotrophic lateral sclerosis
b. Alzheimer's disease
c. Huntington disease
d. multiple sclerosis
e. Parkinson disease

Match the etiology with the correct disease.

11. _____ Unknown cause; the immune system destroys the myelin sheath

12. _____ Caused by an inherited genetic defect

13. _____ No known cause but in about 10% of the cases, a there is a genetic component

14. _____ Caused by a combination of lifestyle, genetics, and environmental factors that affect the brain

15. _____ Unknown cause, but genetics and environmental triggers can increase the risk of the disease

a. amyotrophic lateral sclerosis
b. Alzheimer's disease
c. Huntington disease
d. multiple sclerosis
e. Parkinson disease

Match the signs and symptoms with the correct disease.

16. _____ Starts slowly with difficulty remembering recent activities or the names of people the person knows; affects thinking, reasoning, making judgments and decisions, memory, performing familiar tasks, personality, and behavior

17. _____ Tremors, pill-rolling tremors, bradykinesia, shuffling gait, loss of automatic movement, speech changes, and drooling

18. _____ The muscle weakness starts in the hands and feet and spreads throughout the body, leading to an inability to move the legs and arms and difficulty with eating, speaking, and breathing

19. _____ Behavioral disturbances, hallucinations, psychosis, paranoia, facial grimacing, jerky movements, slow and uncontrolled movements, and dementia

20. _____ Tingling, numbness, or weakness in the extremities, partial or complete loss of vision, double vision, slurred speech, fatigue, and lack of coordination

a. amyotrophic lateral sclerosis
b. Alzheimer's disease
c. Huntington disease
d. multiple sclerosis
e. Parkinson disease

Match the diagnostic measures and treatments with the correct disease.

21. _____ An examination will show abnormalities and tests are ordered to rule out other conditions; Riluzole, physical therapy, assistive devices, and a feeding tube can be used for treatments.

22. _____ Evaluation of the mental and language functions along with movement and coordination, imaging tests, cerebrospinal fluid analysis, and an evoked potential test; treatment is focused on slowing the progression of the disease and corticosteroids can be given.

23. _____ No specific tests; medications such as Sinemet and Mirapex are used to treat the condition.

24. _____ Neurologic tests, CT, MRI, positron emission tomography, psychiatric evaluation, and cognitive and neuropsychological tests; treatment is focused on keeping symptoms from getting worse and medications such as cholinesterase inhibitors and memantine can be used.

25. _____ Psychological testing, head CT or MRI, and a PET scan of the brain; the goal of treatment is to slow symptoms and dopamine blockers can be used.

a. amyotrophic lateral sclerosis
b. Alzheimer's disease
c. Huntington disease
d. multiple sclerosis
e. Parkinson disease

G. Functional Diseases and Disorders of the Nervous System
Select the correct answer.

1. Which of the following is the cause of migraines?
    a. Stress and anxiety
    b. Hormone changes
    c. Strong smells
    d. Bright lights
    e. All of the above

Match the description with the condition.

2. _____ A sudden increase of electrical activity in one or more parts of the brain; also called a *convulsion*

3. _____ A disorder that causes recurring seizures

4. _____ A seizure that affects both sides of the brain

5. _____ A seizure with its effect on the brain unknown

6. _____ A seizure that affects one area of the brain

7. _____ An emergency condition; occurs when a seizure lasts longer than 10 minutes or if the person has three or more seizures without regaining consciousness between them

8. _____ The sciatic nerve becomes compressed by a herniated disk, spinal stenosis, or a bone spur on the vertebrae

9. _____ A neurologic disorder that causes tics

10. _____ A neurologic disorder with an unknown cause that affects the transmission of signals from the nervous system and the body, causing motor dysfunction and sensory dysfunction

11. _____ A chronic neurologic disorder that affects the brain's ability to control the sleep-wake cycle, thus causing extreme daytime sleepiness

a. seizures
b. general onset seizure
c. focal onset seizure
d. unknown onset seizure
e. status epilepticus
f. epilepsy
g. narcolepsy
h. sciatica
i. Tourette syndrome
j. functional neurologic disorder

H. Infections

Match the description with the condition.

1. _____ Inflammation of the meninges surrounding the brain and spinal cord

2. _____ Inflammation of the brain

3. _____ Another name for shingles

a. encephalitis
b. meningitis
c. herpes zoster

Match the etiology with the correct disease.

4. _____ Caused by a viral, bacterial, or fungal infection

5. _____ Caused by a viral or bacterial infection and certain types can be spread by mosquitoes

6. _____ Caused by the varicella zoster virus

a. encephalitis
b. meningitis
c. herpes zoster

Match the signs and symptoms with the correct disease.

7. _____ Flulike symptoms, severe headache, drowsiness, vomiting, confusion, seizures, and a sudden fever

8. _____ Tingling, pain, or itchiness on one side of the body or face, and a rash with fluid-filled blisters develops

9. _____ A sudden high fever, severe headache, stiff neck, nausea, vomiting, hearing loss, brain damage, and stroke

a. encephalitis
b. meningitis
c. herpes zoster

Match the diagnostic measures and treatments with the correct disease.

10. _____ History and physical examination; treated with antiviral medications and analgesics

11. _____ Blood test, imaging tests, and a cerebrospinal fluid analysis; treatment includes medications such as antibiotics, corticosteroids, and antifungals, bedrest, and fluids

12. _____ Cerebrospinal fluid analysis, blood tests, and CT; treated with IV or oral medications and physical, speech, and occupational therapies

    a. encephalitis
    b. meningitis
    c. herpes zoster

I. Structural Diseases and Disorders
Match the description with the condition.

1. _____ A rare autoimmune disorder in which the immune system attacks the peripheral nervous system causing weakness that spreads through the body, making the person almost paralyzed

2. _____ A chronic pain condition that affects the trigeminal nerve; also called *tic douloureux*

3. _____ Most common cause of facial paralysis that affects one side of the face

4. _____ A common malignant tumor that begins in the meninges; the risk increases with age

    a. Bell's palsy
    b. Guillain-Barré syndrome
    c. trigeminal neuralgia
    d. meningioma

J. Injuries
Select the correct answer or fill In the blank.

1. Traumatic brain injuries (TBI) can result from
    a. falls.
    b. motor vehicle accidents.
    c. violence and service in military combat zones.
    d. sports injuries.
    e. all of the above.

2. A(n) _____ is a mild form of a TBI and is the most common type of sports injury.

3. A(n) _____ is bruising or swelling of the brain that occurs when small cerebral blood vessels bleed into brain tissue.

4. _____ is the leading cause of child abuse deaths.

5. The cause of peripheral neuropathy is
    a. physical injuries.
    b. diseases such as diabetes mellitus and lupus.
    c. exposure to toxins.
    d. all of the above.

6. Signs and symptoms of peripheral neuropathy include
    a. tingling, numbness, and paresthesia.
    b. weakness, increased sensitivity to stimuli, and burning pain.
    c. muscle wasting, paralysis, and organ dysfunction.
    d. all of the above.

K. Congenital Diseases and Disorders

Fill in the blank or select the correct answer.

1. _____ are a group of conditions that occur to a person whose mother drank alcohol during pregnancy and the deficiencies will last for life.

2. The alcohol in the mother's bloodstream crosses the _____ and can interfere with _____ and nutrient delivery in the growing baby, causing harm with the development of tissues and organs.

3. Which are common signs and symptoms of fetal alcohol spectrum disorder?
   a. Poor memory, hyperactive behavior, and difficulty with attention and math concepts
   b. Speech and language delays
   c. Poor reasoning and judgment skills
   d. Vision or hearing problems
   e. All of the above

Match the description with the condition.

4. _____ Includes a malformation of the fat, bone, or meninges associated with the spinal cord

5. _____ The most serious type because the spinal canal is open along several vertebrae and the sac contains fluid, part of the spinal cord, and nerves

6. _____ Mildest form; one or more vertebrae are malformed, and the only indication is an abnormal cluster of hair, a small dimple, or birthmark on the infant's back

7. _____ The meninges protrude through an abnormal vertebral opening, creating a sac and the sac is filled with fluid

8. _____ A group of nonprogressive disorders caused by abnormal brain development or brain injury, resulting in muscle weakness or problems with using the muscles

9. _____ A rare genetic disease that causes benign tumors to grow in major organs

10. _____ A person is born with an extra copy of chromosome 21 and the complications can include intellectual disabilities, dementia, heart disease, hearing and visual issues, thyroid disease, and musculoskeletal complications

11. _____ The infant is born without parts of the brain and the remaining part of the brain may not be covered by the cranium or skin

12. _____ A small head size compared to the rest of the body

a. spina bifida occulta
b. closed neural tube defect
c. meningocele
d. myelomeningocele
e. microcephaly
f. tuberous sclerosis
g. Down syndrome
h. cerebral palsy
i. anencephaly

L. Vascular Diseases and Disorders

Fill in the blank or select the correct answer.

1. A(n) _____ stroke, the most common type of stroke, occurs when the arterial blood flow to part of the brain is blocked.

2. A(n) _____ stroke occurs when an artery in the brain leaks or ruptures.

3. A(n) _____ is also called a "ministroke" and lasts for only a few minutes.

4. Which of the following are signs and symptoms of a stroke?
   a. Confusion, mental changes, and speech difficulties
   b. Facial drooping and numbness of the face, arm, or leg
   c. Problem seeing in one or both eyes
   d. Trouble walking, lack of coordination
   e. All of the above

5. A collection of blood between the skull and the dura mater is a(n) _____.

6. A collection of blood between the dura mater and the arachnoid mater that causes pressure on the brain is a(n) _____.

M. The Medical Assistant's Role with Examinations, Diagnostic Procedures, and Treatments
Select the correct answer.

1. Which of the following is a part of the neurologic examination?
   a. Mental status
   b. Functioning of the cranial nerves
   c. Motor function, balance, and coordination
   d. Sensory functions and reflexes
   e. All of the above

Match the description with the correct diagnostic test.

2. _____ The removal of a small piece of the nerve for examination

3. _____ Used to see how the blood flows through the brain

4. _____ Used to test the health of nerves and muscles; uses fine needles and electrodes to record the activity

    a. cerebral angiography
    b. electromyography
    c. nerve biopsy

Match the description with the correct treatment.

5. _____ Surgical incision into the skull

6. _____ A catheter is inserted into the brain and drains extra fluid from the brain ventricles into the abdominal cavity

7. _____ Surgery of the nerve

8. _____ Surgical removal of a portion of the cranium

9. _____ Surgical removal of part or all of a nerve

    a. craniectomy
    b. craniotomy
    c. neurectomy
    d. neuroplasty
    e. ventriculoperitoneal shunt

Match the indication for use and desired effect with the correct medication classification.

10. _____ Reduces inflammation and is used to treat chronic inflammatory disease and acute conditions

11. _____ Reduces the frequency and severity of seizures by reducing excessive stimulation of the brain; treats epilepsy and trigeminal neuralgia

12. _____ Increases naturally occurring substances in the brain and is used to treat Alzheimer's disease

13. _____ Alters circulation to the brain and is used to treat or prevent migraine headaches

14. _____ Reduces the sensory function of the brain; blocks pain receptors and relieves pain

15. _____ Blocks nerve impulses to the brain and produces insensibility to pain or the sensation of pain

a. analgesic
b. anesthetic
c. anti-Alzheimer
d. anticonvulsant and mood stabilizer
e. antimigraine
f. corticosteroid

Match the side effects and adverse reactions with the correct medication classification.

16. _____ Confusion, psychomotor slowing, difficulty concentrating, memory problems, rare but serious cardiac events

17. _____ GI distress, liver and kidney disorders, and tinnitus

18. _____ Headache, mood changes, difficulty falling asleep or staying asleep, increased sweating, vision problems, depression, and weight gain

19. _____ Hypotension, cardiopulmonary depression, sedation, nausea, vomiting, headaches

20. _____ GI distress, frequent urination, muscle cramps, confusion, bradycardia, angina, bloody vomit or stools

21. _____ Sedation, vertigo, visual disturbances, GI disturbances, liver complications

a. analgesic
b. anesthetic
c. anti-Alzheimer
d. anticonvulsant and mood stabilizer
e. antimigraine
f. corticosteroid

CERTIFICATION PREPARATION

Circle the correct answer.

1. The central nervous system contains which structure(s)?
   a. Cranial nerves
   b. Brain
   c. Spinal cord
   d. Both b and c

2. Which subsystem is part of the autonomic nervous system?
   a. Somatic nervous system
   b. Parasympathetic nervous system
   c. Central nervous system
   d. Peripheral nervous system

3. The nervous system works in partnership with which other system to help the body maintain homeostasis?
   a. Endocrine system
   b. Cardiovascular system
   c. Respiratory system
   d. None of the above

4. Which structure of a nerve cell carries impulses away from the cell body?
   a. Glia
   b. Dendrite
   c. Myelin sheath
   d. Axon

5. A chemical that helps a nerve cell communicate with another nerve cell or muscle is
   a. a synapse.
   b. the cerebrospinal fluid.
   c. a neurotransmitter.
   d. the myelin sheath.

6. The pons is located in the
   a. cerebrum.
   b. cerebellum.
   c. brainstem.
   d. spinal cord.

7. Which could be a sign or symptom of a cerebrovascular accident?
   a. Numbness of the face, leg, or arm
   b. Difficulty speaking
   c. Loss of balance or coordination
   d. All of the above

8. Alzheimer's disease is most commonly diagnosed in which age group?
   a. 40-50
   b. 50-60
   c. After age 60
   d. None of the above

9. Which term is defined as a fold or convolution on the surface of the cerebral hemisphere?
   a. Gyri
   b. Sulci
   c. Fissure
   d. Tract

10. Which condition can be detected before birth?
    a. Spina bifida
    b. Cerebral palsy
    c. ADHD
    d. All of the above

WORKPLACE APPLICATIONS

1. Tia goes into the waiting room and starts to call back the next patient, Charlie Wayne-Thomas. Charlie is a regular patient at Walden-Martin Family Medical (WMFM) Clinic. He is 62 years old and in good health. When Tia calls him, he looks at her but only mumbles, he is pointing to his right leg and shaking his head back and forth as if to say "no." Tia tries to talk to Charlie, but she cannot understand his mumbling. Given this limited information, answer the questions below.

   a. What condition or conditions could be causing Charlie's signs and symptoms? _____

   _____

   b. Would this situation be considered a medical emergency? _____

   _____

2. Tia is reviewing nervous system diseases and disorders as part of a continuing education course. Briefly describe the nervous system conditions below and include five common signs and symptoms.

   a. Huntington disease or Huntington chorea _____

   _____

   _____

   b. Fetal alcohol syndrome (FAS) _____

   _____

   _____

   c. Bell's palsy _____

   _____

   _____

3. Sherman Potter was recently diagnosed with migraine headaches.

   a. What is the cause of migraine headaches? _____

   _____

   _____

   b. Briefly describe the aura stage for migraines. _____

   _____

   _____

   _____

   _____

INTERNET ACTIVITIES

1. Using online resources, research a test used for diagnosing a nervous system disease. Create a poster presentation, a PowerPoint presentation, or a written paper summarizing your research. Include the following points in your project:
   a. Description of the test
   b. Any contraindications for the test
   c. Patient preparation for the test
   d. What occurs during the test

2. Using online resources, research a nervous system disease or disorder. Create a poster presentation, a PowerPoint presentation, or a written paper summarizing your research. Include the following points in your project:
   a. Description of the disease
   b. Etiology
   c. Signs and symptoms
   d. Diagnostic procedures
   e. Treatments

3. Using online resources, research the effect that diet can have on the management of multiple sclerosis. In a one-page paper, summarize the information that you found.

4. Using Table 37.6, Medication Classifications, select two medications from each of the following classifications: analgesic, anesthetic, anticonvulsant, and antimigraine. Using the information in Table 37.6, identify for each medication:
   a. Indication for use
   b. Desired effects
   c. Side effects
   d. Adverse reactions

   Write a short paper addressing each of these four areas for each medication.

Procedure 37.1   Perform a Neurologic Status Exam

Name _____   Date _____   Score _____

Tasks: Administer and score a neurologic status exam.

Scenario: Dr. David Kahn has ordered a neurologic status exam form to be completed on Robert Caudill (DOB 10/31/19XX). Mr. Caudill is accompanied by his caregiver.

Directions: Role-play this scenario with two other peers. One will play the patient and the other will be the caregiver.

Equipment and Supplies:
- Patient's health record
- Order for the neurologic status exam
- Neurologic Status Exam Form (Work Product 37.1) or SimChart for the Medical Office (SCMO).

Standard: Complete the procedure and all critical steps in _____ minutes with a minimum score of 85% within two attempts (*or as indicated by the instructor*).

Scoring: Divide the points earned by the total possible points. Failure to perform a critical step, indicated by an asterisk (*), results in grade no higher than an 84% (*or as indicated by the instructor*).

Time: Began_____ Ended_____ Total minutes: _____

Steps:	Point Value	Attempt 1	Attempt 2
1. Wash hands or use hand sanitizer.	10		
2. **SCMO:** Click on the Form Repository and select the Neurological Status Exam on the INFO PANEL. Read the form. **Paper form:** Read the directions for the test.	10		
3. Greet the patient. Identify yourself. Verify the patient's identity with full name and date of birth. Explain the procedure to be performed in a manner that the patient understands. Answer any questions the patient may have about the procedure.	10		
4. **SCMO:** Click on Patient Search. Select the patient and verify the DOB. Click Select and the patient's name and DOB will autofill into the form field. Key in the information for the performed by and the date fields. **Paper form:** The patient information needs to be completed on the form. Your name and the date also need to be completed.	10		
5. Ask for the caregiver's name and clearly ask the caregiver-related questions from the form. Accurately document the information obtained.	15		
6. Perform the patient interview, following the directions on the form. Clearly provide the patient with the directions and the questions. Accurately document the information obtained from the patient.	30		
7. Accurately score the test as indicated by the directions. **SCMO:** Key the scores in the total fields. Save the form when completed. **Paper form:** Write the scores on the total line. Give the completed form to the provider.	15*		
Total Points	100		

Comments

CAAHEP Competencies	Step(s)
I.P.9. Assist provider with a patient exam	Entire procedure
X.P.3. Document patient care accurately in the medical record	4-7
ABHES Competencies	**Step(s)**
4. Medical Law and Ethics a. Follow documentation guidelines	4-7

Work Product 37.1 Neurologic Status Exam

Name _____ Date _____ Score _____

WALDEN-MARTIN
FAMILY MEDICAL CLINIC
1234 ANYSTREET | ANYTOWN, ANYSTATE 12345
PHONE 123-123-1234 | FAX 123-123-5678

Neurological Status Exam

The Neurological Status Examination tests the individual's sense of cognitive functions and quickly allows the provider to screen for cognitive impairment and/or loss. In addition to testing language recall and motor skills, the NSE also allows you to test an individual's orientation to time, detail, and attention.

There are five sections. Each section of the test involves relating a series of questions or commands to a patient; the patient should receive one point for each correct answer. Conduct the test without interruptions in a well-lit, private exam room. Instruct the patient to listen carefully and to answer each question as accurately as possible. In the event that there is a caregiver accompanying the patient, ask the Caregiver Questions and record the responses (these are not part of the final score).

Read each question once and document the patient's response. Do not time the patient's answers or duration of the test overall; once completed, score the test immediately. To do so, add only the number of correct responses. The individual can receive a maximum score of 10 points; a score below 4 indicates cognitive impairment.

Patient Name: _____   **Date of Birth:** _____

Performed By: _____   **Date:** _____

Caregiver Questions (if available): (Yes, No, Not Aware)

Name of Caregiver: _____	Yes	No	Not Aware
• Does the patient have difficulty remembering recent events or conversions?	☐	☐	☐
• Does the patient have difficulty performing activities of daily living (bath, driving, cooking, etc.)	☐	☐	☐
• Have you noticed changes to speech patterns?	☐	☐	☐

Patient Interview

Sequencing:

Read the following statement to the patient three consecutive times: **"Drive the red car to Washington Street"**. Then ask the patient to restate the sentence; you will ask the patient to recall the statement later in the test.

	Yes	No
The patient was able to repeat the exact statement to you.	☐	☐

Total: _____

Time Orientation:

Ask the patient the following questions:

	Correct	Incorrect
• What is today's date?	☐	☐
• What season is it?	☐	☐

- What is the day of the week?

☐ ☐

Total: _____

- -

Drawing:

Give the individual a piece of paper and ask him/her to copy a design of the two intersecting shapes. One point is awarded for correctly copying the shapes. All angles on both figures must be present, and the figures must have one overlapping angle.

Correct   **Incorrect**

☐ ☐

Total: _____

- -

Information:

Ask the patient the following questions:

Correct   **Incorrect**

- Who is president of the United States?   ☐ ☐
- How many stars are on the American flag?   ☐ ☐

Total: _____

- -

Recall:

Ask the patient to restate the sentence that you asked him/her at the beginning of the procedure. One point is given for repeating each of the following words.

Correct   **Incorrect**

- Drive   ☐ ☐
- Red Car   ☐ ☐
- Washington Street   ☐ ☐

Total: _____

- -

Total Exam Score: _____

Procedure 37.2 Assist with the Neurologic Exam

Name _____ **Date** _____ **Score** _____

Tasks: Set up for a neurologic exam and prepare a patient for the procedure. Assist the provider and the patient during the neurologic exam.

Equipment and Supplies:
- Patient's health record
- Patient gown
- Drape
- Otoscope
- Ophthalmoscope
- Percussion hammer
- Disposable pinwheel or other disposable sharp per provider
- Penlight
- Tuning fork
- Cotton ball
- Tongue depressor
- Small vials of warm, cold, sweet, and salty liquids
- Small vials of substances with distinct odors (e.g., spices, coffee, vanilla)
- Gloves
- Disinfecting wipes
- Biohazard sharps container
- Waste container

Standard: Complete the procedure and all critical steps in _____ minutes with a minimum score of 85% within two attempts (*or as indicated by the instructor*).

Scoring: Divide the points earned by the total possible points. Failure to perform a critical step, indicated by an asterisk (*), results in grade no higher than an 84% (*or as indicated by the instructor*).

Time: Began_____ Ended_____ Total minutes: _____

Steps:	Point Value	Attempt 1	Attempt 2
1. Wash hands or use hand sanitizer.	10		
2. Assemble supplies and equipment in the exam room.	25		
3. Greet the patient. Identify yourself. Verify the patient's identity with full name and date of birth. Explain the procedure to be performed in a manner that the patient understands. Answer any questions the patient may have about the procedure.	15		
4. Instruct the patient to change into the gown. The opening should be in the back. Ask the patient if assistance is needed. If so, help. If not, leave the room and allow the patient time to change. When reentering the room, provide a courtesy knock on the door.	10		
5. During the examination, be prepared to assist the patient in changing positions as necessary. Have the necessary examination instruments ready for the provider at the appropriate time during the examination. Record all results from the examination as indicated by the provider.	20		

6.	After the exam, put on gloves and clean the exam room. Discard sharps in the biohazard sharps container. Discard other waste in the appropriate waste containers. Disinfect equipment and surfaces (e.g., exam table). Remove gloves and discard.	10		
7.	Wash hands or use hand sanitizer.	10		
	Total Points	100		

Comments

CAAHEP Competencies	Step(s)
I.P.9 Assist provider with a patient exam	Entire procedure
ABHES Competencies	**Step(s)**
8.e. Perform specialty procedures, including but not limited to minor surgery, cardiac, respiratory, OB-GYN, neurological, and gastroenterology	Entire procedure

Procedure 37.3   Assist with a Lumbar Puncture

Name _____   Date _____   Score _____

Tasks: Set up for a lumbar puncture and prepare a patient for the procedure. Assist the provider during the lumbar puncture procedure. Document the procedure in the patient's health record.

Equipment and Supplies:
- Patient's health record
- Patient gown
- Drape
- Local anesthetic vial
- Syringe and needle
- Alcohol wipes
- Sterile, disposable lumbar puncture kit with specimen tubes
- Mayo stand
- Permanent marker or printed patient labels
- Laboratory requisition and specimen transport bag
- Gloves
- Biohazard waste container
- Biohazard sharps container
- Waste container
- Consent form
- Lumbar puncture instructions (optional)

Standard: Complete the procedure and all critical steps in _____ minutes with a minimum score of 85% within two attempts (*or as indicated by the instructor*).

Scoring: Divide the points earned by the total possible points. Failure to perform a critical step, indicated by an asterisk (*), results in grade no higher than an 84% (*or as indicated by the instructor*).

Time: Began_____ Ended_____ Total minutes: _____

Steps:	Point Value	Attempt 1	Attempt 2
1. Wash hands or use hand sanitizer.	5		
2. Assemble supplies and equipment in the treatment room.	5		
3. Greet the patient. Identify yourself. Verify the patient's identity with full name and date of birth. Explain the procedure to be performed in a manner that the patient understands. Answer any questions the patient may have about the procedure. Encourage the patient to use the restroom before the procedure.	5		
4. Check if the consent form was signed. If the consent was not signed, ask the patient if they have any questions. If there are no questions, explain the consent form and have the patient sign the form. If the patient has questions, let the provider know.	5*		
5. Instruct the patient to change into the gown. The opening should be in the back. Ask the patient if assistance is needed. If so, help. If not, leave the room and allow the patient time to change. When reentering the room, provide a courtesy knock on the door.	5		

6.	Assist the patient into a left side-lying position with the knees drawn up to the chest, or into a sitting position leaning forward on a stable surface. Support the patient's head with a pillow as necessary and provide a pillow for between the knees if needed.	**5**		
7.	Prepare the skin preparation for the provider to use. Open the sterile disposable lumbar puncture kit on a Mayo stand. Without contaminating the supplies, add a sterile needle and sterile syringe to the sterile field.	**10***		
8.	If needed, help the patient remain in the proper position. Use the drape to cover the patient. Give verbal encouragement to the patient during the procedure.	**5**		
9.	Assist the provider as needed during the procedure. When the provider is ready for the anesthetic, wipe the top of the vial with alcohol. Show the label to the provider and then hold the vial upside down as the provider withdraws the medication needed.	**10**		
10.	Attach the printed labels to the specimen tubes or using the permanent marker label the specimens #1, #2, #3, and so on in the order in which they are collected.	**5***		
11.	Complete the laboratory requisition form and prepare the CSF specimens for transport to the laboratory.	**5***		
12.	Put on gloves. Discard the needle/syringe in a biohazard sharps container. Make sure to put the needle in first. Clean up the area. Discard the waste in the appropriate waste container. Remove gloves and discard.	**5**		
13.	Wash hands or use hand sanitizer.	**5**		
14.	Monitor the patient and give liquids as directed by the provider. When the patient is ready to leave, instruct the patient to get dressed. Ask the patient if assistance is needed. If so, help. If not, leave the room and allow the patient time to change.	**5**		
15.	After the patient leaves, put on gloves and clean the room. Disinfect surfaces and discard waste. Remove gloves and discard.	**5**		
16.	Wash hands or use hand sanitizer.	**5**		
17.	Document the procedure in the patient's health record. Include the provider's name, the samples obtained, how the patient tolerated the procedure, and any instructions given.	**10**		
	Total Points	**100**		

Documentation

Comments

CAAHEP Competencies	Step(s)
I.P.8. Instruct and prepare a patient for a procedure or a treatment	3, 5, 6, 8
X.P.3. Document patient care accurately in the medical record	17
ABHES Competencies	**Step(s)**
4. Medical Law and Ethics a. Follow documentation guidelines	17
8.e. Perform specialty procedures, including but not limited to minor surgery, cardiac, respiratory, OB-GYN, neurological, and gastroenterology	Entire procedure

Procedure 37.4   Coach a Patient for an Electroencephalogram

Name _____   Date _____   Score _____

Tasks: Coach a patient on the preparation needed for an electroencephalogram (EEG). Document in the patient's health record.

Order: Provide EEG instructions.

Patient Instructions
Purpose of the EEG:
- An EEG is done to check for changes in the brain activity and can be helpful when diagnosing different disorders.

Patient preparation:
- Avoid caffeine on the day of the test.
- Take daily medications unless the provider indicates to hold medications until after the test.
- Wash hair the night before or the morning of the test, but do not use conditioners or any other hair care products.
- If you are to sleep through the EEG test, stay up later the night before the test or avoid sleeping.

During the test:
- Electrodes (patches with wires) will be attached to your head either with adhesive or by using a special cap.
- There will be little or no discomfort during the test.
- The technician may ask you questions during the test.

After the test:
- The technician will remove the electrodes.
- If sedation was used, you cannot drive after the test and for the rest of the day. Plan to have someone bring you home. Rest for the remaining part of the day.

Directions: Role-play the scenario with a peer, who is the patient. Your instructor is the provider. Make up the location, date, and time of the procedure.

Equipment and Supplies:
- Patient's health record
- Patient instructions for EEG

Standard: Complete the procedure and all critical steps in _____ minutes with a minimum score of 85% within two attempts (*or as indicated by the instructor*).

Scoring: Divide the points earned by the total possible points. Failure to perform a critical step, indicated by an asterisk (*), results in grade no higher than an 84% (*or as indicated by the instructor*).

Time: Began_____ Ended_____ Total minutes: _____

Steps:	Point Value	Attempt 1	Attempt 2
1. Wash hands or use hand sanitizer.	5		
2. Greet the patient. Identify yourself. Verify the patient's identity with full name and date of birth. Explain the procedure to be performed in a manner that the patient understands. Answer any questions the patient may have about the procedure.	10		
3. Explain the purpose of an EEG.	15		

4.	Explain how the patient should prepare for the test.	**20**		
5.	Explain what the patient should expect during and after the test.	**15**		
6.	Ask the patient to teach back the preparation to you. Clarify any misconceptions or inaccuracies. Answer any questions the patient may have. Give the patient a phone number to call if he has questions.	**15**		
7.	Let the patient know when to anticipate the results from the EEG. Also, give the patient the appointment information for the EEG, including the location and time.	**10**		
8.	Document the teaching in the patient's health record. Include the provider's name, what was taught, how the patient responded, and any written directions (including appointment information) sent home with the patient.	**10**		
	Total Points	**100**		

Documentation

Comments

CAAHEP Competencies	Step(s)
I.P.8. Instruct and prepare a patient for a procedure or a treatment	2-7
X.P.3. Document patient care accurately in the medical record	8
ABHES Competencies	**Step(s)**
4. Medical Law and Ethics a. Follow documentation guidelines	8

Behavioral Health

CAAHEP Competencies	Assessment
I.C.6. Identify structure and function of the human body across the life span	Skills and Concepts – C. 3-5
I.C.8.a. Identify common pathology related to each body system including: signs	Skills and Concepts – C. 2, D. 13-18, E. 7, F. 1-6, H. 1-4, 12, I. 1 ; Internet Activity – 2
I.C.8.b. Identify common pathology related to each body system including: symptoms	Skills and Concepts – C. 2, D. 13-18, E. 1-2, 7, F. 1-6, H. 1-4, 12, I. 1 ; Certification Preparation – 7; Internet Activity – 2
I.C.8.c. Identify common pathology related to each body system including: etiology	Skills and Concepts – D. 7-12, H. 10; Internet Activity – 2
I.C.8.d. Identify common pathology related to each body system including: diagnostic measures	Skills and Concepts – D. 19-24, E. 8, K. 2-3, H. 14; Internet Activity – 1, 2
I.C.8.e. Identify common pathology related to each body system including: treatment modalities	Skills and Concepts – D. 19-24, E. 9; Certification Preparation – 8; Internet Activity – 2, 4
V.C.8.a. Identify the following related to body systems: medical terms	Vocabulary Review – A. 1-7, B. 1-8
V.C.8.b. Identify the following related to body systems: abbreviations	Abbreviations – 1-26
ABHES Competencies	**Assessment**
2. Anatomy and Physiology b. Describe common diseases, symptoms, and etiologies as they apply to each system	Skills and Concepts – C. 2, D. 1-18, E. 1-7, F. 1-6, G. 1-4, H. 1-13, 15, I. 1, 3; Certification Preparation – 7; Internet Activity – 2
2.c. Identify diagnostic and treatment modalities as they relate to each body system	Skills and Concepts – D. 19-24, E. 8-9, K. 2-3, L. 1-13; Certification Preparation – 8; Internet Activity – 1-2, 4
3. Medical Terminology c. Apply medical terminology for each specialty	Vocabulary Review – A. 1-7, B. 1-8
3.d. Define and use medical abbreviations when appropriate and acceptable	Abbreviations – 1-26

VOCABULARY REVIEW

Using the word pool on the right, find the correct word to match the definition. Write the word on the line after the definition.

Group A

1. A small mass of gray matter found in each temporal lobe of the cerebrum; involved with memories, emotions, and activating the fight-or-flight response _____

2. Abnormally elated mental state; the person may have feelings of euphoria, lack of inhibitions, sleeplessness, talkativeness, risk-taking behaviors, and irritability _____

3. Unshakable belief in something untrue; maybe accompanied by hallucinations and/or paranoia _____

4. The relative frequency of deaths in a specific population

   _____

5. A sensory experience (e.g., a smell, sound, sight, touch, or taste) involving something that is not present _____

6. A treatment of behavioral health disorders which encourage communication of conflicts and insights into the person's problems; goals include symptoms relief, changes in behavior, improved social and vocational function, and personality growth

   _____

7. The rate of the disease in a population _____

Word Pool
- amygdala
- delusions
- hallucinations
- mania
- morbidity
- mortality
- psychotherapy

Group B

1. Alternative perception of the self; a person's own reality is lost; people feel they are not in control of their own actions or speech

   _____

2. An unfounded or excessive suspicion of the motives of others

   _____

3. Patient-provider details from private, group, or family therapy, including what the patient stated and the provider's analysis of the statements and situation _____

4. Memory loss _____

5. Loss of sensation of the reality of one's surroundings

   _____

6. The external expression of emotion _____

7. Awareness of one's environment, with reference to people, place, and time _____

8. An exaggerated sense of physical and mental well-being

   _____

Word Pool
- affect
- amnesia
- depersonalization
- derealization
- euphoria
- orientation
- paranoia
- psychotherapy notes

ABBREVIATIONS

Write out what each of the following abbreviations stands for.

1. LCSW _____

2. LICSW _____

3. LSW _____

4. DSM _____

5. ICD _____

6. GAD _____

7. CBT _____

8. OCD _____

9. HD _____

10. SSRI _____

11. SNRI _____

12. ASD _____

13. ADHD _____

14. ODD _____

15. CD _____

16. PTSD _____

17. EMDR _____

18. AUD _____

19. WAIS _____

20. IQ _____

21. DAP test _____

22. MMPI _____

23. TAT _____

24. IPT _____

25. DBT _____

26. SOB _____

SKILLS AND CONCEPTS
Answer the following questions. Write your answer on the line or in the space provided.

A. Introduction
Fill in the blank.

1. _____ encompasses our psychological, emotional, and social welfare.

2. _____ is the healthcare specialty that studies the brain and its effects on the body.

3. _____ is used to refer to mental health, substance use, and associated physical disorders.

B. Behavioral Health
Match the behavioral health professional with the correct description.

1. _____ Trained as a medical doctor and had four years of residency training in psychiatry, usually in a hospital setting

2. _____ Studied personality development, psychological problems, and how to diagnose mental and emotional disorders; must obtain a PhD or PsyD doctoral degree; most cannot prescribe medications

3. _____ Has a similar educational background to a psychologist; cannot provide psychological testing but can provide psychotherapy

4. _____ Specializes in cognitive behavioral therapy and helping people change the way they think and behave to help manage their condition (e.g., depression, relationship issues)

5. _____ A registered nurse who has advance training (e.g., master's or doctoral degree) in assessing and treating behavioral health issues

6. _____ Has specialized training to treat patients with substance use disorders and other addictions

7. _____ Trained to treat patients with behavioral health disorders (e.g., depression, anxiety)

a. substance abuse (or addiction) therapist or counselor
b. psychologist
c. cognitive behavioral therapist
d. psychiatrist
e. mental health therapist or counselor
f. social worker
g. psychiatric nurse

Fill in the blank.

8. The DSM-5 contains the International Classification of Disease (ICD) codes required for insurance reimbursement and for monitoring the _____ and _____ statistics.

C. Behavioral Health Disorders
Fill in the correct answer or select the correct answer.

1. Behavioral health disorders are conditions that cause changes in the _____, _____, or _____ of an individual.

2. Which of the following are signs or symptoms of behavioral health disorders?
   a. Withdrawing from others, isolating oneself
   b. Feeling helpless, hopeless, numb, or as if nothing matters
   c. Smoking, drinking alcohol, or using drugs more than usual
   d. All of the above

3. Behavioral health disorders in children
    a. cause changes in the way children learn, behave, or handle their emotions.
    b. can cause problems daily.
    c. can include anxiety, depression, oppositional defiant disorder, conduct disorder, ADHD, OCD, and PTSD.
    d. all of the above.

4. About _____% of the adult population in the U.S. lives with a serious behavioral health condition.

5. Research has shown that _____ is more prevalent in older adults who have been diagnosed with heart disease, diabetes, and stroke.

D. Anxiety Disorders
Match the disorder with the correct description.

1. _____ Causes different worries and the person finds it difficult to control the anxiety; can affect a person at any age and is more common in females

2. _____ Causes recurrent unexpected panic attacks or sudden feelings of terror without real dangers being present

3. _____ Causes a person to have frequent, upsetting thoughts, and then to control the thoughts, the person has an overwhelming urge to repeat certain behaviors

4. _____ Causes a persistent difficulty getting rid of personal possessions

5. _____ Causes a persistent and irrational fear of social situations

6. _____ Causes a strong, irrational fear of something that causes little to no danger

a. obsessive-compulsive disorder
b. phobia
c. social anxiety disorder
d. generalized anxiety disorder
e. panic disorder
f. hoarding disorder

Match the disorder with the correct etiology.

7. _____ Caused by negative experiences, genetics, changes in brain function, and the environment

8. _____ The cause unknown, but genetics may be a factor; stress also contributes to the development of this disease

9. _____ The cause is unknown, but genetics, major stress, sensitivity to stress, and certain changes in brain function may play a factor

10. _____ May be related to overprotective parents or limited social opportunities. Other possible causes include genetics, learning behaviors early in life, and an overactive amygdala

11. _____ The cause is not completely understood, but it may relate to changes in brain function, genetics, and environmental factors. Risk factors include a family history of this disease, other behavioral health disorders, and/or a traumatic event

12. _____ The cause is unknown. Risk factors include being indecisive, family history of this disorder, and stressful life events

a. obsessive-compulsive disorder
b. phobia
c. social anxiety disorder
d. generalized anxiety disorder
e. panic disorder
f. hoarding disorder

Match the disorder with the signs and symptoms of the disorder.

13. _____ The main symptom is excessive worrying for over 6 months about multiple issues without a clear reason. Other signs and symptoms include restlessness, fatigue, irritability, difficulty concentrating, difficulty stopping or controlling the anxiety, muscle tension, and sleep problems.

14. _____ Causes blushing, an increased heart rate, trembling, sweating, nausea, dizziness, lightheadedness, shortness of breath (SOB), and muscle tension. Elevated afternoon cortisol levels have also been reported.

15. _____ Signs and symptoms include fear of touching items others have touched, doubts about locking the door, avoidance of events that trigger problems, and frequent handwashing.

16. _____ May excessively acquire items that are not needed and has difficulty throwing out items. A person may feel the need to save items.

17. _____ Can cause panic, persistent and unreasonable fear, an increase in the heart rate, SOB, trembling, and a strong desire to get away.

18. _____ May experience a sense of impending doom, abdominal cramping, nausea, dizziness, lightheadedness, and numbness. Sweating, trembling, chills, hot flashes, chest pain, and a rapid and pounding heart rate can also occur.

a. obsessive-compulsive disorder
b. phobia
c. social anxiety disorder
d. generalized anxiety disorder
e. panic disorder
f. hoarding disorder

Match the disorder with the diagnostic tests and treatments.

19. _____ Psychological evaluation is done, and treatment includes psychotherapy and medications (e.g., antidepressants, antianxiety medications, and beta blockers).

20. _____ Psychological evaluation is done, and treatment includes psychotherapy and medications (e.g., antidepressants and sedative-hypnotics).

21. _____ A physical exam and a medical history are done. Often, treatments include psychotherapy, exposure therapy, and medication.

22. _____ The provider may review pictures of the patient's living conditions and talk with family members. Treatment consists of cognitive behavioral therapy.

23. _____ Psychological evaluation is done and treatment includes psychotherapy and medications.

24. _____ The provider will do a physical exam, laboratory tests, and a psychological evaluation. Treatment consists of psychotherapy and antidepressants.

a. obsessive-compulsive disorder
b. phobia
c. social anxiety disorder
d. panic disorder
e. hoarding disorder
f. generalized anxiety disorder

E. Depression and Other Mood Disorders
Match the type of depression with the description.

1. _____ Episodes of psychosis occur with severe depression. The person experiences delusions and hallucinations.

2. _____ Occurs after giving birth. The person has feelings of extreme sadness, exhaustion, and anxiety. These feelings interfere with daily life and caring for the new baby.

3. _____ Also called *dysthymia*; depression that lasts for at least 2 years.

4. _____ Depression occurs during the winter months when there is less sunlight. The depression usually lifts in the spring.

5. _____ Causes people to go from mania to depression.

a. persistent depressive disorder
b. postpartum depression
c. psychotic depression
d. bipolar disorder
e. seasonal affective disorder

Fill in the blank or select the correct answer.

6. The cause of _____ is not known, but many factors may be involved, including changes in the brain and the functioning of neurotransmitters, hormone changes, and genetics.

7. Which of the following are signs and symptoms of depression?
   a. Feeling sad, very tired, hopeless, irritable, anxious, or guilty
   b. Loss of interest in favorite activities (e.g., hobbies) and thoughts of death or suicide
   c. Pain, headaches, cramps, digestive issues, anorexia, and overeating
   d. All of the above

8. To diagnose depression, the provider will do a(n) _____ to gather more information on the patient's symptoms, thoughts, feelings, and behaviors.

9. Which medication may be used to treat depression?
   a. Selective serotonin reuptake inhibitors (SSRI) antidepressants
   b. Serotonin and norepinephrine reuptake inhibitor (SNRI) antidepressants
   c. Tricyclic and atypical antidepressants
   d. Monoamine oxidase inhibitors (MAOIs)
   e. All of the above

F. Behavioral Disorders
Fill in the blank or select the correct answer.

1. Disruptive behavior disorder involves _____ or _____ action patterns of behavior.

2. A person with disruptive behavior disorder may have temper tantrums, _____, demonstrate _____ and _____ behaviors, and fight with others.

3. People with disruptive behavioral disorder have problems controlling their _____ and _____, leading to issues at school and home.

4. Which of the following is *not* an inattentive sign or symptom of ADHD?
    a.   Fails to pay close attention and has problems staying focused
    b.   Fidgets
    c.   Appears not to listen and is easily distracted
    d.   Has difficulty following directions

5. Which of the following is *not* a hyperactive and impulsive sign or symptom of ADHD?
    a.   Trouble with organizational skills
    b.   Constantly moving
    c.   Talking too much
    d.   Problems doing quiet activities
    e.   Fidgets

6. Which of the following is a sign or symptom of oppositional defiant disorder?
    a.   Angry and irritable mood
    b.   Argumentative and defiant behaviors
    c.   Vindictiveness
    d.   All of the above

G. Eating Disorders
Match the descriptions with the correct disorder.

1. _____ Causes a person to eat non-food materials.

2. _____ Occurs when people regularly eat unusually large amounts of food in a short amount of time.

3. _____ Causes people to lose more weight than is healthy. Individuals have an intense fear of gaining weight.

4. _____ Overeating that leads to purging and can be life-threatening. To prevent weight gain, self-induced vomiting, laxative use, weight-loss supplements, and enemas may be used.

a.   anorexia nervosa
b.   binge eating disorder
c.   bulimia nervosa
d.   pica

H. Other Types of Behavioral Health Disorders
Select the correct answer or fill in the blank.

1. What are the signs and symptoms of autism spectrum disorder?
    a.   Social communication and interaction behavior issues
    b.   Restrictive and repetitive behaviors
    c.   Sleeping issues
    d.   All of the above

2. _____ cause a person to involuntarily escape from reality and the person may have a disconnection among memories, thoughts, actions, identity, and surroundings.

3. Dissociative disorder can cause a variety of conditions, such as _____ and _____.

4. Memory loss without an explained medical condition and no recollection of self, events, and familiar people is _____.

5. Multiple personality disorder is now called _____.

6. Cluster _____ personality disorders cause odd, eccentric thinking and behavior.

7. Cluster _____ personality disorders cause anxiety and fearful thinking and behaviors.

8. Avoidance personality disorder is part of Cluster _____ personality disorders.

9. Narcissistic personality disorder is part of Cluster _____ personality disorders.

10. _____ is a condition that occurs after experiencing or witnessing a traumatic or terrifying event.

11. Reliving the trauma is called _____.

12. A person with PTSD may
    a. be easily frightened.
    b. do self-destructive activities.
    c. have trouble concentrating and sleeping.
    d. have aggressive behaviors.
    e. all of the above.

13. _____ causes disruptions in thought processes, perceptions, emotional responsiveness, and social interactions.

14. Schizophrenia is usually diagnosed in the _____ to the early thirties.

15. Schizophrenia is more common in _____.

I. Substance Use Disorders and Other Addictions
Select the correct answer or fill in the blank.

1. What are general signs and symptoms of substance abuse or dependence?
    a. Confusion, violence, and hostility
    b. Making excuses to use drugs, lack of control over use, and the need for regular/daily use
    c. Missing work and school
    d. Neglecting self-care
    e. All of the above

2. For the following alcoholic drinks, indicate how many fluid oz make up one "standard" drink?

    a. Regular beer: _____

    b. Table wine: _____

    c. Distilled spirits: _____

    d. Malt liquor: _____

3. Which is *not* an effect of alcohol on the body?
    a. Changes in mood and behavior
    b. Makes it easier to think clearly and move with coordination
    c. High blood pressure, stroke, arrhythmias, and cardiomyopathy
    d. Liver inflammation, fatty liver, alcoholic hepatitis, fibrosis, and cirrhosis

4. Which is *not* an effect of alcohol on the body?
   a. Pancreatitis
   b. Cancer of the mouth, esophagus, throat, liver, and breast
   c. A strong immune system

5. Which of the following is an addiction?
   a. Exercise
   b. Gambling and gaming
   c. Internet
   d. Shopping
   e. All of the above

J. Suicidal Behavior
Select the correct answer or fill in the blank.

1. _____ is death caused by a self-inflicted injury with an intent to die as a result of the behavior.

2. Which of the following a warning sign of suicide?
   a. Looking for a way to kill oneself
   b. Talking about killing oneself or wanting to die; feelings of hopelessness, feeling trapped or in unbearable pain; having no reason to live or being a burden on others
   c. Increased use of drugs or alcohol
   d. All of the above

3. Which of the following a warning sign of suicide?
   a. Socially withdrawn and isolated
   b. Sleeping too much or too little
   c. Extreme mood swings
   d. All of the above

K. Assisting with Behavioral Health Examinations and Diagnostic Procedures
Select the correct answer.

1. What is *not* part of the medical assistant's role with health examinations?
   a. Obtain and document the patient's vital signs, weight, and medical histories.
   b. Prescribe medications.
   c. Prepare prescription refills for the provider to complete and sign.

2. Which is *not* an area on the mental status exam?
   a. Physical appearance, behavior, and motor activity
   b. Mood and affect
   c. Friends and family
   d. Emotional state

3. Which is an area on the mental status exam?
   a. Attention span and concentration
   b. Orientation
   c. Language and communication skills
   d. Judgment and intelligence
   e. All of the above

L. Assisting with Behavioral Health Treatments

Match the medication category with the correct use.

1. _____ Used to reduce anxiety, produce calmness, and release muscle tension

2. _____ Used to treat mania and mixed episodes (mania and depression) with bipolar disorder

3. _____ Used to treat depression, anxiety, and other behavioral health disorders

4. _____ Used to treat schizophrenia and bipolar disorder

5. _____ Used to treat insomnia

6. _____ Used to treat ADHD

a. antidepressants
b. stimulants
c. anticonvulsants and mood stabilizer
d. sedative–hypnotics
e. antipsychotics
f. antianxiety

Match the type of psychotherapy with the description.

7. _____ Used to treat behavioral health disorders, such as eating disorders and major depression by helping the person understand the relationship between symptoms and social interactions.

8. _____ Used to process and resolve traumatic memories (e.g., PTSD). During the therapy, the person concentrates on the memory while focusing on controlled stimuli.

9. _____ Used to treat depression, addictions, social anxiety disorder, and eating disorders. It focuses on helping the patient recognize, express, and overcome negative feelings and repressed emotions.

10. _____ Produces changes in behavior by helping the person face fears, role-play situations, and learn problem-solving skills to cope with difficult issues.

11. _____ Used to help people process their traumatic experiences or feared situations. The person revisits and recounts the memories, which gradually helps the person emotionally process the experience or situation.

12. _____ Used for children who are experiencing behavioral, emotional, social, or relational disorders.

13. _____ Used for individuals who are diagnosed with personality disorders, are suicidal, or engage in self-harm behaviors.

a. cognitive behavioral therapy
b. dialectical behavioral therapy
c. exposure therapy
d. eye movement desensitization and reprocessing
e. interpersonal psychotherapy
f. play therapy
g. psychodynamic therapy

CERTIFICATION PREPARATION

Circle the correct answer.

1. Which term means an unreal sensory perception that occurs with no external cause?
   a. Hallucination
   b. Delusion
   c. Psychosis
   d. Dysphoria

2. Which term describes the rate of a disease in a population?
   a. Mortality
   b. Morbidity
   c. Orientation
   d. Affect

3. Which term means an unshakable belief in something untrue?
   a. Hallucination
   b. Mania
   c. Delusion
   d. Affect

4. Brontophobia is the fear of
   a. flying.
   b. computers.
   c. blood or injury.
   d. thunder.

5. Drugs of abuse include
   a. cocaine.
   b. heroin.
   c. prescription opioids.
   d. all of the above.

6. Which anxiety disorder is described as a persistent difficulty getting rid of personal possessions?
   a. GAD
   b. HD
   c. OCD
   d. None of the above

7. Which is *not* a symptom of depression?
   a. Feeling sad
   b. Loss of interest in hobbies
   c. Mania
   d. Thoughts of death or suicide

8. ADHD is often treated with what type of medication?
   a. Stimulants
   b. Antidepressants
   c. Mood stabilizers
   d. All of the above

9. Amnesia is defined as
   a. loss of hope for the future.
   b. memory loss.
   c. inability to cope.
   d. both a and c.

10. Which behavioral health professional is a trained medical doctor with 4 years of residency?
    a. Psychiatrist
    b. Psychologist
    c. Social worker
    d. Cognitive behavioral therapist

WORKPLACE APPLICATIONS

1. Mike is taking Celeste back to an examination room to see the provider. Celeste has been diagnosed with anorexia nervosa.

   a. Mike has Celeste step on the scale to take her weight. How might Mike ensure an accurate weight is obtained?

   _____

   _____

   b. Should Mike position Celeste at the scale any differently than any other patient? If yes, explain why.

   _____

   _____

   c. Should Mike tell Celeste her weight at the time of her weigh-in? Explain your answer._____

   _____

   _____

2. Mike is preparing Celeste's medical records to be sent to another provider. How should Celeste's psychotherapy notes be treated in this situation? Should they be included with all of her health records?

_____

_____

_____

3. Susan is a medical assistant working in behavioral health. She often needs to coach patients on the use of medication for their conditions. Medication compliance is an important factor for a behavioral health patient. What types of information should Susan emphasize when coaching a patient on medication compliance?

_____

_____

_____

_____

INTERNET ACTIVITIES

1. Using online resources, research a test used for diagnosing mental and behavioral health disorders. Create a poster presentation, a PowerPoint presentation, or a written paper summarizing your research. Include the following points in your project:
   a. Description of the test
   b. Any contraindications for the test
   c. Patient preparation for the test
   d. What occurs during the test

2. Using online resources, research a mental or behavioral health disorder. Create a poster presentation, a PowerPoint presentation, or an infographic summarizing your research. Include the following points in your project:
   a. Description of the disease
   b. Etiology
   c. Signs and symptoms
   d. Diagnostic procedures
   e. Treatments

3. Using online resources, research the three different types of eating disorders covered in this chapter: anorexia nervosa, binge eating disorder, bulimia nervosa. In a one-page paper, describe each eating disorder and describe how it is treated.

4. Using Table 38.4, Medication Classifications, select two medication from each of the following classifications: antianxiety and antipsychotic. Using online resources, identify the following information specific to each medication:
   a. Reasons for use
   b. Desired effects
   c. Side effects
   d. Adverse reactions

   Write a short paper addressing each of these four areas for each medication. Include the Internet sites used.

Endocrinology

CAAHEP Competencies	Assessment
I.C.4. Identify major organs in each body system	Skills and Concepts – A. 6, B. 1, C. 1, D. 1, 3, E. 20-23; Certification Preparation – 1
I.C.5. Identify the anatomical location of major organs in each body system	Skills and Concepts – A. 7, B. 2, 18-25, C. 1, D. 1; Certification Preparation – 5, 6
I.C.6. Identify structure and function of the human body across the life span	Skills and Concepts – F. 5-7; Certification Preparation – 8, 10
I.C.7. Identify the normal function of each body system	Skills and Concepts – A. 8, 9, B. 1-17, C. 2-12, D. 3-15, E. 1-19, F. 1-4; Certification Preparation – 2-3
I.C.8.a. Identify common pathology related to each body system including: signs	Skills and Concepts – G. 1-10, 19-22, H. 5-8, I. 3, J. 10; Certification Preparation – 7, 9; Internet Activity – 2
I.C.8.b. Identify common pathology related to each body system including: symptoms	Skills and Concepts – G. 1-10, 19-22, H. 5-8, I. 3, J. 10; Certification Preparation – 7, 9; Internet Activity – 2
I.C.8.c. Identify common pathology related to each body system including: etiology	Skills and Concepts – G. 15-18, H. 1-4, J. 1-3; Workplace Application – 3; Internet Activity – 2
I.C.8.d. Identify common pathology related to each body system including: diagnostic measures	Skills and Concepts – G. 23-26, H. 9-12, K. 1-8; Certification Preparation – 4; Workplace Application – 1; Internet Activity – 1, 2
I.C.8.e. Identify common pathology related to each body system including: treatment modalities	Skills and Concepts – G. 23-26, H. 9-12, J. 5-6, K. 9-22; Internet Activity – 2-4
1.C.9. Identify Clinical Laboratory Improvement Amendments (CLIA) waived tests associated with common diseases	Skills and Concepts –K. 2, 4-8; Certification Preparation – 4
I.C.10.a. Identify the classifications of medications, including indications for use	Skills and Concepts – K. 14-17
I.C.10.b. Identify the classifications of medications, including desired effects	Skills and Concepts – K. 14-17
I.C.10.c. Identify the classifications of medications, including side effects	Skills and Concepts – K. 18-22
I.C.10.d. Identify the classifications of medications, including adverse reactions	Skills and Concepts – K. 18-22

CAAHEP Competencies	Assessment
V.C.8.a. Identify the following related to body systems: medical terms	Skills and Concepts – G. 1-10, K. 9-13
V.C.8.b. Identify the following related to body systems: abbreviations	Abbreviations – 1-23
V.P.3.b. Coach patients regarding: medical encounters	Procedure 39.1
X.P.3. Document patient care accurately in the medical record	Procedure 39.1

ABHES Competencies	Assessment
2. Anatomy and Physiology a. List all body systems and their structures and functions	Skills and Concepts – A. 6-9, B. 1-17, C. 1-12, D. 1, 3-15, E. 1-23; Certification Preparation – 1, 5, 6
2.b. Describe common diseases, symptoms, and etiologies as they apply to each system	Skills and Concepts – G. 1-22, H. 1-8, I. 1-3, J. 1-3, 10; Certification Preparation – 7, 9; Workplace Application – 1-3; Internet Activities – 2
2.c. Identify diagnostic and treatment modalities as they relate to each body system	Skills and Concepts – G. 23-26, H. 9-12, J. 5-6, K. 1-22; Certification Preparation – 4; Workplace Application – 1; Internet Activity – 1, 4
3. Medical Terminology c. Apply medical terminology for each specialty	Skills and Concepts – G. 1-10, K. 9-13
3. d. Define and use medical abbreviations when appropriate and acceptable	Abbreviations – 1-23
4. Medical Law and Ethics a. Follow documentation guidelines	Procedure 39.1
8. Clinical Procedures d. Assist provider with specialty examination, including cardiac, respiratory, OB-GYN, neurological, and gastroenterology procedures.	Procedure 39.1
8. e. Perform specialty procedures, including but not limited to minor surgery, cardiac, respiratory, OB-GYN, neurological, and gastroenterology	Procedure 39.1

VOCABULARY REVIEW

Using the word pool on the right, find the correct word to match the definition. Write the word on the line after the definition.

Group A

1. Result when fats are broken down; used by the body for energy and tissue development _____

2. The space in the thoracic cavity that lies between the lungs; contains the heart, trachea, and esophagus _____

3. A naturally occurring element that is necessary for many body functions, including strong bones and teeth, proper blood clotting, nerve conduction, and muscle contractions _____

4. A test to measure the amount and concentration of urine produced when water is withheld from a patient for a period of time

   _____

5. A process in which a change from the normal ranges causes a response that opposes or decreases the change, thus helping to maintain homeostasis _____

6. Structures or sites on or in a cell that bind with substances such as hormones, antigens, or drugs _____

7. A cell selectively affected by a specific agent such as a drug, hormone, or virus _____

8. A chemical substance that separates into ions in solution (water) and is capable of conducting an electric current _____

9. The internal environment of the body that is compatible with life; steady state that is created to provide a consistent and unvarying internal environment _____

Word Pool
- calcium
- electrolyte
- fatty acids
- homeostasis
- mediastinum
- negative feedback loop
- receptors
- target cell
- water deprivation test

Group B

1. Increase in the fluid pressure in the eye, can lead to blindness if not treated _____

2. Clouding of the lens, leading to decreased vision

   _____

3. Sexual drive or instinct _____

4. Diabetes mellitus (DM) damages the blood vessels in the retina leading to loss of vision and eventual blindness _____

5. A specialized organelle of a cell that is encased in a membrane and directs growth, metabolism, and reproduction of the cell

   _____

6. A structure within a cell that performs a specific function

   _____

7. To spread, scatter, disperse, or move _____

8. A form of toxemia during pregnancy characterized by high blood pressure, fluid retention, and protein in the urine

   _____

Word Pool
- cataract
- diabetic retinopathy
- diffuse
- glaucoma
- libido
- nucleus
- organelle
- preeclampsia

ABBREVIATIONS

Write out what each of the following abbreviations stands for.

1. ACTH _____

2. FSH _____

3. GH _____

4. LH _____

5. PRL _____

6. TSH _____

7. ADH _____

8. OT _____

9. T_3 _____

10. T_4 _____

11. PTH _____

12. GHRL _____

13. PG _____

14. DI _____

15. RAIU _____

16. DM _____

17. A1c _____

18. DKA _____

19. CKD _____

20. SIADH _____

21. FBG _____

22. OGTT _____

23. TFT _____

SKILLS AND CONCEPTS

Answer the following questions.

A. Introduction

Fill in the blank or select the correct answer.

1. _____ is the healthcare specialty that deals with endocrine disorders.

2. A(n) _____ is a specialist involved in the diagnosis, treatment, and prevention of endocrine disorders.

3. The endocrine system is composed of _____ glands throughout the body.

4. Hormones control
   a. metabolism and growth.
   b. mood.
   c. sexual maturity and reproduction.
   d. water and electrolyte balance.
   e. all of the above.

5. The _____ system and endocrine system work together to perform communication functions and maintain homeostasis.

6. When the _____ detects rising levels of a target organ's hormones, it sends a signal to the pituitary gland to release or prevent the pituitary hormone production.

7. The hypothalamus is located in the middle of the _____.

8. The hypothalamus is responsible for the production of _____ and _____.

9. Antidiuretic hormone (ADH) and oxytocin are stored and secreted by the _____ of the pituitary gland.

B. Anatomy of the Pituitary Gland

1. The pituitary gland is also known as the _____ or the "master gland."

2. The pituitary gland is connected to the hypothalamus by the _____.

Match the action of the hormone with the correct hormones. Answers may be used more than once.

3. _____ Stimulates interstitial cells in the testes to develop and secrete testosterone

4. _____ Stimulates the development of ova (eggs) through ovulation in females

5. _____ Causes the adrenal cortex to produce and release steroids (e.g., cortisol)

6. _____ Stimulates the thyroid gland to release T_3 and T_4

7. _____ Simulates the ovaries to produce estrogen, ova to mature, and the production of progesterone

8. _____ Stimulates breast tissue development and milk production toward the end of pregnancy and after childbirth

9. _____ Involved with glucose metabolism in the body

10. _____ Initiates ovulation and signals the corpus luteum to develop

11. _____ Stimulates growth of the long bones and muscles in children and teens

12. _____ Also called *interstitial cell–stimulating hormone*

13. _____ Called *somatotropin* or *somatotropic hormone*

14. _____ Stimulates the seminiferous tubules to produce sperm in males

15. _____ Also called *vasopressin*

16. _____ Stimulates the uterine muscles to contract and helps with releasing breast milk

17. _____ Stimulates the kidney tubules to reabsorb water, which concentrates the urine

a. adrenocorticotropic hormone
b. follicle-stimulating hormone
c. growth hormone
d. luteinizing hormone
e. prolactin
f. thyroid-stimulating hormone
g. antidiuretic hormone
h. oxytocin

Match the lobe of the pituitary gland with the hormones it secretes. Answers may be used more than once.

18. _____ Adrenocorticotropic hormone

19. _____ Antidiuretic hormone

20. _____ Follicle-stimulating hormone

21. _____ Growth hormone

22. _____ Luteinizing hormone

23. _____ Oxytocin

24. _____ Prolactin

25. _____ Thyroid-stimulating hormone

a.   anterior lobe
b.   posterior lobe

C. Anatomy of the Thyroid and Parathyroid Glands
Fill in the blank.

1.   The thyroid gland and the parathyroid glands are located in the _____.

Match the action of the hormone with the correct hormone. Answers may be used more than once.

2.   _____ Supports the activities of growth hormone

3.   _____ Lowers blood calcium levels by inhibiting osteoclast activity

4.   _____ Regulates metabolism and increases the basal metabolic rate

5.   _____ Regulates calcium and phosphate levels in the blood

6.   _____ Regulates metabolism and increases the basal metabolic rate

7.   _____ Regulates calcium and phosphorus levels in the body

8.   _____ Works against the parathyroid hormone action

a.   triiodothyronine
b.   thyroxine
c.   calcitonin
d.   parathyroid hormone

Match the glands with the hormones they secrete. Answers may be used more than once.

9.   _____ Triiodothyronine

10. _____ Thyroxine

11. _____ Calcitonin

12. _____ Parathyroid hormone

a.   thyroid gland
b.   parathyroid gland

D. Anatomy of the Adrenal Glands
Fill in the blank.

1.   The adrenal glands are located on the top of each _____.

2.   The outer part of the gland is the _____, and the inner part is called the _____.

3.   The _____ and the anterior lobe of the pituitary gland regulate corticosteroids secreted by the adrenal cortex.

Match the action of the hormone with the correct hormones. Answers may be used more than once.

4. _____ It increases the heart rate and strength of the contractions, blood pressure, and blood glucose level.

5. _____ Includes aldosterone, which regulates the sodium and water balance in the body.

6. _____ It relaxes the smooth muscles in the bronchioles.

7. _____ Regulate the electrolytes in the body.

8. _____ It increases the blood glucose level, heart rate, and the force of the heart's contractions.

9. _____ Responsible for some of the secondary sexual characteristics in both males and females during puberty.

10. _____ Regulate protein, fat, and carbohydrate metabolism.

a. mineralocorticoids
b. glucocorticoids
c. gonadocorticoids
d. epinephrine
e. norepinephrine

Match the glands with the hormones they secrete. Answers may be used more than once.

11. _____ Norepinephrine

12. _____ Mineralocorticoids

13. _____ Glucocorticoids

14. _____ Gonadocorticoids

15. _____ Epinephrine

a. adrenal cortex
b. adrenal medulla

E. Anatomy of Other Endocrine Glands

Match the action of the hormone with the correct hormones. Answers may be used more than once.

1. _____ Stimulate the production and maturity of T cells

2. _____ Helps maintain a pregnancy

3. _____ Regulate waking and sleeping patterns

4. _____ Helps move the blood glucose from the blood to the cells

5. _____ Works in the brain to regulate body weight, glucose metabolism, and food intake

6. _____ Stimulates the development of male secondary sexual characteristics

7. _____ Stimulates the stored glycogen in the liver to be converted into glucose

8. _____ Stimulates the development of breasts and other female secondary sexual characteristics

9. _____ Regulates other pancreatic hormones and also inhibits the secretion of growth hormone

10. _____ Stimulates fatty acids and amino acids in the liver to be converted into glucose

a. glucagon
b. insulin
c. somatostatin
d. ghrelin
e. thymosin
f. testosterone
g. estrogen
h. progesterone
i. melatonin

Match the glands with the hormones they secrete. Answers may be used more than once.

11. _____ Glucagon

12. _____ Ghrelin

13. _____ Thymosin

14. _____ Progesterone

15. _____ Testosterone

16. _____ Insulin

17. _____ Estrogen

18. _____ Melatonin

19. _____ Somatostatin

a. pancreas
b. thymus gland
c. gonads
d. pineal gland

Match the gland with its location.

1. _____ Located deep within the brain

2. _____ Located in the mediastinum behind the sternum

3. _____ Located in the testes and ovaries

4. _____ Located inferior and posterior to the stomach

a. pancreas
b. thymus gland
c. gonads
d. pineal gland

F. Physiology of the Endocrine System

Fill in the blank.

1. The target cells have _____ that attract only certain hormones, thus only selected hormones pass into the cell and affect cellular action.

2. _____ hormones are made up of protein or amino acids and attach to target cell membranes.

3. _____ hormones are same lipid-soluble molecules that attach to a target cell.

4. _____, also known as *tissue hormones*, are substances found in many body tissues and affect cells in their local area.

5. Declining levels of _____ leads to menopause.

6. _____ levels gradually decrease with age.

7. _____ decreases with age and causes a loss of normal sleep/wake cycles.

G. Pituitary Gland Disease and Disorders

Match the medical term with the correct definition.

1. _____ The presence of ketones in the urine
2. _____ A low blood calcium level
3. _____ Excessive eating
4. _____ Excessive thirst
5. _____ The swelling of the neck and visible enlargement of the thyroid gland
6. _____ The presence of glucose in the urine
7. _____ Excess urine volume
8. _____ Excessive facial or body hair growth in women
9. _____ A noticeable protrusion of the eyeball
10. _____ A low blood glucose (sugar) level

a. exophthalmia
b. glucosuria
c. goiter
d. hirsutism
e. hypocalcemia
f. hypoglycemia
g. ketonuria
h. polydipsia
i. polyphagia
j. polyuria

Match the description with the correct disease.

11. _____ Also known as "short stature"
12. _____ A rare condition in which there is too much growth hormone in the body during childhood
13. _____ A rare condition in which there is too much growth hormone in the body during adulthood
14. _____ Caused by a hyposecretion of ADH

a. acromegaly
b. gigantism
c. dwarfism
d. diabetes insipidus

Match the etiology with the correct disease.

15. _____ Most types are caused by a genetic mutation.
16. _____ The pituitary gland makes too much growth hormone during childhood.
17. _____ The causes include genetics, a tumor, trauma, or pituitary gland surgery.
18. _____ The pituitary gland makes too much growth hormone during adulthood.

a. acromegaly
b. gigantism
c. dwarfism
d. diabetes insipidus

Match the signs and symptoms with the correct disease.

19. _____ Double vision, gaps between teeth, joint pain, and prominent forehead and jaw
20. _____ Short extremities in comparison to the head and trunk
21. _____ Excessive sweating, body odor, and decreased muscle strength; large bones of the face, jaw, feet, and hands; hirsutism; and decreased peripheral vision
22. _____ Polydipsia, polyuria, nocturia, trouble sleeping, fussiness, fever, vomiting, and delayed growth and weight loss in children

a. acromegaly
b. gigantism
c. dwarfism
d. diabetes insipidus

Match the diagnostic measures and treatments with the correct disease.

23. _____ Laboratory tests, water deprivation test, and imaging tests; treatment includes synthetic ADH hormone and diuretics

24. _____ Laboratory tests including growth hormone and blood glucose, MRI, and spinal x-ray; treatment consists of surgery to remove the tumor, radiation, and medication to block the production of growth hormone

25. _____ Measurements, imaging technology, genetic testing, and hormone testing; treatment is focused on maximizing functioning and independence.

26. _____ CT or MRI scan; treated with surgery

a. acromegaly
b. gigantism
c. dwarfism
d. diabetes insipidus

H. Thyroid Gland and Parathyroid Glands Diseases and Disorders

Match the etiology with the correct disease.

1. _____ Results from thyroidectomy and radiation therapy

2. _____ Caused by an adenoma or a hyperplasia

3. _____ Caused by Graves' disease, thyroid nodules, pituitary disorders and tumors, and thyroiditis

4. _____ Caused by injury or damage to the parathyroid gland

a. hyperthyroidism
b. hypothyroidism
c. hyperparathyroidism
d. hypoparathyroidism

Match the signs and symptoms with the correct disease.

5. _____ Muscle pain and atrophy, vomiting, anorexia, cardiac arrhythmias, renal calculi, and bone tenderness

6. _____ Numbness, tingling, spasms, confusion, irritability, tetany, and laryngospasm

7. _____ Fatigue, slowed heart rate, hoarseness, sensitivity to cold, and thinning hair

8. _____ Fatigue, muscle weakness, increased sweating, rapid and irregular heart rate, goiter, and exophthalmia

a. hyperthyroidism
b. hypothyroidism
c. hyperparathyroidism
d. hypoparathyroidism

Match the diagnostic measures and treatments with the correct disease.

9. _____ Laboratory blood test, electrocardiogram, and imaging tests (e.g., radioimmunoassay studies); treated with calcium and vitamin D supplements

10. _____ Thyroid function test and a radioactive iodine uptake scan; treatment includes radioactive iodine therapy, antithyroid medication, and a thyroidectomy

11. _____ Laboratory blood tests and imaging tests; treatment may consist of minimally invasive surgery to remove the tumor or gland(s) and medications to increase the calcium excretion

12. _____ Thyroid function test and a thyroid ultrasound; treatment consists of administration of synthetic thyroid hormone

a. hyperthyroidism
b. hypothyroidism
c. hyperparathyroidism
d. hypoparathyroidism

I. Adrenal Glands Diseases and Disorders
Fill In the blank.

1. _____ is a malfunction of the adrenal cortex, leading to adrenal insufficiency (hypo-secretion) of cortisol.

2. _____ is a malfunction of the cortex of the adrenal gland, causing increased levels of cortisol.

3. _____ can cause high blood pressure, weight gain, abdominal stretch marks, slow-healing wounds, severe fatigue, depression, and anxiety.

J. Pancreatic Diseases and Disorders
Fill in the blank or select the correct answer.

1. Type 1 DM and LADA are _____ conditions.

2. _____ signs and symptoms include polydipsia, polyuria, polyphagia, weight loss, fatigue, blurred vision, frequent infections, and slow-healing wounds.

3. With _____, the pancreas produces very little to no insulin.

4. With _____, insulin resistance occurs or the pancreas does not make enough insulin to meet the body's needs.

5. Treatment for _____ includes insulin injections; regular exercise; frequent blood glucose monitoring; and dietary changes including carbohydrate, fat, and protein counting.

6. Treatment for _____ includes healthy eating, regular exercise, weight loss if obese, medications (e.g., antihyperglycemics, insulin), and glucose monitoring.

7. Complications of DM include
   a. cardiovascular disease.
   b. blindness and eye conditions.
   c. neuropathy.
   d. poor wound healing.
   e. all of the above

8. _____ develops during pregnancy and the hyperglycemia can affect the health of the pregnancy and the baby.

9. Complications of gestational diabetes can include
   a. excessive growth in utero.
   b. death.
   c. hypoglycemia shortly after birth.
   d. risk of developing obesity and type 2 DM later in life.
   e. all of the above.

10. Signs and symptoms of diabetic ketoacidosis include
    a. decreased alertness and headache.
    b. nausea, vomiting, abdominal pain, and dry mouth.
    c. muscle aches, flushed face, and frequent urination.
    d. fruity-smelling breath.
    e. all of the above.

K. The Medical Assistant's Role with Examinations, Diagnostic Procedures, and Treatments

Match the description with the correct diagnostic modality and laboratory test.

1. _____ Uses a radioactive iodine tracer to measure the uptake of iodine in the thyroid

2. _____ Measures the amount of ketones in the urine sample; some CLIA-waived tests are available

3. _____ Uses a radioactive iodine tracer to examine the thyroid gland

4. _____ Measures the amount of glucose in the urine sample; some CLIA-waived tests are available

5. _____ Used to evaluate the thyroid function; some CLIA-waived tests are available

6. _____ Measures the glucose level in the blood after fasting; some CLIA-waived tests are available

7. _____ Measures the glucose level in the blood without fasting; some CLIA-waived tests are available

8. _____ Measures the average blood glucose level over the past 3 months; some CLIA-waived tests are available

a. thyroid scan
b. radioactive iodine uptake scan
c. HbA_{1c} test
d. fasting blood glucose test
e. urine glucose test
f. urine ketone test
g. random blood glucose test
h. thyroid function tests

Match the medical term with the correct description.

9. _____ Surgical removal of part or all of the thyroid gland

10. _____ Surgical removal of one or more of the parathyroid glands

11. _____ Surgical removal of one or both of the adrenal glands

12. _____ Surgical removal of the pituitary gland

13. _____ Surgical removal of part or all of the pancreas

a. adrenalectomy
b. hypophysectomy
c. pancreatectomy
d. parathyroidectomy
e. thyroidectomy

Match the indication for use and desired effect with the correct medication classification.

14. _____ Maintains adequate hormone levels by replacing thyroid hormone or compensating for hormone deficiency

15. _____ Treats Type 1 and Type 2 DM by replacing insulin, which lowers the blood glucose level

16. _____ Manages DM by reducing blood glucose level

17. _____ Maintains adequate hormone levels by replacing ADH hormone or compensating for hormone deficiency

a. antihyperglycemics
b. insulin
c. thyroid hormone
d. vasopressin

Match the side effects and adverse reactions with the correct medication classification.

18. _____ Weight loss, tremor, headache, chest pain, and arrhythmias

19. _____ Restlessness, seizures, hallucinations, slowed reflexes, and tiredness

20. _____ Shortness of breath, blurred vision, tachycardia, sweating, weakness, muscle cramps, arrhythmias, and other hypoglycemic symptoms

21. _____ Hot flashes, decreased sex drive, nausea, and vomiting

22. _____ GI irritation, fatigue, hypoglycemia, vertigo; possible hypersensitivity reaction

a. antihyperglycemics
b. estrogen
c. insulin
d. thyroid hormone
e. vasopressin

CERTIFICATION PREPARATION

Circle the correct answer.

1. Which is *not* an endocrine gland?
   a. Thymus
   b. Thyroid
   c. Spleen
   d. Pancreas

2. Which hormone is produced by the anterior pituitary gland?
   a. Testosterone
   b. Follicle-stimulating hormone
   c. Cortisol
   d. Melatonin

3. What specific cells of the pancreas produce insulin?
   a. Beta islet cells
   b. Alpha islet cells
   c. Adrenal cortex cells
   d. Both a and b

4. Which is a CLIA-waived test?
   a. A1c
   b. Fasting blood glucose
   c. Ketones urine test
   d. All of the above

5. Which gland is located in the brain?
   a. Adrenal gland
   b. Parathyroid gland
   c. Pineal gland
   d. Thymus

6. The pancreas is located in which body cavity?
   a. Thoracic cavity
   b. Pelvic cavity
   c. Abdominal cavity
   d. None of the above

7. Which could be a sign or symptom of a Type 2 DM?
   a. Polydipsia
   b. Night sweats
   c. Polyuria
   d. Both a and c

8. Gestational diabetes is more common in women with
   a. history of prediabetes.
   b. being overweight.
   c. being younger than 25 years of age.
   d. both a and b.

9. Hyperparathyroidism causes blood calcium levels to
   a. increase.
   b. decrease.
   c. stay the same.
   d. parathyroid hormone does not affect blood calcium.

10. Which condition would most likely be diagnosed in an older adult patient?
    a. Type 1 DM
    b. Gigantism
    c. Type 2 DM
    d. Gestational diabetes

WORKPLACE APPLICATIONS

1. Lexie greets her patient, Mr. Ironsides, and takes him back to the exam room. Mr. Ironsides is coming in for a follow-up visit for his Type 2 DM. Once vital signs are completed, Lexie checks his fasting blood glucose. His blood glucose is 122 mg/dL. Is Mr. Ironsides' 122 mg/dL blood glucose within the normal range? Explain your answer.

   _____

   _____

2. Lexie is reviewing endocrine diseases and disorders as part of a continuing education course. Briefly define the following endocrine disorders.

   a. Gigantism _____

   _____

   b. Growth hormone deficiency _____

   _____

   c. Cretinism_____

   _____

   d. Myxedema _____

   _____

   e. Hashimoto thyroiditis_____

   _____

3. Lisa Tenivoldi has been diagnosed with hyperthyroidism. What are the possible causes of hyperthyroidism?

   _____

   _____

INTERNET ACTIVITIES

1. Using online resources, research a test used for diagnosing an endocrine system disease. Create a poster presentation, a PowerPoint presentation, or a written paper summarizing your research. Include the following points in your project:
   a. Description of the test
   b. Any contraindications for the test
   c. Patient preparation for the test
   d. What occurs during the test

2. Using online resources, research an endocrine system disease or disorder. Create a poster presentation, a PowerPoint presentation, or a written paper summarizing your research. Include the following points in your project:
   a. Description of the disease
   b. Etiology
   c. Signs and symptoms
   d. Diagnostic procedures
   e. Treatments

3. Using online resources, research the effect that diet can have on the management of Type II DM. In a one-page paper, summarize the information that you found.

4. Using Table 39.6, Medication Classifications, select one medication from each of the following classifications: antihyperglycemics, estrogen, insulin, and thyroid hormone. Using a reliable online drug resource, identify for each medication:
   a. Indication for use
   b. Desired effects
   c. Side effects
   d. Adverse reactions
   Write a short paper addressing each of these four areas for each medication.

Procedure 39.1 Perform a Monofilament Foot Exam

Name _____ Date _____ Score _____

Tasks: Perform a monofilament foot exam to screen for peripheral neuropathy. Provide health maintenance coaching by giving the patient foot care instructions. Document test results in the patient's health record.

Equipment and Supplies:
- 10 g monofilament tool
- Gloves
- Paper towel
- Provider's order or standing order
- Patient's health record

Standing Order: For all patients with diabetes:
- Monofilament foot exam bilateral for all physical exam appointments.
- Coach patient on foot care.

Standard: Complete the procedure and all critical steps in _____ minutes with a minimum score of 85% within two attempts (*or as indicated by the instructor*).

Scoring: Divide the points earned by the total possible points. Failure to perform a critical step, indicated by an asterisk (*), results in grade no higher than an 84% (*or as indicated by the instructor*).

Time: Began_____ Ended_____ Total minutes: _____

Steps:	Point Value	Attempt 1	Attempt 2
1. Wash hands or use hand sanitizer.	5		
2. Read the provider's order. Assemble equipment.	5		
3. Greet the patient. Identify yourself. Verify the patient's identity with full name and date of birth. Explain the procedure to be performed in a manner that is understood by the patient. Answer any questions the patient may have on the procedure.	10		
4. Ask the patient to remove socks and shoes and rest the feet on the paper towel. The paper towel should be placed under the person's feet either on the floor or on the exam table step.	10		
5. Using your hand, demonstrate that the monofilament is flexible and not sharp. Also demonstrate the monofilament on the patient's hand. Put gloves on.	10		
6. Instruct the patient to close their eyes. Tell the patient to say "yes" when they feel the monofilament on the foot.	10		
7. Start with the great toe and place the monofilament perpendicular to the skin. Press the monofilament until it bends, hold for 1 second, and release. Pause to give the patient an opportunity to confirm it was felt. A confirmation is a positive or normal response. The test result is abnormal if the patient cannot feel in one area.	10		

8.	Do not cue the patient if no confirmation is given. Just move to the next location. Randomly test 9 to 12 locations on the anterior and posterior side of each foot or as the provider indicates. If a patient does not feel the site, check it three times randomly. Make sure to space out testing times (e.g., the time between each check).	**15**		
9.	Discard supplies in waste container. Remove gloves and wash hands or use hand sanitizer.	**5**		
10.	Coach the patient on proper foot care to prevent sores. Include when to check the feet, what to look for, and how to care for the feet daily. Suspicious areas need to be watched carefully and reported to the provider if they do not return to normal.	**10***		
11.	Document the test results in the patient's health record. Include the provider's name, the order, and the results of the test. For the test, the first number indicates the total number of sites felt, and the last number indicates the total times done. Indicate all sites where the patient did not feel the test. If the provider indicates specific areas to test, documentation should reflect these areas. Include any teaching done.	**10***		
	Total Points	**100**		

Documentation

Comments

CAAHEP Competencies	Step(s)
V.P.3.b. Coach patients regarding: medical encounters	6, 10
X.P.3. Document patient care accurately in the medical record	11
ABHES Competencies	**Step(s)**
8. Clinical Procedures d. Assist provider with specialty examination, including cardiac, respiratory, OB-GYN, neurological, and gastroenterology procedures.	Entire procedure
e. Perform specialty procedures, including but not limited to minor surgery, cardiac, respiratory, OB-GYN, neurological, and gastroenterology.	Entire procedure

Cardiology

CAAHEP Competencies	Assessment
I.C.4. Identify major organs in each body system	Skills and Concepts – B. 2-3, D. 12-20; Certification Preparation – 1
I.C.5. Identify the anatomical location of major organs in each body system	Skills and Concepts – B. 4-5; Certification Preparation – 2
I.C.6. Identify structure and function of the human body across the life span	Skills and Concepts – C. 8-11, G. 1-5; Certification Preparation – 6
I.C.7. Identify the normal function of each body system	Skills and Concepts – B. 1. 15-17, C. 1-7, 9-11, E. 1-8, F. 1-9; Certification Preparation – 3-5, 7-8
I.C.8.a. Identify common pathology related to each body system including: signs	Skills and Concepts – G. 6, 8-10, 13-14, H. 18-21, J. 10-12, K. 1-6; Internet Activities – 2-3
I.C.8.b. Identify common pathology related to each body system including: symptoms	Skills and Concepts – G. 7, 11-12, H. 18-21, J. 10-12; Internet Activities – 2-3
I.C.8.c. Identify common pathology related to each body system including: etiology	Skills and Concepts – H. 14-17, J. 7-9; Internet Activities – 2
I.C.8.d. Identify common pathology related to each body system including: diagnostic measures	Skills and Concepts – H. 22-25, J. 13-15. L. 1-5; Certification Preparation – 10; Internet Activities – 1-2
I.C.8.e. Identify common pathology related to each body system including: treatment modalities	Skills and Concepts – H. 22-25, J. 13-15, L. 6-21; Certification Preparation – 9; Workplace Applications – 1; Internet Activities – 2-4
1.C.9. Identify Clinical Laboratory Improvement Amendments (CLIA) waived tests associated with common diseases	Skills and Concepts – L. 3, 5; Certification Preparation – 10
I.C.10.a. Identify the classifications of medications, including indications for use	Skills and Concepts – L. 6-13; Internet Activities – 4
I.C.10.b. Identify the classifications of medications, including desired effects	Skills and Concepts – L. 6-13; Internet Activities – 4
I.C.10.c. Identify the classifications of medications, including side effects	Skills and Concepts – L. 14-21; Internet Activities – 4
I.C.10.d. Identify the classifications of medications, including adverse reactions	Skills and Concepts – L. 14-21; Internet Activities – 4
V.C.8.a. Identify the following related to body systems: medical terms	Skills and Concepts – G. 6-14, K. 1-6

CAAHEP Competencies	Assessment
V.C.8.b. Identify the following related to body systems: abbreviations	Abbreviations – 1-27
I.P.1.a. Accurately measure and record: blood pressure	Procedure 40.1
I.P.1.c. Accurately measure and record: pulse	Procedure 40.1
I.P.8. Instruct and prepare a patient for a procedure or treatment	Procedure 40.1
X.P.3. Document patient care accurately in the medical record	Procedure 40.1

ABHES Competencies	Assessment
2. Anatomy and Physiology a. List all body systems and their structures and functions	Skills and Concepts – B. 1-5, 15-17, C. 1-7, 9-11, D. 12-20, E. 1-8, F. 1-9; Certification Preparation – 1, 3-5, 7-8
2.b. Describe common diseases, symptoms, and etiologies as they apply to each system	Skills and Concepts – H. 1-21, I. 1-6, J. 1-12, K. 1-17; Workplace Applications – 2-3; Internet Activities – 2-3
2.c. Identify diagnostic and treatment modalities as they relate to each body system	Skills and Concepts – H. 22-25, J. 13-15, Certification Preparation – 7-10; Workplace Application – 2; Internet Activities – 1-4
3. Medical Terminology c. Apply medical terminology for each specialty	Skills and Concepts – G. 6-14, K. 1-6
3. d. Define and use medical abbreviations when appropriate and acceptable	Abbreviations – 1-27
4. Medical Law and Ethics a. Follow documentation guidelines	Procedure 40.1
8. Clinical Procedures d. Assist provider with specialty examination, including cardiac, respiratory, OB-GYN, neurological, and gastroenterology procedures.	Procedure 40.1
8.e. Perform specialty procedures, including but not limited to minor surgery, cardiac, respiratory, OB-GYN, neurological, and gastroenterology.	Procedure 40.1

VOCABULARY REVIEW

Using the word pool on the right, find the correct word to match the definition. Write the word on the line after the definition.

Group A

1. Strong, stretchy, thick-walled vessels that carry blood from the heart _____

2. Thin-walled vessels that allow for exchange of substances _____

3. Collect blood from the venules and return blood to the heart _____

4. Smaller arteries that move blood to the capillaries _____

5. Pointed tip _____

6. Collect blood from capillaries _____

7. Area of the chest wall anterior to the heart and lower thorax _____

8. Oxygen-deficient _____

9. Tendon-like cords that attach the papillary muscle to the heart valve _____

10. Another name for the cardiovascular system _____

Word Pool
- apex
- arteries
- arterioles
- capillaries
- chordae tendineae
- circulatory system
- deoxygenated
- precordium
- veins
- venules

Group B

1. A simple sugar that is absorbed by the intestines and found in the blood _____

2. A liquid that is able to dissolve other substances _____

3. High blood pressure _____

4. Undifferentiated cells that can become specialized cells in the body _____

5. The process of changing a liquid to a solid _____

6. The cells create and discharge the electrical impulse _____

7. The cells respond to the electrical impulse _____

8. The cells transmit electrical impulses to other cells _____

9. Curved inward on both sides _____

10. Complete heartbeat _____

Word Pool
- automaticity
- biconcave
- cardiac cycle
- coagulation
- conductivity
- excitability
- glucose
- hypertension
- solvent
- stem cells
- coagulation

Group C

1. Amount of blood that is pushed out of the left ventricle compared to the total volume of blood that filled the ventricle

   _____

2. Resistance to flow _____

3. Inner opening of arteries _____

4. A condition caused by an abnormally large number of RBCs in the blood _____

5. Tissue death _____

6. An air bubble, blood clot, or foreign body that travels through the bloodstream and blocks a blood vessel _____

7. Inflammatory condition of a valve that results in valve stenosis and obstructed blood flow _____

8. A blood clot that blocks the flow of the blood

   _____

9. A waxy lesion made up of cholesterol, fat, calcium, cells, and other substances that builds up on the inner wall of an artery

   _____

10. Excessive fluid in the intercellular spaces in the tissue; when external pressure (e.g., socks, finger pressure) is relieved, a depression is seen in the tissue _____

11. Occurs when the heart valve flaps are stiff or fused together, thus narrowing the valve _____

12. The valve does not close completely and allows blood to leak backward across the valve into the prior chamber

    _____

Word Pool
- atheroma
- embolus
- infarction
- insufficiency
- lumen
- pitting edema
- polycythemia
- stenosis
- stroke volume
- thrombus
- valvulitis
- viscosity

ABBREVIATIONS

Write out what each of the following abbreviations stands for.

1. RBC _____

2. SA node _____

3. BP _____

4. SOB _____

5. CABG _____

6. CHF _____

7. CAD _____

8. DVT _____

9. PE _____

10. CBC _____

11. MI _____

12. CPK _____

13. PT _____

14. POTS _____

15. HDL _____

16. CTA _____

17. TEE _____

18. LDL _____

19. ICD _____

20. CHD _____

21. PAD _____

22. ASD _____

23. PFO _____

24. PDA _____

25. CLL _____

26. CML _____

27. LDH _____

SKILLS AND CONCEPTS

Answer the following questions. Write your answer on the line or in the space provided.

A. Introduction

Match the description with the correct term.

1. _____ A physician who specializes in internal medicine and hematology
2. _____ A physician who specializes in vascular diseases
3. _____ A physician who specializes in internal medicine and cardiology
4. _____ A physician who specializes in surgical procedures involving the lungs, heart, esophagus, and other organs in the chest
5. _____ The healthcare specialty that deals with cardiovascular diseases and disorders
6. _____ The branch of medicine that focuses on the diagnosis and treatment of diseases related to blood and blood-forming organs

a. cardiology
b. hematology
c. cardiologist
d. vascular surgeon
e. cardiothoracic surgeon
f. hematologist

B. Anatomy of the Cardiovascular System

Select the correct answer or fill in the blank.

1. The cardiovascular system
   a. brings oxygen, nutrients, salts, and hormones to the cells.
   b. carries wastes away from the cells.
   c. secretes hormones to help with homeostasis.
   d. all of the above.
   e. a and b.

2. The cardiovascular system includes
   a. blood vessels.
   b. the heart.
   c. the blood.
   d. all of the above.

3. When tracing the blood leaving the heart to the blood returning to the heart, which of the following is the correct order for blood vessels?
   a. Arterioles, arteries, capillaries, veins, venules
   b. Arterioles, capillaries, arteries, veins, venules
   c. Arteries, arterioles, capillaries, venules, veins
   d. Arteries, arterioles, capillaries, veins, venules
   e. Arterioles, arteries, capillaries, venules, veins

4. The heart is located in the mediastinum of the thoracic cavity, slightly left of the midline. The apex of the heart rests just above the diaphragm.
   a. Both statements are correct.
   b. Both statements are incorrect.
   c. The first statement is correct, but the second statement is incorrect.
   d. The first statement is incorrect, but the second statement is correct.

5. The _____ is the space in the thoracic cavity that lies between the lungs, containing the heart, trachea, and esophagus.

6. The two upper chambers of the heart are called _____ and the _____ are the lower chambers.

7. The _____ is the thick muscular wall that divides the heart into right and left sections.

8. The _____ is the inner layer of the heart, the _____ is the middle layer, and the epicardium is the outer layer.

9. The _____ valves are found between each atrium and ventricle.

10. _____ is the AV valve located between the right atrium and ventricle.

11. _____ or mitral valve is the AV valve located between the left atrium and ventricle.

12. _____ is the SL valve located between the left ventricle and the aorta.

13. _____ is the SL valve located between the right ventricle and the pulmonary artery.

14. _____, or "leaky" valves, do not close completely and allow blood to leak backward into the prior chamber.

15. A complete heartbeat or _____ can be divided into the diastole and systole phases.

16. During the _____ phase, the heart is at rest and the atria fill with blood.

17. The _____ phase occurs when the heart is contracting.

C. Anatomy of the Blood Flow
Match the description with the correct type of circulation.

1. _____ Blood flows through the heart tissues.

2. _____ Oxygenated blood is pumped from the left side of the heart, moves through the body, and returns to the heart.

3. _____ Blood flow of a baby in utero.

4. _____ Deoxygenated blood is pumped from the right side of the heart to the lungs and returns to the heart.

5. _____ Veins from the spleen, gallbladder, pancreas, stomach, and intestines dump the blood into the hepatic portal vein, which takes the blood to the liver. Eventually, the blood drains into the hepatic veins before emptying into the inferior vena cava.

a. pulmonary circulation
b. systemic circulation
c. coronary circulation
d. fetal circulation
e. hepatic portal circulation

Fill in the blank or select the correct answer.

6. The right and left _____ arteries are the first branches off the ascending aorta bring nutrients and oxygen to the heart tissue.

7. The advantage of the hepatic portal system includes
   a. the glucose absorbed can be filtered and stored in the liver as glycogen.
   b. toxic substances can be partially filtered before moving to the rest of the body.
   c. all of the above.

8. The _____ contains two umbilical arteries and one umbilical vein.

9. The _____ shifts the majority of the blood from the umbilical vein and empties it into the inferior vena cava, bypassing the liver.

10. The _____, a small flaplike opening in the interatrial septum, allows blood to move from the right atrium to the left atrium, bypassing the immature lungs.

11. The _____ is a short vessel that connects the pulmonary artery with the aorta, bypassing the immature lungs.

D. Anatomy of the Blood

Match the description with the correct term.

1. _____ Clump together
2. _____ Controlling the blood flow
3. _____ Include fibrinogen and prothrombin, which are important in the coagulation process
4. _____ Liquid portion of the blood
5. _____ Proteins produced by cells in the immune system in response to a specific antigen
6. _____ Special proteins that speed up a chemical reaction in the body
7. _____ Most abundant protein in the plasma; normally stays in the blood vessel and attracts water
8. _____ Undifferentiated cells that can become specialized cells in the body
9. _____ Another name for platelets
10. _____ A liquid that can dissolve other substances
11. _____ Plasma and the formed elements of blood in a free-flowing liquid form

a. plasma
b. albumin
c. clotting factors
d. antibodies
e. enzymes
f. thrombocytes
g. stem cells
h. agglutinate
i. hemostasis
j. solvent
k. whole blood

Match the description with the correct term.

12. _____ Another name for white blood cells
13. _____ Jellylike substance that surrounds the nucleus and fills the cells
14. _____ Have granules within the cytoplasm and include neutrophils, eosinophils, and basophils
15. _____ Lack granules in the cytoplasm and include monocytes and lymphocytes
16. _____ Include T cells and B cells; involved in the immune response and destroy pathogens
17. _____ The type of WBCs that respond to an allergic reaction by releasing histamine
18. _____ Very aggressive phagocytic cells; transform into macrophages when in lymphatic tissue
19. _____ The most abundant white blood cells; phagocytic
20. _____ The type of WBCs that increase in number when the body is defending against allergens and parasites

a. leukocytes
b. granulocytes
c. agranulocytes
d. cytoplasm
e. neutrophils
f. eosinophils
g. basophils
h. lymphocytes
i. monocytes

Match the description with the correct term.

21. _____ Another name for red blood cells

22. _____ A reddish-yellow pigment that results from the breakdown of red blood cells in the liver

23. _____ The formation of blood cells

24. _____ A hormone produced in the kidneys that stimulates the production of RBCs

25. _____ A molecule on the RBC capable of binding, transporting, and releasing oxygen and carbon dioxide

26. _____ Substances on the surface of cells, viruses, bacteria, fungi, and nonliving substances

a. erythrocytes
b. hemoglobin
c. hematopoiesis
d. erythropoietin
e. bilirubin
f. antigens

Fill in the blank.

27. Red blood cells have a life span of approximately _____ days.

28. RBCs are broken down in the _____ and the iron is mainly stored in the _____ and recycled into new RBCs.

29. Type _____ blood contains A antigen and B antibodies and can receive Type A and O blood.

30. Type _____ blood contains A and B antibodies and can receive Type O blood.

31. Type _____ blood contains B antigen and A antibodies and can receive Type B and O blood.

32. Type _____ blood contains A and B antigens and can receive Type A, B, AB, and O blood.

33. Type _____ blood is considered the universal recipient.

34. Type _____ blood is considered the universal donor.

E. Physiology of the Conduction System
Match the description with the correct term.

1. _____ Final conduction system structure; transmit the impulse quickly and efficiently to the ventricular myocardial cells

2. _____ Called the "pacemaker of the heart"

3. _____ Fourth conduction system structure; located in the lower interventricular septum

4. _____ Second conduction system structure; located at the base of the interatrial septum

5. _____ Third conduction system structure; also called the *atrioventricular (AV) bundle* and is located in the upper interventricular septum

6. _____ The "waiting" stage of the cardiac cell cycle

7. _____ The cardiac cell cycle stage when the impulse hits the cell

8. _____ The "recovery" stage of the cardiac cell cycle

a. atrioventricular (AV) node
b. right and left bundle branches
c. bundle of His
d. sinoatrial (SA) node
e. Purkinje fibers
f. depolarized state
g. polarized state
h. repolarized state

F. Physiology of the Blood

Fill in the blank or select the correct answer.

1. Which is correct regarding the coagulation process?
    a. A platelet plug is formed over the injury.
    b. Platelets release clotting factors.
    c. Fibrin is formed and traps RBCs.
    d. All of the above.

2. _____ can be defined as the resulting force of blood against the walls of the arteries.

3. _____ pressure is measured when the heart is contracting and pumping out the blood.

4. _____ pressure is measured when the heart is resting between contractions.

5. _____, or the amount of circulating blood, has a direct influence on blood pressure.

6. Which is correct regarding the blood volume?
    a. Blood, plasma, and intravenous transfusions increase blood volume and the blood pressure.
    b. Increased sodium increases the blood volume and the blood pressure.
    c. Hemorrhaging, dehydration, and diuretic medications can decrease the blood volume and the blood pressure.
    d. All of the above.
    e. Both a and b.

7. The greater the force of the contraction, the more blood is pumped into the arteries, which _____ the blood pressure.

8. What factors affect the blood pressure?
    a. Blood volume
    b. Strength of ventricular contraction
    c. Resistance to blood flow
    d. All of the above

9. Which factor increases the blood pressure?
    a. Narrowed arterial lumen
    b. Loss of vessel elasticity due to aging and plaque
    c. Increased blood viscosity
    d. All of the above

G. Life Span Changes of the Cardiovascular System

Fill in the blank or select the correct answer.

1. As a child grows and matures, the heart rate _____.

2. The resistance for blood flow decreases with age. The blood pressure increases with age.
    a. Both statements are correct.
    b. Both statements are incorrect.
    c. The first statement is correct, and the last statement is incorrect.
    d. The first statement is incorrect, and the last statement is correct.

3. Which change occurs with pregnancy?
   a. The cardiac input decreases.
   b. Extracellular fluid volume increases, thus increasing the blood volume.
   c. Total peripheral resistance increases, thus reducing the blood pressure.
   d. Blood pressure decreases in the third trimester.
   e. All of the above.

4. Which change occurs in older adults?
   a. SA node loses some cells.
   b. The left ventricle may increase in size, thus reducing the amount of blood it can hold.
   c. Normal ECG changes can occur with age.
   d. Valves can become thicker and stiffer, causing a heart murmur.
   e. All of the above.

5. With age, the baroreceptors become less sensitive, making older people more at risk for _____ when changing positions.

Match the description with the correct sign or symptom.

6. _____ A bluish discoloration of the skin, lips, and nail beds
7. _____ Difficulty breathing
8. _____ A pulse greater than 100 bpm
9. _____ Fainting or loss of consciousness and postural tone caused by diminished blood flow to the brain.
10. _____ Profuse sweating
11. _____ Breathlessness
12. _____ Chest pain
13. _____ A pulse less than 60 beats per minute
14. _____ Fast, strong, or irregular heartbeats

a. angina pectoris
b. palpitations
c. bradycardia
d. tachycardia
e. cyanosis
f. diaphoresis
g. dyspnea
h. shortness of breath
i. syncope

H. Heart Diseases and Disorders
Match the description with the correct disease.

1. _____ Also called *heart failure*; occurs when the heart does not efficiently pump blood
2. _____ The blood flow is limited or blocked, and the heart muscle cells die due to the lack of oxygen
3. _____ An abnormal heart rate or rhythm
4. _____ The heart muscle becomes abnormal; thin and weakened, enlarged and thick, or rigid
5. _____ Ductus arteriosus does not close soon after birth, causing too much blood to move into the pulmonary circulation
6. _____ A congenital defect that causes a narrowing of the aorta, resulting in blood flowing back into the left ventricle, high blood pressure, and weakened pulses in the legs
7. _____ A congenital defect caused by a hole in the interatrial septum allows oxygen-rich blood from the left atrium to flow into the right atrium

a. arrhythmias
b. cardiomyopathy
c. congestive heart failure
d. myocardial infarction
e. atrial septal defect
f. coarctation of the aorta
g. patent foramen ovale
h. patent ductus arteriosus
i. mitral valve prolapse
j. aortic insufficiency
k. pericarditis
l. metabolic syndrome
m. rheumatic fever

8. _____ Foramen ovale does not close during infancy but remains patent

9. _____ The aortic valve does not close tightly, and blood backs up into the left ventricle

10. _____ Occurs when one or both cusps of the mitral valve protrude back into the left atrium during ventricular systole

11. _____ An inflammatory reaction that affects the heart valves (valvulitis) and causes swelling and scarring of the valves

12. _____ A group of factors that increase a person's risk for heart disease, type 2 diabetes, and stroke

13. _____ Inflammation of the pericardium

Match the etiology with the correct disease.

14. _____ Caused by coronary artery disease, high blood pressure, congenital problems, heart attack, faulty valves, arrhythmias, and infections

15. _____ Caused by an issue with the heart's conduction system from diseases, stress, substances, and electrolyte imbalance

16. _____ A result of other diseases or can be inherited

17. _____ Caused by a blood clot or plaque buildup in the coronary arteries

a. arrhythmias
b. cardiomyopathy
c. congestive heart failure
d. myocardial infarction

Match the signs and symptoms with the correct disease.

18. _____ SOB especially after activity; edema in the legs, feet, ankles, abdomen; distention of neck veins; and fatigue

19. _____ Angina pectoris, upper body discomfort, SOB, cold sweats, tiredness without a reason, nausea and vomiting, dizziness, lightheadedness, arrhythmias, and palpitations

20. _____ Cough, SOB with reclining or activity, fatigue, faintness, weakness, loss of appetite, palpitations, pitting edema in the feet and legs, swollen liver and abdomen, and weight gain

21. _____ Fast or slow heart rate; irregular, skipping, or uneven heartbeats; lightheadedness, dizziness, SOB, pallor, angina, sweating

a. arrhythmias
b. cardiomyopathy
c. congestive heart failure
d. myocardial infarction

Match the diagnostic measures and treatments with the correct disease.

22. _____ Echocardiography, imaging tests, and blood tests; treatment includes healthy lifestyle changes (limiting dietary cholesterol, salts, and fluids), medications, a pacemaker, an implantable defibrillator, or heart transplantation

23. _____ Chest x-ray, an ECG, ECHO, a stress test, cardiac catheterization, coronary angiography, or myocardial biopsy; treated with healthy lifestyle changes, medications, surgery, a heart transplantation, and an implanted device

24. _____ ECG, heart monitoring, ECHO, coronary angiography, and an electrophysiology study; treatment may include defibrillation, antiarrhythmic medications, and cardiac ablation

25. _____ ECG and blood tests (i.e., troponin, creatine kinase, creatine kinase–MB, and serum myoglobin tests); treated with aspirin, nitroglycerin, oxygen therapy, and thrombolytic medications

a. arrhythmias
b. cardiomyopathy
c. congestive heart failure
d. myocardial infarction

I. Blood Vessel Diseases and Disorders
Match the description with the correct disease.

1. _____ A bulging of the arterial wall that can burst, causing bleeding and possible death of the blood vessel wall

2. _____ With cold temperatures or stress, the blood vessels narrow, and blood cannot get to the surface of the skin of the toes and fingers

3. _____ Swollen, twisted veins seen under the skin, usually in the legs or rectum

4. _____ Enlarged veins in the esophagus that can rupture

5. _____ A condition in which plaque buildup narrows the arteries

6. _____ Occurs when a thrombus forms in a vein deep in the body, usually in the legs

a. deep vein thrombosis
b. varicose veins
c. aneurysm
d. esophageal varices
e. Raynaud disease
f. atherosclerosis

J. Blood Pressure Related Diseases and Disorders
Match the description with the correct disease.

1. _____ Occurs when there is not enough blood and oxygen getting to the organs and tissues

2. _____ Lower than normal blood pressure

3. _____ Also called *essential hypertension*; most common type with no identifiable cause

4. _____ An abnormal condition of the autonomic nervous system; the ANS does not control the blood pressure or heart rate when a person is standing up

5. _____ Very high blood pressure that causes organ damage

6. _____ High blood pressure is caused by another disease, condition, or medication

a. primary hypertension
b. secondary hypertension
c. hypotension
d. postural orthostatic tachycardia syndrome
e. shock
f. malignant hypertension

Match the etiology with the correct disease.

7. _____ The cause is unknown

8. _____ Caused by severe allergic reaction, heart attack, hemorrhage, neurologic injury or disorder, and an overwhelming infection

9. _____ Caused by genetics, environmental factors, kidney fluid and salt balance, and changes in blood vessels

a. hypertension
b. postural orthostatic tachycardia syndrome
c. shock

Match the signs and symptoms with the correct disease.

10. _____ Hypovolemia, tachycardia, hypotension, fatigue, exercise intolerance, lightheadedness, blurred vision, syncope, and heart palpitations

11. _____ A high blood pressure reading

12. _____ Weak, rapid pulse and rapid, shallow respirations, changes in the level of consciousness, dizziness, lightheadedness, faintness, sweaty pale skin, cool hands and feet, bluish lips and fingernails, and reduced or no urine output

a. hypertension
b. postural orthostatic tachycardia syndrome
c. shock

Match the diagnostic measures and treatments with the correct disease.

13. _____ Diagnosed based on the history, exam, and vital signs of the patient; treated by increasing the cardiac output and blood pressure with medications, blood transfusions, and IV fluids

14. _____ Diagnostic testing includes tilt table test and orthostatic vital signs; treatment includes heart and blood pressure medications, fluids, a high-salt low-carbohydrate diet, exercise; and compression stockings

15. _____ Diagnosed by high blood pressure readings; treatment involves a low-salt or heart-healthy diet, maintaining a healthy weight, stopping smoking, exercise, and limiting alcohol intake

a. hypertension
b. postural orthostatic tachycardia syndrome
c. shock

K. Blood Diseases and Disorders

Match the description with the correct sign or symptom.

1. _____ A deficiency of RBCs

2. _____ A deficiency of platelets

3. _____ An elevated number of RBCs

4. _____ A deficiency in WBCs

5. _____ An elevated number of platelets

6. _____ An elevated number of WBCs

a. leukopenia
b. leukocytosis
c. anemia
d. erythrocytosis
e. thrombocytopenia
f. thrombocytosis

Match the description with the correct disease.

7. _____ A rare autoimmune disease that results in the destruction of platelets

8. _____ A cancer of the blood-forming tissues, such as the bone marrow and the lymphatic system

9. _____ Most common cause of cancer in children; causes an increase in large, immature lymphocytes

10. _____ Genetic bleeding disorder that can lead to spontaneous bleeding

11. _____ Most common type of acute leukemia in adults; causes an elevated level of myeloblasts

12. _____ A type of vitamin B$_{12}$–deficiency anemia

13. _____ Inherited disorder that causes the RBCs to form a sickle shape, get stuck in the blood vessels, and break apart

14. _____ Also described as *chronic granulocytic*; a slow-growing cancer that causes an increase in myeloblasts

15. _____ Most common form of anemia, treated with iron supplements

16. _____ A mismatch between the fetus and the mother involving the Rh factor causes the baby's blood to break down at a faster rate

17. _____ Second most common type of leukemia in adults; a slow-growing cancer that causes a gradual increase in B lymphocytes

a. hemophilia
b. idiopathic thrombocytopenic purpura
c. leukemia
d. iron-deficiency anemia
e. sickle cell anemia
f. pernicious anemia
g. acute lymphocytic leukemia
h. acute myeloid leukemia
i. chronic lymphocytic leukemia
j. chronic myeloid leukemia
k. hemolytic disease of the fetus and newborn

L. The Medical Assistant's Role with Examinations, Diagnostic Procedures, and Treatments

Match the description with the correct diagnostic modality and laboratory test.

1. _____ The catheter is inserted in an artery in the groin and threaded to the heart; a contrast medium is injected and narrowed or blocked arteries can be observed.

2. _____ Insulated electric catheters are threaded through a vein from the thigh to the heart; used to test the conduction system of the heart when a patient has arrhythmias.

3. _____ CLIA-waived blood test used to measure the cholesterol and triglycerides in the circulating blood.

4. _____ A sonographic test that uses sound waves to create pictures of the heart structures.

5. _____ CLIA-waived test used to measure the number of seconds it takes a clot to form after reagents are added to the blood sample.

a. echocardiography
b. cardiac catheterization
c. electrophysiology study
d. lipid profile
e. prothrombin test

Match the indication for use and desired effect with the correct medication classification.

6. _____ Reduces low-density lipoprotein and triglycerides and increases high-density lipoprotein by preventing the absorption of cholesterol in the intestine

7. _____ Inhibits reabsorption of sodium and chloride in the kidneys; promotes excretion of excess fluid in the body, which increases urinary output and lowers the blood pressure

8. _____ Controls acute or chronic blood-clotting disorder; promotes formation of absorbable, artificial clot

9. _____ Reduces and controls the blood pressure

10. _____ Inhibits the function of platelets and is used for post-treatment of stroke, heart attack or angina

11. _____ Treats low neutrophil levels and anemia by promoting neutrophil and red blood cell production

12. _____ Treats arrhythmias by helping the heart work better and controls the heart rate

13. _____ Decreases blood clotting ability, thus prevents blood clots from forming

a. antiarrhythmic
b. anticoagulant
c. antihypertensive
d. antiplatelet
e. cholesterol-lowering agent
f. diuretic
g. hematopoietic
h. hemostatic

Match the side effects and adverse reactions with the correct medication classification.

14. _____ Arrhythmias, weight gain, difficulty breathing, swelling of hands and feet.

15. _____ Dehydration, muscle weakness, fatigue, electrolyte imbalance.

16. _____ GI distress, bleeding, weakness, or numbness

17. _____ GI discomfort, muscle pain and weakness, liver complications, hypersensitivity, cataracts, and myopathy

18. _____ Increased bleeding, blood irregularities, and hypersensitivity

19. _____ Hypersensitivity reactions, transient flushing, dizziness, and newborn hyperbilirubinemia

20. _____ Headache, vertigo, GI disturbances, rash, hypotension, and a nonproductive cough

21. _____ Pain in the arms and legs, bone pain, injection site reaction, headache, weight loss, and insomnia

a. antiarrhythmic
b. anticoagulant
c. antihypertensive
d. antiplatelet
e. cholesterol-lowering agent
f. diuretic
g. hematopoietic
h. hemostatic

CERTIFICATION PREPARATION
Circle the correct answer.

1. Which are components of the cardiovascular system?
   a. Blood
   b. Vessels
   c. Heart
   d. All of the above

2. What is the anatomic location of the heart?
   a. In the abdominal cavity, slightly left of the midline
   b. In the thoracic cavity, slightly left of the midline
   c. In the abdominal cavity, slightly right of the midline
   d. In the thoracic cavity, slightly right of the midline

3. What is the function of the cardiovascular system?
   a. Brings oxygen to the cells and carries carbon dioxide away from the cells
   b. Brings nutrients, water, and other substances (e.g., salts and hormones) to the cells
   c. Carries waste products (e.g., metabolic waste) away from the cells to be excreted
   d. All of the above

4. The pulmonary veins bring oxygenated blood back to the _____.
   a. left atrium
   b. left ventricle
   c. right atrium
   d. right ventricle

5. Which arteries bring oxygenated blood to the heart tissue?
   a. Pulmonary arteries
   b. Aorta
   c. Coronary arteries
   d. Carotid arteries

6. In unborn babies, which structure shifts most of the blood from the umbilical vein to the inferior vena cava, bypassing the immature liver?
   a. Foramen ovale
   b. Ductus arteriosus
   c. Ductus venosus
   d. Both b and c

7. Which conduction system structure is considered the pacemaker of the heart?
   a. Bundle of His (AV bundle)
   b. Right and left bundle branches
   c. Atrioventricular (AV) node
   d. Sinoatrial (SA) node

8. What factor influences blood pressure?
   a. Blood volume
   b. Ventricular contraction strength
   c. Resistance to blood flow
   d. All of the above

9. Which treatment procedure is used to destroy abnormal tissue that causes arrhythmias?
   a. Percutaneous transluminal coronary angioplasty
   b. Cardiac ablation
   c. Pericardiocentesis
   d. Left ventricular assist device

10. Which CLIA-waived test is used for anticoagulant therapy and heart disease?
    a. Cardiac enzymes test
    b. Cholesterol test
    c. Lipid profile
    d. Prothrombin test

WORKPLACE APPLICATIONS

1. Ken Thomas asked Lizzy how a low-sodium diet helps lower the blood pressure. How would you respond to this question?

   _____

   _____

2. You are working with a patient who was just diagnosed with tricuspid stenosis. The patient has a sibling with tricuspid insufficiency. She asks you to explain the difference between stenosis and insufficiency. Describe how you would explain the difference between these two conditions.

   _____

   _____

   _____

3. You are working with a patient who has a sibling that was just diagnosed with POTS. The patient asks you to explain this condition. Describe how you would explain POTS.

_____

_____

INTERNET ACTIVITIES

1. Using online resources, research a test used for diagnosing cardiovascular diseases. Create a poster presentation, a PowerPoint presentation, or write a paper summarizing your research. Include the following points in your project:
   a. Description of the test
   b. Any contraindications for the test
   c. Patient preparation for the test
   d. What occurs during the test

2. Using online resources, research a cardiovascular disease. Create a poster presentation, a PowerPoint presentation, or write a paper summarizing your research. Include the following points in your project:
   a. Description of the disease
   b. Etiology
   c. Signs and symptoms
   d. Diagnostic procedures
   e. Treatments

3. Using online resources, research right-sided heart failure and left-sided heart failure. In a one-page paper, describe each type of heart failure including the signs, symptoms, and possible treatments.

4. Using Table 40.12, Medication Classifications, select a generic medication from each of the following classifications: antiarrhythmic, anticoagulant, antihypertensive, antiplatelet, cholesterol-lowering agent, diuretic, hematopoietic, and hemostatic. Using a reliable online drug resource, identify for each medication:
   a. Reasons for use
   b. Desired effects
   c. Side effects
   d. Adverse reactions
   Write a short paper addressing each of these four areas for each medication.

Procedure 40.1   Measuring Orthostatic Vital Signs

Name _____   Date _____   Score _____

Tasks: Obtain orthostatic vital signs and document in the patient's health record.

Equipment and Supplies:
- Patient's health record
- Sphygmomanometer and stethoscope
- Watch with a second hand
- Alcohol wipes
- Exam table

Standard: Complete the procedure and all critical steps in _____ minutes with a minimum score of 85% within two attempts (*or as indicated by the instructor*).

Scoring: Divide the points earned by the total possible points. Failure to perform a critical step, indicated by an asterisk (*), results in grade no higher than an 84% (*or as indicated by the instructor*).

Time: Began_____ Ended_____ Total minutes: _____

Steps:	Point Value	Attempt 1	Attempt 2
1. Wash hands or use hand sanitizer.	5		
2. Assemble the equipment and supplies needed. Clean the earpieces and diaphragm of the stethoscope with alcohol wipes.	5		
3. Greet the patient. Identify yourself. Verify the patient's identity with full name and date of birth. Explain the procedure to be performed in a manner that the patient understands. Answer any questions the patient may have about the procedure.	10		
4. Help the patient lie comfortably in a supine position on the examination table. Pull out the table extender, if necessary, for them to rest their feet. Allow the patient to rest in this position for 5 minutes.	5		
5. Take the patient's pulse and blood pressure with the patient lying down. Do not remove the cuff from the arm.	10		
6. Help the patient into a sitting position and ask the patient if they are experiencing any dizziness, weakness, or visual changes with the position change. Watch for any change in skin coloring or in the patient's behavior.	10*		
7. Once the patient has been sitting for 1 minute, repeat the pulse and blood pressure. *Note:* If the patient has symptoms associated with the position change or if the sitting blood pressure is less than 90 systolic and/or 60 diastolic, have the patient lay back down and immediately notify the provider.	10*		
8. Assist the patient to stand. Ask the patient about dizziness, weakness, or visual changes associated with the position change. Note any change in the patient's appearance or behavior.	5*		
9. Immediately repeat the blood pressure and pulse readings after the patient has stood up.	10*		
10. Ask the patient to continue standing and repeat the pulse and blood pressure measurements after 3 minutes.	10*		

11. Clean the earpieces and the head of the stethoscope with an alcohol wipe and return both the cuff and the stethoscope to storage.	5			
12. Wash hands or use hand sanitizer.	5			
13. Clearly document each blood pressure and pulse reading along with the position and any symptoms the patient experienced in the patient's health record.	10			
Total Points	100			

Documentation

Comments

CAAHEP Competencies	Step(s)
I.P.1.a. Accurately measure and record: blood pressure	5, 7, 9
I.P.1.c. Accurately measure and record: pulse	5, 7, 9
I.P.8. Instruct and prepare a patient for a procedure or a treatment	3
X.P.3. Document patient care accurately in the medical record	13
ABHES Competencies	**Step(s)**
4. Medical Law and Ethics a. Follow documentation guidelines	13
8. Clinical Procedures d. Assist provider with specialty examination, including cardiac, respiratory, OB-GYN, neurological, and gastroenterology procedures.	Entire procedure
8.e. Perform specialty procedures, including but not limited to minor surgery, cardiac, respiratory, OB-GYN, neurological, and gastroenterology.	Entire procedure

Pulmonology

CAAHEP Competencies	Assessment
I.C.4. Identify major organs in each body system	Skills and Concepts – B. 5-11, C. 1-11; Certification Preparation – 1
I.C.5. Identify the anatomical location of major organs in each body system	Skills and Concepts – B. 6-7, 10-11, C. 6-7; Certification Preparation – 2
I.C.6. Identify structure and function of the human body across the life span	Skills and Concepts – E. 1-5; Certification Preparation – 8
I.C.7. Identify the normal function of each body system	Skills and Concepts – A. 3, B. 2, 5, D. 1-9; Certification Preparation – 3
I.C.8.a. Identify common pathology related to each body system including: signs	Skills and Concepts – F. 1-2, 9, G. 9-12, I. 14-18; Workplace Applications – 2; Internet Activities – 2
I.C.8.b. Identify common pathology related to each body system including: symptoms	Skills and Concepts – F. 3-8, 10-13, G. 9-12; Workplace Applications – 2; Internet Activities – 2
I.C.8.c. Identify common pathology related to each body system including: etiology	Skills and Concepts – G. 5-8, H. 2-3, I. 9-13; Certification Preparation – 7; Internet Activities – 2, 3
I.C.8.d. Identify common pathology related to each body system including: diagnostic measures	Skills and Concepts – G. 13-16, I. 19-23, J. 1-6; Certification Preparation – 4, 9; Workplace Application – 4; Internet Activities – 1-2
I.C.8.e. Identify common pathology related to each body system including: treatment modalities	Skills and Concepts – G. 13-16, H. 4-7, J. 7-13; Certification Preparation – 5-6, 10; Workplace Applications – 1; Internet Activities – 2, 4
1.C.9. Identify Clinical Laboratory Improvement Amendments (CLIA) waived tests associated with common diseases	Skills and Concepts – J. 6; Certification Preparation – 4
I.C.10.a. Identify the classifications of medications, including indications for use	Skills and Concepts – J. 7-13
I.C.10.b. Identify the classifications of medications, including desired effects	Skills and Concepts – J. 7-13
I.C.10.c. Identify the classifications of medications, including side effects	Skills and Concepts – J. 14-20
I.C.10.d. Identify the classifications of medications, including adverse reactions	Skills and Concepts – J. 14-20

CAAHEP Competencies	Assessment
V.C.8.a. Identify the following related to body systems: medical terms	Skills and Concepts – F. 1-13, H. 4-7
V.C.8.b. Identify the following related to body systems: abbreviations	Abbreviations – 1-34
I.P.2.d. Perform the following procedures: Pulmonary function testing	Procedures 41.1, 41.2
I.P.4.a. Verify the rules of medication administration: right patient	Procedure 41.3
I.P.4.b. Verify the rules of medication administration: right medication	Procedure 41.3
I.P.4.c. Verify the rules of medication administration: right dose	Procedure 41.3
I.P.4.d. Verify the rules of medication administration: right route	Procedure 41.3
I.P.4.e. Verify the rules of medication administration: right time	Procedure 41.3
I.P.4.f. Verify the rules of medication administration: right documentation	Procedure 41.3
I.P.8. Instruct and prepare a patient for a procedure or treatment	Procedures 41.1, 41.2, 41.3
X.P.3. Document patient care accurately in the medical record	Procedures 41.1, 41.2, 41.3, 41.4

ABHES Competencies	Assessment
2. Anatomy and Physiology a. List all body systems and their structures and functions	Skills and Concepts – B. 5-11, C. 1-11, E. 1-5; Certification Preparation – 1-2, 8
2.b. Describe common diseases, symptoms, and etiologies as they apply to each system	Skills and Concepts – F. 1-13, G. 1-12, 17, H. 1-3, I. 1-18; Workplace Applications – 2-3; Internet Activities – 2, 3
2.c. Identify diagnostic and treatment modalities as they relate to each body system	Skills and Concepts – G. 13-16, H. 4-7, J. 7-13; Internet Activities – 2, 4
3. Medical Terminology c. Apply medical terminology for each specialty	Skills and Concepts – F. 1-13, H. 4-7
3. d. Define and use medical abbreviations when appropriate and acceptable	Abbreviations – 1-34
4. Medical Law and Ethics a. Follow documentation guidelines	Procedures 41.1, 41.2, 41.3, 41.4
8. Clinical Procedures d. Assist provider with specialty examination, including cardiac, respiratory, OB-GYN, neurological, and gastroenterology procedures.	Procedures 41.1, 41.2
8. e. Perform specialty procedures, including but not limited to minor surgery, cardiac, respiratory, OB-GYN, neurological, and gastroenterology	Procedures 41.1, 41.2, 41.3, 41.4

VOCABULARY REVIEW

Using the word pool on the right, find the correct word to match the definition. Write the word on the line after the definition.

Group A

1. Insufficient oxygen in the blood _____
2. An increase in the depth of breathing _____
3. Hollow, air-filled cavities in the skull and facial bones; lighten the weight of the skull and increase the tone, or resonance, of speech

   _____
4. Stoppage of breathing _____
5. Exhaling _____
6. Inhaling _____
7. Greater-than-normal level of carbon dioxide in the blood

   _____
8. Muscles located between the ribs that help with quiet respiration

   _____
9. Muscles in the neck, abdomen, and back that assist in breathing

   _____
10. Temporary absence of breathing _____

Word Pool
- apnea
- accessory muscle
- expiration
- hypercapnia
- hyperpnea
- hypoxemia
- inspiration
- intercostal muscles
- paranasal sinuses
- respiratory arrest

Group B

1. Abnormal enlargement of the distal phalanges associated with chronic tissue hypoxia due to cyanotic heart disease or advanced chronic pulmonary disease _____
2. A group of steroid hormones produced in the body or given as a medication _____
3. A cough that produces phlegm or mucus

   _____
4. A drug that relaxes smooth muscle contractions in the bronchioles to improve lung ventilation _____
5. A drug that is used to reduce a fever _____
6. A drug that reduces or eliminates pain _____
7. Aspiration of a fluid from the pleural cavity

   _____
8. A drug that is used for nasal congestion _____

Word Pool
- analgesic
- antipyretic
- bronchodilator
- clubbing
- corticosteroids
- decongestant
- productive cough
- thoracentesis

ABBREVIATIONS

Write out what each of the following abbreviations stands for.

1. O_2 _____
2. CO_2 _____

3. COPD _____

4. CBC _____

5. MDI _____

6. AAT _____

7. SIDS _____

8. CF _____

9. RV _____

10. OSA _____

11. CPAP _____

12. PE _____

13. ECG _____

14. TB _____

15. TST _____

16. PPD _____

17. QFT-Plus _____

18. RSV _____

19. TLC _____

20. SOB _____

21. ABG _____

22. CXR _____

23. VQ scan _____

24. TV _____

25. FVC _____

26. FEV_1 _____

27. ERV _____

28. IRV _____

29. VC _____

30. IC _____

31. FRC _____

32. MVV _____

SKILLS AND CONCEPTS
Answer the following questions.

A. Introduction
Fill in the blank.

1. _____ is the healthcare specialty that deals with respiratory diseases and disorders.

2. A(n) _____ is a specialist involved in the diagnosis, treatment, and prevention of disorders of the respiratory system.

3. The _____ respiratory tract structures are considered passageways for the air, whereas the _____ respiratory tract structures are involved in gas exchange.

B. Anatomy of the Upper Respiratory Tract
Fill in the blank or select the correct answer.

1. The upper respiratory tract structures start with the _____ and end with the _____, and they are all located outside of the _____ cavity.

2. The main function of the upper respiratory tract includes
   a. warming and cleaning the inspired air.
   b. serving as a passageway for air.
   c. providing the sense of smell.
   d. all of the above.

3. The nasal septum separates the _____, also called the *nostrils*, and _____ are the small hairs in the nasal cavity.

4. The nasal cavity is connected to four pairs of _____.

Match the descriptions with the correct structure.

5. _____ Equalizes the pressure in the ear with the air pressure outside the body

6. _____ A flap of cartilage at the larynx opening

7. _____ Located behind the nasal cavity

8. _____ Throat

9. _____ Vocal cords

10. _____ Located behind the mouth and part of the respiratory and digestive systems.

11. _____ Located between the epiglottis and the esophagus

a. pharynx
b. nasopharynx
c. oropharynx
d. laryngopharynx
e. epiglottis
f. larynx
g. eustachian tube

C. Anatomy of the Lower Respiratory Tract
Fill in the blank.

1. The lower respiratory tract consists of the _____, _____, and _____.

Match the descriptions with the correct term.

2. _____ A thin serous membrane found in the thoracic cavity

3. _____ Covers the lungs and adjoining structures

4. _____ The bronchi divide into these smaller branches

5. _____ The space between the visceral and parietal pleurae

6. _____ A broad, dome-shaped muscle used for breathing; separates the thoracic and abdominopelvic cavities

7. _____ Windpipe; lies in the mediastinum

8. _____ The outer portion of the pleura; lines the thoracic cavity and covers the diaphragm and mediastinum

9. _____ A mixture of protein and fats that lines the alveoli and prevents the tissues from sticking together and collapsing during exhalation.

10. _____ The space between the lungs

11. _____ Air sacs

a. trachea
b. mediastinum
c. bronchioles
d. alveoli
e. surfactant
f. pleura
g. visceral pleura
h. parietal pleura
i. diaphragm
j. pleural cavity

D. Physiology of the Respiratory System

Select the correct answer.

1. The function of the respiratory system is to
   a. exchange oxygen from the atmosphere for CO_2 waste.
   b. maintain the acid-base balance in the body.
   c. all of the above.

Match the description with the correct term.

2. _____ Occurs when oxygenated air moves into the alveoli

3. _____ Occurs when O_2 is exchanged for CO_2 between the cells in the body and the blood

4. _____ Includes the process of inspiration and expiration

a. ventilation
b. external respiration
c. internal respiration

Fill in the blank or select the correct answer.

5. A healthy person breathes when the blood _____ level increases.

6. For a person with chronic obstructive pulmonary disease (COPD), their breathing is triggered by a decreased blood _____ level.

7. The respiratory center is located in the _____, which is found in the brainstem.

8. Which is correct regarding expiration?
   a. The diaphragm and intercostal muscles relax, which causes the diaphragm to move upward into the thoracic cavity.
   b. Requires very little energy.
   c. The accessory muscles are needed to help with complete exhalation.
   d. All of the above.

9. Which is correct regarding the acid-base balance in the body?
   a. The respiratory system regulates the amount of CO_2 in the blood.
   b. Hyperventilation can result in respiratory acidosis.
   c. Hypoventilation can result in respiratory alkalosis.
   d. All of the above

E. Life Span Changes
Fill in the blank or select the correct answer.

1. Which is correct regarding the respiratory system in infants?
   a. They have a narrow airway and a shorter, softer trachea.
   b. They are abdominal breathers and have immature respiratory muscles.
   c. Their risk for airway obstruction is minimal.
   d. All of the above.
   e. Both a and b.

2. Lung function starts to decline by age _____.

3. Chest wall and thoracic spine deformities cause _____ work of breathing.

4. The diaphragm grows weaker, leading to a(n) _____ ability to inhale and exhale.

5. _____ lose their shape, which causes air to be trapped in the lungs.

F. Respiratory Diseases
Fill in the blank.

1. _____ is defined as difficulty breathing.

2. The medical term for breathlessness is _____.

3. The medical term for nosebleed is _____.

4. The medical term for nasal discharge is _____.

5. The medical term for the temporary absence of breathing is _____.

6. The medical term for abnormally slow breathing is _____.

7. An increase in the depth and rate of breathing, followed by a decrease in breathing, and then a period of apnea is called _____.

8. The medical term for an abnormal increase in breathing is _____.

9. Difficulty breathing unless in an upright position is _____.

10. The medical term for rapid, shallow breathing is _____.

11. The lack of oxygen in the blood, causing a bluish color in the skin, nail beds, and lips is _____.

12. Inspiratory auscultatory sounds resembling crackles or popping sounds caused by fluid in the airway or alveoli is _____.

13. A high-pitched sound produced by a narrowed airway is called _____.

G. Chronic Respiratory Diseases

Match the description with the correct disease.

1. _____ A chronic disease that causes bronchospasms and narrowing of the airway; severe attacks are life-threatening

2. _____ A life-threatening disease that causes mucus to build up in the lungs, pancreas, and other organs

3. _____ A chronic disease caused by an allergy to dust, animal dander, pollen, and/or food

4. _____ A disease that develops slowly, making it hard for the affected person to breathe

a. allergic rhinitis
b. asthma
c. COPD
d. cystic fibrosis

Match the etiology with the correct disease.

5. _____ Allergens

6. _____ A genetic disease

7. _____ Smoking tobacco, secondhand smoke, air pollution, dust, chemical fumes, and an alpha-1 antitrypsin (AAT) deficiency

8. _____ Allergens, environmental causes, strong emotional states, and strenuous physical exercise

a. allergic rhinitis
b. asthma
c. COPD
d. cystic fibrosis

Match the signs and symptoms with the correct disease.

9. _____ Shortness of breath, chest tightness, breathlessness, wheezing, cyanosis of the lips and nail beds, and clubbing

10. _____ Itchy nose, sneezing, watery eyes, nasal congestion, coughing, and decreased sense of smell

11. _____ Higher-than-normal levels of salt in the sweat, persistent cough that produces a thick, sticky sputum, poor growth and weight gain, breathlessness, shortness of breath, and wheezing

12. _____ Shortness of breath, chest tightness or pain, coughing or wheezing attacks, and early morning or nighttime coughing

a. allergic rhinitis
b. asthma
c. COPD
d. cystic fibrosis

Match the diagnostic measures and treatments with the correct disease.

13. _____ Sweat tests and genetic testing; treatment includes antibiotics, bronchodilators, mucus-thinning medications, and oral pancreatic enzymes

14. _____ Allergy testing and CBC; treatment includes allergen exposure, nasal wash, antihistamines, decongestants, and corticosteroids

15. _____ Peak flow monitoring, oxygen saturation measurement, and spirometry; treatments include inhaled corticosteroids, leukotriene modifiers, long-acting beta agonists, and quick-relief medications such as inhaled albuterol

16. _____ Lung function tests, chest x-ray, and chest computed tomography; treatment includes bronchodilators, corticosteroids, low-level oxygen therapy, lung volume reduction surgery and lung transplantation

a. allergic rhinitis
b. asthma
c. COPD
d. cystic fibrosis

Select the correct answer.

17. Chronic obstructive pulmonary disease includes which two conditions?
    a. Emphysema and asthma
    b. Acute bronchitis and asthma
    c. Acute bronchitis and emphysema
    d. Emphysema and chronic bronchitis

H. Respiratory System Cancers
Fill in the blank.

1. _____ cancer is throat cancer, and it affects the vocal cords and larynx.

2. The causes of laryngeal cancer include _____ and _____ use.

3. The leading cause of lung cancer is _____.

4. The removal of a small portion of the lung tissue, including the tumor and the healthy tissue on the edge of the tumor is called a(n) _____.

5. The removal of a larger portion or segment of the lung is called a(n) _____.

6. The removal of a lobe of the lung is called a(n) _____.

7. The removal of the entire lung is called a(n) _____.

I. Acute Respiratory Diseases
Fill in the blank.

1. Acute bronchitis _____ is an inflammation of the lining of the bronchial tubes usually caused by a lower respiratory viral infection.

2. _____, an upper respiratory system disease, is a life-threatening inflammation of the epiglottis.

3. _____, also called whooping cough, is a contagious disease caused by *Bordetella pertussis*.

Match the description with the correct disease.

4. _____ An inflammation of the trachea and larynx and usually affects children ages 3 months to 5 years of age

5. _____ A bacterial infection of the lungs

6. _____ A highly contagious bacterial infection of the throat

7. _____ An infection of the lungs and can range from mild to life-threatening

8. _____ A medical emergency and a life-threatening condition in which one of the pulmonary arteries is blocked

a. croup
b. pneumonia
c. pulmonary embolism
d. pulmonary tuberculosis
e. strep throat

Match the etiology with the correct disease.

9. _____ Caused by bacteria, viruses, fungi, and chemicals

10. _____ A clot blocks the pulmonary artery

11. _____ Caused by bacteria and viruses, such as parainfluenza RSV, adenovirus, and influenza

12. _____ Caused by group A streptococcal bacteria

13. _____ Caused by *Mycobacterium tuberculosis*

a. croup
b. pneumonia
c. pulmonary embolism
d. pulmonary tuberculosis
e. strep throat

Match the signs and symptoms with the correct disease.

14. _____ Causes a mild cold, low-grade fever, barking cough, hoarseness, inspiratory stridor, wheezing, and chest retractions

15. _____ Causes unexplained shortness of breath, rapid breathing, chest pain, coughing or coughing up blood, arrhythmias, lightheadedness, and fainting

16. _____ Bad cough that lasts 3 or more weeks, pain in the chest, blood in the sputum, weakness, no appetite, weight loss, chills, fever, and night sweats

17. _____ Causes a rash, nausea, vomiting, fever, headache, painful swallowing, sore throat, tiny red spots at the back of the throat, and white pus patches

18. _____ Causes high fever, chills, productive cough, shortness of breath, and chest pain with coughing or breathing

a. croup
b. pneumonia
c. pulmonary embolism
d. pulmonary tuberculosis
e. strep throat

Match the diagnostic measures and treatments with the correct disease.

19. _____ Physical examination and chest x-ray; treatment includes antipyretics, humidifier, bed rest, and increase fluid intake

20. _____ Mantoux tuberculin skin test or a TB blood test, chest x-ray, and sputum smear/culture; treatment may include isoniazid, rifampin, ethambutol, or pyrazinamide

21. _____ Chest x-rays, a CBC, a sputum culture, and pulse oximetry; treatment depends on the cause of the disease and may include antibiotics, antivirals, antipyretics, and analgesics

22. _____ A rapid antigen test and a throat culture; treatment consists of antibiotics, antipyretics, and over-the-counter analgesics

23. _____ Ultrasound, CT scan with contrast, lung ventilation perfusion scan, pulmonary angiography, and chest x-ray; treatment includes anticoagulants, thrombolytics, and compression stockings

a. croup
b. pneumonia
c. pulmonary embolism
d. pulmonary tuberculosis
e. strep throat

J. The Medical Assistant's Role with Examinations, Diagnostic Procedures, and Treatments

Match the description with the correct diagnostic modality and laboratory test.

1. _____ Measures the volume of inhaled and exhaled air, and the time required for each

2. _____ A handheld device that measures the exhaled air; can be used at home

3. _____ A noninvasive test used to measure the oxygen saturation level in blood

4. _____ The insertion of a bronchoscope through the mouth to visualize the trachea and bronchi

5. _____ A procedure in which a catheter is inserted into the pulmonary blood vessels, dye is injected, and x-ray pictures show the blood flow through the pulmonary vessels

a. pulmonary angiography
b. peak flow monitor
c. pulse oximetry
d. spirometry test
e. bronchoscopy

Select the correct answer.

6. Which of the following are CLIA-waived tests?
   a. Legionella urinary antigen test
   b. Influenza A & B test
   c. Rapid strep A test
   d. RSV test
   e. All of the above

Match the indication for use and desired effect with the correct medication classification.

7. _____ Relieves nasal and sinus congestion caused by common cold, hay fever, or upper respiratory tract disorders

8. _____ Treats asthma and bronchospasm by relaxing the smooth muscle of the bronchi

9. _____ Treats viral infections by inhibiting the growth or reducing the spread of viral cells

10. _____ Treats asthma and exercise-induced bronchospasms by blocking the action of substances that cause asthma and allergic rhinitis

11. _____ Reduces airway inflammation and bronchial resistance and is used for long-term relief of asthma symptoms

12. _____ Relieves allergies by blocking the action of histamine, which causes allergic symptoms

13. _____ Relieves upper respiratory tract congestion by thinning the secretions in the bronchial tubes to make it easier to cough up the mucus

a. antihistamine
b. antiviral
c. bronchodilator
d. corticosteroid (nasal and inhaled)
e. decongestant
f. expectorant
g. leukotriene receptor antagonist

Match the side effects and adverse reactions with the correct medication classification.

14. _____ GI distress

15. _____ CNS depression, muscle weakness, GI distress, and dry mouth

16. _____ Headache, pharyngitis, myalgia, hypersensitivity, oral candidiasis

17. _____ Confusion, diarrhea, headache, kidney disease, urticaria, and vomiting

18. _____ Headache, dizziness, heartburn, stomach pain, tiredness, hypersensitivity, numbness in arms and legs, and swelling of the sinuses

19. _____ CNS stimulation, tremors, tachycardia, increased blood glucose level, and hypertension

20. _____ Arrhythmias, hypertension, headache, nausea, dry mouth

a. antihistamine
b. antiviral
c. bronchodilator
d. corticosteroid (nasal and inhaled)
e. decongestant
f. expectorant
g. leukotriene receptor antagonist

CERTIFICATION PREPARATION

Circle the correct answer.

1. Which are components of the respiratory system?
   a. Nasal cavity
   b. Trachea
   c. Lungs
   d. All of the above

2. What is the anatomic location of the lungs and trachea?
   a. Cranial cavity
   b. Spinal cavity
   c. Thoracic cavity
   d. Abdominopelvic cavity

3. What is the function of the respiratory system?
   a. Maintain the acid-base balance in the body
   b. Carry waste products away from the cells to be excreted in the urine
   c. Exchange oxygen from the atmosphere for carbon dioxide waste
   d. Both a and c

4. Which test is a CLIA-waived test?
   a. VQ scan
   b. Arterial blood gas
   c. Sputum cytology
   d. Rapid strep A test

5. What medication is considered a quick-relief asthma medication?
   a. Fluticasone
   b. Montelukast
   c. Albuterol
   d. Budesonide

6. Which is surgical removal of the entire lung?
   a. Wedge resection
   b. Lobectomy
   c. Segmental resection
   d. Pneumonectomy

7. Which disease caused by a bacterial infection of the respiratory tract is also called *whooping cough*?
   a. Influenza
   b. Pertussis
   c. Croup
   d. Pleurisy

8. Which are characteristics of an infant's respiratory system?
   a. Airway collapses if the neck is overextended.
   b. Trachea is shorter and softer than in adults.
   c. Airway is narrow.
   d. All of the above.

9. What is the maximum volume of air that can be as forcefully and rapidly exhaled as possible after taking in a full inhalation?
   a. TLC
   b. FVC
   c. RV
   d. FRC

10. What is true regarding oxygen delivery?
    a. A nasal cannula has a flow range between 1 and 6 L/min.
    b. The soft nasal cannula prongs must curve downwards when placed in the nose.
    c. A mask has a flow range of 5-10 L/min.
    d. All of the above are true.

WORKPLACE APPLICATIONS

1. Ken Thomas has COPD. He asks Renée why he needs to be on low levels of oxygen instead of higher levels. Describe how you would answer this question.

   _____

   _____

   _____

2. A mother calls and states her son is having difficulty breathing. Explain how you would ask her to check if he was using accessory muscles when breathing.

   _____

   _____

   _____

3. You are working with a patient who has a sibling who was just diagnosed with latent TB infection. The patient asks you to explain this condition. Describe how you would explain latent TB infection.

   _____

   _____

   _____

   _____

4. Read the peak flow meter measurements and label your answer.

    A. _____

    B. _____

    C. _____

    D. _____

    E. _____

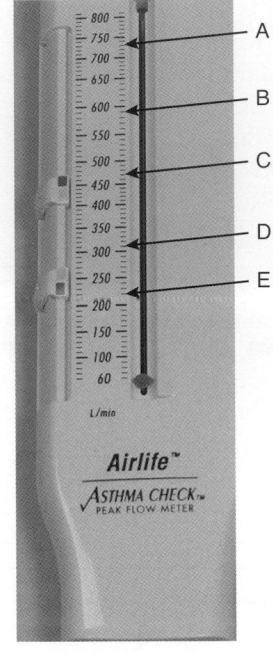

INTERNET ACTIVITIES

1. Using online resources, research a test used for diagnosing respiratory diseases. Create a poster presentation, a PowerPoint presentation, or write a paper summarizing your research. Include the following points in your project:
    a. Description of the test
    b. Any contraindications for the test
    c. Patient preparation for the test
    d. What occurs during the test

2. Using online resources, research a respiratory disease. Create a poster presentation, a PowerPoint presentation, or write a paper summarizing your research. Include the following points in your project:
    a. Description of the disease
    b. Etiology
    c. Signs and symptoms
    d. Diagnostic procedures
    e. Treatments

3. Using online resources, research the health risks attributed to smoking. Create a poster or a PowerPoint presentation summarizing the health risks associated with smoking and smokeless tobacco. Cite two online resources used.

4. Using Table 41.6, Medication Classifications, select a generic medication from each of the following classifications: antihistamines, antivirals, antitussives, bronchodilators, corticosteroids (oral), corticosteroids (nasal and inhaled), decongestants, and expectorant. Using a reliable online drug resource, identify for each medication:
    a. Reasons for use
    b. Desired effects
    c. Side effects
    d. Adverse reactions
    Write a short paper addressing each of these four areas for each medication.

Procedure 41.1 Measure a Peak Flow Rate

Name _____ Date _____ Score _____

Tasks: Perform a peak flow. Document the procedure in the patient's health record.

Equipment and Supplies:
- Peak flow meter
- Disposable mouthpiece
- Disinfection wipes
- Gloves
- Waste container
- Paper towel or denture cup (optional)
- Patient's health record

Standard: Complete the procedure and all critical steps in _____ minutes with a minimum score of 85% within two attempts (*or as indicated by the instructor*).

Scoring: Divide the points earned by the total possible points. Failure to perform a critical step, indicated by an asterisk (*), results in grade no higher than an 84% (*or as indicated by the instructor*).

Time: Began_____ Ended_____ Total minutes: _____

Steps:	Point Value	Attempt 1	Attempt 2
1. Wash hands or use hand sanitizer.	5		
2. Assemble equipment and supplies needed for the peak flow procedure. Place the mouthpiece on the peak flow meter. Move the indicator to the bottom of the calibration scale (if not using a digital meter).	5		
3. Greet the patient. Identify yourself. Verify the patient's identity with full name and date of birth. Explain the procedure to be performed in a manner that the patient understands. Answer any questions the patient may have on the procedure.	10		
4. Ask the patient to loosen any restrictive clothing. Have the patient remove any gum and loose dentures. Make sure to provide a paper towel or denture cup if needed.	10		
5. With the patient in the seated position, ensure that their feet are flat on the floor and the legs uncrossed. The patient should sit straight up and against the back of the chair.	10		
6. Describe how the patient should do the test. "Take the deepest breath possible. Seal your lips around the mouthpiece. Blow as hard and as fast as you can." Encourage the patient to state when they are ready to start the test. Tell patients to seal their lips around the mouthpiece.	15*		
7. Coach the patient during the test. After the patient has blown through the meter, read the number next to the indicator. Write the number down. Reset the indicator to the bottom of the scale (if it's not a digital meter).	15		
8. Make any adjustments as needed. Repeat the test two additional times. Write down the last two numbers.	10		

9. Put on gloves and remove the mouthpiece. Discard the mouthpiece in the waste container. Disinfect the peak flow meter. Remove your gloves and dispose of them in the waste container. Wash your hands or use hand sanitizer.	10*		
10. Notify the provider of the readings and document the readings in the patient's health record. Indicate the name of the provider who ordered the test, the name of the test, the results of the test, and how the patient tolerated the test.	10		
Total Points	**100**		

Documentation

Comments

CAAHEP Competencies	Step(s)
I.P.2.d. Perform: pulmonary function testing	Entire procedure
I.P.8. Instruct and prepare a patient for a procedure or a treatment	4, 5, 6
X.P.3. Document patient care accurately in the medical record	10
ABHES Competencies	**Step(s)**
4. Medical Law and Ethics a. Follow documentation guidelines	10
8.d. Assist provider with specialty examination, including cardiac, respiratory, OB-GYN, neurological, and gastroenterology procedures	Entire procedure
8.e. Perform specialty procedures, including but not limited to minor surgery, cardiac, respiratory, OB-GYN, neurological, and gastroenterology	Entire procedure

Procedure 41.2   Perform Spirometry Testing

Name _____ Date _____ Score _____

Tasks: Perform a spirometry test. Document the procedure in the patient's health record.

Equipment and Supplies:
- Spirometry machine with paper (and users' guide if applicable)
- Disposable mouthpiece and tubing (if applicable)
- Nose clip
- Calibration equipment
- Disinfection wipes
- Gloves
- Waste container
- Paper towel or denture cup (optional)
- Patient's health record
- Scale (if no height and weight measurements were taken earlier that day)

Standard: Complete the procedure and all critical steps in _____ minutes with a minimum score of 85% within two attempts (*or as indicated by the instructor*).

Scoring: Divide the points earned by the total possible points. Failure to perform a critical step, indicated by an asterisk (*), results in grade no higher than an 84% (*or as indicated by the instructor*).

Time: Began_____ Ended_____ Total minutes: _____

Steps:	Point Value	Attempt 1	Attempt 2
1. Wash hands or use hand sanitizer.	5		
2. Assemble the equipment and supplies needed for the spirometry procedure. Calibrate the machine according to the users' guide and the facility's procedures.	5		
3. Greet the patient. Identify yourself. Verify the patient's identity with full name and date of birth. Make sure the patient's information matches the order and the record. Explain the procedure in a manner that the patient understands. Answer any questions the patient may have about the procedure.	10		
4. Enter the patient's name, medical record number, age (or date of birth), race, sex, weight, and height into the machine. Enter any additional required information.	10		
5. Ask the patient to loosen any restrictive clothing. Have the patient remove gum and loose dentures (if applicable). Make sure to provide a paper towel or denture cup if needed..	10		
6. With the patient in the seated position, ensure that the feet are flat on the floor and the legs are uncrossed. The patient should sit straight up and against the back of the chair.	10*		
7. Describe how the patient should do the test. "Take the deepest breath possible. Seal your lips around the mouthpiece. Blow as hard and as fast as you can. Blow until you empty the air from your lungs."	10*		

8.	Attach the mouthpiece to the machine. Explain the purpose of the nose clip to the patient. Apply the nose clip to the patient. Have the patient state when they are ready to start. Start the test as directed by the users' guide.	10		
9.	During the test, encourage the patient to empty the lungs. Repeat until three acceptable tests have been done. Allow the patient to rest between tests, if needed, and to indicate when they are ready for next test.	10		
10.	Put on gloves and remove the mouthpiece. Discard the mouthpiece in the waste container. Disinfect the spirometer as indicated in the users' guide. Remove your gloves and dispose of them in the waste container. Wash your hands or use hand sanitizer.	10		
11.	Document that the test was performed. Indicate the name of the provider who ordered the test, the name of the test, how the patient tolerated the test, and what you did with the test results. Any patient instructions regarding follow-up can also be documented.	10		
	Total Points	**100**		

Documentation

Comments

CAAHEP Competencies	Step(s)
I.P.2.d. Perform: pulmonary function testing	Entire procedure
I.P.8. Instruct and prepare a patient for a procedure or a treatment	5, 6, 7
X.P.3. Document patient care accurately in the medical record	11
ABHES Competencies	**Step(s)**
4. Medical Law and Ethics a. Follow documentation guidelines	11
8.d. Assist provider with specialty examination, including cardiac, respiratory, OB-GYN, neurological, and gastroenterology procedures	Entire procedure
8.e. Perform specialty procedures, including but not limited to minor surgery, cardiac, respiratory, OB-GYN, neurological, and gastroenterology	Entire procedure

Procedure 41.3 Administer a Nebulizer Treatment

Name _____ Date _____ Score _____

Tasks: Perform a nebulizer treatment. Document the medication administration in the patient's health record.

Order: Levalbuterol 0.63 mg by nebulization.

Equipment and Supplies:
- Nebulizer machine
- Disposable nebulizer patient kit (tubing, medication cup, mouthpiece or mask, flexible tube, and tee)
- Medication as ordered
- Provider's order
- Normal saline (as ordered or according to the facility's protocol)
- Disinfection wipes
- Gloves
- Waste container
- Patient's health record

Standard: Complete the procedure and all critical steps in _____ minutes with a minimum score of 85% within two attempts (*or as indicated by the instructor*).

Scoring: Divide the points earned by the total possible points. Failure to perform a critical step, indicated by an asterisk (*), results in grade no higher than an 84% (*or as indicated by the instructor*).

Time: Began_____ Ended_____ Total minutes: _____

Steps:	Point Value	Attempt 1	Attempt 2
1. Wash hands or use hand sanitizer. Using the drug reference information and the order, review the information on the medication if needed. Clarify any questions you have with the provider.	5		
2. Select the right medication from the storage area. Check to see if the medication is concentrated and requires normal saline to dilute it. Check the medication label (and normal saline label, if used) against the order. Check for the right name, form, and route. Check the expiration date to make sure the drug has not expired. Verify that it is the right dose and time.	5*		
3. Assemble the equipment and supplies needed for the nebulizer treatment.	5		
4. Perform the second medication check. Check the medication and normal saline label(s) against the order. Check for the right name, form, and route.	5*		
5. Add the medication, and if required, the normal saline to the medication cup. Secure the cover on the cup.	5		
6. Perform the third medication check. Check the medication label and normal saline label (if used) against the order. Check for the right name, form, and route. Verify that the amount of medication in the cup is correct with according to the order. Clean up the area.	5*		

7. Prior to entering the exam room, provide courtesy knock on the door. Greet the patient. Identify yourself. Verify the patient's identity with full name and date of birth. Make sure the patient's information matches the order and the record.	10*		
8. Provide the right education to the patient. Explain the medication ordered, the desired effect, and common side effects; also identify the provider who ordered it. Explain the procedure in a manner that the patient understands. Answer any questions the patient may have about the procedure. Ask the patient if they have any allergies. If the patient refuses the medication, notify the provider.	10*		
9. Attach the mouthpiece (or mask). Attach the tubing to the medication cup and the machine.	5		
10. Perform the right technique. The patient should be sitting upright on a chair. Instruct the patient to hold the mouthpiece between the teeth and seal the lips around the mouthpiece. Encourage the patient to take slow, deep breaths through the mouth. The patient should hold each breath 2 to 3 seconds before exhaling.	10*		
11. Turn on the nebulizer and give the medicine cup and mouthpiece to the patient to start the treatment. Instruct patients to put it into their mouth. If using a mask, position it securely and comfortably over the patient's nose and mouth.	10		
12. Continue the treatment until the mist is no longer produced (approximately 10 minutes). Turn off the nebulizer. Encourage the patient to take several deep breaths and cough.	10		
13. Put on gloves and dispose of the used supplies. Disinfect the nebulizer machine. Remove your gloves and dispose of them in the waste container. Wash your hands or use hand sanitizer.	5		
14. Document the procedure in the patient's health record. Include the name of the provider ordering the treatment, what was administered, how the patient tolerated the medication, and any follow-up assessments (e.g., vital signs).	10		
Total Points	100		

Documentation

Comments

CAAHEP Competencies	Step(s)
I.P.4.a. Verify the rules of medication administration: right patient	7
I.P.4.b. Verify the rules of medication administration: right medication	2, 4, 6
I.P.4.c. Verify the rules of medication administration: right dose	2, 6
I.P.4.d. Verify the rules of medication administration: right route	2, 4, 6
I.P.4.e. Verify the rules of medication administration: right time	2
I.P.4.f. Verify the rules of medication administration: right documentation	14
I.P.8. Instruct and prepare a patient for a procedure or a treatment	8, 10
X.P.3. Document patient care accurately in the medical record	14
ABHES Competencies	**Step(s)**
4. Medical Law and Ethics a. Follow documentation guidelines	14
8.e. Perform specialty procedures, including but not limited to minor surgery, cardiac, respiratory, OB-GYN, neurological, and gastroenterology	Entire procedure

Procedure 41.4   Administer Oxygen per Nasal Cannula or Mask

Name _____ **Date** _____ **Score** _____

Tasks: Administer oxygen per nasal cannula or mask. Document the oxygen administration in the patient's health record.

Order 1: Administer 2 LPM of oxygen per nasal cannula.

Order 2: Administer 6 LPM of oxygen per simple mask.

Equipment and Supplies:
- Oxygen cylinder with oxygen regulator or oxygen flowmeter (wall unit)
- Adult nasal cannula or simple mask
- Provider's order
- Patient's health record
- Mannequin (optional)

Standard: Complete the procedure and all critical steps in _____ minutes with a minimum score of 85% within two attempts (*or as indicated by the instructor*).

Scoring: Divide the points earned by the total possible points. Failure to perform a critical step, indicated by an asterisk (*), results in grade no higher than an 84% (*or as indicated by the instructor*).

Time: Began_____ Ended_____ Total minutes: _____

Steps:	Point Value	Attempt 1	Attempt 2
1. Wash hands or use hand sanitizer.	10		
2. Assemble the equipment and supplies needed for the provider's order. If an oxygen cylinder is used, identify the amount of oxygen left in the cylinder.	10		
3. Verify the order if you have any questions.	10		
4. Greet the patient. Identify yourself. Verify the patient's identity with full name and date of birth. Make sure the patient's information matches the order and the record. Explain the procedure in a manner that the patient understands. Answer any questions the patient may have about the procedure.	10		
5. Connect the nasal cannula or mask to the regulator or flow meter. Turn on the oxygen and adjust the flow rate to the correct amount per the provider's order. The ball should be centered on the number of liters ordered.	20		
6. Apply the mask or nasal cannula: a. Place the mask over the patient's nose, mouth, and chin. Place the elastic over the head. Adjust the elastic strap to tighten the mask on the face. Adjust the metal nasal bridge clamp, making sure it fits without obstructing the nose. Ensure that the mask fits tightly on the face. b. Insert the tips of the cannula into the nostrils. If the tips are curved, the curves face downward towards the bottom of the nose. Adjust the tubing around the back of the ears and then under the chin. Encourage the patient to breathe through the nose with the mouth closed.	20		

7.	Make sure the patient is comfortable. Answer any questions they may have. Sanitize your hands.	**10**		
8.	Document the procedure in the patient's health record. Include the name of the ordering provider, the number of liters of oxygen administered, the device used for administering the oxygen, and the patient's condition.	**10**		
	Total Points	**100**		

Documentation

Comments

CAAHEP Competencies	Step(s)
X.P.3. Document patient care accurately in the medical record	8
ABHES Competencies	**Step(s)**
4. Medical Law and Ethics a. Follow documentation guidelines	8
8.e. Perform specialty procedures, including but not limited to minor surgery, cardiac, respiratory, OB-GYN, neurological, and gastroenterology	Entire procedure

Urology and Male Reproduction

CAAHEP Competencies	Assessment
I.C.4. Identify major organs in each body system	Skills and Concepts – B. 1, F. 1; Certification Preparation – 1
I.C.5. Identify the anatomical location of major organs in each body system	Skills and Concepts – B. 7, 19
I.C.6. Identify structure and function of the human body across the life span	Skills and Concepts – D. 1-4, H. 1-3; Certification Preparation – 4-5
I.C.7. Identify the normal function of each body system	Skills and Concepts – B. 2-5, 20, C. 1-8, F. 1-4, 6, G. 1-5; Certification Preparation – 6
I.C.8.a. Identify common pathology related to each body system including: signs	Skills and Concepts – E. 1, 3, 6, 18-22, H. 1; Internet Activities – 2
I.C.8.b. Identify common pathology related to each body system including: symptoms	Skills and Concepts – E. 2, 4-5, 7, 18-22, H. 1; Internet Activities – 2
I.C.8.c. Identify common pathology related to each body system including: etiology	Skills and Concepts – E. 13-17, I. 1; Internet Activities – 2
I.C.8.d. Identify common pathology related to each body system including: diagnostic measures	Skills and Concepts – E. 23-27, J. 1-6; Certification Preparation – 7-8; Internet Activities – 1-2
I.C.8.e. Identify common pathology related to each body system including: treatment modalities	Skills and Concepts – E. 23-27, H.1, K. 1-24; Certification Preparation – 9-10; Workplace Application – 3; Internet Activities – 2, 4
1.C.9. Identify Clinical Laboratory Improvement Amendments (CLIA) waived tests associated with common diseases	Skills and Concepts – J. 2; Certification Preparation – 8
I.C.10.a. Identify the classifications of medications, including indications for use	Skills and Concepts – K. 13-18; Internet Activities – 4
I.C.10.b. Identify the classifications of medications, including desired effects	Skills and Concepts – K. 13-18; Internet Activities – 4
I.C.10.c. Identify the classifications of medications, including side effects	Skills and Concepts – K. 19-24; Internet Activities – 4
I.C.10.d. Identify the classifications of medications, including adverse reactions	Skills and Concepts – K. 19-24; Internet Activities – 4
V.C.8.a. Identify the following related to body systems: medical terms	Skills and Concepts – I. 2-5, K. 1-10

CAAHEP Competencies	Assessment
V.C.8.b. Identify the following related to body systems: abbreviations	Abbreviations – 1-23
I.P.8. Instruct and prepare a patient for a procedure or treatment	Procedures 42.2, 42.3
V.P.3.b. Coach patient regarding: medical encounters	Procedure 42.1
X.P.3. Document patient care accurately in the medical record	Procedures 42.1, 42.2, 42.3

ABHES Competencies	Assessment
2. Anatomy and Physiology a. List all body systems and their structures and functions	Skills and Concepts – B. 1-5, 17, 19-20, C. 1-8, F. 1-4, 6, G. 1-5; Certification Preparation – 1, 6
2.b. Describe common diseases, symptoms, and etiologies as they apply to each system	Skills and Concepts – E. 1-22, I. 1-7; Internet Activities – 2
2.c. Identify diagnostic and treatment modalities as they relate to each body system	Skills and Concepts – E. 23-27, I. 1, 6, J. 1-6, K. 1-24; Certification Preparation – 7-10; Workplace Application – 3; Internet Activities – 1-2, 4
3. Medical Terminology c. Apply medical terminology for each specialty	Skills and Concepts – I. 2-5, K. 1-10
3. d. Define and use medical abbreviations when appropriate and acceptable	Abbreviations – 1-23
4. Medical Law and Ethics a. Follow documentation guidelines	Procedures 42.1, 42.2, 42.3
8. Clinical Procedures e. Perform specialty procedures, including but not limited to minor surgery, cardiac, respiratory, OB-GYN, neurological, and gastroenterology	Procedures 42.2, 42.3

VOCABULARY REVIEW
Using the word pool on the right, find the correct word to match the definition. Write the word on the line after the definition.

Group A
1. Small arteries _____
2. A very small vein _____
3. Pertaining to carrying toward a structure _____
4. Fluid and substances that are filtered out of the blood in the Bowman capsule _____
5. Pertaining to carrying away from a structure _____
6. A serous membrane lining of the abdominal cavity, which folds inward to enclose the viscera (internal organs) _____
7. Folds in the wall of the organ _____
8. Sensory nerve ending that responds to a stretch stimulus

   _____
9. Blood capillaries surrounding the proximal and distal convoluted tubules in the kidneys _____
10. A type of cell found in the lining of hollow organs; it has ability to stretch with the contraction and distention of the organ

    _____

Word Pool
- afferent
- arterioles
- efferent
- filtrate
- peritoneum
- peritubular capillaries
- rugae
- stretch receptor
- transitional epithelium
- venule

Group B
1. A quality or characteristic of a material that allows another substance to pass through it _____
2. Stones formed in the kidneys, gallbladder, and other parts of the body _____
3. An abnormal joining of an artery and vein _____
4. A synthetic tube that connects an artery to a vein

   _____
5. A hollow, flexible tube that can be inserted into a vessel, organ, or cavity of the body to withdraw or instill fluid, monitor information, and visualize a vessel or cavity _____
6. Between the cells _____
7. Testosterone-secreting cells of testes that are found in the spaces between the seminiferous tubules _____
8. Byproducts of drug metabolism _____
9. A decreased level of albumin (protein) in the blood

   _____
10. A surgical procedure that creates a vein to remove and return blood during the hemodialysis procedure _____
11. A temporary or permanent surgically created opening used for drainage (i.e., urine, stool) _____
12. A surgically created opening on the abdominal wall used to drain urine _____

Word Pool
- arteriovenous fistula
- arteriovenous graft
- calculi
- catheter
- hypoalbuminemia
- interstitial
- interstitial cells
- metabolites
- permeability
- stoma
- urostomy
- vascular access

ABBREVIATIONS

Write out what each of the following abbreviations stands for.

1. ADH _____

2. NH_3 _____

3. K^+ _____

4. H^+ _____

5. RAAS _____

6. UTI _____

7. VCUG _____

8. ESRD _____

9. BUN _____

10. ESR _____

11. RCC _____

12. PKD _____

13. IVP _____

14. PSA _____

15. DRE _____

16. ESWL _____

17. UI _____

18. UPJ _____

19. VUR _____

20. BPH _____

21. TURP _____

22. TSE _____

23. ED _____

SKILLS AND CONCEPTS
Answer the following questions.

A. Introduction
Match the description with the correct term.

1. _____ A specialist who diagnoses and treats kidney conditions
2. _____ The healthcare specialty that deals with most urinary diseases and disorders
3. _____ The healthcare subspecialty that focuses on kidney function and disorders
4. _____ A specialist involved in the diagnosis, treatment, and prevention of disorders of the urinary system and the male reproductive system

a. urology
b. nephrology
c. urologist
d. nephrologist

B. Anatomy of the Urinary System
Select the correct answer or fill in the blank.

1. The urinary system is composed of
   a. two kidneys.
   b. two ureters.
   c. one urinary bladder.
   d. one urethra.
   e. all of the above.

2. The _____ filter the blood and eliminate waste through the passage of urine.

3. The _____ move urine from the kidneys to the bladder.

4. The _____ stores the urine until it is excreted.

5. The _____ is the tube that conducts the urine out of the bladder.

6. The _____ is the indentation on the kidney.

7. The kidneys are located _____ to the peritoneum, the muscles of the back, and between the T12 and L3 vertebrae.

8. Each kidney contains tissue with millions of microscopic units called _____, which are the functional units of the kidneys.

Match the description with the correct structure.

9. _____ The outer portion of the kidney

10. _____ The inner portion that extends from the end of the cortex to the calyces

11. _____ A cup-shaped structure of the nephron that surrounds the glomerulus

12. _____ The first section of the renal tubule that is attached to the Bowman capsule

13. _____ The fibrous outer covering of the kidney

14. _____ Multiple distal tubules join and form this straight collecting duct, which empties into the calyx

15. _____ An extension of the cortex that dips down between the medullary pyramids

16. _____ A cluster of capillaries inside of the Bowman capsule

17. _____ Follows the proximal convoluted tubule and includes a straight descending section, a loop, and then a straight ascending section

18. _____ Follows the ascending section of the Henle loop

a. Bowman capsule
b. glomerulus
c. capsule
d. cortex
e. renal column
f. medulla
g. proximal convoluted tubule
h. Henle loop
i. distal convoluted tubule
j. collecting duct

Fill in the blank.

19. The urinary bladder is in the _____ cavity.

20. The _____ relaxes when the bladder fills, and it contracts to push urine out of the bladder and into the urethra.

Match the description with the term.

21. _____ A sensory nerve ending that responds to a stretch stimulus

22. _____ Urine that remains in the bladder after urination

23. _____ Folds in the wall of the bladder

24. _____ The point where the ureter enters the bladder

25. _____ The distal end of the urethra

26. _____ A type of cell found in the lining of hollow organs that has the ability to stretch with the contraction and distention of the organ

27. _____ Urination

a. ureterovesical junction
b. rugae
c. urinary meatus
d. stretch receptors
e. micturition
f. residual urine
g. transitional epithelium

C. Physiology of the Urinary System
Select the correct answer.

1. What is a role of the urinary system?
   a. Maintains fluid volume and adequate blood pressure
   b. Maintains the normal composition of body fluids
   c. Activates vitamin D
   d. Controls red blood cell production
   e. All of the above

Match the description with the correct term. Answers can be used more than once.

2. _____ Substances move from the blood to the filtrate

3. _____ Substances move from the filtrate back into the blood in the peritubular capillaries

4. _____ First step in urine formation; a continual process that involves the renal corpuscle

5. _____ During this process, urea moves back to the filtrate in the Henle loop; ammonia, certain drugs, hydrogen, and potassium move from the blood into the filtrate

a. filtration
b. reabsorption
c. secretion

Fill in the blank.

6. _____ hormone helps increase the water permeability of the walls of the distal tubule and collecting duct and water moves out of the filtrate and into the bloodstream.

7. _____ is secreted by the adrenal cortex and increases the movement of sodium out of the filtrate in the distal tubule and collecting duct.

8. _____, a hormone released from the kidney cells, stimulates the marrow to make more red blood cells.

D. Life Span Changes of the Urinary System
Select the correct answer or fill in the blank.

1. The nephrons are immature and reach maturity by age _____.

2. Females are at more risk for _____ than are males, which is attributed to the anatomical differences.

3. During pregnancy, the
   a. filtration rate increases.
   b. filtration surface increases.
   c. bladder may be twice as big later in pregnancy.
   d. all of the above.

4. In older adults, the
   a. kidney tissue and number of nephrons are reduced by up to 40%.
   b. renal arteries can harden.
   c. kidneys filter blood slower.
   d. all of the above.
   e. both b and c.

E. Urinary System Diseases and Disorders

Match the description to the correct sign or symptom.

1. _____ Excessive excretion of urine
2. _____ The sudden, almost uncontrollable need to urinate
3. _____ Inability to release urine
4. _____ Painful or difficult urination
5. _____ Urination at short periods without an increase in the daily volume of urine output
6. _____ Inability to hold urine
7. _____ Urination at night

a. dysuria
b. nocturia
c. polyuria
d. frequency
e. urgency
f. urinary incontinence
g. urinary retention

Match the description with the correct disease.

8. _____ A urinary tract infection of one or both kidneys
9. _____ Cysts form in the kidneys, causing the kidneys to become enlarged
10. _____ Kidney stone
11. _____ An inflammation of the bladder
12. _____ Advanced-stage chronic kidney disease; occurs when the kidneys are no longer filtering waste from the blood

a. polycystic kidney disease
b. pyelonephritis
c. acute cystitis
d. end-stage renal disease
e. renal calculi

Match the etiology with the correct disease.

13. _____ Caused by a bacterium or virus
14. _____ Caused by diabetes mellitus, hypertension, glomerulonephritis, polycystic kidney disease, and recurrent kidney infections
15. _____ Inherited condition
16. _____ Caused by a bacterial infection, medications, radiation therapy, spermicidal jellies, and long-term catheterization
17. _____ Can occur when high levels of certain minerals such as calcium, oxalate, and uric acid collect in the kidney

a. polycystic kidney disease
b. pyelonephritis
c. acute cystitis
d. end-stage renal disease
e. renal calculi

Match the signs and symptoms with the correct disease.

18. _____ Fever, chills, nausea, vomiting, dysuria, frequency, hematuria, foul-smelling urine, and low back, side (flank), or groin pain
19. _____ Nocturia, dysuria, urgency, frequency, urinary retention; cloudy, bloody, or strong/foul-smelling urine; low abdominal pressure or cramping, low-grade fever; and for older adults, confusion and mental changes
20. _____ Nausea, vomiting, loss of appetite, weakness, fatigue, muscle cramps, twitching, pruritus, hypertension, decreased amounts of urine, sleep issues, and a reduction in mental sharpness
21. _____ Dysuria, nausea, vomiting, fever, chills, and severe constant pain on either side of the lower back
22. _____ Pain in the flank, abdomen, and joints; nocturia, hematuria, drowsiness, nail abnormalities, pain or tenderness over the liver, an enlarged liver, heart murmur, and hypertension

a. polycystic kidney disease
b. pyelonephritis
c. acute cystitis
d. end-stage renal disease
e. renal calculi

Match the diagnostic measures and treatments with the correct disease.

23. _____ A urinalysis, urine culture, blood culture, blood work, voiding cystourethrogram, and a dimercaptosuccinic acid scan; treated with antibiotics and for severe infections, intravenous fluids and antibiotics are given

24. _____ A urinalysis, blood tests, and imaging tests; treatment may consist of analgesics, extra fluids, extracorporeal shock wave lithotripsy, ureteroscopy, and nephrolithotomy

25. _____ A urinalysis and a urine culture and sensitivity test; treated with antibiotics

26. _____ CT, MRI, and ultrasound; treatment often includes antihypertensive medications, diuretics, and a low-salt diet

27. _____ Blood work and a bone density test; treated with dialysis or kidney transplant

a. polycystic kidney disease
b. pyelonephritis
c. acute cystitis
d. end-stage renal disease
e. renal calculi

F. Anatomy of the Male Reproductive System
Fill in the blank.

1. The _____ produce spermatozoa and are suspended together in a sac called the scrotum.

2. The spermatozoa are formed in a series of tightly coiled tiny tubes in each testis called the _____.

3. In the _____, the spermatozoa mature and are stored.

4. Each _____ is a muscular tunnel that connects to the base of the epididymis and passes along the side of the testis and travels into the pelvic cavity to just behind the bladder.

5. The _____ is found below the bladder in males and surrounds part of the urethra.

6. The _____ is found within the penis and transports the semen to the outside of the body.

G. Physiology of the Male Reproductive System
Match the description with the hormone. Answers can be used more than once.

1. _____ Produced by the interstitial cells in the testicles at puberty

2. _____ Produced by the pituitary gland, stimulates the interstitial cells to produce testosterone

3. _____ Responsible for maintaining reproductive structures and the development of sperm cells

4. _____ Secreted by the pituitary gland, promotes the formation of spermatozoa

5. _____ Helps with the development of secondary sex characteristics

a. testosterone
b. follicle-stimulating hormone
c. luteinizing hormone

H. Life Span Changes of the Male Reproductive System

Select the correct answer or fill in the blank.

1. The _____ develops in the abdomen and starts its descent into the scrotum in utero around the seventh month.

2. Male secondary sex characteristics include
    a. a deep voice.
    b. broad shoulders and narrow hips.
    c. additional body hair.
    d. all of the above.

3. Which of the following occurs in the older adult male?
    a. The testicular tissue mass decreases.
    b. Testosterone levels gradually increase.
    c. The testes continue to create sperm at a faster rate.
    d. All of the above.

I. Male Reproductive System Disorders

Fill in the blank or select the correct answer.

1. Prostate cancer
    a. is caused when cells in the prostate gland mutate.
    b. can cause frequency, nocturia, hematuria, and hip and back pain.
    c. treatments depend on the type and may include a prostatectomy and radiation.
    d. all of the above.

2. _____ is the absence of one or both testes at birth.

3. _____ is also called *undescended testicle* and occurs when the testicle fails to descend into the scrotum.

4. _____ is a congenital malformation causing the urethra to open on the underside of the penis.

5. _____ is the inflammation of the epididymis and is often caused by a bacterial infection that starts in the bladder, prostate, or urethra.

6. Benign prostatic hyperplasia
    a. is a benign condition that causes the prostate gland to enlarge.
    b. causes urgency, frequency, difficulty starting urination, and hematuria.
    c. can be diagnosed with a digital rectal exam, blood tests, transrectal biopsy, and a cystoscopy.
    d. is treated with medications to shrink the prostate and surgery to remove part of the prostate.
    e. all of the above.

7. _____ is an enlargement of breast tissue in males caused by an estrogen and testosterone imbalance.

J. Assisting with an Examination and Diagnostic Procedures

Match the description with the correct diagnostic modality and laboratory test.

1. _____ Blood test used as a screening tool for prostate cancer

2. _____ CLIA-waived test used to analyze urine for abnormal levels of substances

3. _____ A procedure used to examine the urethra and bladder and to remove small tumors

4. _____ A renal scan that uses the radioisotope technetium-99m DMSA to evaluate the kidneys

5. _____ A procedure used to examine the ureters

6. _____ Measures the amount of urine in the bladder after urination

a. cystoscopy
b. ureteroscopy
c. dimercaptosuccinic acid scan
d. postvoid residual urine test
e. prostate-specific antigen
f. urinalysis

K. Assisting with Treatments for Urinary and Male Reproductive Disorders

Match the description with the correct treatment.

1. _____ Removal of the kidney

2. _____ Removal of the kidney, adrenal gland, surrounding tissue, and local lymph nodes

3. _____ A technique in which filtration through a semipermeable membrane is used to remove metabolic wastes and extra fluid from the blood

4. _____ Surgical removal of the cancer and surrounding tissue; kidney remains functional

5. _____ Nonsurgical approach using shock waves to break up stones in the ureters and kidneys

6. _____ Surgical removal of the kidney and ureter

7. _____ A surgical incision of the kidney to remove a stone

a. dialysis
b. extracorporeal shock wave lithotripsy
c. simple nephrectomy
d. partial nephrectomy
e. radical nephrectomy
f. nephrolithotomy
g. nephroureterectomy

Match the description with the correct treatment.

8. _____ A surgical procedure in which the vasa deferentia are cut, tied, and cauterized for the purpose of male sterilization

9. _____ Surgical removal of the prostate

10. _____ Surgical removal of the testicle

11. _____ A lighted scope is inserted into the urethra, and all but the outer part of the prostate is removed

12. _____ Surgical removal of the foreskin (or prepuce) of the penis

a. circumcision
b. prostatectomy
c. orchidectomy
d. transurethral resection of the prostate surgery
e. vasectomy

Match the indication for use and desired effect with the correct medication classification.

13. _____ Parasympathetic blocking agents; reduce spasms in smooth muscles

14. _____ Facilitates an erection in patients with impotence and symptoms of benign prostatic hypertrophy

15. _____ Treats overactive bladder by relaxing the bladder muscles

16. _____ Mineral supplement used to maintain normal electrolyte level

17. _____ Treats bacterial infections by killing or inhibiting bacterial growth

18. _____ Increases urinary output and lower the blood pressure by inhibiting the reabsorption of sodium and chloride in the kidneys

a. antibiotic
b. anticholinergic
c. antimuscarinic
d. diuretic
e. electrolyte
f. erectile dysfunction

Match the side effects and adverse reactions with the correct medication classification.

19. _____ Hypersensitivity reaction and GI distress

20. _____ Depends on the type; confusion, listlessness, gray skin, and black stools

21. _____ Dehydration, muscle weakness, fatigue, and electrolyte imbalance

22. _____ Blurred vision, confusion, reduced GI and genitourinary motility, dilation of pupils, fever, flushing, headache, and increased heart rate

23. _____ Headache, flushing, nasal congestion, myalgia, prolonged erections, cerebrovascular accident (CVA), and myocardial infarction (MI)

24. _____ Blurred vision, dry mouth and eyes, GI disturbances, headache, confusion, and arrhythmias

a. antibiotic
b. anticholinergic
c. antimuscarinic
d. diuretic
e. electrolyte
f. erectile dysfunction

CERTIFICATION PREPARATION
Circle the correct answer.

1. What statement is correct?
   a. The body has two urethras and one ureter.
   b. The kidneys are between T12 and L3 vertebrae.
   c. Urine moves from the bladder to the ureter and out of the body.
   d. The kidneys are anterior to the peritoneum.

2. The liquid in the renal tubule is called _____.
   a. electrolytes
   b. urine
   c. water
   d. filtrate

3. The point where the ureter enters the bladder is called _____.
   a. ureteral junction
   b. trigone
   c. ureterovesical junction
   d. rugae

4. During pregnancy, the filtration rate _____ and the number of nephrons _____.
   a. decreases; decreases
   b. increases; remains the same
   c. remains the same; increases
   d. increases; increases

5. The urinary system changes as a person ages. Which statement is *not* correct regarding older adults?
   a. Kidney tissue and the number of nephrons decrease.
   b. Renal arteries become hardened.
   c. Kidneys filter the blood faster.
   d. The bladder wall becomes less stretchy.

6. What is the normal role of the urinary system?
   a. Maintains fluid volume
   b. Controls red blood cell production
   c. Maintains an adequate blood pressure
   d. All of the above are normal roles of the urinary system

7. Which test measures the amount of urine left in the bladder after urination?
   a. Voiding cystourethrogram
   b. Ultrasound
   c. Postvoid residual urine test
   d. Intravenous pyelogram

8. What is a commonly used CLIA-waived test used to identify abnormal substances in the urine?
   a. Urinalysis
   b. Urine culture
   c. Cystoscopy
   d. Both a and c

9. Which medication is *not* an oral erectile dysfunction agent?
   a. Avanafil
   b. Sildenafil
   c. Warfarin
   d. Vardenafil

10. Which medication relaxes bladder muscles and decreases bladder contractions?
    a. Anticholinergic
    b. Antimuscarinic
    c. Alpha blockers
    d. Beta-3 adrenergic agonist

WORKPLACE APPLICATION

1. When Mrs. Williams was diagnosed with a urinary tract infection (UTI), she asked Hannah why females are more at risk for UTIs. Describe how you explain this to the patient.

   _____

   _____

2. You are working with a pediatric patient who was just diagnosed with diabetes insipidus. The child's mother asks you if it is "sugar diabetes." Describe how you would explain diabetes insipidus.

   _____

   _____

3. You are working with a patient who is confused about peritoneal dialysis and hemodialysis. Briefly explain both types of dialysis using words that a patient could understand.

   _____

   _____

   _____

INTERNET ACTIVITIES

1. Using online resources, research a test used for diagnosing urinary diseases. Create a poster presentation, a PowerPoint presentation, or write a paper summarizing your research. Include the following points in your project:
   a. Description of the test
   b. Any contraindications for the test
   c. Patient preparation for the test
   d. What occurs during the test

2. Using online resources, research a disorder of the urinary or male reproductive system. Create a poster presentation, a PowerPoint presentation, or write a paper summarizing your research. Include the following points in your project:
   a. Description of the disease
   b. Etiology
   c. Signs and symptoms
   d. Diagnostic procedures
   e. Treatments

3. Using online resources, research the different types of incontinence. In a one-page paper, describe each type of incontinence and how it is treated.

4. Using Table 42.6, Medication Classifications, select a generic medication from each of the following classifications: antibiotics, anticholinergics, antimuscarinics, diuretics, electrolytes, and erectile dysfunction agents. Using a reliable online drug resource, identify for each medication:
   a. Indication for use
   b. Desired effects
   c. Side effects
   d. Adverse reactions

   Write a short paper addressing each of these four areas for each medication.

Procedure 42.1   Coach a Patient on Testicular Self-Exam

Name _____ Date _____ Score _____

Tasks: Coach a patient to do a testicular self-exam (TSE) while considering the patient's developmental life stage. Document your teaching in the patient's health record.

Equipment and Supplies:
- Testicular self-examination brochure (optional)
- Testicular model
- Provider's order
- Patient's health record

Scenario: You are working with Dr. David Kahn. For Truong Tran (DOB 05/30/19XX), he ordered: testicular self-exam (TSE) coaching.

Directions: Role-play this scenario with a peer.

Standard: Complete the procedure and all critical steps in _____ minutes with a minimum score of 85% within two attempts (*or as indicated by the instructor*).

Scoring: Divide the points earned by the total possible points. Failure to perform a critical step, indicated by an asterisk (*), results in grade no higher than an 84% (*or as indicated by the instructor*).

Time: Began_____ Ended_____ Total minutes: _____

Steps:	Point Value	Attempt 1	Attempt 2
1. Wash hands or use hand sanitizer.	10		
2. Read the provider's order. Assemble the equipment.	10		
3. Greet the patient. Identify yourself. Verify the patient's identity with full name and date of birth. Explain the procedure to be performed in a manner that the patient understands. Answer any questions the patient may have about the procedure.	10		
4. Ask the patient what he knows about the self-exam. Clarify any inaccuracies. Build on the patient's prior knowledge of the topic during the session. Identify the patient's motivating factor for learning about the self-exam. Listen to the patient's concerns.	10		
5. Explain to the patient that the best time to do the self-exam is after a warm shower or bath.	10		
6. Demonstrate on the model while discussing the technique. Instruct the patient to examine each testicle gently with both hands. Roll the testicle between the thumb and fingers. Show the patient the epididymis, the soft curved structure behind and on top of the testicle. Then show the patient how to examine the vas deferens, which is the tube that runs up the epididymis.	10		
7. Instruct the patient to feel for any abnormalities and lumps. These could be painless or painful. Instruct the person to look for changes in the size, texture, or shape.	10		
8. Have the patient demonstrate the technique on the model. Coach the patient on ways to improve the exam if needed.	10		

9.	Answer any questions the patient may have. Provide the patient with a brochure to take home (optional).	**10**		
10.	Document the patient education in the patient's health record. Include the provider's name, the order, what was taught, how the patient responded, how the patient did the demonstration, and any handouts provided.	**10**		
	Total Points	**100**		

Documentation

Comments

CAAHEP Competencies	Step(s)
V.P.3.b. Coach patient regarding: medical encounters	Entire procedure
X.P.3. Document patient care accurately in the medical record	10

Procedure 42.2 Urinary Catheterization: Insertion of an Indwelling Foley Catheter

Name _____ Date _____ Score _____

Tasks: Insert an indwelling catheter with a drainage bag using sterile technique. Remove an indwelling catheter. Document the procedures.

Equipment and Supplies:
- Catheterization training model
- Patient's health record
- Gloves
- Waterproof pad (optional)
- Provider's order
- Straight catheterization tray kit containing the following items:
    - Waterproof pad
    - Fenestrated drape
    - Sterile gloves
    - Presaturated antiseptic applicators or antiseptic solution (povidone-iodine or chlorhexidine), sterile cotton balls, and sterile forceps
    - Water-soluble lubrication jelly packet or syringe
    - Indwelling urethral catheter connected to a urine drainage bag
    - Prefilled syringe with fluid
- Mayo stand
- Biohazard waste container
- Waste container
- Disinfectant wipes for cleaning

Provider's order: Insert Foley catheter.

Standard: Complete the procedure and all critical steps in _____ minutes with a minimum score of 85% within two attempts (*or as indicated by the instructor*).

Scoring: Divide the points earned by the total possible points. Failure to perform a critical step, indicated by an asterisk (*), results in grade no higher than an 84% (*or as indicated by the instructor*).

Time: Began_____ Ended_____ Total minutes: _____

Steps:	Point Value	Attempt 1	Attempt 2
1. Wash your hands or use hand sanitizer. Read the provider's order. Assemble the necessary supplies.	3		
2. Greet the patient. Identify yourself. Verify the patient's identity with full name and date of birth. Explain the procedure to be performed in a manner that is understood by the patient. Answer any questions the patient may have on the procedure.	3		
3. Place a waterproof pad on the lower part of the examination table. Provide a drape for the patient. Instruct the person to remove clothing from the waist down and sit on the examination table with the drape covering the patient's lap. Give the patient privacy.	3		
4. Before entering the room, give a courtesy knock. Ensure adequate lighting.	3		

5.	Position the patient. Place a drape to cover the patient and expose only the required anatomical areas. • Female patient: On the back with the knees flexed and the thighs relaxed so that the hips rotate to expose the perineal area. • Male patient: Supine with the legs extended and slightly apart	3		
6.	Put on gloves. Open the outer kit wrap.	3		
7.	Cleanse the perineal area with wipes from the kit or a with a washcloth, warm water, and soap or a perineal cleanser, according to facility policy.	3		
8.	Remove and dispose of gloves. Use hand sanitizer to perform hand hygiene.	3		
9.	Carefully open the catheterization kit, avoiding contaminating the sterile interior.	3		
10.	Put on sterile gloves using sterile technique.	3		
11.	Using the waterproof pad from the kit, wrap the edges of the pad around your sterile gloved hands. Place it between the patient's legs, creating a sterile field.	3		
12.	Place the fenestrated drape on the patient, only exposing the perineum or penis.	3		
13.	Working in the sterile field, prepare supplies. Open antiseptic applicators or open the antiseptic solution and pour it over the cotton balls. Open the lubricant packet or use the lubricant jelly syringe and place the water-soluble jelly on the tray. Remove the plastic upper tray from the bottom tray and place it nearby.	3		
14.	In the lower tray, place the water-filled syringe to the inflation port on the catheter. If required by the facility's procedures, check the Foley catheter's balloon. Push the plunger of the syringe, filling the balloon. Make sure the balloon fills correctly and there are no leaks or tears. Withdraw the fluid from the balloon. Keep the syringe attached to the catheter. Make sure the tubing to empty and the Foley bag is closed.	3		
15.	Lubricate the tip of the catheter about 1.5 to 2 inches. Make sure to keep the catheter sterile.	5*		

16. Clean the perineal area:
• Female patient
  – Separate the labia with the fingers of the nondominant hand; this will contaminate the hand, and it can no longer be used in the sterile field. This hand will continue to hold the labia until the catheter is inserted.
  – With the dominant hand, pick up an applicator or use the forceps and pick up a cotton ball. Wipe down the left side of the vagina, from top to bottom. Discard the applicator or cotton ball.
  – Repeat the above procedure but wipe down the right side of the vagina. Lastly, repeat the same action, but wipe down the center over the urinary meatus towards the rectum.
• Male patient
  – Gently grasp the penis shaft and hold it at a right angle to the body with the nondominant hand. If the patient is uncircumcised, use this hand to gently retract the foreskin. (After the catheter is inserted, make sure to push the foreskin back to the original position.) This will contaminate the hand. This hand will continue to hold the penis until the catheter is inserted.
  – With the dominant hand, pick up an applicator or use the forceps and pick up a cotton ball. Using the applicator or cotton ball, wipe the center of the urinary meatus and work outward in a circular manner. Discard the applicator or cotton ball. Repeat this cleaning technique two additional times, using a new applicator or cotton ball each time.
	5*		

17. Pick up the catheter and the lower tray with the sterile dominant hand. Place the bottom tray between the patient's legs. Make sure to hold the catheter approximately 2 to 3 inches from the tip.	3		

18. Insert the catheter. If you meet resistance while inserting the catheter, do not force the catheter. Discontinue the procedure if continued resistance is met or if the patient is having unusual discomfort or pain. Talk with the provider.
  • Female patient
    – Ask the patient to bear down gently to help expose the urethral meatus.
    – Insert the catheter 2 to 3 inches into the meatus until urine starts to flow. Then advance the catheter an additional 1 to 2 inches to ensure it is in the bladder.
    – Release the labia with the nondominant hand and hold the catheter in place as the dominant hand inflates the balloon. Disconnect the syringe and gently pull on the catheter until you feel resistance.
Note: If urine does not appear, the catheter may be in the patient's vagina. You may leave the catheter in place as a landmark and insert another sterile catheter into the urinary meatus. The catheter in the vagina is no longer sterile. Do not reuse that catheter. Do not allow the new catheter to come into contact with the previous catheter.
  • Male patient
    – With the nondominant hand (which is holding the penis at a right angle to the body), pull up slightly on the shaft.
    – Ask the patient to bear down gently and slowly insert the catheter through the urethral meatus. Advance the catheter 6 to 8 inches until urine flows. Then advance the catheter an additional 1 to 2 inches to ensure it is in the bladder.
    – Hold the catheter in place with the nondominant hand while the dominant hand inflates the balloon. Disconnect the syringe and gently pull on the catheter until you feel resistance.
Note: If the catheter does not advance in the male patient, do not force it. The patient may have an enlarged prostate or urethral obstruction.
	10*		

19. Secure the catheter on the thigh with tape or a catheter holder. Allow enough slack to prevent tension. Ensure the catheter is not secured too tightly, affecting movement or blocking urine drainage.	**3**		
20. Discard all biohazardous waste in the biohazardous waste container. Discard all other waste in the waste container. Remove your gloves and discard them in the biohazardous waste container. Wash your hands. After the patient has dressed and left the room, put on gloves and disinfect the examination table and Mayo stand.	**3**		
21. Remove the gloves and dispose of them appropriately. Wash your hands or use hand sanitizer.	**3**		
22. Using the patient's health record, document the procedure. Include the ordering provider's name, size of the catheter inserted, how the patient tolerated the procedure, and the urine output.	**3**		
Scenario update: The patient returns for removal of the indwelling Foley catheter. 23. Wash your hands or use hand sanitizer. Read the provider's order. Assemble the necessary supplies. Place a waterproof pad on the lower part of the examination table.	**3**		

24. Greet the patient. Identify yourself. Verify the patient's identity with full name and date of birth. Explain the procedure to be performed in a manner that is understood by the patient. Answer any questions the patient may have on the procedure. Instruct the person to remove clothing from the waist down and sit on the examination table; provide a drape for them to place over their lap. Put on nonsterile gloves.	3			
25. Measure the contents of the catheter bag. Empty urine from the bag. Remove any securement or anchor device from the patient's thigh.	3			
26. If indicated by the facility's procedures, clean around the meatus and catheter using soap and water or an antiseptic solution. Always wipe away from the urethral meatus and use a new cloth or swab with each wipe.	3			
27. Attach a syringe to the inflation port on the catheter. Verify the balloon size on the catheter. Withdraw that amount of fluid from the balloon.	5*			
28. Remove the catheter by pulling out slowly and smoothly. If resistance is met, it might mean that fluid is still in the balloon. Reattach the syringe and pull back any remaining fluid. Continue to remove the catheter and wrap the used catheter in the waterproof pad.	3			
29. Discard waste in the appropriate waste containers. Wash or sanitize your hands. Using the patient's health record, document the procedure.	3			
Total Points	100			

Documentation

Comments

CAAHEP Competencies	Step(s)
I.P.8. Instruct and prepare a patient for a procedure or treatment	2, 24
X.P.3. Document patient care accurately in the medical record	22, 29
ABHES Competencies	**Step(s)**
4. Medical Law and Ethics a. Follow documentation guidelines	22, 29
8. Clinical Procedures e. Perform specialty procedures, including but not limited to minor surgery, cardiac, respiratory, OB-GYN, neurological, and gastroenterology	Entire procedure

Procedure 42.3 Urinary Catheterization: Insertion of a Straight Catheter to Obtain a Urine Specimen

Name _____ Date _____ Score _____

Tasks: Place a urinary catheter to collect a urine specimen using sterile technique and document the procedure.

Equipment and Supplies:
- Catheterization training model
- Patient's health record
- Gloves
- Waterproof pad (optional)
- Provider's order
- Straight catheterization tray kit, containing:
  - Waterproof pad
  - Fenestrated drape
  - Sterile gloves
  - Presaturated antiseptic applicator, swab sticks, or antiseptic solution (povidone-iodine or chlorhexidine), sterile cotton balls, and sterile forceps
  - Water-soluble lubrication jelly packet
  - Specimen container with lid
  - Urethral catheter (properly sized)
  - Outer basin tray
- Specimen label, laboratory requisition, and biohazard specimen bag
- Mayo stand
- Biohazard waste container
- Waste container
- Disinfectant wipes for cleaning

Provider's order: UA using a straight catheter for specimen collection.

Standard: Complete the procedure and all critical steps in _____ minutes with a minimum score of 85% within two attempts (*or as indicated by the instructor*).

Scoring: Divide the points earned by the total possible points. Failure to perform a critical step, indicated by an asterisk (*), results in grade no higher than an 84% (*or as indicated by the instructor*).

Time: Began_____ Ended_____ Total minutes: _____

Steps:	Point Value	Attempt 1	Attempt 2
1. Wash your hands or use hand sanitizer. Read the provider's order. Assemble the necessary supplies.	5		
2. Greet the patient. Identify yourself. Verify the patient's identity with full name and date of birth. Explain the procedure to be performed in a manner that is understood by the patient. Answer any questions the patient may have on the procedure.	5		
3. Place a waterproof pad on the lower part of the examination table. Provide a drape for the patient. Instruct the person to remove clothing from the waist down and sit on the examination table with the drape covering the patient's lap. Give the patient privacy.	5		

4.	Before entering the room, give a courtesy knock. Ensure adequate lighting.	**5**		
5.	Position the patient. Place a drape to cover the patient and expose only the required anatomical areas. • Female patient: On the back with the knees flexed and the thighs relaxed so that the hips rotate to expose the perineal area. • Male patient: Supine with the legs extended and slightly apart	**5**		
6.	Open the kit. Put on sterile gloves using sterile technique.	**5**		
7.	Using the waterproof pad from the kit, wrap the edges of the pad around your sterile gloved hands. Place the pad between the patient's legs, creating a sterile field.	**5**		
8.	Working in the sterile field, prepare supplies. Open the antiseptic applicators or open the antiseptic solution and pour it over the cotton balls. Open the lubricant packet. Lubricate the tip of the catheter about 1.5 to 2 inches.	**10**		

9.	Clean the perineal area:
	• Female patient
	  – Separate the labia with the fingers of the nondominant hand; this will contaminate the hand, and it can no longer be used in the sterile field. This hand will continue to hold the labia until the catheter is inserted.
	  – With the dominant hand, pick up an applicator or use the forceps and pick up a cotton ball. Wipe down the left side of the vagina, from top to bottom. Discard the applicator or cotton ball.
	  – Repeat the above but wipe down the right side of the vagina. Lastly, repeat the same action, but wipe down the center over the urinary meatus towards the rectum.
	• Male patient
	  – Gently grasp the penis shaft and hold it at a right angle to the body with the nondominant hand. If the patient is uncircumcised, use this hand to gently retract the foreskin. (After the catheter is inserted, make sure to push the foreskin back to the original position.) This will contaminate the hand. This hand will continue to hold the penis until the catheter is inserted.
	  – With the dominant hand, pick up an applicator or use the forceps and pick up a cotton ball. Using the applicator or cotton ball, wipe the center of the urinary meatus and work outward in a circular manner. Discard the applicator or cotton ball. Repeat this cleaning technique two additional times, using a new applicator or cotton ball each time.
		10*		

10.	Place the sterile collection cup in the sterile tray. Place the tray between the patient's legs. Place the end of the catheter in the sterile collection cup. Pick up the catheter with the sterile dominant hand approximately 2 to 3 inches from the tip.	**5**		

11. Insert the catheter. If you meet resistance while inserting the catheter, do not force the catheter. Discontinue the procedure if continued resistance is met or if the patient is having unusual discomfort or pain. Talk with the provider.
   • Female
     – Ask the patient to bear down gently to help expose the urethral meatus.
     – Insert the catheter 2 to 3 inches into the meatus until urine starts to flow.
Note: If urine does not appear, the catheter may be in the patient's vagina. You may leave the catheter in place as a landmark and insert another sterile catheter into the urinary meatus. The catheter in the vagina is no longer sterile. Do not reuse that catheter. Do not allow the new catheter to come into contact with the previous catheter.
   • Male
     – With the nondominant hand (which is holding the penis at a right angle to the body), pull up slightly on the shaft.
     – Ask the patient to bear down gently and slowly insert the catheter through the urethral meatus. Advance the catheter 6 to 8 inches until urine flows.
Note: If the catheter does not advance in the male patient, do not force it. The patient may have an enlarged prostate or urethral obstruction.
	10*		

12. Once the specimen is obtained, secure the cover on the container. Make sure not to touch the inside of the container or cover. Set the specimen container on the Mayo stand.	5		
13. Remove the catheter by pulling out slowly and smoothly. Wrap the used catheter in the waterproof pad.	5		
14. Discard all biohazard waste in the biohazard waste container. Discard all other waste in the waste container. Remove your gloves and discard them in the biohazard waste container. Wash or sanitize your hands.	5		
15. After the patient has dressed and left the room, put on gloves and disinfect the examination table and Mayo stand. Label the urine specimen.	5		
16. Remove the gloves and dispose of them appropriately. Wash your hands or use hand sanitizer.	5		
17. Using the patient's health record, document the procedure. Include the ordering provider's name, the size of the catheter inserted, how the patient tolerated the procedure, and the urine output.	5		
Total Points	100		

Documentation

Comments

CAAHEP Competencies	Step(s)
I.P.8. Instruct and prepare a patient for a procedure or treatment	2
X.P.3. Document patient care accurately in the medical record	17
ABHES Competencies	**Step(s)**
4. Medical Law and Ethics a. Follow documentation guidelines	17
8. Clinical Procedures e. Perform specialty procedures, including but not limited to minor surgery, cardiac, respiratory, OB-GYN, neurological, and gastroenterology	Entire procedure

Obstetrics and Gynecology

CAAHEP Competencies	Assessment
I.C.4. Identify major organs in each body system	Skills and Concepts – A. 1, 2, 3
I.C.5. Identify the anatomical location of major organs in each body system	Skills and Concepts – A. 1-12
I.C.6. Identify structure and function of the human body across the life span	Skills and Concepts – B. 1-4
I.C.7. Identify the normal function of each body system	Skills and Concepts – A. 13-18
I.C.8.a. Identify common pathology related to each body system including: signs	Skills and Concepts – C. 6-10
I.C.8.b. Identify common pathology related to each body system including: symptoms	Skills and Concepts – C. 6-18
I.C.8.c. Identify common pathology related to each body system including: etiology	Skills and Concepts – C. 1-5
I.C.8.d. Identify common pathology related to each body system including: diagnostic measures	Skills and Concepts – C. 11-15
I.C.8.e. Identify common pathology related to each body system including: treatment modalities	Skills and Concepts – C. 11-15, Workplace Applications – 1
V.C.8.a. Identify the following related to body systems: medical terms	Vocabulary Review
V.C.8.b. Identify the following related to body systems: abbreviations	Abbreviations
I.P.8. Instruct and prepare a patient for a procedure or a treatment	Procedures 43.1, 43.2
I.P.9. Assist provider with a patient exam	Procedure 43.1
V.P.3.b. Coach patients regarding: medical encounters	Procedure 43.2
X.P.3. Document patient care accurately in the medical record	Procedure 43.2
A.5. Respect diversity	Procedure 43.2

ABHES Competencies	Assessment
2. Anatomy and Physiology a. List all body systems and their structures and functions	Skills and Concepts – B. 1, 2, 3; C. 8
2. b. Describe common diseases, symptoms, and etiologies as they apply to each system	Skills and Concepts – C. 4, 7, 8
2. c. Identify diagnostic and treatment modalities as they relate to each body system	Skills and Concepts – C. 5
3. Medical Terminology c. Apply medical terminology for each specialty	Vocabulary Review
3. d. Define and use medical abbreviations when appropriate and acceptable	Vocabulary Review, Abbreviations
8. Clinical Procedures d. Assist provider with specialty examination, including cardiac, respiratory, OB-GYN, neurological, and gastroenterology procedures	All procedures
8. e. Perform specialty procedures, including but not limited to minor surgery, cardiac, respiratory, OB-GYN, neurological, and gastroenterology	All procedures

VOCABULARY REVIEW

Using the word pool on the right, find the correct word to match the definition. Write the word on the line after the definition.

Group A

1. The area between the opening of the vagina and the anus
   _____

2. The larger external folds of skin surrounding the opening of the vagina _____

3. Sensitive erectile tissue _____

4. Removal of a breast tumor and a small amount of the surrounding tissue _____

5. A mature sexual reproductive cell; spermatozoa or ovum
   _____

6. Removal of the entire breast _____

7. The release of the ovum from the ovarian follicle
   _____

8. Organs that produce sex cells in both males and females
   _____

9. The smaller inner folds of skin surrounding the opening of the vagina _____

10. The vaginal opening _____

Word Pool
- gonads
- gamete
- orifice
- labia majora
- labia minora
- clitoris
- perineum
- ovulation
- lumpectomy
- mastectomy

Group B

1. Painful menstrual flow, cramps _____
2. A high-frequency electrical current running through a wire is used to remove abnormal tissue from both the cervix and the endocervical canal _____
3. Bands of scar tissue that can bind anatomic structures together _____
4. Removal of a limited number of lymph nodes to determine if the cancer has spread to the lymph nodes _____
5. Surgical removal of the fallopian tube and ovary _____
6. A sample of abnormal tissue from the cervix using a small spoon-shaped instrument called a *curette* _____
7. Surgical removal of the uterus and cervix _____
8. Painful or difficult intercourse _____
9. An extensive cervical biopsy during which a wedge of tissue is removed from the cervix and examined under a microscope _____
10. Using a microscope with a light source, the vagina and cervix are visually examined to locate and evaluate abnormal cells _____

Word Pool
- sentinel node biopsy
- curettage
- colposcopy
- loop electrosurgical excision procedure
- cone biopsy
- hysterectomy
- salpingo-oophorectomy
- adhesions
- dysmenorrhea
- dyspareunia

Group C

1. A fluid-filled cyst in one of the vestibular glands located on either side of the vaginal orifice _____
2. Excessive menstrual flow and uterine bleeding other than that caused by menstruation _____
3. Lack of menstrual flow _____
4. Tissue death _____
5. Failure of the ovaries to release an ovum at the time of ovulation _____
6. A procedure used to visually examine the abdomen _____
7. Abnormal thinning of the bone structure, causing bones to become brittle and weak _____
8. Abnormally heavy menstrual flow or prolonged menstrual periods _____
9. Similarity in size, form, and arrangement of parts on opposite sides of the body _____
10. Pus-like _____

Word Pool
- menorrhagia
- menometrorrhagia
- laparoscopy
- purulent
- amenorrhea
- osteoporosis
- symmetry
- Bartholin cysts
- anovulation
- necrosis

Group D

1. A condition in which the spinal column has an abnormal opening that allows protrusion of the meninges and/or the spinal cord

   _____

2. A deficiency in the enzyme phenylalanine hydroxylase, which is responsible for converting phenylalanine into tyrosine

   _____

3. An abnormal condition of pregnancy of unknown cause, marked by hypertension, edema, and proteinuria

   _____

4. Congenital absence of part or all of the brain

   _____

5. Implantation of the embryo in any location other than the uterus

   _____

6. A disorder that affects all the exocrine cells but affects the respiratory system the most; mucus is abnormally thick and blocks the alveoli, causing dyspnea _____

7. A genetic disorder in which abnormal cell division results in an extra chromosome 21 _____

8. An inherited anemia characterized by crescent-shaped red blood cells _____

9. Ability to live _____

10. A group of inherited blood disorders characterized by a deficiency of one of the factors necessary for the coagulation of blood _____

11. The protrusion of the meninges through an opening in the spinal column or skull _____

Word Pool

- viability
- ectopic pregnancy
- preeclampsia
- Down syndrome
- spina bifida
- meningocele
- anencephaly
- hemophilia
- sickle cell anemia
- cystic fibrosis
- phenylketonuria

ABBREVIATIONS

Write out what each of the following abbreviations stands for.

1. OB/GYN _____

2. hCG _____

3. STI _____

4. HIV _____

5. GN-RH _____

6. AIDS _____

7. PID _____

8. HRT _____

9. DUB _____

10. PMDD _____

11. PMS _____

12. MRI _____

13. HPV _____

14. Pap _____

15. LEEP _____

16. CA-125 _____

17. ACOG _____

18. LMP _____

19. OSHA _____

20. OCP _____

21. IUD _____

22. ASC _____

23. ASC-US _____

24. ASC-H _____

25. HSIL _____

26. LSIL _____

27. CIS _____

28. ACG _____

29. AIS _____

30. KOH _____

31. EDD _____

32. IUFD _____

33. PID _____

34. CF _____

35. PKU _____

36. HDN _____

37. CPR _____

38. WIC _____

39. cm _____

40. PPD _____

41. EPDS _____

42. AFP _____

43. BMI _____

44. IV _____

45. CVS _____

SKILLS AND CONCEPTS

Answer the following questions. Write your answer on the line or in the space provided.

A. Anatomy and Physiology of the Female Reproductive System

1. Label the structures in the following figure.

    a. _____

    b. _____

    c. _____

    d. _____

    e. _____

    f. _____

    g. _____

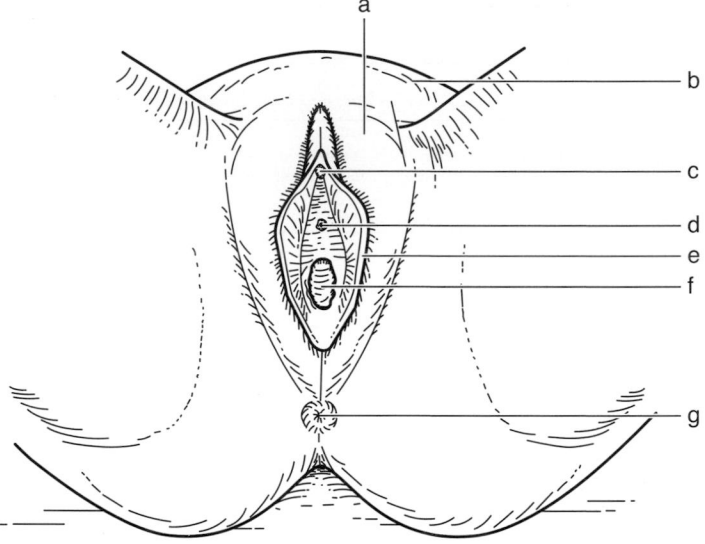

2. Label the structures in the following figure.

a. _____

b. _____

c. _____

d. _____

e. _____

f. _____

g. _____

h. _____

i. _____

j. _____

k. _____

l. _____

3. Which body cavity contains the ovaries, fallopian tubes, and uterus?_____

Match the term to the correct definition.

4. _____ Perimetrium

5. _____ Myometrium

6. _____ Endometrium

7. _____ Corpus or body

8. _____ Fundus

9. _____ Cervix

   a. middle, muscle layer of the uterus
   b. narrowed lower area of the uterus
   c. large central area of the uterus
   d. outer layer of the uterus
   e. raised area at the top of the uterus between the outlets for the fallopian tubes
   f. inner lining of the uterus

10. The _____ serves as the passageway for the endometrium during menstruation, receives the penis during intercourse, and is the birth canal during the delivery of a baby.

11. The external female genitalia are called the _____.

12. In addition to the pelvic organs, the _____ are also part of the female reproductive system.

13. The term for the beginning of the menstrual cycle is _____.

Match the phase of the menstrual cycle with the correct description.

14. _____ Follicular phase

15. _____ Luteal phase

16. _____ Menstrual phase

a. Lasts about 5 days. Menstrual discharge is made up of necrotic endometrial tissue, mucus, and blood from the endometrial engorgement. The uterus contracts to shed the excess tissue.

b. Begins once ovulation is complete. Progesterone is secreted by the corpus luteum, causing extensive growth of the endometrium as it prepares for a possible pregnancy. If conception occurs, the corpus luteum continues to secrete progesterone until the placenta is well established. The corpus luteum can secrete progesterone and hCG to maintain the pregnancy. If conception does not occur, hCG is not secreted, and the corpus luteum atrophies, the endometrium breaks down, and menstruation begins.

c. The hypothalamus secretes gonadotropin-releasing hormone stimulating the anterior pituitary to release FSH and LSH to mature the Graafian follicle. The follicle secretes estrogen which stimulates the growth of the endometrium. Ends with the expulsion of the ovum.

17. Put the steps of the zygote's journey in the correct order.

_____ Moves from the fallopian tube to the uterus.

_____ Is called a *morula*.

_____ Divides as it moves through the fallopian tube to the uterus.

_____ Implants into the uterine wall.

_____ Is called a *blastocyst*.

18. From weeks 3 through 8 of development, the organism is called a(n) _____; from weeks 9 through 38, it is called a(n) _____.

B. Life Span Changes

1. Which of the following hormones stimulates the production of sex hormones?
   a. Luteinizing hormone
   b. Follicle-stimulating hormone
   c. Estrogen
   d. All of the above
   e. A and B only

2. Primary amenorrhea is when a girl who is _____years old has never had a period.

3. Changes in hormone levels can cause which of the following physical changes in the reproductive tract of women?
   a. Vaginal walls become thinner, dryer, and less elastic.
   b. Sex can become painful.
   c. There is a greater risk for vaginal yeast infections.
   d. All of the above.
   e. Only b and c.

4. Older women are most often seen for neoplasms of the _____, _____, _____, and _____.

C. Diseases and Disorders of the Female Reproductive System

Match the etiology with the correct condition.

1. _____ Caused by *Candida albicans*

2. _____ End of ovarian function, occurring between the ages of 45 and 55

3. _____ Functional endometrial tissue located outside of the uterus

4. _____ Any acute or chronic infection of the reproductive system that ascends from the vagina, cervix, uterus, fallopian tubes, and ovaries

5. _____ Inflammation caused by an invading organism caused by sexually transmitted infections, all allergic reaction, or bacterial overgrowth

a. endometriosis
b. candidiasis
c. cervicitis
d. pelvic inflammatory disease
e. menopause

Match the signs and symptoms with the correct disease.

6. _____ Asymptomatic, fever, abdominal or pelvic pain, vaginal discharge, dysuria, dyspareunia

7. _____ Dysmenorrhea, pain with bowel movements or urination, menorrhagia, menometrorrhagia, infertility, fatigue, diarrhea, constipation, bloating, and nausea

8. _____ Thick, purulent discharge with odor, dysuria, dyspareunia, vaginal bleeding

9. _____ Vulvovaginal itching; dry, bright red vaginal tissue; an odorless, white, "cottage cheese" like vaginal discharge

10. _____ Twelve months of amenorrhea; hot flashes, concentration problems, mood swings, vaginal dryness, urinary incontinence, dry skin, sleep disorders

a. endometriosis
b. candidiasis
c. cervicitis
d. pelvic inflammatory disease
e. menopause

Match the diagnostic measures and treatments with the correct disease.

11. _____ Pelvic examination and testing of the vaginal secretions; antifungal medications, cream, ointments, tablets, and suppositories

12. _____ Pelvic examination and testing of the vaginal secretions; treatment not needed unless caused by an STI, then both patient and partner must be treated

13. _____ Ultrasound, laparoscopy; medication or surgery

14. _____ No periods for 12 months; very low-dose contraceptives, short-term hormone replacement therapy, soy products or soy supplements, vitamin E, Vitamin B_6, antidepressants, gabapentin, clonidine

15. _____ Pelvic examination and test of the vaginal secretions; antibiotics for the patient and partner, analgesics

a. endometriosis
b. candidiasis
c. cervicitis
d. pelvic inflammatory disease
e. menopause

Match the description with the correct disease or condition.

16. _____ Placenta that is positioned in the uterus so that it covers the opening of the cervix.

17. _____ Extremely serious form of hypertension secondary to pregnancy. Patients are at risk for coma, convulsions, and death.

18. _____ Bilateral presence of numerous cysts, caused by a hormonal abnormality leading to the secretion of androgens. Can cause acne, facial hair, and infertility.

19. _____ Poorly understood group of symptoms that occur in some women on a cyclical basis: breast pain, irritability, fluid retention, headache, and a lack of coordination are some of the symptoms.

20. _____ Excessive vomiting that causes weakness, dehydration, and fluid and electrolyte imbalance.

21. _____ Abnormal uterine bleeding not caused by a tumor, inflammation, or pregnancy.

22. _____ Premature separation of the placenta from the uterine wall; may result in a severe hemorrhage that can threaten both infant and maternal lives.

23. _____ The cessation of menses.

24. _____ A mosquito-borne virus that typically causes a mild fever, rash, and joint pain. The virus can be passed to a fetus and is associated with certain birth defects such as microcephaly.

25. _____ Mood disorder that includes depression, irritability, fatigue, changes in appetite or sleep, and difficulty in concentrating; occurs 1 to 2 weeks before the onset of the menstrual flow.

26. _____ Smooth muscle tumors of the uterus. They are usually nonpainful growths that may be removed surgically. Theses tumors may also be referred to as *myomas.*

27. _____ Abnormal condition of pregnancy with unknown cause, marked by hypertension, edema, and proteinuria.

28. _____ A mother with Rh− blood will develop antibodies to an Rh+ fetus during the first pregnancy. If another pregnancy occurs with an Rh+ fetus, the antibodies can destroy the fetal blood cells.

29. _____ Benign, fluid-filled sac that can be either a follicular cyst, which occurs when a follicle does not rupture at ovulation, or a cyst of the corpus luteum, which is caused when it does not continue its transformation.

a. abruptio placenta
b. dysfunctional uterine bleeding
c. eclampsia
d. fibroids
e. hemolytic disease of the newborn
f. hyperemesis gravidarum
g. menopause
h. ovarian cyst
i. placenta previa
j. polycystic ovary syndrome
k. preeclampsia
l. premenstrual dysphoric disorder
m. premenstrual syndrome
n. Zika virus

30. _____ or _____ are the most frequent causes of PID.

31. The condition where functional endometrial tissue is located outside of the uterus is called _____.

32. The vaginal infection commonly called a *yeast infection* is caused by what organism? _____

D. Cancers of the Female Reproductive System

Match the etiology with the correct cancer.

1. _____ Cause is not known; risk factors include age, inherited gene mutation, estrogen hormone replacement therapy, menarche at a young age, menopause at an older age, having never been pregnant, fertility treatment, smoking, use of an IUD, polycystic ovary syndrome.

2. _____ Cause is not known; risk factors include being female, family history, inherited genes, radiation exposure, obesity, menarche at a young age.

3. _____ Almost all are caused by HPV; risk factors include many sexual partners, early sexual activity, having other STIs, a weak immune system, and smoking.

a. breast cancer
b. cervical cancer
c. ovarian cancer

Match the signs and symptoms with the correct cancer.

4. _____ Initially asymptomatic, advanced stages vaginal bleeding after intercourse, between periods, or after menopause; watery, bloody vaginal discharge that may be heavy and have a foul odor, pelvic pain or pain during intercourse

5. _____ Initially asymptomatic, advanced stages abdominal bloating, quickly feeling full when eating, weight loss, discomfort in the pelvis area, changes in bowel habits, and a frequent need to urinate

6. _____ Thickening or lump, change is size, shape or appearance; changes to the skin such as dimpling, peeling, scaling, or flaking, redness or pitting

a. breast cancer
b. cervical cancer
c. ovarian cancer

Match the diagnostic measures and treatments with the correct disease.

7. _____ Pelvic examination, ultrasound or CT, CA-125 blood test, biopsy; hysterectomy, unilateral or bilateral salpingo-oophorectomy, chemotherapy, targeted drug therapy

8. _____ Examination by the provider, mammogram, ultrasound, biopsy, MRI; lumpectomy, mastectomy, or sentinel node biopsy, radiation, chemotherapy, and/or hormone therapy

9. _____ Pap test, punch biopsy, endocervical curettage, colposcopy, and LEEP; in addition, LEEP treatment can include cone biopsy, hysterectomy, radiation, and chemotherapy

a. breast cancer
b. cervical cancer
c. ovarian cancer

E. The Medical Assistant's Role with Examinations, Diagnostic Procedures, and Treatments

1. When setting up for a gynecologic examination, which of the following would be included if the provider is going to do a direct smear method for the Pap test?
   a. Microscope slides
   b. Plastic-fronded broom
   c. Fixative
   d. Liquid preparation container
   e. Both a and c

2. When the patient schedules an appointment for a gynecologic examination, she should be advised not to _____ or have _____ for 24 hours before the examination.

3. Which of the following would *not* be included in the gynecologic history?
    a. Age at menarche
    b. Childhood diseases
    c. Date of last menstrual period
    d. Number of times pregnant
    e. All of the above would be included in the gynecologic history

4. Which of the following are ways that a medical assistant can help prevent embarrassment for the patient when assisting with a gynecologic examination?
    a. Behave in a professional manner.
    b. Explain what is going to happen.
    c. Show genuine interest in the patient's concerns.
    d. All of the above.

5. For the breast examination, the patient starts in the _____ position and then is placed in the _____ position.

6. The patient remains in the _____ position for the abdominal examination and then is placed in the _____ position for the pelvic examination.

Match the type of contraceptive to the correct characteristic.

7. _____ Flexible plastic implant inserted under skin of upper arm; releases progestin to prevent ovulation, thickens cervical secretions to block semen, thins endometrial wall; effective for up to 3 years

8. _____ Must be fitted by clinician; requires instruction on how to insert and remove; spermicide must be used each time; must be left in place for 6 hours after intercourse

9. _____ Suppress ovulation; atrophy of the endometrium

10. _____ No prescription or examination needed, easily available, and inexpensive

11. _____ Requires 150-mg intramuscular injection every 3 months

12. _____ Copper type releases copper, which slows sperm in the cervix; hormonal type releases progestin, which reduces sperm mobility and prevents thickening of the endometrial wall

a. male or female condom
b. diaphragm, cervical cap, cervical sponge
c. intrauterine device
d. birth control implants
e. depo-provera
f. oral contraceptives, hormonal patch, vaginal ring

13. With the direct smear method of obtaining a specimen for a Pap test, a fixative must be applied immediately to the slide before it is sent to the laboratory. With the liquid-based method of obtaining a specimen for a Pap test, a cervical spatula is used.
    a. The first statement is true, and the second statement is false.
    b. The first statement is false, and the second statement is true.
    c. Both statements are true.
    d. Both statements are false.

14. A(n) _____ is an endocrine evaluation that can assist in the diagnosis and treatment of infertility issues, amenorrhea, menopause, or postmenopausal bleeding.

15. When testing for candidiasis, the provider will add a drop of _____ to the slide that will dissolve other cellular debris so that the provider can see the yeast buds.

16. When testing for trichomoniasis, the provider will add a drop of _____ to the slide.

F. Obstetrics

1. When obtaining the pregnancy history for the first prenatal visit, _____ refers to the number of pregnancies regardless of weeks; _____ refers to the number of pregnancies that have gone to the age of viability; _____ refers to the termination of a pregnancy before the age of viability.

2. A patient relates that she has had five pregnancies, three have gone to term, one was a premature birth at 32 weeks, and she had one miscarriage. Her gravida, para, and abortion numbers would be:
   a. Gravida 4, para 2, abortion 1
   b. Gravida 5, para 2, abortion 0
   c. Gravida 5, para 4, abortion 1
   d. Gravida 4, para 4, abortion 0

3. The _____ history will help to determine if additional testing may be needed during the prenatal period. The _____ history will help determine patient education as it relates to the pregnancy.

4. Blood tests done during the first prenatal visit include which of the following?
   a. Hemoglobin and hematocrit
   b. Rubella titer
   c. Hepatitis B screening
   d. Blood type and Rh
   e. All of the above

5. Return prenatal visits are scheduled every 4 weeks through 28 weeks gestation. Return prenatal visits are scheduled every 2 weeks through 35 weeks gestation.
   a. The first statement is true, the second statement is false.
   b. The first statement is false, the second statement if true.
   c. Both statements are true.
   d. Both statements are false.

6. Fetal heart tones can be heard between _____ weeks gestation. The fetal heart rate should be between _____ beats per minute.

7. The postpartum visit occurs at about _____ after delivery.

8. The 10-question tool to identify patients at risk for depression is called _____.

9. Instructions for the patient who has been scheduled for an ultrasound include drinking _____ 8-ounce glasses of water _____ before the scheduled ultrasound.

10. The triple screen test to detect any risk of fetal and chromosomal disorders include tests for which of the following?
    a. Alpha-fetoprotein
    b. Human chorionic gonadotropin
    c. Estriol
    d. All of the above

CERTIFICATION PREPARATION

Circle the correct answer.

1. The _____ starts the follicular phase of the menstrual cycle.
   a. hypothalamus
   b. pituitary gland
   c. ovary
   d. medulla

2. During implantation, the zygote functions as an endocrine gland by secreting which hormone?
   a. FSH
   b. hCG
   c. LSH
   d. GnRH

3. According to the American Cancer Society, what is the risk of a woman developing breast cancer?
   a. 1 in 2
   b. 1 in 8
   c. 1 in 20
   d. 1 in 100

4. What position is used for a pelvic examination?
   a. Supine
   b. Prone
   c. Sims
   d. Lithotomy

5. When testing for candidiasis, a drop of what solution is added to the slide?
   a. Sterile water
   b. Potassium hydroxide
   c. Saline
   d. Nothing is added to the slide

6. During a pelvic examination, what occurs after the provider has collected the specimen for a Pap test?
   a. Breast examination
   b. Bimanual examination
   c. Digital rectal examination
   d. Abdominal examination

7. A maturation index can assist in the diagnosis and treatment of which condition?
   a. Infertility issues
   b. Amenorrhea
   c. Menopause
   d. All of the above

8. What method of contraception either kills sperm or prevents them from entering the cervical os?
   a. Barrier methods
   b. Hormonal contraceptives
   c. Intrauterine devices
   d. None of the above

9. What procedure uses a microscope with a light source and magnifying lens?
   a. Cryotherapy
   b. Pap test
   c. LEEP
   d. Colposcopy

10. What term refers to the number of pregnancies that have gone to the age of viability?
    a. Gravida
    b. Multigravida
    c. Para
    d. Primipara

WORKPLACE APPLICATIONS

1. Anna Richardson is scheduled for a loop electrosurgical excision procedure (LEEP) today because of an abnormal Pap test. Explain to Anna how the procedure is performed and why Dr. Walden has ordered it.

   _____

   _____

   _____

   _____

2. Julia Berkley is in for her first prenatal visit. When taking her history, she tells you that she has a 2-year-old, 4-year-old twins, and had a miscarriage last year. What is her gravida, para, and abortion information?

   _____

   _____

3. Dr. Walden has asked you to prepare a patient for a bimanual examination. How should the patient be gowned and draped? How should you position the patient? What type of supplies will Dr. Walden need to complete the examination? What is assessed during this examination?

   _____

   _____

   _____

   _____

   _____

INTERNET ACTIVITIES

1. IUDs are a highly recommended form of birth control. Research the types of IUDs online. Create a poster presentation, a PowerPoint presentation, or write a paper summarizing your research. Include the following points in your project:
   a. Describe the different types of IUDs and how they work.
   b. How are they inserted and removed?
   c. What are their potential complications?

2. Search the Internet for resources for pregnant and breastfeeding women. Develop a resource guide for these patients in an obstetric practice.

Procedure 43.1   Setting Up for and Assisting the Provider with a Gynecologic Examination

Name _____ Date _____ Score _____

Task: Prepare equipment for a gynecologic examination and assist the provider by placing the patient in the appropriate positions.

Equipment and Supplies:
- Disposable examination gloves
- Fecal occult blood test kit
- Water-soluble lubricant
- Vaginal speculum
- Slide and fixative or liquid preparation container
- Cervical spatula or plastic-fronded broom
- Laboratory requisition form
- Cotton-tipped applicator
- Patient gown
- Patient drape sheet
- Tray or Mayo stand

Standard: Complete the procedure and all critical steps in _____ minutes with a minimum score of 85% within two attempts (*or as indicated by the instructor*).

Scoring: Divide the points earned by the total possible points. Failure to perform a critical step, indicated by an asterisk (*), results in grade no higher than an 84% (*or as indicated by the instructor*).

Time: Began_____ Ended_____ Total minutes: _____

Steps:	Point Value	Attempt 1	Attempt 2
1. Wash hands or use hand sanitizer.	5		
2. Assemble equipment needed for the gynecologic examination. Place on a tray or Mayo stand in a logical order.	5		
3. Change the table paper if needed.	5		
4. Greet the patient. Identify yourself. Verify the patient's identity with full name and date of birth. Explain the procedure to be performed in a manner that is understood by the patient. Answer any questions the patient may have about the procedure.	10		
5. Ask if the patient needs to empty her bladder and collect a urine specimen if needed.	10		
6. Instruct the patient to undress and put on the gown.	10		
7. Assist the patient onto the examination table and she should remain in the sitting position. Place the drape across her lap.	10		
8. Assist the patient into the supine position, providing a pillow for under her head for comfort. Pull out the leg extension on the examination table.	10		
9. With the stirrups in place on the examination table, assist the patient into the lithotomy position. The leg extension should then be pushed in.	15*		
10. When the examination is complete, assist the patient into the sitting position. Instruct the patient that she can get dressed.	10		

11. After the patient has dressed and left the exam room, clean the room and prepare specimens for transport to the laboratory.	10		
Total Points	100		

Comments

CAAHEP Competencies	**Step(s)**
I.P.8. Instruct and prepare a patient for a procedure or a treatment	4-6
I.P.9. Assist provider with a patient exam	Entire procedure
ABHES Competencies	**Step(s)**
8.d. Assist provider with specialty examination, including cardiac, respiratory, OB-GYN, neurological, and gastroenterology procedures	Entire procedure
8.e. Perform specialty procedures, including but not limited to minor surgery, cardiac, respiratory, OB-GYN, neurological, and gastroenterology	Entire procedure

Procedure 43.2   Coach a Patient on Breast Self-Exam

Name _____   Date _____   Score _____

Tasks: Coach a patient to do BSE while considering the patient's cultural beliefs and developmental life stage. Document teaching in the patient's health record.

Equipment and Supplies:
- Breast self-examination brochure (optional)
- Breast model
- Provider's order
- Patient's health record

Scenario: You are working with Dr. David Kahn. He has ordered you to show Binh, a 17-year-old Vietnamese patient, how to do a breast self-exam. She has a strong family history of breast cancer. The patient can fluently speak and understand English.

Directions: Role-play this scenario with another peer.

Standard: Complete the procedure and all critical steps in _____ minutes with a minimum score of 85% within two attempts (*or as indicated by the instructor*).

Scoring: Divide the points earned by the total possible points. Failure to perform a critical step, indicated by an asterisk (*), results in grade no higher than an 84% (*or as indicated by the instructor*).

Time: Began_____ Ended_____ Total minutes: _____

Steps:	Point Value	Attempt 1	Attempt 2
1. Wash hands or use hand sanitizer.	5		
2. Read the provider's order. Assemble equipment.	5		
3. Greet the patient. Identify yourself. Verify the patient's identity with full name and date of birth. Explain the procedure to be performed in a manner that the patient understands. Answer any questions the patient may have about the procedure.	10		
4. Provide privacy and independence during the session. Encourage the patient to ask questions and discuss her concerns.	5*		
5. Ask the patient if she is familiar with breast self-examinations. Ask about her thoughts on illness and if she does alternative therapies. Explain the importance of doing a self-exam.	5*		

6.   Explain to the patient that she will need to undress and look at her breast in the mirror to identify any changes.
    a. Let her know that she will need to check to see if they are the usual size, shape, and color.
    b. She should also look for swelling, redness, rash, dimpling, puckering, or bulging of the skin.
    c. She should check to see if the nipple position or appearance has changed.
    d. Finally, she should check to see if any fluid is coming from the nipple by placing her thumb and index finger on the tissue by the nipple and pulling outward towards the end of the nipple.
	10		

7.	Instruct the patient that she needs to change positions and continue to check the appearance of the breasts. She needs to place her hands on her hips and press down. This tightens the chest muscle under the breasts. While in this position, she should turn from side to side to see the outer part of the breasts. Instruct her to clasp her hands behind her head or raise her arms and look at the outer part of the breasts again.	**10**		
8.	Instruct the patient to bend forward and roll her shoulders and elbows forward while tightening her chest muscles. While in this position, she can check for changes in the shape of the breasts.	**10**		
9.	Instruct the patient to palpate the breast using one of the two techniques. Use the model as you explain the technique. *Lying-down technique*: Instruct the patient to check the breast while lying down. Have her do the following: Tuck a small pillow under the side being checked. Tuck one arm under the head and with the other hand check the opposite breast (e.g., right hand checks the left breast). Use the first two or three finger pads. With fingers together, use a circular motion and a firm, smooth touch to check the entire breast. Start at the top outer breast tissue and move around the breast in a circular pattern. When the top of the breast is reached again, move in 1 inch towards the nipple and complete another circle around the breast. Repeat until the entire breast from the armpit to the cleavage is checked. Then place fingers flat on the nipple and feel for any changes beneath the nipple. Repeat these steps on the other breast. *Shower technique*: Place the right hand on the right hip. With a soapy left hand, feel for changes in the right axilla area. Use two or three finger pads to press on the breast. Move in an up and down pattern over the breast tissue. Make sure to cover from the bra line to the collarbone. Repeat on the opposite side.	**10**		
10.	Have the patient select a technique that she will use. Encourage the patient to demonstrate the technique on the breast model. Coach the patient on ways to improve the exam if needed.	**10**		
11.	Answer any questions the patient may have. Provide the patient with a brochure to take home (optional).	**10**		
12.	Document the patient education in the patient's health record. Include the provider's name, the order, what was taught, how the patient responded, how the patient did the demonstration, and any handouts provided.	**10**		
	Total Points	**100**		

Documentation

Comments

CAAHEP Competencies	Step(s)
V.P.3.b. Coach patients regarding: medical encounters	Entire procedure
X.P.3. Document patient care accurately in the medical record	12
ABHES Competencies	**Step(s)**
8.e. Perform specialty procedures, including but not limited to minor surgery, cardiac, respiratory, OB-GYN, neurological, and gastroenterology	Entire procedure

Pediatrics

CAAHEP Competencies	Assessment
I.C.6. Identify structure and function of the human body across the life span	Skills and Concepts – A. 2
I.C.13 Identify appropriate vaccinations based on an immunization schedule	Procedure 44.4
II.C.3.a. Identify normal and abnormal results as reported in: graphs	Skills and Concepts – D. 3-5
II.C.3.b. Identify normal and abnormal results as reported in: tables	Skills and Concepts – D. 3-5
V.C.13.b. Understand the basic concepts of the following theories: Erikson	Skills and Concepts – A. 3-7
I.P.1.f. Accurately measure and record: weight (adult and infant)	Procedure 43.2
I.P.1.g. Accurately measure and record: length (infant)	Procedure 44.2
I.P.1.h. Accurately measure and record: head circumference (infant)	Procedure 44.1
I.P.9. Assist provider with a patient exam	Procedures 44.1, 43.2
II.P.3. Document on a growth chart	Procedures 44.1, 44.2
X.P.3. Document patient care accurately in the medical record	Procedures 44.1, 44.2
ABHES Competencies	**Assessment**
5. Human Relations d. Adapt care to address the developmental stages of life	Workplace Applications – 1-3

VOCABULARY REVIEW

Using the word pool on the right, find the correct word to match the definition. Write the word on the line after the definition.

1. A thin, watery serum-like drainage _____

2. The state of being drowsy and dull, listless, and unenergetic

   _____

3. A space covered by thick membranes between the sutures of an infant's skull _____

4. The ability to function independently _____

5. Abnormally small head associated with incomplete brain development _____

6. A disorder that does not have a cause that can be found in the body _____

7. A thin layer of cartilage located at the ends of a long bone where new bone forms _____

8. Weakened or changed _____

9. Inflammation and irritation of the skin _____

10. Hives _____

11. Characterized by the formation and/or discharge of pus

    _____

12. Enlargement of the cranium caused by abnormal accumulation of cerebrospinal fluid in the cerebral system

    _____

Word Pool
- epiphyseal plates
- autonomy
- excoriation
- lethargy
- nonorganic
- serous
- suppurative
- fontanelle
- hydrocephaly
- microcephaly
- attenuated
- urticaria

ABBREVIATIONS

Write out what each of the following abbreviations stands for.

1. CDC_____

2. VIS_____

3. BMI_____

4. OTC_____

5. IV_____

6. OME_____

7. AAP_____

8. AAFP_____

9. ASD_____

10. PDD_____

11. NCVIA_____

12. RSV_____

13. STI _____

14. HPV _____

SKILLS AND CONCEPTS

Answer the following questions. Write your answer on the line or in the space provided.

A. Normal Growth and Development

1. Height and weight are examples of _____. Motor, mental, social, and language skills are examples of _____.

2. What would be the expected growth pattern for the following age groups?

    a. 6 months _____

    _____

    b. 1 year _____

    _____

    c. 2 years _____

    _____

    d. 3 years _____

    _____

    e. 3-6 years _____

    _____

Match Erikson's stage of development with the correct description.

3. _____ Toddlers learn language skills and gain independence; they may have issues if they cannot meet parental expectations or are overprotected.

4. _____ Adolescents face many physical and hormonal changes in this stage. Teenagers work at figuring out who they are and where they fit; they are looking for a direction for their lives.

5. _____ School-age children enjoy finishing projects and receiving recognition; they are feeling inadequate if not accepted by peers or if they cannot please their parents.

6. _____ Infants learn to rely on caregivers; apprehension occurs if needs are not met.

7. _____ Preschoolers actively seek out new experiences; children become hesitant if restrictions or reprimands make them feel guilty or afraid to try more challenging skills.

a. trust vs. mistrust
b. autonomy vs. shame and doubt
c. initiative vs. guilt
d. industry vs. inferiority
e. identity vs. role confusion

B. Pediatric Diseases and Disorders

1. Colic is a condition that is usually seen in infants between _____ weeks and _____ months of age. It involves crying episodes that occur at least _____ times a week and last for longer than _____ hours a day and lasting at least _____ weeks.

Match the signs and symptoms with the correct disease/disorder.

2. _____ An infant or young child whose weight is consistently below the 3rd percentile on growth charts or one who is 20% below the ideal body weight for length

3. _____ Two or more watery or abnormal stools within 24 hours

4. _____ Inflammation of the middle ear, with fluid building up behind the tympanic membrane; child may cry persistently, tug at the ear, have a fever, be irritable, have diminished hearing

5. _____ Crying episodes that occur at least three times a week for longer than 3 hours a day and lasting 3 or more weeks; infant draws up legs, clenches the fists, and cries inconsolably

a. colic
b. diarrhea
c. failure to thrive
d. otitis media

Match the common childhood disease to the correct description.

6. _____ It is caused by the coxsackievirus, which is transmitted by direct contact with nose and throat drainage, saliva, or the stool of an infected individual.

7. _____ Also called *pinkeye*, this is a common infection in children and is highly contagious, especially in day care centers and schools. It can be caused by a bacterial or viral infection that produces white or yellowish pus, which may cause the eyelids to stick shut in the morning.

8. _____ An acute and sometimes fatal illness characterized by fatty invasion of the inner organs, especially the liver, and swelling of the brain.

9. _____ Also called *erythema infectiosum*, parvovirus infection, or slapped cheek disease, is an infection caused by parvovirus B19.

a. conjunctivitis
b. fifths disease
c. hand-foot-and-mouth disease
d. Reye syndrome

10. Autism-specific screenings are recommended for all children at the _____ and _____ month visits.

11. Children with autism often have impaired social interaction, do not respond to their name, avoid eye contact, and show limited interest in their surroundings. Many children with autism have a very low pain tolerance and have no issues with noise, touch, or other sensory stimulation.
    a. The first statement is true, and the second statement is false.
    b. The first statement is false, and the second statement is true.
    c. Both statements are true.
    d. Both statements are false.

12. Nearly _____ of all children and adolescents in the United States are obese.

13. Reasons for childhood obesity include which of the following?
    a. Family history of obesity
    b. Inactivity
    c. High-calorie diet
    d. Metabolic or endocrine disorders
    e. All of the above

C. The Medical Assistant's Role with the Pediatric Examination and Diagnostic Procedures

1. Which of the following is *not* one of medical assistant's responsibilities in a pediatric examination?
    a. Updating patient histories
    b. Administering immunizations
    c. Assessing cognitive skills
    d. Measuring and weighing children
    e. All of the above

2. When assisting with diagnostic procedures the medical assistant should offer reasonable choices when possible. The medical assistant should use a firm, direct approach about expected behavior to gain the cooperation of older children.
    a. The first statement is true, and the second statement is false.
    b. The first statement is false, and the second statement is true.
    c. Both statements are true.
    d. Both statements are false.

D. Assisting with the Examination

1. When measuring the pulse of a child younger than 2, the _____ site should be used.

2. Blood pressure is checked in children ages _____ years and older.

3. By the age of 1, the brain's growth is _____% complete; by the age of 3, it is _____% complete; and by the age of 6, it is _____% complete.

4. The CDC growth charts are _____ specific and there are charts for _____ age range, and _____ age range.

5. Using the growth charts in the textbook (Figures 44.7 and 44.8), plot the measurements and answer the following questions.

    a. Simon Blackstone, 18 months: head circumference, 14.25 inches; 85 cm long; 14 kg.

    What is his height percentile? _____

    What is his weight percentile? _____

    b. Carla Toomis, 9 years old: 50 inches tall and weighs 88 pounds.

    What is her height percentile? _____

    What is her weight percentile? _____

E. Assisting with Diagnostic Procedures

1. The most common method of performing a distance vision screening is to use a(n) _____ chart.

2. Traditionally, the child would need to stand _____ feet away from the chart, but now the chart can be displayed on a tablet computer and require the child to be _____ feet away.

3. A(n) _____ is used to test hearing. It can test hearing at various _____ _____ and _____.

F. Assisting with Treatments

1. List eight details that must be documented when a vaccination is given.

    a. _____

    b. _____

    c. _____

    d. _____

    e. _____

    f. _____

    g. _____

    h. _____

2. List the route of administration for the following vaccines.

    a. Dtap _____

    b. HAV _____

    c. HBV _____

    d. HPV _____

    e. Hib _____

    f. Influenza _____

    g. IPV _____

    h. MMR _____

    i. PCV _____

    j. Varicella _____

3. Nebulizers are used to administer medication in a form that can be _____. It is used to treat respiratory conditions such as _____, _____, respiratory syncytial virus, or reactive airway disease.

4. When using a nebulizer, a(n) _____ works better for younger patients than a mouthpiece.

G. The Adolescent Patient

1. When working with an adolescent patient, the health examination includes which of the following?
   a. Screening for STIs
   b. Pap test for sexually active female adolescents
   c. Assessing for high-risk behaviors
   d. All of the above

2. _____ are the leading cause of death and injury in adolescence, and _____ is the third leading cause of death.

CERTIFICATION PREPARATION

Circle the correct answer.

1. During which period in a child's life do they gain weight the fastest?
   a. First 6 months
   b. Age 6 months to 1 year
   c. Preschool
   d. Adolescence

2. In which illness or condition are dehydration and electrolyte imbalance of particular concern when the disorder occurs in children?
   a. Colic
   b. Influenza
   c. Hepatitis B
   d. Diarrhea

3. The first dose of MMR vaccine should be administered at what age?
   a. 2 months
   b. 4 months
   c. 12 months
   d. 4 years

4. What method of evaluation is used to detect microcephaly?
   a. Culture of infectious material
   b. Developmental screening tests
   c. Laryngoscopy
   d. Measurement of the head circumference

5. Tetanus is part of which immunization?
   a. HBV
   b. Hib
   c. DTaP
   d. MMR

6. Which is a helpful approach to adolescent patients?
   a. The parents should be present for discussions about health problems.
   b. The medical assistant should recognize the importance of personal appearance to adolescents.
   c. The medical assistant should use distraction if painful procedures are performed.
   d. The medical assistant should give the adolescent advice on handling personal problems.

7. The varicella vaccine is usually administered to children in which age group?
   a. Newborns (first dose)
   b. 6 months
   c. 12-18 months
   d. Preschool age

8. Studies have shown that a child who is obese between the ages of _____ has an 80% chance of becoming an obese adult.
   a. 2 and 4
   b. 4 and 8
   c. 8 and 12
   d. 10 and 13

9. The Hib vaccine prevents _____.
   a. measles
   b. varicella
   c. meningitis
   d. hepatitis B

10. One of the primary causes of childhood injuries is _____.
    a. motor vehicle accidents
    b. drowning
    c. burns
    d. all of the above

WORKPLACE APPLICATIONS

1. Based on what you have learned about therapeutic approaches for the pediatric patient, what would be the best way to deal with the following patient situations?

   a. A crying 2-month-old scheduled for the first round of vaccinations _____

   _____

   _____

   b. A 3-year-old who is diagnosed with croup _____

   _____

   _____

   c. An 8-year-old who needs his blood glucose checked with a glucometer _____

   _____

   _____

   d. A 13-year-old who has to receive a penicillin injection in the ventrogluteal site _____

   _____

   _____

2. The grandmother of a 3-year-old patient calls today with concerns about her granddaughter, who has had diarrhea for 2 days. What types of questions should the medical assistant ask about the child's condition? What types of fluids and diet might the provider recommend?

   _____

   _____

   _____

   _____

3. Allison is trying to obtain vital signs on a 4-year-old child who refuses to stand on the scale or cooperate while her temperature is taken. What can Allison do to try to obtain the child's cooperation? What is the best way to take this patient's temperature?

   _____

   _____

   _____

   _____

INTERNET ACTIVITIES

1. Using internet resources, research childhood obesity. Create a poster presentation, a PowerPoint presentation, or write a paper summarizing your research. Include the following points in your project:
   a. Possible reasons for the increase in childhood obesity
   b. Possible solutions
   c. Describe how BMI is determined and used with pediatric patients

2. Using internet resources, research ADHD. Create a poster presentation, a PowerPoint presentation, or write a paper summarizing your research. Include the following points in your project:
   a. Possible causes of ADHD
   b. Treatment options for ADHD including nontraditional options
   c. Techniques a medical assistant can use when working with a patient with ADHD

Procedure 44.1 Measure the Circumference of an Infant's Head

Name _____ Date _____ Score _____

Task: To obtain an accurate measurement of the circumference of an infant's head and plot the result on the patient's growth chart.

Equipment and Supplies:
- Patient's record
- Flexible disposable tape measure
- Age- and gender-specific growth chart
- Pen

Standard: Complete the procedure and all critical steps in _____ minutes with a minimum score of 85% within two attempts (*or as indicated by the instructor*).

Scoring: Divide the points earned by the total possible points. Failure to perform a critical step, indicated by an asterisk (*), results in grade no higher than an 84% (*or as indicated by the instructor*).

Time: Began_____ Ended_____ Total minutes: _____

Steps:	Point Value	Attempt 1	Attempt 2
1. Wash hands or use hand sanitizer.	10		
2. Greet the patient and the parents or caregivers. Identify yourself. Verify the patient's identity with full name and date of birth. Explain the procedure to be performed in a manner the patient (if old enough) or the parent or caregiver understands. Answer any questions the patient may have on the procedure. If he or she is old enough, gain the child's cooperation through conversation.	10		
3. Place an infant in the supine position, or the infant may be held by the parent. An older child may sit on the examination table.	10		
4. Hold the tape measure with the zero mark against the infant's forehead, slightly above the eyebrows and the top of the ears. Ask the parent for assistance if necessary.	15*		
5. Bring the tape measure around the head, just above the ears, until it meets.	15*		
6. Read to the nearest 0.5 cm or 1/4 inch.	10		
7. Record the measurement on the growth chart and in the patient's health record.	10		
8. Dispose of the tape measure.	10		
9. Wash hands or use hand sanitizer.	10		
Total Points	100		

Documentation

Comments

CAAHEP Competencies	Step(s)
I.P.1.h. Accurately measure and record: head circumference (infant)	Entire procedure
II.P.3. Document on a growth chart	7
I.P.9. Assist provider with a patient exam	Entire procedure
X.P.3. Document patient care accurately in the medical record	7
ABHES Competencies	**Step(s)**
5.d. Adapt care to address the developmental stages of life	Entire procedure

Procedure 44.2 Measure an Infant's Length and Weight

Name _____ Date _____ Score _____

Task: To measure an infant's length and weight accurately so that growth patterns can be monitored and recorded.

Equipment and Supplies:
- Patient's record
- Infant scale with paper cover
- Flexible measuring tape
- Examination table paper
- Pen
- Pediatric length board, if available
- Gender-specific infant growth chart
- Waste container

Standard: Complete the procedure and all critical steps in _____ minutes with a minimum score of 85% within two attempts (*or as indicated by the instructor*).

Scoring: Divide the points earned by the total possible points. Failure to perform a critical step, indicated by an asterisk (*), results in grade no higher than an 84% (*or as indicated by the instructor*).

Time: Began_____ Ended_____ Total minutes: _____

Steps for measuring infant length:	Point Value	Attempt 1	Attempt 2
1. Wash hands or use hand sanitizer, assemble the necessary equipment.	5		
2. Greet the patient and parents or caregivers. Identify yourself. Verify the patient's identity with full name and date of birth. Explain the procedure to be performed in a manner the patient (if old enough) or the parent or caregiver understands. Answer any questions the parents or caregivers may have on the procedure.	5		
3. Undress the infant. The diaper may be left on.	5		
4. Cover the examination table with smooth, flat paper. Ask the caregiver to place the infant on his or her back on the examination table. If the table is a pediatric table with a headboard, ask the caregiver to hold the infant's head gently against the headboard while you straighten the infant's leg and note the location of the heel on the measurement area. If there is no headboard, ask the caregiver to gently hold the infant's head still while you draw a line on the paper at the top of the baby's head and at the heel after extending the leg.	10*		
5. Measure the infant's length with the tape measure and record it.	10		
6. Document the results in either inches or centimeters, depending on office policy, on the infant's growth chart, in the progress notes, and in the caregiver's record if requested.	5		
Steps for measuring infant weight:			
7. Wash hands or use hand sanitizer, assemble the necessary equipment, and explain the procedure to the infant's caregiver.	5		
8. Greet the patient and parents or caregivers. Identify yourself. Verify the patient's identity with full name and date of birth. Explain the procedure to be performed in a manner that is understood by the patient. Answer any questions the parents or caregivers may have on the procedure.	5		

9. If the scale is not a digital model, prepare the scale by sliding weights to the left; line the scale with disposable paper to reduce the risk of pathogen transmission.	5			
10. Completely undress the infant. If the diaper is clean and dry, it can remain on.	5			
11. Place the infant gently on the center of the scale, keeping your hand directly above the infant's trunk for safety.	10			
12. If the scale is not a digital model, slide the weights across the scale until balance is achieved. Read the infant's weight while he or she is still.	10*			
13. If the scale is not a digital model, return the weights to the far left of the scale and remove the baby. Discard the paper lining the scale. If the scale became contaminated during the procedure, follow Occupational Safety and Health Administration (OSHA) guidelines for use of gloves and disposal of contaminated waste. Disinfect the equipment according to the manufacturer's guidelines.	10			
14. Wash hands or use hand sanitizer.	5			
15. Document the results in either pounds or kilograms, depending on office policy, on the infant's growth chart, in the progress notes, and in the caregiver's record if requested.	5			
Total Points	100			

Documentation

Comments

CAAHEP Competencies	Step(s)
I.P.1.g. Accurately measure and record: length (infant)	1-6
II.P.3. Document on a growth chart	6, 13
I.P.9. Assist provider with a patient exam	Entire procedure
X.P.3. Document patient care accurately in the medical record	6, 15
ABHES Competencies	**Step(s)**
5.d. Adapt care to address the developmental stages of life	Entire procedure

Procedure 44.3   Document Immunizations

Name _____ Date _____ Score _____

Task: To document accurately the administration of a pediatric immunization.

Equipment and Supplies:
- Patient's record
- Vaccine administration record (VAR) (Work Product 43-1)
- Parent's immunization record (if used in the medical practice)
- Vaccine Information Sheet (VIS) for hepatitis B (a link to the current VIS forms can be accessed at www. cdc.gov/vaccines/hcp/vis/current-vis.html)

Scenario: Samantha Anderson, a 5-week-old infant, has just received her second dose of the hepatitis B (HBV) vaccine. Document the administration of the vaccine.

Standard: Complete the procedure and all critical steps in _____ minutes with a minimum score of 85% within two attempts (*or as indicated by the instructor*).

Scoring: Divide the points earned by the total possible points. Failure to perform a critical step, indicated by an asterisk (*), results in grade no higher than an 84% (*or as indicated by the instructor*).

Time: Began_____ Ended_____ Total minutes: _____

Steps:	Point Value	Attempt 1	Attempt 2
1. Gather the necessary forms.	20		
2. Make sure that the hepatitis B VIS form was given, and that all the parent's questions were answered before the vaccine is dispensed and administered.	20*		
Scenario update: The parent signed the required paperwork and you have the vaccine in the left vastus lateralis and now you need to document. 3. After the vaccine has been given, complete the information required on the VAR, including the name of the vaccine, the date given, the route of administration and site, the vaccine lot number and manufacturer, the date on the VIS form, the date it was given to the parent, and your signature or initials.	20		
4. In the parent's immunization record, record the date of administration, the name and address of the provider's practice, and the type of vaccine administered.	20		
5. After administering the HBV vaccine, record the following details in the child's health record: • Date the vaccine was administered • Vaccine's manufacturer, batch and lot numbers, and expiration date • Type of vaccine administered and dose • Route of administration and exact site if an injection was given • Any reported or observed side effects • Publication date of the VIS form given to the parent (on the bottom of the form) • Parent education about possible side effects of the vaccine • Name and title of the person who administered the vaccine	20*		
Total Points	100		

Documentation

Comments

ABHES Competencies	Step(s)
5.d. Adapt care to address the developmental stages of life	Entire procedure

Work Product 44.1   Vaccine Administration Record

Name _____   Date _____   Score _____

Vaccine Administration Record for Children and Teens

Patient name: _____

Birthdate: _____   Chart number: _____

Clinic name and address

Before administering any vaccines, give copies of all pertinent Vaccine Information Statements (VISs) to the child's parent or legal representative and make sure he/she understands the risks and benefits of the vaccine(s). Always provide or update the patient's personal record card.

Vaccine	Type of Vaccine[1]	Date given (mo/day/yr)	Funding Source (F,S,P)[2]	Route & Site[3]	Vaccine		Vaccine Information Statement (VIS)		Vaccinator[5] (signature or initials & title)
					Lot #	Mfr.	Date on VIS[4]	Date given[4]	
Hepatitis B[6] (e.g., HepB, Hib-HepB, DTaP-HepB-IPV) Give IM.[3]									
Diphtheria, Tetanus, Pertussis[6] (e.g., DTaP, DTaP/Hib, DTaP-HepB-IPV, DT, DTaP-IPV/Hib, Tdap, DTaP-IPV, Td) Give IM.[3]									
Haemophilus influenzae type b[6] (e.g., Hib, Hib-HepB, DTaP-IPV/Hib, DTaP/Hib, Hib-MenCY) Give IM.[3]									
Polio[6] (e.g., IPV, DTaP-HepB-DTaP-IPV/Hib, DTaP-IPV) Give IPV SC or IM.[3] Give all others IM.[3]									
Pneumococcal (e.g., PCV7, PCV13, conjugate; PPSV23, polysaccharide) Give PCV IM.[3] Give PPSV SC or IM.[3]									
Rotavirus (RV1, RV5) Give orally (po).[3]									

See page 2 to record measles-mumps-rubella, varicella, hepatitis A, meningococcal, HPV, influenza, and other vaccines (e.g., travel vaccines).

How to Complete This Record

1. Record the generic abbreviation (e.g., Tdap) or the trade name for each vaccine (see table at right).

2. Record the funding source of the vaccine given as either F (federal), S (state), or P (private).

3. Record the route by which the vaccine was given as either intramuscular (IM), subcutaneous (SC), intradermal (ID), intranasal (IN), or oral (PO) and also the site where it was administered as either RA (right arm), LA (left arm), RT (right thigh), or LT (left thigh).

4. Record the publication date of each VIS as well as the date the VIS is given to the patient.

5. To meet the space constraints of this form and federal requirements for documentation, a healthcare setting may want to keep a reference list of vaccinators that includes their initials and titles.

6. For combination vaccines, fill in a row for each antigen in the combination.

Abbreviation	Trade Name and Manufacturer
DTaP	Daptacel (sanofi); Infanrix (GlaxoSmithKline [GSK]); Tripedia (sanofi pasteur)
DT (pediatric)	Generic DT (sanofi pasteur)
DTaP-HepB-IPV	Pediarix (GSK)
DTaP/Hib	TriHIBit (sanofi pasteur)
DTaP-IPV/Hib	Pentacel (sanofi pasteur)
DTaP-IPV	Kinrix (GSK)
HepB	Engerix-B (GSK); Recombivax HB (Merck)
HepA-HepB	Twinrix (GSK), can be given to teens age 18 and older
Hib	ActHIB (sanofi pasteur); Hiberix (GSK); PedvaxHIB (Merck)
Hib-HepB	Comvax (Merck)
Hib-MenCY	MenHibrix (GSK)
IPV	Ipol (sanofi pasteur)
PCV13	Prevnar 13 (Pfizer)
PPSV23	Pneumovax 23 (Merck)
RV1	Rotarix (GSK)
RV5	RotaTeq (Merck)
Tdap	Adacel (sanofi pasteur); Boostrix (GSK)
Td	Decavac (sanofi pasteur); Generic Td (MA Biological Labs)

Technical content reviewed by the Centers for Disease Control and Prevention

For additional copies, visit www.immunize.org/catg.d/p2022.pdf • Item #P2022 (4/14)

This form was created by the Immunization Action Coalition • www.immunize.org • www.vaccineinformation.org

Procedure 44.4   Complete an Immunization Schedule for a Patient

Name _____   Date _____   Score _____

Task: Complete an immunization schedule for a patient by reviewing a patient immunization record and determine what vaccines are needed. Document all vaccines given.

Equipment and Supplies:
- CDC Immunization Schedule (Fig. 44.11)
- Vaccine Information Sheet (VIS)
- Electronic health record or SimChart for the Medical Office (SCMO)

Scenario: In preparation for Daniel Miller's 2-year-old well-child visit tomorrow, you review his immunization record and see that he was up to date with his immunizations through 9 months of age, including the third dose of hepatitis B and inactivated poliovirus. His record doesn't show any immunizations since that time. A review of the statewide vaccination record system doesn't show any additional vaccines given elsewhere.

Standard: Complete the procedure and all critical steps in _____ minutes with a minimum score of 85% within two attempts (*or as indicated by the instructor*).

Scoring: Divide the points earned by the total possible points. Failure to perform a critical step, indicated by an asterisk (*), results in grade no higher than an 84% (*or as indicated by the instructor*).

Time: Began_____ Ended_____ Total minutes: _____

Steps:	Point Value	Attempt 1	Attempt 2
1. Using the CDC Immunization Schedule, determine the vaccines needed to bring Daniel up to date with all of his vaccinations.	20*		
Scenario Update: Daniel and his father have arrived for his well-child visit. The provider has discussed the needed vaccines with Daniel's father, and he has agreed that Daniel should get the missing vaccinations. He has given his consent. You provide Daniel's father with the required VIS and he has no further questions or concerns. You administer the vaccines that were identified with the CDC Schedule review per the provider's orders and now need to document the vaccines.			
2. Utilizing EHR software or SCMO (using the Simulation Playground), locate Daniel Miller's record (DOB 03/21/20XX). Create an office visit encounter for today's visit with Dr. Angela Perez.	20		
3. Document that the patient has no allergies to drugs, food, or environmental items.	20		
4. Using the Immunization screen, document the immunizations that were given today as per Dr. Perez's orders. All of the following information should be documented: • Dose • Date (today's date) • Provider • Route/site (IM or SUBQ/vastus lateralis or anterolateral thigh) • Manufacturer (Elsevier) • Expiration date (one year from today's date) • Reaction - None • VIS edition (document in the Reaction field of SCMO)	20*		
5. Log out of EHR or SCMO.	20*		
Total Points	100		

Comments

CAAHEP Competencies	Step(s)
I.C.13 Identify appropriate vaccinations based on an immunization schedule	1

Geriatrics

CAAHEP Competencies	Assessment
I.C.6. Compare structure and function of the human body across the life span	Skills and Concepts – A. 1, 2, 3, 5, 7, 9, 11, 12, 15, 18, 22, 25-28, 30; Workplace Application – 2; Internet Activities – 2, 3
I.P.9. Assist provider with a patient exam	Procedure 45.1
A.3. Demonstrate empathy for patient's concerns	Procedure 45.1

ABHES Competencies	Assessment
5. Human Relations d. Adapt care to address the developmental stages of life	Procedure 45.1

VOCABULARY REVIEW

Using the word pool, find the correct word to match the definition. Write the word on the line after the definition.

Group A

1. Rhythmic contraction of involuntary muscles lining the gastrointestinal tract _____

2. Fully and clearly expressed or demonstrated, leaving nothing merely implied _____

3. The most abundant structural protein found in skin and other connective tissues; provides strength and cushioning to many parts of the body _____

4. Nerve pain that occurs after a shingles outbreak and may become chronic _____

5. A temporary fall in blood pressure when a person rapidly changes from a recumbent position to a standing position

   _____

6. Skin surface areas supplied by a single afferent spinal nerve

   _____

7. The relative frequency of deaths in a specific population

   _____

8. Proceeding in a gradual, subtle way, but with harmful effects

   _____

Word Pool
- mortality
- orthostatic hypotension
- insidious
- explicit
- peristalsis
- collagen
- dermatome
- postherpetic neuralgia

Group B

1. A medicine or substance capable of damaging cranial nerve VIII or the organs of hearing and balance _____

2. A highly elastic protein in connective tissue that allows tissues to resume their shape after stretching or contracting; found abundantly in the dermis of the skin _____

3. Frequent urination at night _____

4. Chronic disease of the inner ear causing recurrent episodes of vertigo, progressive sensorineural hearing loss, and tinnitus

   _____

5. The secretion or discharge of tears _____

6. Surgical removal of the ovaries _____

7. Sores that develop over a bony prominence as the result of ischemia from prolonged pressure _____

8. Abnormal thinning of the bone structure causing bones to become brittle and weak _____

Word Pool
- osteoporosis
- oophorectomy
- pressure injury
- nocturia
- elastin
- lacrimation
- Meniere's disease
- ototoxic

ABBREVIATIONS

Write out what each of the following abbreviations stands for.

1. CHF _____
2. DVT _____
3. DM _____
4. GERD _____
5. IV _____
6. CVA _____
7. OTC _____
8. AD _____
9. CNS _____
10. CT _____
11. MRI _____
12. PET _____
13. FDA _____
14. REM _____
15. PLMD _____
16. COPD _____

SKILLS AND CONCEPTS

Answer the following questions.

A. Changes in Anatomy, Physiology, and Diseases of the Cardiovascular and Pulmonary Systems

1. The most common reason for hospitalization among older adults is _____.

2. Which of the following factors contribute to making the myocardial wall stiffer and increases the time needed for the relaxation phase of the cardiac cycle?
   a. Hypertension increases the workload; valves tend to thicken and become more rigid.
   b. Myocardial cells enlarge; deposits of fat and connective tissue increase.
   c. Walls of the veins weaken and stretch; valves of the veins are damaged.
   d. All of the above.

3. Hypertension increases the workload of the _____ of the heart. This can result in _____ of the chamber and weakening in of the _____ wall.

4. Which of the following is *not* a sign of orthostatic hypotension?
   a. A drop of 20 mm Hg or more in the systolic pressure
   b. An increase of 10 mm Hg or more in the diastolic pressure
   c. Experiencing lightheadedness or dizziness
   d. All of the above

5. As we age, the rate of airflow through the bronchi slowly declines after age _____.

6. Which factors put the older adult at greater risk for pneumonia?
   a. Sleep apnea and sleep disorders
   b. Respiratory muscles become weaker
   c. The alveoli enlarge and their walls become thinner
   d. All of the above
   e. Both a and c

B. Changes in Anatomy, Physiology, and Diseases of the Endocrine and Gastrointestinal Systems

1. The most common endocrine system disorder seen in aging patients is _____.

2. What are the classic symptoms of diabetes mellitus? _____

   _____

3. Sensory abnormalities associated with DM type 2 include _____ or problems with _____.

4. Due to the fact that many older people are unable to chew and lubricate their food as well as younger people, _____ is a common age-related problem.

5. Common gastrointestinal diseases in aging individuals include which of the following?
   a. GERD
   b. Diverticulosis
   c. Celiac disease
   d. Irritable bowel syndrome
   e. Both a and b

C. Changes in Anatomy, Physiology, and Diseases of the Integumentary and Musculoskeletal Systems

1. Exposure to UV light from the sun may frequently cause what skin conditions with aging? _____

   _____

   _____

2. List the three layers of the skin. _____

   _____

3. Loss of what substance in the skin causes it to sag and wrinkle? _____

4. The dermis loses _____ of its mass during the aging process.

5. Which of the following is *not* a suggestion to help older people prevent or treat dry skin?
   a. Use a room humidifier to moisten the air
   b. Use hot water when bathing
   c. Use a mild soap or cleansing cream
   d. Wear protective clothing in cold weather
   e. All of the above

6. The term for hair loss is _____.

7. Another term for age spots is _____.

8. Shingles is caused by the same virus that causes _____.

9. Osteoarthritis is caused by _____ loss and degeneration, and commonly occurs in the _____ joints.

10. Muscular changes in the aging patient are directly related to the individual's _____.

11. List five risk factors for osteoporosis. _____

    _____

    _____

12. When an aging individual falls, the possible complications include which of the following?
    a. Pressure injuries
    b. Pneumonia
    c. Placement in long-term care facilities
    d. Death
    e. All of the above

13. List five measures that can be taken to prevent falls. _____

    _____

    _____

    _____

D. Changes in Anatomy, Physiology, and Diseases of the Nervous System and Sensory Organs

1. The best way to ensure mental functioning in later life is to remain _____ and _____ stimulated.

2. Risk factors for cognitive decline include all of the following *except*
   a. low stress.
   b. sedentary lifestyle.
   c. smoking and substance abuse.
   d. hypertension, diabetes, and heart disease.
   e. all of the above.

3. Alzheimer's disease typically begins after the age of 60. Research shows that 1 in 4 Americans older than 65 have AD.
   a. The first statement is true, and the second statement is false.
   b. The first statement is false, and the second statement is true.
   c. Both statements are true.
   d. Both statements are false.

4. List five conditions that can interfere with sleep. _____

   _____

Match the structure of the eye to the age-related change.

5. _____ Thickens, curve decreases
6. _____ Decrease in size and volume
7. _____ Decrease in number of rods and cones
8. _____ Affects pupil constriction and dilation
9. _____ Thickens, becomes more opaque

   a. lens
   b. anterior chamber
   c. ciliary muscles
   d. cornea
   e. retina

10. List eye diseases and disorders that occur frequently in older patients. _____

    _____

    _____

11. The decreased ability to hear high frequencies and discriminate sounds associated with aging is

    _____.

12. The hearing disorder that is associated with a ringing or buzzing in the ear is known as

    _____.

13. During the aging process, the abilities to _____ and _____ decline subtly. The ability to taste _____ and _____ flavors is reduced, but the ability to detect _____ and _____ flavors remains the same.

E. Changes in Anatomy, Physiology, and Diseases of the Urinary and Reproductive Systems

1. Between the ages of _____, the kidney loses about _____ of its mass.

2. As we age, the kidneys require less water to excrete the same amount of waste. Older adults are at increased risk for toxic levels of medication in the bloodstream.
   a. The first statement is true, and the second statement is false.
   b. The first statement is false, and the second statement is true.
   c. Both statements are true.
   d. Both statements are false.

3. What term is defined as the involuntary loss of urine? _____

4. Aging decreases the female hormones _____ and _____, and increases _____. Aging men can experience a change in _____ levels, which can affect the _____.

F. The Medical Assistant's Role in Caring for the Older Patient

1. To be sensitive to the needs of older patients, what accommodations should an ambulatory care clinic make?

   _____

   _____

   _____

   _____

2. What are general guidelines for effective patient education with older adults? _____

   _____

   _____

   _____

   _____

   _____

   _____

   _____

CERTIFICATION PREPARATION

Circle the correct answer.

1. The most common disorder of the endocrine system is
   a. hyperthyroidism.
   b. diabetes mellitus.
   c. Alzheimer's disease.
   d. Meniere's disease.

2. The relative frequency of deaths in a specific population is the definition for
   a. insidious.
   b. explicit.
   c. mortality.
   d. exploitation.

3. Indications that a patient may be a victim of elder abuse may include
   a. recurrent injuries caused by accident.
   b. poor general appearance and hygiene.
   c. bruising, dehydration, and pressure injuries.
   d. all of the above.

4. Which taste buds decline as a person ages?
   a. Sweet
   b. Salty
   c. Bitter
   d. Both a and b

5. Hearing loss associated with normal aging is
   a. Meniere's disease.
   b. presbycusis.
   c. otosclerosis.
   d. ototoxic.

6. A condition that makes it difficult to focus in detail on objects close at hand is
   a. glaucoma.
   b. cataracts.
   c. macular degeneration.
   d. presbyopia.

7. Which medical condition does *not* interfere with sleep?
   a. Congestive heart failure
   b. Otosclerosis
   c. Parkinson's disease
   d. Joint and bone pain

8. The formation of amyloid plaques in the brain would be found in a patient with which disease or disorder?
   a. Congestive heart failure
   b. Macular degeneration
   c. Alzheimer's disease
   d. Depression

9. Risk factors for cognitive decline include
   a. hypertension.
   b. diabetes mellitus.
   c. sedentary lifestyle.
   d. all of the above.

10. The primary cause of hip fractures is
    a. osteoporosis.
    b. dementia.
    c. stroke.
    d. Parkinson's disease.

WORKPLACE APPLICATIONS

1. Patricia is a 75-year-old patient who has a cataract in her right eye. Patricia is going to have a phaco-emulsification of her right eye. How would you explain this procedure to Patricia in language that would help her understand the procedure? Write your answer below.

_____

_____

_____

_____

2. Gracie, a 68-year-old patient, has an appointment for a physical today. As the medical assistant talks to her, she mentions that her skin has become very dry over the last few years. How could the medical assistant coach her about maintaining the health of her skin as she ages?

_____

_____

_____

_____

3. Juan is reviewing the medications used to treat osteoporosis for a continuing education course he is taking. List the medications used below. List the generic, brand names, and brief action of the medication.

_____

_____

_____

_____

INTERNET ACTIVITIES

1. Using online resources, research an imaging test used for diagnosing Alzheimer's disease. Create a poster presentation, a PowerPoint presentation, or a written paper summarizing your research. Include the following points in your project:
   a. Description of the test
   b. Any contraindications for the test
   c. Patient preparation for the test
   d. What occurs during the test

2. Using online resources, research a disease or disorder that occurs in older patient populations. Create a poster presentation, a PowerPoint presentation, or a written paper summarizing your research. Include the following points in your project:
   a. Description of the disease
   b. Etiology
   c. Signs and symptoms
   d. Diagnostic procedures
   e. Treatments
   f. Prognosis
   g. Prevention

3. Using online resources, research the effect that diet can have on the aging process. In a one-page paper, summarize the information that you found.

Procedure 45.1 Understand the Sensorimotor Changes of Aging

Name _____ Date _____ Score _____

Task: To role-play an older adult to better understand the needs of aging people.

Equipment and Supplies:
- Yellow-tinted glasses, ski goggles, or laboratory goggles
- Pink, white, yellow "pills" (e.g., various colors of Tic Tacs)
- Petroleum jelly (e.g., Vaseline)
- Cotton balls
- Eye patches
- Tape
- Utility gloves
- Tongue depressors
- Elastic bandages
- Medical forms in small print
- Pennies
- Button shirts
- Walker

Standard: Complete the procedure and all critical steps in _____ minutes with a minimum score of 85% within two attempts (*or as indicated by the instructor*).

Scoring: Divide the points earned by the total possible points. Failure to perform a critical step, indicated by an asterisk (*), results in grade no higher than an 84% (*or as indicated by the instructor*).

Time: Began_____ Ended_____ Total minutes: _____

Steps:	Point Value	Attempt 1	Attempt 2
1. Role-play vision and hearing loss. • Put two cotton balls in each ear and an eye patch over one eye. Follow your partner's instructions. • *Partner:* Stand out of the line of vision (to prevent lip-reading). Without using gestures or changing your voice volume, tell your partner to cross the room and pick up a book.	10		
2. Role-play yellowing of the lens of the eye. • Line up "pills" of different pastel colors. • *Partner:* Pick out the different colors while wearing the yellow-tinted glasses.	10		
3. Role-play difficulty focusing. • Put on goggles smeared with petroleum jelly and follow your partner's directions. • *Partner:* Stand at least 3 feet in front of your partner and motion for him or her to come to you (your partner is deaf, so talking will not help).	10		
4. Role-play loss of peripheral vision. • Put on goggles with black paper taped to the sides. • *Partner:* Stand to the side, out of the field of vision, and motion for your patient to follow you.	10		

5. Role-play aphasia and partial paralysis. • You are unable to use your right arm or leg. Place tape over your mouth. Let your partner know you need to go to the bathroom. • *Partner:* Stand at least 3 feet away with your back to your partner and wait for instructions.	**10**			
6. Role-play problems with dexterity. • Put thick gloves on your hands and try to sign your name, button a shirt, tie your shoes, and pick up pennies.	**10**			
7. Role-play problems with mobility. • Use the walker to cross the room. • *Partner:* After your partner starts to use the walker, hand him or her a book to carry.	**10**			
8. Role-play changes in sensation. • Put a rubber utility glove on; turn on very warm water; test the difference in temperature between the gloved hand and the ungloved hand.	**10**			
9. Summarize and share with the group your impressions of the effect of age-related sensorimotor changes. *(Refer to the Checklist for Affective Behaviors)*	**20***			
Total Points	**100**			

Affective Behavior	**Affective Behaviors Checklist** **Directions:** *Check behaviors observed during the role-play.*					
Empathy	**Negative, Unprofessional Behaviors**	**Attempt**		**Positive, Professional Behaviors**	**Attempt**	
		1	**2**		**1**	**2**
	Did not acknowledge the age-related sensorimotor changes in the older population			Acknowledged the age-related sensorimotor changes in the older population		
	Failed to reassure patient; did not respond to the patient's concerns			Discussed the difficulty of doing the tasks; how it felt not being able to do what was asked when being the "older person"		
	Failed to identify ways to adapt interactions when working with older people that could accommodate the age-related sensorimotor changes			Verbalized ways to adapt interactions when working with older people while considering age-related sensorimotor changes		
	Other:			Other:		

Grading Rubric for the Affective Behaviors Checklist **Directions:** *Based on checklist results, identify the points received for the procedure checklist. Indicate how the behaviors demonstrated met the expectations.*		Point Value	Attempt 1	Attempt 2
Does not meet Expectation	• Response lacks empathy. • Student demonstrated more than 2 negative, unprofessional behaviors during the interaction.	0		
Needs Improvement	• Response lacks empathy. • Student demonstrated 1 or 2 negative, unprofessional behaviors during the interaction.	0		
Meets Expectation	• Response was empathetic; no negative, unprofessional behaviors observed. • Responses where limited, more thought/consideration is needed.	20		
Occasionally Exceeds Expectation	• Response was empathetic; no negative, unprofessional behaviors observed. • Response provided more insights, more thought/ consideration is needed.	20		
Always Exceeds Expectation	• Response empathetic; no negative, unprofessional behaviors observed. • Student's response showed a depth understanding that is consistent with a professional medical assistant.	20		

Comments

CAAHEP Competencies	Step(s)
A.3. Demonstrate empathy for patients' concerns	9
I.P.9. Assist provider with a patient exam	Entire procedure
ABHES Competencies	**Step(s)**
5. Human Relations d. Adapt care to address the developmental stages of life	Entire procedure

Introduction to the Clinical Laboratory

CAAHEP Competencies	Assessments
I.C.11. Identify quality assurance practices in healthcare	Skills and Concepts – D. 2-3, 4-11
II.C.3.a. Identify normal and abnormal results as reported in: graphs	Skills and Concepts – D. 20-21
II.C.3.b. Identify normal and abnormal results as reported in: tables	Skills and Concepts – D. 24-26
XII.C.1. Identify workplace safeguards	Skills and Concepts – E. 7-11, 16
XII.C.2.a. Identify safety techniques that can be used in responding to accidental exposure to: blood	Skills and Concepts – E. 20-23
XII.C.2.b. Identify safety techniques that can be used in responding to accidental exposure to: other body fluids	Skills and Concepts – E. 20-23
XII.C.2.c. Identify safety techniques that can be used in responding to accidental exposure to: needle sticks	Skills and Concepts – E. 20, 23
XII.C.2.d. Identify safety techniques that can be used in responding to accidental exposure to: chemicals	Skills and Concepts – E. 12-14
XII.C.3. Identify fire safety issues in an ambulatory healthcare environment.	Skills and Concepts – E. 24-26
XII.C.5. Identify the purpose of Safety Data Sheets (SDS) in a healthcare setting	Skills and Concepts – E. 3, 12; Workplace Application – 3
XII.C.6.a. Identify processes for disposal of: biohazardous waste	Skills and Concepts – E. 16-19
XII.C.6.b. Identify processes for disposal of: chemicals	Skills and Concepts – E. 6
I.P.10. Perform a quality control measure	Procedure 46.1
III.P.2. Select appropriate barrier/personal protective equipment (PPE)	Procedure 46.1
XII.P.1. Comply with safety practices	Procedures 46.1, 46.3
XII.P.2.a. Demonstrate proper use of: eyewash equipment	Procedure 46.2

CAAHEP Competencies	Assessments
I.C.11. Identify quality assurance practices in healthcare	Skills and Concepts – D. 2-3, 4-11
XII.P.4. Evaluate an environment to identify unsafe conditions	Procedure 46.3

ABHES Competencies	Assessments
9. Medical Laboratory Procedures a. Practice quality control	Procedure 46.1
b. Perform selected CLIA-waived tests that assist with diagnosis and treatment	Procedure 46.1
c. Dispose of biohazardous materials	Procedure 46.1

VOCABULARY REVIEW

Using the word pool, find the correct word to match the definition. Write the word on the line after the definition.

Group A

1. A biological sample such as blood, urine, body fluids, feces, or tissue collected for analysis and evaluation

   _____

2. A physician specially trained in the nature and cause of disease

   _____

3. Free from living pathogenic organisms _____

4. Free from all living organisms _____

5. The substance or chemical being analyzed or detected in a specimen _____

6. Latin term meaning "in glass" _____

7. Also called *prothrombin time*; used to test the effectiveness of blood-thinning medication _____

8. A substance for use in a chemical reaction

   _____

9. Capable of burning, corroding, or damaging tissue by chemical action _____

10. Causing or tending to cause the gradual destruction of a substance by chemical action _____

Word Pool
- analyte
- aseptically
- caustic
- corrosive
- in vitro
- International Normalized Ratio (INR)
- pathologist
- reagent
- specimen
- sterile

Group B

1. A blood sample in which the red blood cells have ruptured
   _____

2. A portion of a well-mixed sample removed for testing
   _____

3. Medical term for devices with points or edges that can puncture or cut skin; examples include needles, scalpels, or broken glass
   _____

4. Scientific tests or techniques used for the detection or evidence of a crime _____

5. Fluids with high concentrations of protein and cellular debris that have escaped from the blood vessels and have been deposited in tissues or on tissue surfaces _____

6. To withdraw fluid using suction _____

7. Category of medication or a chemical that prevents clotting of blood _____

Word Pool
- aliquot
- aspirate
- anticoagulant
- exudates
- forensic
- hemolyzed
- sharps

ABBREVIATIONS

Write out what each of the following abbreviations stands for.

1. POL _____

2. UTI _____

3. MT _____

4. MLT _____

5. AMT _____

6. ASCP _____

7. CLS _____

8. CLT _____

9. MLA _____

10. CMLA _____

11. CPT _____

12. RBC _____

13. WBC _____

14. INR _____

15. LDL _____

16. HDL _____

17. CSF _____

18. CLIA _____

19. CMS _____

20. FDA _____

21. CDC _____

22. HIV _____

23. SOP _____

24. QA _____

25. QC _____

26. OSHA _____

27. HCS _____

28. SDS _____

29. PPE _____

30. OPIM _____

31. HBV _____

32. HCV _____

33. C _____

34. F _____

35. SI _____

36. WHO _____

37. PPMP _____

38. KOH _____

39. CAP _____

40. HIPAA _____

41. RPM _____

42. TSH _____

SKILLS AND CONCEPTS
Answer the following questions.

A. Introduction
Select the correct answer.

1. Laboratory tests are used to
   a. document the good health of a patient.
   b. screen patients for diseases and conditions.
   c. to help the provider diagnose a medical disease, disorder, or condition.
   d. to help the provider decide the most appropriate treatment, to monitor the effects of medications and treatments, and to monitor a disease process.
   e. all of the above.

2. The medical assistant can
   a. provide the patient with specimen collection instructions.
   b. collect and label patient specimens.
   c. assist with preparing specimens to be transported to a laboratory for testing.
   d. perform CLIA-waived testing.
   e. all of the above.

B. Organization of the Clinical Laboratory
Fill in the blank.

1. A(n) _____ is a laboratory that performs testing for another laboratory; also called *reference, diagnostic,* or *commercial testing laboratories.*

2. A laboratory director is either a(n) _____ or clinical laboratory scientist with a(n) _____.

3. In an ambulatory care facility, the lab director may be a(n) _____; this type of laboratory is referred to as a(n) _____.

4. A change in the internal environment of the body often results in _____ that are outside the population's _____.

5. A(n) _____ is a substance or chemical being analyzed or detected in a specimen.

6. A(n) _____ examines a specimen for the presence of an analyte that may indicate a disease state.

7. _____ test results are reported as positive or negative and do not contain a numeric value.

8. _____ test results do not indicate a precise amount of a substance present, but an estimate of how much is present.

9. _____ test result is expressed as a number, usually with units of measure attached to numeric values.

Match the definition with the correct term.

10. _____ The study of tissues

11. _____ The study of cells using microscopic methods

12. _____ The study and science that deal with the effects, antidotes, and detection of poisons or drugs

13. _____ The study of blood cells and coagulation

14. _____ The study of very small, infectious organisms such as bacteria, fungi, yeasts, parasites, and viruses

a. cytology
b. toxicology
c. histology
d. microbiology
e. hematology

Fill in the blank.

15. Urine is tested with a multiple test strip, also called a(n) _____.

16. A(n) _____ is a solid, liquid, or semisolid medium designed to support the growth of microorganisms, especially bacteria and fungus.

17. The growth of only one microorganism in a culture or on a nutrient surface is called a(n) _____.

18. _____ is performed on organisms to establish an appropriate antibiotic therapy for specific bacterium or fungi.

C. Government Legislation Affecting Clinical Laboratory Testing

Select the correct answer or fill in the blank.

1. Clinical Laboratory Improvement Amendments (CLIA)
   a. was passed by Congress in 1988.
   b. established quality standards for all clinical laboratory testing.
   c. was designed to ensure the accuracy, precision, reliability, and timeliness of patient test results, regardless of which laboratory performed the testing.
   d. requires all laboratories to register with the Centers for Medicare and Medicaid Services (CMS) and meet certain federal requirements.
   e. all of the above.

2. The U.S. Food and Drug Administration (FDA) is responsible for categorizing commercially marketed tests performed _____, based on the CLIA guidelines.

3. _____ tests are generally performed in a hospital or reference laboratory.

Match the terms with the correct description.

4. _____ A process to ensure the reliability of test results, often using manufactured samples with known values

5. _____ The laboratory must test samples provided by an approved proficiency-testing agency and results are reported to the proficiency-testing agency, and the accuracy of testing is verified

6. _____ A set of step-by-step instructions to help employees carry out routine operations with efficiency, high quality, and uniformity of performance

7. _____ Laboratory tests and procedures that have been approved by the FDA for home use or that are simple laboratory tests and procedures to perform

8. _____ Written policies and procedures that ensure monitoring of all of the processes involved before, during, and after a laboratory test is performed to produce reliable patient test results

a. standard operating procedures
b. quality assurance
c. quality control
d. proficiency testing
e. CLIA-waived

D. Quality Assurance and Quality Control
Select the correct answer.

1. Quality assurance
   a. includes a comprehensive set of policies developed to ensure excellent documentation and reliability of laboratory testing.
   b. benefits the provider by reducing the liability for inaccurate reporting of test results.
   c. focuses on establishing a series of operating procedures for the benefit of the patient and the medical assistant who does the laboratory testing.
   d. enables the laboratory to assess, verify, and document the quality of the laboratory process.
   e. all of the above.

2. Quality assurance monitors
   a. specimen collection.
   b. specimen processing.
   c. specimen testing.
   d. reporting steps.
   e. all of the above.

3. Quality assurance includes
   a. quality control.
   b. personnel orientation and knowledge of laboratory instrumentation.
   c. laboratory documentation.
   d. proficiency testing program.
   e. all of the above.

Match the activity with the correct stage of quality assurance. Answers can be used more than once.

4. _____ Controls are run and analyzed for each test method.

5. _____ Specimens are properly discarded.

6. _____ Instruments are maintained and calibrated.

7. _____ The provider interprets and signs all lab reports.

8. _____ The provider orders a test to screen, monitor, or diagnose a patient's condition.

9. _____ The specimen is collected, labeled, and processed.

10. _____ The test results are logged and documented in the patient's health record.

11. _____ Analyses of control results are compared over time.

a. preanalytic stage
b. analytic stage
c. postanalytic stage

Fill in the blank.

12. _____ involves determining the accuracy of an instrument by comparing its output with that of a known standard or another instrument known to be accurate.

13. _____ is the process used to ensure the reliability of test results, often using manufactured samples with known values.

14. _____ are manufacturer-prepared samples that have a known quantity of a specific analyte. Used for quality control purposes. Testing results should fall within a manufacturer-defined range of results.

15. _____ is regularly scheduled care of equipment that will decrease the likelihood of failure.

16. _____ is a measure of how close a test result is to the true value of the control material, as established by the manufacturer.

17. _____ is the ability to consistently reproduce a test result.

18. When a series of control results show both _____ and _____, the test is considered reliable and may be used for testing patients.

19. Every day that patient tests are performed, _____ must also be performed, and the results entered onto a paper or electronic graph or flow sheet.

Use Fig. 46.1, Glucose QC Graph, to answer the following questions.

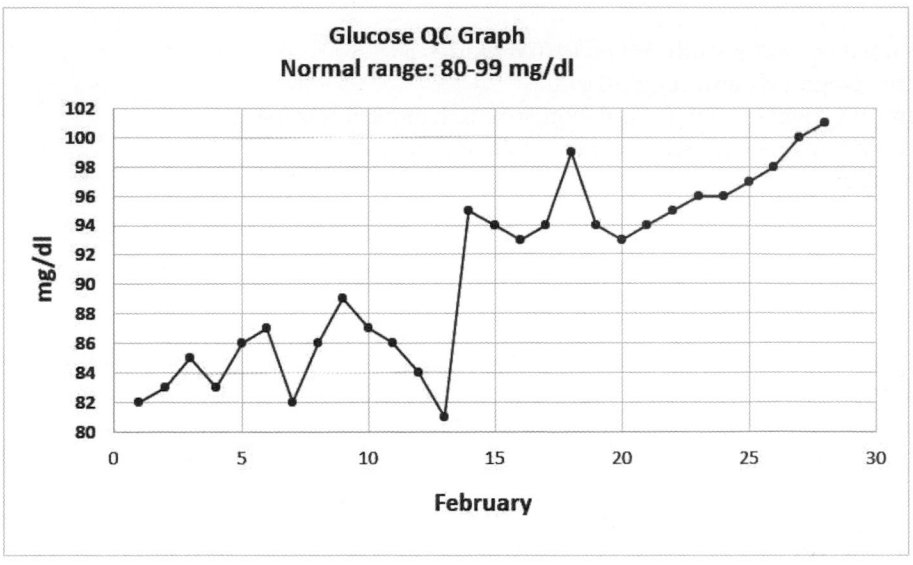

20. On what dates were the values within the normal range? Indicate the date range(s).
    _____

21. On what dates were the values abnormal or outside the normal range? Indicate the date range(s).
    _____

22. Is there any shifts in the data? If so, indicate the date range(s). _____

23. Is there any trends in the data? If so, indicate the date range(s). _____

Use Fig. 46.2 Glucose QC Table to answer the following questions. The normal range is between 80-99 mg/dL.

24. On what dates were the values within the normal range? Indicate the date range(s). _____

25. On what dates were the values abnormal higher than the normal range? Indicate the date range(s).
    _____

26. On what dates were the values abnormal lower than the normal range? Indicate the date range(s). _____

Glucose QC Table	
March	mg/dL
1	92
2	89
3	105
4	103
5	72
6	76
7	78
8	72
9	88
10	89
11	86
12	84
13	81
14	95
15	94

E. Laboratory Safety

Select the correct answer or fill in the blank.

1. Occupational Safety and Health Act of 1970 includes a
   a. system of safeguards and regulations.
   b. program that covers occupational exposure to chemical hazards.
   c. program that covers exposure to blood-borne pathogens.
   d. all of the above.

2. _____, also called the employee "right to know" rule, ensures that laboratory workers are made fully aware of the hazards associated with their workplace.

3. The Safety Data Sheet
   a. is created by the manufacturer to communicate information on the chemical safety and hazards of the chemical.
   b. must be available in the laboratory for each chemical.
   c. includes information on the handling, storage, stability, reactivity, disposal, and transport of the chemical.
   d. includes first aid and fire-fighting measures.
   e. all of the above.

4. Which of the following guidelines is used to reduce the risks associated with handling and storage of chemicals in the clinical laboratory?
   a. Date the chemical containers are first opened.
   b. Date the chemical containers are first received.
   c. Keep the laboratory doors open at all times.
   d. All of the above.
   e. Both a and b

5. Which of the following guidelines is used to reduce the risks associated with handling and storage of chemicals in the clinical laboratory?
   a. Only use chemicals that you have been trained to use.
   b. Store large bottles of acids on low shelves.
   c. Store flammable substances away from sources of ignition.
   d. If a chemical produces toxic or flammable vapors, work under a fume hood that exhausts air to the outside.
   e. All of the above.

6. When disposing of chemical waste, what must the medical assistant do?
   a. Check the Safety Data Sheet for disposal considerations.
   b. Keep chemical separated.
   c. Ensure the chemical waste is correctly identified and labeled.
   d. Contact the disposal company.
   e. All of the above.

7. On chemicals, a hazard identification system provides information at a glance on the
   a. potential health hazards.
   b. flammability hazard.
   c. chemical reactivity hazard.
   d. all of the above.

For the hazard identification system, match the description with the correct diamond.

8. _____ Provides special hazard information, including recommended PPE

9. _____ Indicates the health hazard

10. _____ Indicates a reactivity or stability hazard

11. _____ Indicated the flammability

    a. top (red) diamond
    b. left (blue) diamond
    c. bottom (white) diamond
    d. right (yellow) diamond

Select the correct answer or fill in the blank.

12. The _____ provides first-aid measures that should be given by untrained responders to individuals with a chemical exposure.

13. With an accidental exposure of the skin, rinse the affected area under running water for at least _____ minutes and remove any contaminated clothing.

14. If chemicals are splashed in the eyes, flush the eyes with water from an eyewash station for a minimum of _____ minutes.

15. Write the definition for each warning symbol in the spaces provided.

    A. _____

    B. _____

16. Biohazardous waste
    a. disposal must be done according to state and federal guidelines.
    b. disposal methods include treatment by heat, incineration, steam sterilization, and chemical treatments to render the waste inactive.
    c. must be collected in impermeable red polyethylene or polypropylene biohazard-labeled bags or containers and sealed.
    d. All of the above

17. Blood and potentially infectious materials mixed with chemicals are considered _____waste.

18. Mixed waste should be _____ and the disposal should follow the chemical disposal procedure.

19. Sharps containers should be replaced when they are about _____ filled and the lid should be securely closed.

20. Which of the following is correct regarding a needlestick and a blood or OPIM exposure to a cut or a body surface?
    a. Wash the area with soap and warm running water as soon as possible after the exposure.
    b. Wash the area for 10 to 15 minutes.
    c. Chlorine-based antiseptics and 10% iodine solution can also be used to clean the area.
    d. All of the above.

21. For blood or OPIM splashes to the nose or mouth, flush the area with _____.

22. For a blood or OPIM exposure in the eyes, continuously flush with water as soon as possible for a minimum of _____ minutes using an eyewash station.

23. Report needlesticks and blood or OPIM exposures to the _____ and immediately seek medical treatment.

24. Which of the following is correct?
    a. Fires may be ignited by smoking, heating elements, and sparks from electrical connections.
    b. Flammable materials should be stored near any source of ignition.
    c. If clothing is on fire, wrap the person in a fire blanket.
    d. All of the above.

25. To prevent electrical hazards
    a. use surge protectors.
    b. do not overload circuits and never use extension cords.
    c. inspect all cords and plugs frequently.
    d. all of the above.

26. _____ extinguishers can be used on all types of fires.

F. Specimen Collection, Processing, and Storage

1. Which of the following specimens are collected less frequently in the ambulatory care environment?
   a. Swab samples collected from wounds or mucous membranes
   b. Feces
   c. Blood
   d. Urine
   e. Both b and d

2. If the patient is not _____ properly, the laboratory results that are generated will be useless.

3. Collection in an incorrect colored tube may result in a(n) _____ specimen.

4. If a specimen will be tested for the presence of microorganisms, a(n) _____ container must be used.

5. What information is needed on a specimen label?
   a. Patient name and identification number
   b. Date and time of collection
   c. Specimen type
   d. Collector's initials
   e. All of the above

6. Forensic specimens are also called _____ specimens.

7. _____ refers to the stepwise method used to collect, process, and test a specimen.

G. Laboratory Mathematics and Measurement

Express the following Greenwich times as military times. Use Table 46.5 for reference.

1. 8:10 AM = _____

2. 2:15 PM = _____

3. 6:30 PM = _____

4. 5:50 AM = _____

Express the following temperatures in Celsius.

5. 98.6° F = _____

6. 32° F = _____

7. 212° F = _____

8. 72° F = _____

9. What systems of measurement are used in the clinical laboratory? _____

_____

Determine the type of specimen by which metric units of measure are used for the following.

10. 20 mL of reagent   volume   weight   length

11. 9.45 kg of tissue   volume   weight   length

12. 327 mcg of reagent   volume   weight   length

13. 41.5 cm of tubing   volume   weight   length

14. 7.25 cc of reagent   volume   weight   length

15. 10.5 mm of specimen   volume   weight   length

16. When liquids are measured into test tubes, the most common piece of glassware used is the

_____.

H. Laboratory Equipment

1. Which instrument is used to view objects too small to be seen with the naked eye?_____

_____

2. Which medical personnel *cannot* make a final analysis of a microscope slide?
   a. Physician
   b. Nurse practitioner and physician's assistant
   c. Medical assistant
   d. Dentist
   e. Trained laboratory professional with CLIA moderate- or high-complexity training

3. An instrument used to separate blood cells from serum or plasma is called a(n) _____.

4. Cabinets that maintain constant temperatures are called _____, and are used most frequently in the _____ department of a clinical laboratory.

CERTIFICATION PREPARATION
Circle the correct answer.

1. Which term is defined as the substance or chemical being analyzed or detected in a specimen?
   a. Electrolyte
   b. Reagent
   c. Analyte
   d. Identifiers

2. Which laboratory department studies tissues?
   a. Cytology
   b. Histology
   c. Toxicology
   d. Chemistry

3. Which laboratory department does sensitivity testing?
   a. Microbiology
   b. Chemistry
   c. Urinalysis
   d. Hematology

4. Which is a CLIA-waived test?
   a. Fasting blood glucose
   b. Dipstick urinalysis
   c. Rapid strep testing
   d. All of the above

5. Which government agency is responsible for determining the CLIA complexity of all laboratory tests?
   a. CMS
   b. HHS
   c. FDA
   d. OSHA

6. Which CLIA complexity tests can a medical assistant always perform?
   a. Waived tests
   b. Moderate-complexity tests
   c. High-complexity tests
   d. All of the above

7. Which term is defined as the ability to consistently reproduce a test result?
   a. Accuracy
   b. Reliability
   c. Trend
   d. Precision

8. According to the CDC, the single most effective means of preventing infection is
   a. wearing proper PPE during patient contact.
   b. always wearing gloves when working with blood specimens.
   c. proper and frequent hand sanitation.
   d. all of the above.

9. An example of a blood-borne pathogen is
   a. HIV.
   b. influenza.
   c. HBV.
   d. a and c.

10. Which piece of laboratory equipment is defined as a cabinet that maintains a constant temperature?
    a. Microscope
    b. Centrifuge
    c. Incubator
    d. Rotor

WORKPLACE APPLICATIONS

1. Greg is helping train a student medical assistant today and he is responsible for going through the following competency: Evaluate the work environment to identify unsafe working conditions. He has set up a number of items on a benchtop and is asking the student to review each environment.

   Evaluate each statement below and determine if the work environment described would be safe or unsafe. Circle your answer for each environment.

   - Two unopened rapid strep kits enclosed in their boxes sitting on a countertop at room temperature

     SAFE   UNSAFE

   - Two pipets containing an unknown yellow liquid, laying on absorbent laboratory paper

     SAFE   UNSAFE

   - A disinfectant wipes container that is open, and two wipes look like they have been used to clean up a pinkish-red spill, and are now laying on the counter

     SAFE   UNSAFE

   - A bottle of urinalysis dipsticks that are properly closed, sitting on the counter

     SAFE   UNSAFE

   - A countertop sharps container that has a few used pipets in it

     SAFE   UNSAFE

   - A pipet and bulb sitting on the counter, with a few small pieces of broken glass nearby

     SAFE   UNSAFE

   - An unlabeled beaker with a blue liquid inside of it

     SAFE   UNSAFE

2. Greg is giving a laboratory tour to a small group of new clinic employees. Greg meets them in the waiting area of the laboratory. A few people have water bottles with them and one person is checking their phone in the waiting room until the tour starts.

   Read each scenario below and answer each question at the end of the statement by circling YES or NO.

   - There is a sign on the door leading into the laboratory that states, "No food or drink beyond this point." To comply with the sign, should people bring their water bottles into the lab?

     YES   NO

   - Once inside the lab, there is a symbol showing a cell phone with a big red X over it. To comply with the symbol, should people bring their cell phones into the lab?

     YES   NO

- Once inside the lab, there are lab coats with safety glasses in the pockets hanging on a coat rack. Each lab coat has a label on the sleeve that reads "guest." Above the coat rack a sign reads "Lab coats and safety glasses must be worn beyond this point." To comply with the wall sign and coat label, should each person put on a lab coat and safety glasses?

  YES   NO

- As they finish their tour of the lab, there are two boxes—one labeled "lab coats here" the other labeled "safety glasses here." To comply with the labels on the boxes, can the people take the lab coats and safety glasses out of the laboratory?

  YES   NO

3. Greg is unpacking supplies that he ordered for the laboratory. One box contains a chemical reagent and the accompanying SDS. Briefly explain the purpose of SDS in a healthcare setting.

_____

_____

_____

_____

INTERNET ACTIVITIES

1. Using online resources, research one department of the laboratory. Create a poster presentation, a PowerPoint presentation, or a written paper summarizing your research. Include the following points in your project:
   a. Name of the department
   b. General overview of the testing performed in the department
   c. Common specimens tested
   d. Common disease states tested for in the department
   e. Common CLIA-waived tests performed in the department

2. Go to the website for the CDC (https://www.cdc.gov/) and research a blood-borne pathogen of your choice. Create a poster presentation, a PowerPoint presentation, or a written paper summarizing your research. Include the following points in your project:
   a. Description of the pathogen
   b. Testing used to identify the blood-borne pathogen
   c. CLIA-waived testing available for the blood-borne pathogen
   d. Personal protective equipment (PPE) needed during testing procedures

3. Using online resources, research the preventive maintenance routinely performed on a microscope, centrifuge, or incubator. In a one-page paper, summarize the information that you found.

4. Go to https://www.cdc.gov/ or https://www.fda.gov/ and research protocols or guidelines for laboratory waste disposal. In a one-page paper, summarize the information that you found.

Procedure 46.1 Perform a Quality Control Measure on a Glucometer and Record the Results on a Flow Sheet

Name _____ Date _____ Score _____

Tasks: Test and analyze the results of glucometer controls to see whether a glucometer is producing reliable test results and record the results on the laboratory flow sheet.

Equipment and Supplies:
- Fluid-impermeable lab coat, gloves, and protective eyewear
- Glucometer
- Coded test strips designed for the glucometer used
- Control solution provided by the manufacturer
- Package insert showing directions on how to run the glucometer
- Biohazard waste container
- Waste container
- Glucose test control flow sheet

Standard: Complete the procedure and all critical steps in _____ minutes with a minimum score of 85% within two attempts (*or as indicated by the instructor*).

Scoring: Divide the points earned by the total possible points. Failure to perform a critical step, indicated by an asterisk (*), results in grade no higher than an 84% (*or as indicated by the instructor*).

Time: Began_____ Ended_____ Total minutes: _____

Steps:	Point Value	Attempt 1	Attempt 2
1. Put on a lab coat. Wash your hands or use hand sanitizer. Put on gloves and eye protection. Comply with safety practices during the procedure.	10*		
2. Take a coded strip out of the bottle and note the control level and range listed on the control bottle or the strip container. Close the coded strip bottle.	10		
3. Review the directions on the glucometer package insert. Calibrate the meter by inserting the precoded test strip into the monitor or by manually inserting the code number into the monitor.	10		
4. Check the expiration date on the liquid control bottle and mix well by inverting and rolling the bottle between the palms of your hands.	10*		
5. Complete the top portion of the control log sheet with the test name, control lot number, expiration date, and the control's reference range based on whether it is a low-level, normal, or high-level control.	10*		
6. Insert the strip into the glucometer and apply a drop of the liquid control to the strip according to the directions.	10		
7. Record the result on the glucose test control flow sheet and note whether it falls within the manufacturer's reference range. If not, the test should be repeated with a new strip.	10*		
8. When you have finished running the controls, properly dispose of the strips as recommended by the manufacturer.	10*		
9. Remove your gloves and eyewear. Dispose of the gloves in the waste container. Wash your hands or use hand sanitizer.	10*		

10. Review the control results for the following: • Accuracy: Did all the results fall near the middle of the reference range? • Precision: Were the results consistently close to each other (without extreme highs and lows)? • Reliability: If both of the previous points are affirmed, the test is reliable and the glucometer may be used to test patient samples.	10		
Total Points	100		

GLUCOSE TEST CONTROL FLOW SHEET

Control Lot #: _____			Expiration Date: _____		
Control Range: _____			Level: Low/Normal/High		
Date	Student/MA Initials	Result	Accept	Reject	Corrective Action

Comments

CAAHEP Competencies	**Step(s)**
I.P.10. Perform a quality control measure	Entire procedure
III.P.2. Select appropriate barrier/personal protective equipment (PPE)	1
XII.P.1. Comply with safety practices	1
ABHES Competencies	**Step(s)**
9. Medical Laboratory Procedures a. Practice quality control	Entire procedure
b. Perform selected CLIA-waived tests that assist with diagnosis and treatment	Entire procedure
c. Dispose of biohazardous materials	8

Procedure 46.2 Use of the Eyewash Equipment: Perform an Emergency Eyewash

Name _____ Date _____ Score _____

Task: To minimize the risk of occupational exposure to pathogens if body fluids contact the eyes.

Equipment and Supplies:
* Plumbed or self-contained eyewash unit

Standard: Complete the procedure and all critical steps in _____ minutes with a minimum score of 85% within two attempts (*or as indicated by the instructor*).

Scoring: Divide the points earned by the total possible points. Failure to perform a critical step, indicated by an asterisk (*), results in grade no higher than an 84% (*or as indicated by the instructor*).

Time: Began _____ Ended _____ Total minutes: _____

Steps:	Point Value	Attempt 1	Attempt 2
1. If a hazardous substance enters the eye, immediately go to the eyewash station and push the activation lever to discharge water into both eyes. If using an eyewash unit, follow the manufacturer's directions.	25*		
2. Quickly remove your gloves once irrigation has begun and is in uninterrupted flow. Then hold the eyelids open with the thumb and index finger to ensure adequate rinsing of the entire eye and eyelid surface. If you have contacts in, gently remove during the flushing process.	25*		
3. Flush the eyes and eyelids for a minimum of 15 minutes, rolling the eyes periodically to ensure complete removal of the foreign material.	25*		
4. After completion of the eyewash, wash your hands and complete the postexposure follow-up procedures.	25*		
Total Points	**100**		

Comments

CAAHEP Competencies	Step(s)
XII.P.2.a. Demonstrate proper use of: eyewash equipment	Entire procedure

Procedure 45-2   Use of the Radiation Equipment Platform on Emergency Run with

Procedure 46.3   Evaluate the Laboratory Environment

Name _____   Date _____   Score _____

Tasks: Evaluate the laboratory environment and identify unsafe working conditions. Identify compliance with safety practices, such as safety signs, symbols, and labels.

Equipment and Supplies:
- Laboratory environment evaluation form (Work Product 46.1)
- Pen

Standard: Complete the procedure and all critical steps with a minimum score of 85% within two attempts (*or as indicated by the instructor*).

Scoring: Divide the points earned by the total possible points. Failure to perform a critical step, indicated by an asterisk (*), results in grade no higher than an 84% (*or as indicated by the instructor*).

Steps:	Point Value	Attempt 1	Attempt 2
1. Observe the use of workplace safeguards, such as safety signs, symbols, and labels, in the laboratory setting. Document what each sign, symbol, and label means. Document your findings on the work environment evaluation form (Work Product 46.1).	25*		
2. Explain if the laboratory personnel are complying with the safety signs, symbols, and labels.	25*		
3. Observe the environment for safety risks. Document your findings.	25*		
4. Based on your observations, summarize your findings. If risks are present, create a list of issues that need to be addressed. Describe what needs to be done for each risk.	25*		
Total Points	**100**		

Comments

CAAHEP Competencies	Step(s)
XII.P.1. Comply with safety practices	1, 2
XII.P.4. Evaluate an environment to identify unsafe conditions	Entire procedure

Work Product 46.1   Work Environment Evaluation Form

Name _____   **Date** _____   **Score** _____

To be used with Procedure 46.3.

Directions: Check either in the "Yes" or "No" column for each question. Check "NA" if it is not applicable. Include any issues in the comment column. Summarize your findings for each area, using the space indicated.

Complying with Safety Signs, Symbols, and Labels	**Yes**	**No**	**NA**	**Comments**
• Refrigerator displays a biohazard symbol.				
• Refrigerator displays a sign indicating "not for storage of food or medication."				
• Biohazard waste containers display a biohazard symbol.				
• Biohazard waste containers use a red biohazard bag.				
• Chemicals and reagents labeled with original manufacturer's label and a hazard identification system label (by the National Fire Protection Association).				
• Sign on the door indicating "No food or drink beyond this point."				
• A sign in the lab indicates no cell phones are allowed.				
• A sign at the entrance of the lab indicates that lab coats and safety glasses must be worn.				
Safety of the Laboratory Environment	**Yes**	**No**	**NA**	**Comments**
• Chemicals and reagents are sealed.				
• Safety Data Sheets are available for all chemicals used in the laboratory.				
• If using a chemical that produces toxic or flammable vapors, the person works under a fume hood that exhausts air to the outside.				
• Disinfection wipes available in work area				
• A fire extinguisher is available in the laboratory.				
• Ceiling sprinkler system is present.				
• A sink with running water is available for emergencies.				
• Eye wash station is present.				
• Are electrical cords and plugs free from cracks, fraying, or other damage?				
• Are power strips overloaded?				
• Are flammable chemicals and supplies stored according to manufacturers' guidelines?				
• Are combustibles (e.g., paper, cardboard, cloth, flammable chemicals) away from heat sources?				
Observations of unsafe practices:				

Are the laboratory personnel complying with the safety signs, symbols, and labels? Explain why or why not based on your observations.

If risks are present, create a list of issues that need to be addressed. Describe what needs to be done for each risk.

Procedure 46.4   Perform Routine Maintenance on a Microscope

Name _____ Date _____ Score _____

Tasks: Focus the microscope properly using a prepared slide under low power, high power, and oil immersion. Then perform routine maintenance on the microscope before storing it.

Equipment and Supplies:
- Microscope
- Lens cleaner
- Lens tissue
- Slide containing specimen
- Immersion oil
- Waste container

Standard: Complete the procedure and all critical steps in _____ minutes with a minimum score of 85% within two attempts (*or as indicated by the instructor*).

Scoring: Divide the points earned by the total possible points. Failure to perform a critical step, indicated by an asterisk (*), results in grade no higher than an 84% (*or as indicated by the instructor*).

Time: Began _____ Ended _____ Total minutes: _____

Steps:	Point Value	Attempt 1	Attempt 2
1. Wash hands or use hand sanitizer.	5*		
2. Gather the needed materials.	5		
3. Clean the lenses with lens tissue and lens cleaner.	5*		
4. Adjust the seating to a comfortable height.	5		
5. Plug the microscope into an electrical outlet and turn on the light switch.	5		
6. Place the slide specimen on the stage and secure it.	5		
7. Turn the revolving nosepiece to engage the 4× or 10× lens.	5		
8. Carefully raise the stage while observing with the naked eye from the side.	5		
9. Focus the specimen using the coarse adjustment knob.	5*		
10. Adjust the amount of light by closing the iris diaphragm, by bringing the condenser up or down, or by adjusting the light from the source.	5		
11. Switch to the 40× lens. Use the fine adjustment knob to focus on the specimen in detail.	5		
12. Turn the revolving nosepiece to the area between the high-power objective and oil immersion. Place a small drop of oil on the slide.	5		
13. Carefully rotate the oil immersion objective into place. The objective will be immersed in the oil. Adjust the focus with the fine adjustment knob.	5*		
14. Increase the light by opening the iris diaphragm and raising the condenser.	5		
15. Identify the specimen.	5		
16. Return to low power, but do not drag the 40× lens through the oil. Remove the slide and dispose of it in a biohazard sharps container.	5		
17. Lower the stage. Center the stage.	5		

18. Switch off the light and unplug the microscope. Clean the lenses with lens tissue and remove oil with lens cleaner.	5*		
19. Wipe the microscope with a cloth. Cover the microscope.	5*		
20. Place the trash in the waste container. Sanitize the work area. Wash hands or use hand sanitizer.	5		
Total Points	100		

Comments

Urinalysis

CAAHEP Competencies	Assessments
I.P.10. Perform a quality control measure	Procedure 47.4
I.P.11.c. Collect specimens and perform: CLIA-waived urinalysis	Procedures 47.1 through 47.3, 47.5, 47.7, 47.8
II.P.2. Record laboratory test results into the patient's record	Procedures 47.3, 47.5, 47.7, 47.8
III.P.2. Select appropriate barrier/personal protective equipment (PPE)	Procedure 47.2 through 47.8
XII.P.1. Comply with safety practices	Procedures 47.1 through 47.8
A.2. Reassure patients	Procedure 47.9
A.4. Demonstrate active listening	Procedure 47.9
ABHES Competencies	Assessments
3.d. Define and use medical abbreviations when appropriate and acceptable	Abbreviations – 1-21
9.a. Practice quality control	Procedure 47.4
9 b. Perform selected CLIA-waived tests that assist with diagnosis and treatment 1) Urinalysis	Procedures 47.3, 47.5, 47.7, 47.8
9.c. Dispose of biohazardous materials	Procedures 47.3, 47.5, 47.7, 47.8
9.d. Collect, label, and process a specimen	Procedures 47.1, 47.2
9.e. Instruct patients in the collection of 1) clean-catch midstream urine specimens	Procedure 47.2

VOCABULARY REVIEW

Using the word pool, find the correct word to match the definition. Write the word on the line after the definition

Group A

1. Microorganisms (mostly bacteria and yeast) that live on or in the body _____

2. A procedure for evaluating the glomerular filtration rate of the kidneys _____

3. Hollow, flexible tube that can be inserted into a vessel, organ, or cavity of the body to withdraw or instill fluid, monitor information, and visualize a vessel or cavity

   _____

4. A narrow, tube-shaped container marked with horizontal lines to represent units of measurement; used to precisely measure the volume of liquids _____

5. A body opening or passage, especially the external opening of a structure _____

6. Insoluble material that settles to the bottom of a urine specimen and to the bottom of centrifuged urine _____

7. A kidney disease affecting the glomeruli of the nephron; characterized by albumin in the urine, edema, and high blood pressure _____

8. A test result is expressed as a number, usually with units of measure attached to numeric values _____

9. The internal environment of the body that is compatible with life; steady state that is created by all the body systems working together _____

10. An essential amino acid found in milk, eggs, and other foods

    _____

Word Pool
- catheter
- creatinine clearance rates
- glomerulonephritis
- graduated cylinder
- homeostasis
- meatus
- normal flora
- phenylalanine
- quantitative
- sediment

Group B

1. Any enzyme that breaks down esters (a type of organic molecule) into alcohols and acids _____

2. Yellow discoloration of the skin, whites of the eyes, and mucous membranes, due to an increase of bilirubin in the blood

   _____

3. An electrically charged atom or the smallest component of an element _____

4. A dilute urine concentration _____

5. A hormone secreted by the anterior pituitary gland; it stimulates the growth of ovum (eggs) in the ovary and induces the formation of sperm in the testis _____

6. A blood flow deficiency to the kidney(s) _____

7. A concentrated urine _____

8. Damaging or destructive to the kidneys _____

Word Pool
- adulterated
- artificial insemination
- esterase
- follicle-stimulating hormone
- hypertonic
- hypotonic
- ion
- jaundice
- lateral flow immunoassay
- luteinizing hormone
- nephrotoxic
- protozoa
- renal ischemia

9. The injection of semen into the vagina or uterus using a catheter or syringe; nonsexual _____

10. A hormone produced by the anterior pituitary gland; stimulates ovulation and the development of the corpus luteum in females and the production of testosterone in males

_____

11. A laboratory technique that uses the specific binding between an antigen and antibody to identify and quantify a substance in a sample; the sample in this technique moves in a sideways motion, usually on an absorbent paper

_____

12. Single-celled organisms that are the most primitive form of animal life; most are microscopic _____

13. The intentional manipulation of a urine sample that allows someone to falsely pass a drug screening test

_____

ABBREVIATIONS

Write out what each of the following abbreviations stands for.

1. POL _____

2. C&S _____

3. FSH _____

4. LH _____

5. PKU _____

6. UTI _____

7. UA _____

8. CCMS _____

9. CPT _____

10. PPE _____

11. Na+ _____

12. K+ _____

13. RBC _____

14. WBC _____

15. FDA _____

16. PPMPs _____

17. CLSI _____

18. hCG _____

19. OTC_____

20. SAMHSA _____

21. NIDA _____

SKILLS AND CONCEPTS
Answer the following questions.

A. Introduction
Fill in the blank or select the correct answer.

1. _____ is the second most common specimen analyzed in the laboratory.

2. Urine is analyzed to detect
   a. abnormal substances excreted by the kidneys.
   b. diseases or disorders of the kidneys or urinary tract.
   c. medications or drugs that are excreted by the kidneys.
   d. all of the above.

B. Urine Formation and Elimination
Fill in the blank or select the correct answer.

1. Which of the following statements is *incorrect*?
   a. In the nephrons, blood is filtered to form urine.
   b. Selective reabsorption and secretion occur in the renal tubules.
   c. The composition of the filtrate is adjusted in the renal tubules.
   d. The urinary tract consists of 2 kidneys, 2 ureters, 1 bladder, and 1 urethra.

2. The largest component of urine is _____.

3. What is an abnormal waste product found in urine?
   a. Urea
   b. Uric acid
   c. Creatinine
   d. Glucose

4. What is an abnormal waste product found in urine?
   a. Sodium
   b. Nitrites
   c. Chloride
   d. Potassium

5. What is a normal waste product found in urine?
   a. Protein
   b. Ketones
   c. Red blood cells
   d. White blood cells
   e. None of the above

C. Collecting and Handling of a Urine Specimen

Fill in the blank or select the correct answer.

1. Which type of specimen is collected in nonsterile containers?
   a. Routine UA tests
   b. Pregnancy tests
   c. Abnormal analyte tests
   d. All of the above

2. Urine samples required for a culture are collected in a(n) _____ container.

3. The label on all specimens must include the
   a. patient's name.
   b. date and time of collection.
   c. type of specimen.
   d. all of the above.

Match the description with the correct type of urine specimen. Answers may be used more than once.

4. _____ The second void of the day is collected for testing.
5. _____ This type of specimen is more concentrated.
6. _____ The specimen is collected 2 hours after a meal.
7. _____ Most tests use this type of specimen.
8. _____ This specimen is required for diabetes screening and for home diabetes testing programs.
9. _____ A sterile tube is inserted in the bladder to collect the specimen.
10. _____ A urine specimen is collected when the patient first wakes up in the morning.

a. random specimen
b. first morning specimen
c. second-voided specimen
d. 2-hour postprandial urine specimen
e. catheterized specimen

Fill in the blank or select the correct answer.

11. A 24-hour urine specimen is collected over 24 hours to provide a(n) _____ chemical analysis.

12. What is correct regarding the storage of a 24-hour urine specimen?
    a. Place the covered container in the freezer.
    b. The collection container should remain at room temperature.
    c. The collection container should remain cool.
    d. The temperature does not matter with the specimen.

13. A(n) _____ specimen is ordered when the provider suspects a urinary tract infection.

14. The _____ and _____ components of urine change if the urine warms to room temperature

15. Urine specimens should be kept refrigerated and should be processed within _____ hour(s) of collection.

16. Evacuated transport tubes for urine
    a. contain preservatives that prevent the overgrowth of bacteria.
    b. contain preservatives that will prevent chemical changes.
    c. look like blood collection tubes.
    d. all of the above.

17. Chemical reagent strip testing can be performed on preserved specimens within _____ hour(s).

18. Culture and sensitivity testing should be performed within _____ hour(s).

D. Routine Urinalysis
Fill in the blank or select the correct answer.

1. The color depends on the concentration of the pigment _____.

2. _____ may be caused by cells, bacteria, yeast, vaginal contaminants, or crystals.

3. _____ consists of small bubbles that persist for a long time after the specimen has been swirled to mix.

4. White foam can indicate the presence of increased _____.

5. Greenish-yellow foam may indicate _____ in the urine.

6. A(n) _____ or a putrid smell in the urine can be caused by an infection.

7. _____ is defined as the weight of a substance compared with the weight of an equal volume of distilled water.

8. The normal specific gravity of urine ranges from _____ to _____.

9. The analysis that uses a reagent strip, also called a *urine dipstick*, is a(n) _____ test.

10. The _____ is a measurement of the acidity or alkalinity of the urine.

11. Normal, freshly voided urine may have a pH range of _____ to _____.

12. Specimens should be tested for glucose within _____ hour(s) of collection or within _____ hour(s) if refrigerated.

13. The cause of proteinuria is
    a. orthostatic proteinuria.
    b. pregnancy.
    c. after heavy exercise.
    d. renal disease.
    e. all of the above.

14. The blood test pad on the reagent strip reacts with
    a. intact red blood cells.
    b. hemoglobin from lysed (broken) red blood cells.
    c. myoglobin.
    d. all of the above.

Match the description with the correct term.

15. _____ The end product of fat metabolism in the body
16. _____ The presence of hemolyzed red blood cells in urine
17. _____ Occurs when muscle tissue is damaged or injured
18. _____ A product of the breakdown of hemoglobin
19. _____ Occurs in urine when bacteria break down nitrate
20. _____ Present in urine when a person has a UTI

a. bilirubin
b. myoglobinuria
c. ketone
d. nitrate
e. hemoglobinuria
f. leukocytes

E. Microscopic Preparation and Examination of Urine Sediment
Fill in the blank.

1. A microscopic examination of urine is categorized as a CLIA-_____ test.

Match the description with the correct term.

2. _____ Created when protein accumulates and precipitates in the kidney tubules and is then washed into the urine
3. _____ Hyaline casts that contain leukocytes
4. _____ Pouring a liquid gently so that it does not disturb the remaining sediment
5. _____ Pale, transparent, cylindric structures that have rounded ends and parallel sides
6. _____ The clear liquid above the sediment in a centrifuged urine specimen
7. _____ Common in urine specimens, particularly if the specimen has been allowed to cool
8. _____ Pale, irregular, threadlike structures with tapered ends, frequently seen in patients with inflammation

a. decanting
b. supernatant
c. cast
d. hyaline casts
e. white blood cell casts
f. mucus threads
g. crystals

F. Additional CLIA-Waived Urine Tests
Fill in the blank.

1. All pregnancy tests detect the presence of _____.

2. Ovulation testing, a CLIA-waived lateral flow urine test, detects _____ in the urine.

3. Menopause testing, a CLIA-waived lateral flow test, detects _____ in the urine.

4. _____ is the study of poisonous substances and drugs, and their effects on the body.

5. The _____ protocol is required for any legal specimen.

6. With the chain of custody rules, the individual being tested must provide a(n) _____.

7. Within 4 minutes of receiving the urine specimen, the temperatures should be between _____° F to _____° F.

CERTIFICATION PREPARATION

Circle the correct answer.

1. Which structure is the functional unit of the urinary system?
   a. Renal tubules
   b. Glomerulus
   c. Kidney
   d. Nephron

2. Which substance is a normal constituent of urine?
   a. Protein
   b. Urea
   c. Glucose
   d. Red blood cells

3. What type of urine specimen should be collected for culture and sensitivity testing?
   a. Random specimen
   b. 2-hour postprandial specimen
   c. Clean-catch midstream specimen
   d. 24-hour specimen

4. Which is a CLIA-waived test?
   a. Ovulation test
   b. Dipstick urinalysis
   c. Urine microscopy
   d. Both a and b

5. Sensitivity limits for drug screening tests are set by which agency?
   a. SAMHSA
   b. NIDA
   c. HHS
   d. All of the above

6. What hormone is being detected in a CLIA-waived urine pregnancy test?
   a. hCG
   b. FSH
   c. LH
   d. Both b and c

7. Which term is defined as pouring a liquid gently so that it does not disturb the remaining sediment?
   a. Supernatant
   b. Turbidity
   c. Decant
   d. Precipitate

8. A positive urine dipstick nitrite test is seen in which condition?
   a. Diabetes mellitus
   b. Glomerulonephritis
   c. Urinary tract infection
   d. All of the above

9. Which medical terminology root below means bend or deflect?
   a. orth/o
   b. morph/o
   c. prot/o
   d. refract/o

10. The definition of the term *cystitis* is
    a. inflammation of the kidney.
    b. infection of the kidney.
    c. inflammation of the bladder.
    d. infection of the bladder.

WORKPLACE APPLICATIONS

1. Becca is looking at the results of a patient dipstick urinalysis. Using the table of results below, indicate if the result is normal or abnormal by checking the appropriate box. Use Table 47.4 as a reference for UA test normal values.

Analyte	Patient Result	Normal	Abnormal
Specific gravity	1.020		
pH	6.0		
Protein (mg/dL)	NEG		
Glucose (mg/dL)	250 mg/dL		
Ketone (mg/dL)	40 mg/dL		
Bilirubin (mg/dL)	NEG		
Blood (mg/dL)	NEG		
Nitrite (mg/dL)	NEG		
Urobilinogen (Ehrlich units)	0.5 Ehrlich units		
White blood cells	NEG		

2. Julie is giving Ethel instructions about how to collect a random urine sample. Ethel is elderly and a little hard of hearing, but Julie is patient and goes through the written instructions with her. Julie then asks Ethel to repeat back some key information so that she is sure Ethel understands the directions. She asks Ethel if she has any questions and Ethel replies "Yes, I do. How do I know this urine test is accurate? I will collect the sample here, and then it goes to the lab. How do I know the results are correct? How do I know they are testing my urine sample?"

   How would you assure Ethel that the testing done in the laboratory is correct? _____

   _____

   _____

   _____

   _____

   _____

   _____

   _____

   _____

INTERNET ACTIVITIES

1. Using online resources, find the list of CLIA-approved provider-performed microscopy procedures (PPMP). (HINT: the http://www.fda.gov/ or https://www.cms.gov/ sites are a great place to start.) What tests in the urinalysis department are CLIA-PPMP tests? Write a one-page paper summarizing your research. Include the following points in your paper:
   a. Name and give a brief description of the tests
   b. List the CPT codes for each test

2. Using online resources, research one drug of abuse. Create a poster presentation, a PowerPoint presentation, or a written paper summarizing your research. Include the following points in your project:
    a. Description of the drug and its effects on the body
    b. Tests available that are used to identify the drug or its metabolites
    c. CLIA-waived testing available for the detection of the drug
    d. How long does the drug remain detectable in the body after use?

3. Using online resources, write a short paper that describes a lateral flow immunoassay procedure. Summarize your research and include the following points in your project.
    a. What substance does the test detect?
    b. What is the antigen and antibody in the test?
    c. What is the CLIA category for the test?
    d. Briefly describe the principle of the test.

Procedure 47.1   Provide Instructions How to Collect a 24-Hour Urine Specimen and Process the Sample

Name _____ Date _____ Score _____

Tasks: Instruct a patient how to collect a urine 24-hour urine specimen. Process a 24-hour specimen for a creatinine clearance test.

Equipment and Supplies:
- Patient's health record
- 2-4 L urine collection container
- Plastic cup or specimen collection pan for collecting urine (which is then poured into the collection container)
- Printed patient instructions
- Laboratory requisition
- Fluid-impermeable lab coat, protective eyewear, and gloves

Standard: Complete the procedure and all critical steps in _____ minutes with a minimum score of 85% within two attempts (*or as indicated by the instructor*).

Scoring: Divide the points earned by the total possible points. Failure to perform a critical step, indicated by an asterisk (*), results in grade no higher than an 84% (*or as indicated by the instructor*).

Time: Began_____ Ended_____ Total minutes: _____

Steps:	Point Value	Attempt 1	Attempt 2
1. Greet the patient. Identify yourself. Verify the patient's identity with full name, ask the patient to spell the first and last name, and give their date of birth. Explain the procedure to be performed in a manner that is understood by the patient. Answer any questions the patient may have on the procedure.	10*		
2. Label the container with the patient's name and the current date; identify the specimen as a 24-hour urine specimen; and include your initials. Check for preservative if needed.	5		
3. Explain the following instructions to adult patients or to the guardians of pediatric patients. *Patient Instructions: Obtaining a 24-Hour Urine Specimen* a. Empty your bladder into the toilet in the morning without saving any of the specimen. Record the time you first emptied your bladder on the label. b. For the next 24 hours, each time you empty your bladder, all the urine should be collected into the plastic cup or collection pan that is placed on the toilet. Then pour all the collected urine directly into the large specimen container. c. Put the lid back on the container after each urination and rinse out the plastic cup or collection pan and store the container in the refrigerator or at room temperature, as directed, throughout the 24 hours of the study. d. If at any time you forget to collect your specimen or if some urine is accidentally spilled, the test must be started over again with a new container and a newly recorded start time.	10		

	e. Collect the final urine specimen at the same time you started the collection process on the previous day. This last collected specimen is placed in the large container. Collection ends with the voided morning specimen on the second day, which completes the 24-hour period. f. As soon as possible after completing collection, return the specimen container to the provider's office or the designated laboratory.			
4.	Give the patient the specimen container and supplies with written instructions to confirm understanding.	**10**		
5.	Document details of the patient education session in the patient's record.	**10**		
Processing a 24-Hour Urine Specimen				
6.	Ask the patient whether he or she collected all voided urine throughout the 24-hour period or whether any problems occurred during the collection process.	**10**		
7.	Complete the laboratory request form. Make sure that all the information is filled out on the container label.	**10**		
8.	Wash hands or use hand sanitizer. Put on a fluid-impermeable lab coat, protective eyewear, and gloves before preparing the specimen for transport. Comply with safety practices.	**10***		
9.	Store the specimen in the refrigerator until it is picked up by the laboratory.	**5**		
10.	Remove gloves and discard appropriately. Remove protective eyewear and lab coat. Wash hands or use hand sanitizer.	**10***		
11.	Document that the specimen was sent to the laboratory, including the type of test ordered, the date and time, the type of specimen, and your initials.	**10***		
	Total Points	**100**		

Documentation

Comments

CAAHEP Competencies	Step(s)
I.P.11.c. Obtain specimens and perform: CLIA-waived urinalysis	Entire procedure
XII.P.1. Comply with safety practices	8
ABHES Competencies	**Step(s)**
9.d. Collect, label, and process a specimen	Entire procedure

Procedure 47.2 Provide Instructions How to Collect a Clean-Catch Midstream Specimen and Process the Sample

Name _____ Date _____ Score _____

Tasks: Instruct a patient how to collect a clean-catch midstream specimen (CCMS). Process the specimen.

Equipment and Supplies:
- Patient's health record
- Patient written instructions
- Sterile container with lid and label
- Antiseptic towelettes
- Laboratory requisition
- Biohazard specimen bag
- Fluid-impermeable lab coat, protective eyewear, and gloves

Standard: Complete the procedure and all critical steps in _____ minutes with a minimum score of 85% within two attempts (*or as indicated by the instructor*).

Scoring: Divide the points earned by the total possible points. Failure to perform a critical step, indicated by an asterisk (*), results in grade no higher than an 84% (*or as indicated by the instructor*).

Time: Began_____ Ended_____ Total minutes: _____

Steps:	Point Value	Attempt 1	Attempt 2
1. Greet the patient. Identify yourself. Verify the patient's identity with full name, ask the patient to spell the first and last name, and give their date of birth. Explain the procedure to be performed in a manner that is understood by the patient. Answer any questions the patient may have on the procedure.	15*		
2. Label the sterile sealed container (not the lid) and give the patient the towelette supplies and written patient instructions form, if needed.	10		

3. Using written directions, explain the following instructions to adult patients or to the guardians of pediatric patients, making sure you show sensitivity to privacy issues.
 	
Patient Instructions: Obtaining a Clean-Catch Midstream Specimen (Female Patient)
 	
  a. Wash your hands and open the towelette packages for easy access.
 	
  b. Remove the lid from the specimen container, being careful not to touch the inside of the lid or the inside of the container. Place the lid, facing up, on a paper towel.
 	
  c. Lower your underclothing and sit on the toilet.
 	
  d. Expose the urinary meatus by spreading apart the labia with one hand
 	
  e. Cleanse each side of the urinary meatus with a front-to-back motion, from the pubis toward the anus. Use a separate antiseptic wipe to cleanse each side of the meatus.
 	
  f. Cleanse directly across the meatus, front to back, using a third antiseptic wipe
	25*		

g. Hold the labia apart throughout this procedure.			
h. Void a small amount of urine into the toilet.			
i. Move the specimen container into position and void the next portion of urine into it. Fill the container halfway. Remember, this is a sterile container. Do not put your fingers on the inside of the container.			
j. Remove the cup and void the last amount of urine into the toilet. (This means that the first part and the last part of the urinary flow have been excluded from the specimen. Only the middle portion of the flow is included.)			
k. Place the lid on the container, taking care not to touch the interior surface of the lid. Wipe in your usual manner, redress. Wash your hands and return the sterile specimen to the place designated by the medical facility.			
Patient Instructions: Obtaining a Clean-Catch Midstream Specimen (Male Patient)			
a. Wash your hands and expose the penis.			
b. Retract the foreskin of the penis (if not circumcised).			
c. Cleanse the area around the glans penis (tip of the penis) and the urethral opening by washing each side of the glans with a separate antiseptic wipe.			
d. Cleanse directly across the urethral opening using a third antiseptic wipe.			
e. Void a small amount of urine into the toilet or urinal.			
f. Collect the next portion of the urine in the sterile container, filling the container halfway without touching the inside of the container with the hands or the penis.			
g. Void the last amount of urine into the toilet or urinal.			
h. Place the lid on the container, taking care not to touch the interior surface of the lid. Wipe in your usual manner, redress. Wash your hands.			
i. Return the sterile specimen to the place designated by the medical facility.			
Processing a Clean-Catch Urine Specimen			
4. Document the date, time, and collection type.	**10**		
5. Wash hands or use hand sanitizer. Put on the fluid-impermeable lab coat, protective eyewear, and gloves. Comply with safety practices.	**15***		
6. Process the specimen according to the provider's orders. Perform urinalysis in the office or prepare the specimen for transport to the laboratory. If it is to be sent to an outside laboratory, complete the following steps: • Make sure the label is properly completed with the patient's information and the date, time, test ordered, and your initials. • Place the specimen in a biohazard specimen bag. • Complete a laboratory requisition and place it in the outside pocket of the specimen bag. • Keep the specimen refrigerated until pickup.	**15***		

7.	Remove gloves, protective eyewear, and lab coat. Dispose of gloves appropriately. Wash hands or use hand sanitizer. Document that the specimen was sent.	**10***		
	Total Points	**100**		

Documentation

Comments

CAAHEP Competencies	Step(s)
I.P.11.c. Obtain specimens and perform: CLIA-waived urinalysis	Entire procedure
III.P.2. Select appropriate barrier/personal protective equipment (PPE)	5
XII.P.1. Comply with safety practices	5
ABHES Competencies	**Step(s)**
9.d. Collect, label, and process a specimen	Entire procedure
9.e. Instruct patients in the collection of 1) clean-catch midstream urine specimens	3

Procedure 47.3 Assess Urine for Color and Turbidity: Physical Test

Name _____ Date _____ Score _____

Tasks: To assess and record the color and clarity of a urine specimen.

Equipment and Supplies:
- Patient's health record
- Urine specimen
- Centrifuge tube
- Fluid-impermeable lab coat, protective eyewear, and gloves
- White piece of paper with thin black lines drawn on it
- Biohazard waste container

Standard: Complete the procedure and all critical steps in _____ minutes with a minimum score of 85% within two attempts (*or as indicated by the instructor*).

Scoring: Divide the points earned by the total possible points. Failure to perform a critical step, indicated by an asterisk (*), results in grade no higher than an 84% (*or as indicated by the instructor*).

Time: Began_____ Ended_____ Total minutes: _____

Steps:	Point Value	Attempt 1	Attempt 2
1. Wash hands or use hand sanitizer. Put on the fluid-impermeable lab coat, protective eyewear, and gloves. Comply with safety practices.	10*		
2. Mix the urine by gently swirling the specimen.	10		
3. Label a centrifuge tube if a complete urinalysis is to be done.	10		
4. Pour the specimen into a standard-sized centrifuge tube.	10		
5. Assess and record the color: • Pale straw or straw • Yellow • Amber or dark amber	15*		
6. Assess the turbidity by placing a piece of white paper with fine, dark black print behind the specimen and see if you can see the print: • Clear—Able to read through the specimen; no cloudiness • Slightly turbid—Can barely see fine lines on white paper through the specimen • Turbid—Cannot see fine print, dark print possibly seen through the tube, or see no print at all through the tube	15*		
7. Clean the work area and dispose of procedure supplies in the biohazard waste container.	10*		
8. Dispose of gloves. Remove lab coat and protective eyewear. Wash hands or use hand sanitizer.	10*		
9. Document the results in the patient's record.	10		
Total Points	100		

Documentation

Comments

CAAHEP Competencies	Step(s)
I.P.11.c. Obtain specimens and perform: CLIA-waived urinalysis	Entire procedure
II.P.2. Record laboratory test results into the patient's record	9
III.P.2. Select appropriate barrier/personal protective equipment (PPE)	1
XII.P.1. Comply with safety practices	1
ABHES Competencies	**Step(s)**
9 b. Perform selected CLIA-waived tests that assist with diagnosis and treatment 1) Urinalysis	Entire procedure
9.c. Dispose of biohazardous materials	7

Procedure 47.4 Perform Quality Control Measures to Determine the Reliability of Chemical Reagent Strips

Name _____ Date _____ Score _____

Tasks: To reconstitute a control sample and test the reliability of the urinalysis chemical testing strip.

Equipment and Supplies:
- Chek-Stix control strips with reference ranges for urinalysis
- Distilled water
- Capped tube with milliliter markings
- Test tube rack
- Forceps
- Timer
- Urine chemical strips for urine testing
- Color chart for interpreting the chemical strip results
- Fluid-impermeable lab coat, protective eyewear, and gloves
- Biohazard waste container
- Control reference sheet and control flow sheet

Standard: Complete the procedure and all critical steps in _____ minutes with a minimum score of 85% within two attempts (*or as indicated by the instructor*).

Scoring: Divide the points earned by the total possible points. Failure to perform a critical step, indicated by an asterisk (*), results in grade no higher than an 84% (*or as indicated by the instructor*).

Time: Began_____ Ended_____ Total minutes: _____

Steps:	Point Value	Attempt 1	Attempt 2
1. Assemble the equipment and supplies. Record the lot number and the expiration date of the Chek-Stix on the control log sheet.	5		
2. Wash hands or use hand sanitizer. Put on the fluid-impermeable lab coat, protective eyewear, and gloves. Comply with safety practices.	10*		
3. Place a conical tube in a test tube rack and remove the cap.	5		
4. Pour 15 mL of distilled water into the tube.	5		
5. Using forceps, remove one strip from the Chek-Stix bottle. Inspect the strips for mottling or discoloration.	5		
6. Place the strip into the water and tightly cap the tube.	5		
7. Invert the tube for 2 minutes.	5		
8. Allow the tube to sit in the rack for 30 minutes.	5		
9. Invert the tube one time and remove the strip with forceps.	5		
10. Discard the strip in the biohazard waste container. Once reconstituted, the control solution is stable for 8 hours at room temperature.	5*		
11. Perform quality control of the chemical reagent strip by dipping it into the control solution.	5		
12. Read and record the results.	10*		
13. Compare the results with the control reference ranges provided on the Chek-Stix package insert.	10		

14. Discard the chemical reagent strip and the control solution in the biohazard waste container.	5*		
15. Clean up the work area and appropriately dispose of supplies and gloves in a biohazard waste container.	5		
16. Remove protective eyewear and lab coat. Wash hands or use hand sanitizer.	10*		
Total Points	100		

Documentation

Comments

CAAHEP Competencies	Step(s)
I.P.10. Perform a quality control measure	Entire procedure
III.P.2. Select appropriate barrier/personal protective equipment (PPE)	2
XII.P.1. Comply with safety practices	2
ABHES Competencies	**Step(s)**
9.a. Practice quality control	Entire procedure

Procedure 47.5   Test Urine with Chemical Reagent Strips

Name _____ Date _____ Score _____

Task: Perform chemical testing on a urine sample.

Equipment and Supplies:
- Patient's health record
- Urine specimen
- Reagent strips
- Timer
- Fluid-impermeable lab coat, protective eyewear, and gloves
- Biohazard waste container

Standard: Complete the procedure and all critical steps in _____ minutes with a minimum score of 85% within two attempts (*or as indicated by the instructor*).

Scoring: Divide the points earned by the total possible points. Failure to perform a critical step, indicated by an asterisk (*), results in grade no higher than an 84% (*or as indicated by the instructor*).

Time: Began_____ Ended_____ Total minutes: _____

Steps:	Point Value	Attempt 1	Attempt 2
1. Wash hands or use hand sanitizer. Put on the fluid-impermeable lab coat, protective eyewear, and gloves. Comply with safety practices.	10*		
2. Check the time of collection, the container, and the mode of preservation.	5		
3. If the specimen has been refrigerated, allow it to warm to room temperature.	5		
4. Check the reagent strip container for the expiration date.	5*		
5. Remove the reagent strip from the container. Hold it in your hand or place it on a clean, dry paper towel. Recap the container tightly.	5		
6. Compare nonreactive test pads with the negative color blocks on the color chart on the container. Discard strips that have discolored pads.	5		
7. Thoroughly mix the specimen by gently swirling the container.	5		
8. Following the manufacturer's directions, note the time, dip the strip into the urine, and then remove it.	5		
9. Quickly remove the excess urine from the strip by pulling the back of the strip across the lip of the specimen container and then blotting the edge of the strip on a clean, dry paper towel or the side of the specimen container.	10*		
10. Hold the strip horizontally. At the required time, compare the strip with the appropriate color chart on the reagent container. Do not touch the strip to the bottle. Alternately, the strip can be placed on a paper towel.	10*		
11. Read and record the first two results 30 seconds after dipping the strip. Compare the two reagent pads closest to your hand with the bottom two rows of the color chart. Continue reading and recording each row of possible results with its appropriate reagent pad at its designated time.	10*		
12. Clean the work area. If a paper towel was used, dispose of it and the reagent strip in an appropriate biohazard waste container.	10		

13. Remove gloves and dispose of appropriately. Remove protective eyewear and lab coat. Wash hands or use hand sanitizer.	10*			
14. Document the results in the patient's health record.	5			
Total Points	100			

Documentation

Comments

CAAHEP Competencies	Step(s)
I.P.11.c. Obtain specimens and perform: CLIA-waived urinalysis	Entire procedure
II.P.2. Record laboratory test results into the patient's record	14
III.P.2. Select appropriate barrier/personal protective equipment (PPE)	1
XII.P.1. Comply with safety practices	1
ABHES Competencies	**Step(s)**
9 b. Perform selected CLIA-waived tests that assist with diagnosis and treatment 1) Urinalysis	Entire procedure
9.c. Dispose of biohazardous materials	13

Procedure 47.6 Prepare a Urine Specimen for Microscopic Examination

Name _____ Date _____ Score _____

Task: To prepare a urine specimen for the provider's microscopic examination to determine the presence of normal and abnormal elements.

Equipment and Supplies:
- Patient's health record
- Urine specimen
- Centrifuge tube
- Centrifuge
- Disposable pipet
- Sedi-Stain
- Microscope slide and coverslip
- Microscope
- Permanent marker
- Fluid-impermeable lab coat, protective eyewear or face shield, and gloves
- Biohazard waste container

Standard: Complete the procedure and all critical steps in _____ minutes with a minimum score of 85% within two attempts (*or as indicated by the instructor*).

Scoring: Divide the points earned by the total possible points. Failure to perform a critical step, indicated by an asterisk (*), results in grade no higher than an 84% (*or as indicated by the instructor*).

Time: Began_____ Ended_____ Total minutes: _____

Steps:	Point Value	Attempt 1	Attempt 2
1. Wash hands or use hand sanitizer. Put on the fluid-impermeable lab coat, protective eyewear, and gloves. Comply with safety practices.	10*		
2. Gently mix the urine specimen by swirling the covered specimen container.	5		
3. Pour 12 mL of urine into a labeled centrifuge tube and cap the tube.	5		
4. Place the tube in the centrifuge.	10		
5. Place another tube containing 12 mL of urine or water in the opposite cup.	10*		
6. Secure the lid and centrifuge for 5 minutes or for the time specified for your instrument.	5		
7. Remove the tube from the centrifuge after the instrument has come to a full stop.	5		
8. Pour off the clear supernatant from the top of the specimen by inverting the centrifuge tube over the sink drain while allowing the running water from the faucet to flush the urine down the drain.	10		
9. Turn the tube upright when the supernatant has been decanted, allowing a small amount to return to the sediment on the bottom of the tube without losing sediment down the drain	10		
10. Thoroughly mix the sediment with a drop of Sedi-Stain by grasping the tube near the top and rapidly flicking it with the fingers of the other hand until all sediment is thoroughly resuspended.	10		

11. Transfer 1 drop of sediment to a clean, labeled slide using a clean, disposable transfer pipet. Transfer pipet should be disposed of in a sharps container.	5			
12. Place a clean coverslip over the drop and place the slide on the microscope stage. Remove eye protection.	5			
13. Focus under low power and reduce the light.	10			
Total Points	100			

Comments

CAAHEP Competencies	Step(s)
III.P.2. Select appropriate barrier/personal protective equipment (PPE)	1
XII.P.1. Comply with safety practices	1

Procedure 47.7   Perform a CLIA-Waived Urinalysis: Perform a Pregnancy Test

Name _____ **Date** _____ **Score** _____

Task: To perform a pregnancy test on urine using the QuickVue pregnancy test method.

Equipment and Supplies:
- Patient's health record
- Urine specimen
- QuickVue test kit
- Fluid-impermeable lab coat, protective eyewear, and gloves
- Biohazard sharps container
- Biohazard waste container

Standard: Complete the procedure and all critical steps in _____ minutes with a minimum score of 85% within two attempts (*or as indicated by the instructor*).

Scoring: Divide the points earned by the total possible points. Failure to perform a critical step, indicated by an asterisk (*), results in grade no higher than an 84% (*or as indicated by the instructor*).

Time: Began_____ Ended_____ Total minutes: _____

Steps:	Point Value	Attempt 1	Attempt 2
1. Wash hands or use hand sanitizer. Put on fluid-impermeable lab coat, protective eyewear, and gloves. Comply with safety practices.	10*		
2. Prepare the testing equipment. Check the expiration date of the kit before proceeding.	10*		
3. Obtain the proper patient specimen (preferably a first morning specimen).	5		
4. Remove the test cassette from the foil pouch.	5		
5. Add 3 drops of urine using the transfer pipet (dropper) that accompanies the kit.	10		
6. Dispose of the pipet in a biohazard sharps container.	10*		
7. Wait 3 minutes and read the test results.	5		
8. Interpret the results: • Negative: A blue control line is next to the letter C; no line is seen next to the letter T. • Positive: A blue control line is next to the letter C; a pink line is next to the letter T. • Invalid: If a blue line does not appear in the C area, the test is invalid, and the specimen must be retested using another kit.	15*		
9. Discard the test cassette in the biohazard waste container, clean up testing area, then remove and discard gloves in a biohazard waste container. Remove lab coat and protective eyewear.	10*		
10. Wash hands or use hand sanitizer.	10*		
11. Document the results in the patient's health record as either positive or negative for pregnancy.	10		
Total Points	**100**		

Documentation

Comments

CAAHEP Competencies	**Step(s)**
I.P.11.c. Obtain specimens and perform: CLIA-waived urinalysis	Entire procedure
II.P.2. Record laboratory test results into the patient's record	11
III.P.2. Select appropriate barrier/personal protective equipment (PPE)	1
XII.P.1. Comply with safety practices	1
ABHES Competencies	**Step(s)**
9 b. Perform selected CLIA-waived tests that assist with diagnosis and treatment 1) Urinalysis	Entire procedure
9.c. Dispose of biohazardous materials	9

Procedure 47.8 Obtain a Specimen and Perform a CLIA-Waived Urinalysis: Perform a Multidrug Screening Test on Urine

Name _____ Date _____ Score _____

Task: To screen a urine specimen for drugs or drug metabolites at their specified cutoff levels.

Equipment and Supplies:
- Patient's health record
- Multi-Drug Screen Urine Test in a sealed container
- Freshly voided urine sample
- Timer
- Fluid-impermeable lab coat, eye protection, and gloves
- Biohazard waste container

Standard: Complete the procedure and all critical steps in _____ minutes with a minimum score of 85% within two attempts (*or as indicated by the instructor*).

Scoring: Divide the points earned by the total possible points. Failure to perform a critical step, indicated by an asterisk (*), results in grade no higher than an 84% (*or as indicated by the instructor*).

Time: Began_____ Ended_____ Total minutes: _____

Steps:	Point Value	Attempt 1	Attempt 2
1. Wash hands or use hand sanitizer. Put on fluid-impermeable lab coat, protective eyewear, and gloves. Comply with safety practices.	10*		
2. Assemble the equipment and specimen. Check the expiration date on the test kit.	5		
3. Determine the temperature of the urine (within 4 minutes of voiding). The temperature should be between 32° and 38° C (90° and 100° F).	10*		
4. Bring the specimen and the testing device to room temperature.	5		
5. Remove the device from the foil pouch and label it with the specimen identification.	10		
6. Apply the specimen to the device by using one of two methods: • *Dip Method*: Remove the cap of the specimen and dip the device into the specimen for 10 seconds, making sure the surface of the urine is above the sample well and below the arrowheads in the window. • *Alternate Method*: Remove the pipet from the pouch and fill it to the line on the barrel with urine. Dispense the entire volume onto the sample well on the testing device.	15*		
7. Recap the urine specimen.	5*		
8. Set the timer for the designated time. Do not read the results until after maximum time as stated in the manufacturer's instructions.	5*		

9. Interpret the results:
  • Positive: If the C line appears but the T line does not, the result is positive for that drug.
  • Negative: If both the C line and the T line appear, the level of the drug or its metabolites is below the cutoff level (i.e., negative for that drug).
  • Invalid: If no C line develops within 5 minutes on any test strip, the assay is invalid. Repeat the assay with a new test device if invalid.
	10*		

10. Discard the urine and the device in the biohazard container.	5		
11. Disinfect the area. Remove your gloves and dispose in biohazard container. Remove lab coat, and wash hand or use hand sanitizer.	10*		
12. Document the results in the patient's health record.	10		
Total Points	100		

Documentation

Comments

CAAHEP Competencies	Step(s)
I.P.11.c. Obtain specimens and perform: CLIA-waived urinalysis	Entire procedure
II.P.2. Record laboratory test results into the patient's record	13
III.P.2. Select appropriate barrier/personal protective equipment (PPE)	1
XII.P.1. Comply with safety practices	1
ABHES Competencies	**Step(s)**
9 b. Perform selected CLIA-waived tests that assist with diagnosis and treatment 1) Urinalysis	Entire procedure
9.c. Dispose of biohazardous materials	9

Procedure 47.9   Reassure a Patient of the Accuracy of the Test Results

Name _____ **Date** _____ **Score** _____

Task: Show empathy and communicate respectfully and professionally with patient. Reassure patient of the accuracy of the test result.

Scenario: Elyse is seeing Jean Burke, NP at WMFM Clinic today. Elyse has been feeling tired and slightly nauseous for the last few weeks. She and her husband use birth control, but her menstrual periods are very irregular. She did a home pregnancy test 2 weeks ago, and it was negative. But she is still feeling poorly. Jean Burke orders a urine pregnancy test. The lab runs a CLIA-waived urine pregnancy test, and it is positive. Elyse doesn't believe the result. You need to reassure her the accuracy of the test result.

Directions: Role-play the scenario with a peer. The peer is the patient, and you are the medical assistant.

Standard: Complete the role-play in _____ minutes with a minimum score of 100% within two attempts (*or as indicated by the instructor*).

Scoring: Divide the points earned by the total possible points. Met competency: 100% (10 points). Not met competency: 0% (0 points).

Time: Began_____ Ended_____ Total minutes: _____

Steps:	Point Value	Attempt 1	Attempt 2
1. Encourage the patient to talk about her concerns and fears. Demonstrate active listening skills. *(Refer to the Affective Behaviors Checklist – Active Listening and the Grading Rubric)*	30*		
2. Address the patient's concerns and notify the provider of any issues that are outside of the medical assistant's scope of practice. Reassure the patient by demonstrating respect and empathy while addressing the concerns. *(Refer to the Affective Behaviors Checklist – Respect and Empathy and the Grading Rubric)*	30*		
Scenario update: The patient indicates that she does not understand how the first test was negative and the second test is positive. 3. Describe the difference between the first and second tests. Use language that the patient can understand.	30		
4. Answer any questions the patient has.	10		
Total Points	100		

Affective Behavior	**Affective Behaviors Checklist** **Directions:** *Check behaviors observed during the role-play.*				
	Negative, Unprofessional Behaviors	**Attempt**		**Positive, Professional Behaviors**	**Attempt**
Active Listening		**1**	**2**		**1**	**2**
	Interrupted			Refrained from interrupting		
	Did not allow for silence or pauses			Allowed for periods of silence		
	Negative nonverbal behaviors (rolled eyes, yawned, frowned, avoided eye contact)			Positive nonverbal behaviors (smiled, nodded head, appropriate eye contact)		
	Distracted (looked at watch, phone)			Focused on patient, avoided distractions		
	Biased, offensive			Remained neutral		
	Other:			Other:		
Respect	Rude, unkind, disrespectful, impolite			Courteous, polite		
	Unwelcoming, brief, abrupt, unpleasant, unapproachable			Welcoming, took time with the patient, personable, and approachable		
	Unconcerned with person's dignity			Maintained person's dignity		
	Poor eye contact with patient			Proper eye contact with patient		
	Negative nonverbal behaviors			Positive nonverbal behaviors		
	Other:			Other:		
Empathy	Didn't listen to the patient, interrupted patient; unsupportive, uninterested, or uncaring			Listened to the patient; supportive and caring		
	Did not acknowledge or respond appropriately to the patient's emotional responses; cold, aloof, insensitive, indifferent, or unfeeling			Acknowledged and responded appropriately to the patient's emotional responses; showed sensitivity		
	Failed to reassure patient; did not respond to the patient's concerns			Reassured patient by repeating and responding to the patient's concerns		
	Used language that is hard to understand (e.g., slang, generational terms, medical terminology, too scientific)			Used language that the patient can understand		
	Failed to address the patient's questions; or answers to patient's questions are inappropriate			Answered the patient's questions appropriately		
	Other:			Other:		

Grading Rubric for the Affective Behaviors Checklist **Directions:** *Based on checklist results, identify the points received for the procedure checklist. Indicate how the behaviors demonstrated met the expectations.*		Point Value	Attempt 1	Attempt 2
Does not meet Expectation	• Response lacked active listening, respect, and/or empathy. • Student demonstrated more than 2 negative, unprofessional behaviors during the interaction.	0		
Needs Improvement	• Response lacked active listening, respect, and/or empathy. • Student demonstrated 1 or 2 negative, unprofessional behaviors during the interaction.	0		
Meets Expectation	• Response demonstrates active listening, respect, and empathy; no negative, unprofessional behaviors observed. • More practice is needed for behavior to appear natural and for student to appear comfortable and at ease.	30		
Occasionally Exceeds Expectation	• Response demonstrates active listening, respect, and empathy; no negative, unprofessional behaviors observed. • At times student appeared comfortable and at ease; but more practice is needed for behavior to become natural and consistent with a professional medical assistant.	30		
Always Exceeds Expectation	• Response demonstrates active listening, respect, and empathy; no negative, unprofessional behaviors observed. • Student's behaviors appeared natural and comfortable. Behaviors are consistent with a professional medical assistant.	30		

Comments

CAAHEP Competencies	Step(s)
A.2. Reassure patients	2
A.4. Demonstrate active listening	1

Blood Collection

CAAHEP Competencies	Assessments
XII.C.2.c. Identify safety techniques that can be used in responding to accidental exposure to: needle sticks	Skills and Concepts – C. 3-4
I.P.2.b. Perform the following procedures: venipuncture	Procedures 48.1, 48.2, 48.3
I.P.2.c. Perform the following procedures: capillary puncture	Procedure 48.4
III.P.2. Select appropriate barrier/personal protective equipment (PPE)	Procedures 48.1, 48.2, 48.3, 48.4
III.P.10.a. Demonstrate proper disposal of biohazardous material: sharps	Procedures 48.1, 48.2, 48.3, 48.4
III.P.10.b. Demonstrate proper disposal of biohazardous material: regulated wastes	Procedures 48.1, 48.2, 48.3, 48.4
X.P.3. Document patient care accurately in the medical record	Procedures 48.1, 48.2, 48.3, 48.4
A.1. Demonstrate critical thinking skills	Procedures 48.1, 48.2, 48.3
A.3. Demonstrate empathy for patients' concerns	Procedure 48.5
A.4. Demonstrate active listening	Procedure 48.5
ABHES Competencies	**Assessments**
3. Medical Terminology c. Apply medical terminology for each specialty	Vocabulary Review – A. 1-10, B. 1-7
d. Define and use medical abbreviations when appropriate and acceptable	Abbreviations – 1-18
9. Medical Laboratory Procedures c. Dispose of biohazardous materials	Procedures 48.1, 48.2, 48.3, 48.4
d. Collect, label, and process a specimen 1) Perform venipuncture	Procedures 48.1, 48.2, 48.3
d. Collect, label, and process a specimen 2) Perform capillary puncture	Procedure 48.4

VOCABULARY REVIEW

Using the word pool, find the correct word to match the definition. Write the word on the line after the definition.

Group A

1. The inner bend in front of the elbow _____

2. Also known as *healthcare-acquired infections* _____

3. A device with a slender barrel and needle used to withdraw blood from a vein or artery _____

4. A device for temporarily constricting blood flow _____

5. The chemical breakdown of carbohydrates (glucose) by enzymes, with the release of energy _____

6. A microbiologic procedure where a blood sample is placed in a nutrient medium and held at body temperature to encourage the growth of the infecting bacteria in the laboratory _____

7. This type of tube top has the advantage of not splattering blood when the cap is removed from the tube _____

8. Obstruction or interruption of normal lymph flow _____

9. The breakdown of red blood cells with the release of hemoglobin _____

10. An abnormal buildup of blood in an organ or tissue of the body, caused by a leak or cut in a blood vessel _____

Word Pool
- antecubital
- blood culture
- glycolysis
- Hemogard
- hemolysis
- hematoma
- lymphostasis
- nosocomial
- syringe
- tourniquet

Group B

1. The production of a partial vacuum by the removal of air to force fluid into a vacant space _____

2. The sole of the foot _____

3. Very small, round hemorrhage in the skin or mucous membrane _____

4. A force acting on an object because of gravity; for example, a centrifuge spinning _____

5. To draw off or remove by suction _____

6. The palm of the hand _____

7. Space between the cells _____

Word Pool
- aspirating
- g-force
- interstitial
- palmar
- petechiae
- plantar
- suction

ABBREVIATIONS

Write out what each of the following abbreviations stands for.

1. PPE _____

2. ASCP _____

3. HBV _____

4. HCV _____

5. HIV _____

6. OSHA _____

7. NPA _____

8. POL _____

9. CLSI _____

10. CBC _____

11. EDTA _____

12. SST _____

13. PST _____

14. PT/INR _____

15. APTT _____

16. FDA _____

17. POCT _____

18. PKU _____

SKILLS AND CONCEPTS
Answer the following questions.

A. Introduction
Fill in the blank.

1. What is the most common specimen tested in the laboratory? _____

2. _____ is the process of acquiring blood from a patient.

3. _____ is defined as taking blood directly from a surface vein.

4. The blood-borne viruses identified as possible blood-borne pathogen risks are _____, _____, and _____.

B. Venipuncture Equipment
Fill in the blank or select the correct answer.

1. Syncope is another term for _____.

2. OSHA requires healthcare workers to wear _____ during venipuncture.

3. James touched the prepared site with his gloved finger just before inserting the needle. Which statement is correct?
   a. The site is not contaminated, and he was correct to insert the needle.
   b. The site was contaminated, and he should have cleansed the site again before inserting the needle.
   c. A and B are incorrect.
   d. A and B are correct.

4. The tourniquet should be tied for no longer than _____ minute(s) at a time.

5. Most venipunctures are done in the _____, or inner bend in front of the elbow.

6. Tourniquets are applied _____ inches above the elbow immediately before the venipuncture procedure begins.

7. _____ is a condition in which the concentration of blood cells is increased in proportion to the plasma.

8. A(n) _____ is a substance that inhibits the growth of microorganisms on living tissue.

9. To be most effective, the alcohol should remain on the skin for _____ seconds and allowed to air dry.

10. Which product *cannot* be used to cleanse the site when collecting a blood alcohol sample?
    a. Alcohol wipe
    b. Sterile soap pads
    c. Benzalkonium chloride
    d. Povidone-iodine
    e. All of the above

Match the description with the correct term. Answers can be used more than once.

11. _____ The liquid portion of a whole blood sample that has not clotted due to an anticoagulant.

12. _____ A synthetic, chemically neutral gel that settles between the plasma/serum and cells during centrifugation

13. _____ The anticoagulant that prevents platelet clumping and preserves the appearance of blood cells for microscopic examination

14. _____ Substances added to a venipuncture tube to enhance and speed up blood clotting

15. _____ Absence of air to create a vacuum in a tube, flask, or reaction vessel

16. _____ The liquid portion of a clotted blood specimen that no longer contains active clotting agents

17. _____ A substance that prevents clotting of blood

a. evacuated
b. anticoagulant
c. clot activators
d. plasma
e. ethylenediaminetetraacetic acid
f. serum
g. thixotropic gel

Match the evacuated tube stopper color with the additive it contains.

18. _____ Light blue
19. _____ Red
20. _____ Gold Hemogard
21. _____ Green
22. _____ Light green
23. _____ Lavender
24. _____ Gray
25. _____ Light blue

a. EDTA
b. heparin
c. lithium heparin and gel
d. potassium oxalate and sodium fluoride
e. silica particles
f. sodium citrate
g. none

Select the correct answer.

26. Which of the following shows the correct order for a draw?
    a. Red top, gray top, lavender top
    b. Red top, green top, light blue top
    c. Red top, lavender top, gray top
    d. Red top, gray top, green top

27. Which of the following shows the correct order for a draw?
    a. Blood culture bottles, lavender top, green top
    b. Green top, light blue top, lavender top
    c. Lavender top, green top, gold top
    d. Light blue top, green top, gray top

28. Which of the following shows the correct order for a draw?
    a. Red top, green top, light blue top
    b. Lavender top, green top, gray top
    c. Green top, lavender top, gray top
    d. Light blue top, gray top, green top

Match the description with the correct term.

29. _____ The bore, or hollow space, inside the needle
30. _____ One end of the shaft is cut at an angle, which creates a very sharp point
31. _____ Lumen size

a. bevel
b. lumen
c. gauge

Fill in the blank.

32. _____ are double-pointed needles that are commonly used when several tubes need to be drawn during a single venipuncture.

33. Double-pointed needles must be firmly placed into a(n) _____.

34. _____ are used if the phlebotomist thinks the vacuum from the stoppered vacuum tube might collapse the vein.

35. _____ are often used to draw veins in the back of the hand or when drawing a pediatric patient.

C. Needle Safety

Fill in the blank or select the correct answer.

1. According to OSHA, the best practice for preventing needlestick injuries after phlebotomy is to use _____ that are activated with one hand immediately after use.

2. OSHA requires employers to establish and maintain a(n) _____ for recording injuries from contaminated sharps.

3. Which statement is correct regarding immediately after a needlestick injury?
   a. The wound is inspected.
   b. The wound is washed for 10 minutes.
   c. The wound is washed with soap, 10% iodine solution, or chlorine-based antiseptic.
   d. all of the above.

4. With a needlestick injury, which is correct?
   a. The injury is reported to the supervisor.
   b. An incident report is completed.
   c. The employee is referred to a provider for confidential assessment and follow-up.
   d. Baseline testing is performed.
   e. All of the above.

D. Routine Venipuncture

Fill in the blank or select the correct answer.

1. According to CLSI, proper identification includes asking outpatients to state
   a. and spell their first and last name.
   b. their birth date.
   c. the city they live in.
   d. all of the above.
   e. both a and b.

2. All of the patient identification information must be compared and verified with the

   _____.

3. According to CLSI standards, the veins in the _____ of the antecubital area should be located as a first choice.

4. The _____ veins generally run at a slight angle to the fold in the antecubital area.

5. The _____ veins are on the thumb side of the antecubital area.

6. The tourniquet should be placed about _____ inches above the patient's elbow.

7. After removing the tourniquet, wait _____ minutes before reapplying it.

8. Insert the needle into the vein at about a _____-degree angle, depending on the depth and position of the vein.

9. Tubes with sodium citrate should be inverted _____ times.

10. Tubes with clot activator should be inverted _____ times.

11. Tubes with anticoagulant should be inverted _____ times

12. After the procedure, observe the site for _____ seconds after releasing pressure and removing the gauze.

E. Problems Associated with Venipuncture
Fill in the blank or select the correct answer.

1. A(n) _____ is caused by blood leaking into the tissue.

2. Which of the following are signs or symptoms of a hematoma?
    a.   Extremity numbness
    b.   Swelling at the puncture site
    c.   Large, painful, bruised area at the puncture site
    d.   All of the above
    e.   Both b and c

3. Which of the following does *not* cause a hematoma?
    a.   Creating too much friction when cleansing the site
    b.   Excessive probing with the needle to locate the vein
    c.   Passing the needle through the vein
    d.   Removing the needle before the tourniquet is removed

4. What action should the medical assistant take if a hematoma starts to form?
    a.   Discontinue the procedure immediately.
    b.   Apply pressure to the area for at least 3 minutes and then apply an ice pack.
    c.   Notify the provider.
    d.   Observe the site to determine whether the bleeding has stopped.
    e.   All of the above.

5. As a rule, it is wise to limit yourself to three venipuncture attempts for a patient. If a third attempt is unsuccessful, ask whether the patient would allow another phlebotomist to look at his or her arms.
    a.   Both statements are correct.
    b.   Both statements are incorrect.
    c.   The first statement is correct, and the second statement is incorrect.
    d.   The first statement is incorrect, and the second statement is correct.

6. When a patient faints, what should the medical assistant do?
    a.   Remove the tourniquet and needle from the arm and dispose of the needle properly, while putting pressure on the site.
    b.   Notify staff members for assistance.
    c.   Lay the patient flat or lower the head if the patient is sitting.
    d.   Apply a cold compress to the patient's forehead.
    e.   All of the above.

F. Pediatric Phlebotomy
Fill in the blank or select the correct answer.

1. Removing large amounts of blood, especially from premature infants, may result in

    _____.

2. Which complication can occur if a deep vein is punctured in a child?
    a.   Cardiac arrest
    b.   Hemorrhage and venous thrombosis
    c.   Damage to surrounding tissues and infection
    d.   All of the above

3. Blood should be collected only by dermal puncture from children younger than age _____ unless the procedure warrants venous collection.

4. Venipuncture on children younger than age _____ should be performed only on surface veins.

5. A _____-gauge winged infusion set coupled to a syringe or a pediatric vacuum tube collection set should be used for children younger than 2 years.

6. _____, such as ethyl chloride spray may be used to reduce pain at the puncture site.

G. Capillary Puncture

Fill in the blank or select the correct answer.

1. Capillaries connect small _____ and small _____.

2. Capillary puncture is warranted for all of the following patients *except*
   a. pediatric patients younger than 2 years.
   b. adults older than 45 years.
   c. patients who require frequent glucose monitoring.
   d. patients with burns or scars in venipuncture sites.
   e. obese patients.

3. Hemoglobin and glucose values are _____ in capillary blood.

4. Potassium, calcium, and total protein are _____ in capillary blood.

5. The device used to perform a dermal puncture is called a(n) _____.

6. Safety lancets only puncture _____.

7. Lancets should always be discarded in a(n) _____ immediately after use.

8. Blood drops are collected into the _____ through a funnel-like device.

9. A(n) _____ is a glass tube surrounded by a protective plastic coating for safety.

10. The blood is pulled into the tube by _____.

11. The _____ is used to test babies for certain metabolic disorders, such as phenylketonuria.

12. In adults and children older than 1 year, capillary puncture sites include the _____ or _____ finger.

13. Punctures should be made _____ to the whorls of the finger, which helps to create a nice drop of blood to collect.

14. For children younger than 2 years, dermal puncture is performed on the _____ or _____ areas of the plantar surface of the heel.

15. After the skin has been punctured, it is important to wipe away the first drop of blood with gauze, since the drop contains _____ that could interfere with test results.

16. Which of the following is the correct order of draws for capillary punctures?
   a. Red top, green top, and blood smear
   b. Green top, lavender top, and red top
   c. Blood smear, lavender top, and green top
   d. Gold top, green top, and red top

H. Handling Specimens After Collection
Fill in the blank.

1. Sample processing may include separation of _____ or _____ from red blood cells.

2. Tubes with clot accelerator should form a dense clot within _____ minutes.

3. Removing the serum from a clot tube requires _____.

4. The College of American Pathologists (CAP) recommends that whole blood for automated blood counts be refrigerated and tested within _____ hours.

5. _____ is a legal term that refers to the ability to guarantee the identity and integrity of the specimen from collection to reporting of test results.

CERTIFICATION PREPARATION
Circle the correct answer.

1. Which vessel type is most frequently used for phlebotomy?
   a. Artery
   b. Vein
   c. Capillary
   d. Both a and c

2. Fainting, or a brief lapse of consciousness, is the definition of what term?
   a. Syncope
   b. Evacuated
   c. Antecubital
   d. None of the above

3. What type of blood collection procedure should be used for a health screening blood glucose test?
   a. Arterial puncture
   b. Capillary puncture
   c. Venipuncture
   d. All of the above

4. Which colored-stopper tube contains EDTA as an anticoagulant?
   a. Green
   b. Light blue
   c. Gray
   d. Lavender

5. Which blood sample contains clotting factors?
   a. Serum
   b. Plasma
   c. Blood collected in a red-topped tube
   d. All of the above

6. The tourniquet should be removed during a routine venipuncture when
   a. blood starts to flow in the first tube.
   b. the last tube has completed filling.
   c. blood starts to flow in the last tube of the draw.
   d. none of the above.

7. Which vein in the antecubital region should not be used for routine venipuncture?
   a. Medial
   b. Cephalic
   c. Basilic
   d. None of the above

8. A substance that prevents clotting of blood is the definition of which term?
   a. Clot activator
   b. Antiseptic
   c. Anticoagulant
   d. Thixotropic gel

9. Which substance listed below is an anticoagulant?
   a. FDA
   b. CBC
   c. ASCP
   d. EDTA

10. The device used to perform a capillary puncture is called a
    a. tourniquet.
    b. lancet.
    c. butterfly assembly.
    d. hematocrit tube.

WORKPLACE APPLICATIONS

1. Maggie is quizzing a medical assistant student about the order of the draw. For each of the tube combinations below, put them in the correct order of the draw.

    a. Light blue, green, red _____

    b. Gray, lavender, green _____

    c. Gold, gray, green _____

    d. Red, light blue, lavender_____

2. Maggie goes to the waiting room to bring back Stella Brown for a capillary puncture. Stella is 9 years old and needs to have a capillary puncture today for red blood cell count. Maggie notices that Stella is anxious and also notices Stella is wearing a necklace with an ice skate charm on it. How can Maggie show awareness of a patient's concerns related to the procedure being performed?

    _____

    _____

    _____

    _____

    _____

    _____

    _____

3. Maggie will be performing a heelstick on a 3-week-old infant girl. The infant needs to have her bilirubin level checked and the mother is very nervous about her baby having the procedure done. The mother really wants to stay with her baby but doesn't like the sight of blood. How can Maggie help the mother with her concerns and still perform the heelstick that needs to be done?

    _____

    _____

    _____

    _____

    _____

    _____

INTERNET ACTIVITIES

1. Go to the OSHA website, https://www.osha.gov/SLTC/bloodbornepathogens/index.html and read through the OSHA Bloodborne Pathogens Standard fact sheet. Summarize the standard fact sheet in a one-page paper.

2. Using online resources, research the possible complications of a venipuncture. Create a poster presentation, a PowerPoint presentation, or an infographic summarizing your research. Include the following points in your project:
   a. Describe at least five complications of a venipuncture.
   b. How are the complications caused during the venipuncture?
   c. How can complications be avoided?
   d. What equipment should or should not be used to avoid complications?

3. Make a poster or infographic about the order of the draw for phlebotomy. Be ready to share your poster and catch-phrase with the class. Include the following information:
   a. Create a unique saying or catch-phrase to help remember the order of the draw.
   b. Explain how you came up with your saying and why it is memorable to you.
   c. Why is the order of the draw needed for a multiple tube venipuncture?

Procedure 48.1   Perform a Venipuncture: Collect a Venous Blood Sample Using the Vacuum Tube Method

Name _____   Date _____   Score _____

Tasks: To collect a venous blood specimen by the vacuum tube technique. Document in the patient's health record.

Equipment and Supplies:
- Patient's health record
- Provider's order and/or lab requisition
- Vacuum tube needle, needle holder, and proper tubes for requested tests
- 70% isopropyl alcohol wipes
- Gauze
- Tourniquet
- Hypoallergenic self-stick wrap, tape, or bandage
- Permanent marking pen and/or printed labels
- Fluid-impermeable lab coat, protective eyewear, and gloves
- Biohazard sharps container
- Biohazard waste container

Standard: Complete the procedure and all critical steps in _____ minutes with a minimum score of 85% within two attempts (*or as indicated by the instructor*).

Scoring: Divide the points earned by the total possible points. Failure to perform a critical step, indicated by an asterisk (*), results in grade no higher than an 84% (*or as indicated by the instructor*).

Time: Began_____ Ended_____ Total minutes: _____

Steps:	Point Value	Attempt 1	Attempt 2
1. Check the provider's order and/or requisition form to determine the tests ordered. Gather the appropriate tubes and supplies. Put on a fluid-impermeable lab coat.	4		
2. Greet the patient. Identify yourself. Verify the patient's identity with full name, ask the patient to spell the first and last name, and give their date of birth. Explain the procedure to be performed in a manner that is understood by the patient. Answer any questions the patient may have on the procedure. Obtain permission for the capillary puncture.	4*		
3. Wash hands or use hand sanitizer, then put on gloves and protective eyewear.	4*		
4. Ask the patient if they have a preference which arm is used for the venipuncture. Have the patient sit with their arm well supported in a slightly downward position.	4		
5. Apply the tourniquet around the patient's arm 3-4 inches above the elbow on the patient's preferred arm. The tourniquet should never be tied so tightly that it restricts blood flow in the artery. Tourniquets should remain in place no longer than 60 seconds.	4		

6.	Select the venipuncture site by palpating the antecubital space. Use your index finger to trace the path of the vein and to judge its depth. Look at both arms and use your critical thinking skills to find the vein that will give you the greatest chance of success for the venipuncture. *(Refer to the Affective Behaviors Checklist – Critical Thinking and the Grading Rubric.)*	4*		
7.	Remove the tourniquet and cleanse the site with a 70% alcohol wipe.	4		
8.	Assemble the equipment and supplies near your nondominant hand, next to the patient's arm for easy access during the procedure. Select an appropriate needle size and method of collection based on your inspection of the patient's veins. Attach the needle firmly to the vacuum tube holder. Keep the cover on the needle.	4		
9.	Reapply the tourniquet when the alcohol is dry.	4		
10.	Hold the vacuum tube assembly in your dominant hand. Your thumb should be on top and your fingers underneath. Remove the needle sheath.	4		
11.	Grasp the patient's arm with the nondominant hand and anchor the vein with your thumb of your nondominant hand.	4		
12.	With the bevel up and the needle aligned parallel to the vein, insert the needle at a 15- to 20-degree angle through the skin and into the vein with a quick but smooth motion.	4*		
13.	Hold the assembly in place with the dominant hand, steady through the venipuncture.	4		
14.	Place two fingers on the flanges of the needle holder and use the thumb to push the tube onto the double-pointed needle. Make sure you do not change the needle's position in the vein.	4*		
15.	Allow the tube to fill to its maximum capacity. Remove the tube by placing the fingers at the end of the tube and pushing on the needle holder with the index finger. Do not to move the needle when removing the tube. Immediately after removing the tube from the needle holder, gently invert the tube to mix the additives and the blood.	4*		
16.	Insert the second tube into the needle holder, following the instructions in the previous steps. Continue filling tubes until the order on the requisition has been filled. Gently invert each tube after removing it from the needle holder.	4		
17.	As the last tube begins filling, release the tourniquet. The tourniquet must be released before the needle is removed from the arm.	4		
18.	Remove the last tube from the holder. Place gauze over the puncture site and quickly remove the needle, engaging the safety device.	4*		
19.	Dispose of the entire needle/holder assembly into the sharps container.	4*		
20.	Apply pressure to the gauze or instruct the patient to do so. The patient may elevate the arm but should not bend the elbow.	4		
21.	While the patient is applying pressure to the site, label the tubes with the patient's name, date, time, and your initials, or affix the preprinted tube labels and print your initials and time on the label.	4		
22.	Check the venipuncture site. Make sure bleeding has stopped. Apply a new folded gauze square to the puncture site. Secure the gauze to the site with a hypoallergenic self stick wrap, tape, or a bandage.	4		
23.	Disinfect the work area. Dispose of blood-contaminated materials in a biohazard waste container. Remove your protective eyewear and gloves.	4*		

24. Wash hands or use hand sanitizer.	4*			
25. Complete the laboratory requisition form and route the specimen to the proper place. Record the procedure in the patient's health record.	4			
Total Points	**100**			

Affective Behavior	**Affective Behaviors Checklist** **Directions:** *Check behaviors observed during the role-play.*					
Critical Thinking	**Negative, Unprofessional Behaviors**	**Attempt**		**Positive, Professional Behaviors**	**Attempt**	
		1	**2**		**1**	**2**
	Coached or told of an issue or problem			Independently identified the problem or issue		
	Failed to consider alternatives; failed to ask questions that demonstrate understanding of principles/concepts			Willing to consider other alternatives; asked appropriate questions that showed understanding of principles/concepts		
	Failed to make an educated, logical judgment/decision; actions or lack of actions demonstrated unsafe practices			Made an educated, logical judgment/decision and actions reflected principles of safe practice		
	Other:			Other:		

Grading Rubric for the Affective Behaviors Checklist **Directions:** *Based on checklist results, identify the points received for the procedure checklist. Indicate how the behaviors demonstrated met the expectations.*		**Point Value**	**Attempt 1**	**Attempt 2**
Does not meet Expectation	• Response fails to show critical thinking. • Student demonstrated more than 2 negative, unprofessional behaviors during the interaction.	0		
Needs Improvement	• Response fails to show critical thinking. • Student demonstrated 1 or 2 negative, unprofessional behaviors during the interaction.	0		
Meets Expectation	• Response demonstrates critical thinking; no negative, unprofessional behaviors observed. • More practice is needed for behavior to appear natural and for student to appear comfortable and at ease.	4		
Occasionally Exceeds Expectation	• Response demonstrates critical thinking; no negative, unprofessional behaviors observed. • At times student appeared comfortable and at ease; but more practice is needed for behavior to become natural and consistent with a professional medical assistant.	4		
Always Exceeds Expectation	• Response demonstrates critical thinking; no negative, unprofessional behaviors observed. • Student's behaviors appeared natural and comfortable. Behaviors are consistent with a professional medical assistant.	4		

Documentation

Comments

CAAHEP Competencies	Step(s)
I.P.2.b. Perform the following procedures: venipuncture	Entire procedure
III.P.2. Select appropriate barrier/personal protective equipment (PPE)	1, 3
III.P.10.a. Demonstrate proper disposal of biohazardous material: sharps	19
III.P.10.b. Demonstrate proper disposal of biohazardous material: regulated wastes	23
X.P.3. Document patient care accurately in the medical record	25
A.1. Demonstrate critical thinking skills	6
ABHES Competencies	**Step(s)**
9.c. Dispose of biohazardous materials	19, 23
9.d. Collect, label, and process a specimen 1) Perform venipuncture	Entire procedure

Procedure 48.2   Perform a Venipuncture: Collect a Venous Blood Sample Using the Syringe Method

Name _____ Date _____ Score _____

Tasks: To collect a venous blood specimen using the syringe technique. Document in the patient's health record.

Equipment and Supplies:
- Patient's health record
- Provider's order and/or lab requisition
- Syringe with 21- or 22-gauge safety needle
- Vacuum tubes appropriate for tests ordered
- 70% isopropyl alcohol wipes
- Gauze
- Tourniquet
- Safety transfer device to transfer blood from syringe to vacuum tubes
- Hypoallergenic self-stick wrap, tape, or bandage
- Permanent marking pen or printed labels
- Fluid-impermeable lab coat, protective eyewear, and gloves
- Biohazard sharps container
- Biohazard waste container

Standard: Complete the procedure and all critical steps in _____ minutes with a minimum score of 85% within two attempts (*or as indicated by the instructor*).

Scoring: Divide the points earned by the total possible points. Failure to perform a critical step, indicated by an asterisk (*), results in grade no higher than an 84% (*or as indicated by the instructor*).

Time: Began_____ Ended_____ Total minutes: _____

Steps:	Point Value	Attempt 1	Attempt 2
1. Check the provider's order and/or requisition form to determine the tests ordered. Gather the appropriate tubes and supplies. Put on a fluid-impermeable lab coat.	5		
2. Greet the patient. Identify yourself. Verify the patient's identity with full name, ask the patient to spell the first and last name, and give their date of birth. Explain the procedure to be performed in a manner that is understood by the patient. Answer any questions the patient may have on the procedure. Obtain permission for the venipuncture.	5*		
3. Wash hands or use hand sanitizer. Put on gloves and protective eyewear.	5*		
4. Ask the patient if they have a preference which arm is used for the venipuncture. Have the patient sit with the arm well supported in a slightly downward position.	3		
5. Apply the tourniquet around the patient's arm 3-4 inches above the elbow on the patient's preferred arm. The tourniquet should never be tied so tightly that it restricts blood flow in the artery. Tourniquets should remain in place no longer than 60 seconds.	5		

6. Select the venipuncture site by palpating the antecubital space. Use your index finger to trace the path of the vein and to judge its depth. Look at both arms and use your critical thinking skills to find the vein that will give you the greatest chance of success for the venipuncture. (*Refer to the Affective Behaviors Checklist – Critical Thinking and the Grading Rubric.*)	5*		
7. Remove the tourniquet and cleanse the site with a 70% alcohol wipe.	3		
8. Assemble the equipment and supplies on the nondominant side of the patient's arm. Use your critical thinking skills to choose the proper syringe barrel size and needle size. This depends on the amount of blood required for the ordered tests and your inspection of the patient's veins.	5*		
9. Attach the needle firmly to the syringe. Pull and depress the plunger several times to loosen it in the barrel while keeping the cover on the needle. The plunger must be pushed in completely after you have loosened in the barrel.	5*		
10. Reapply the tourniquet when the alcohol is dry.	3		
11. Hold the syringe in your dominant hand. Your thumb should be on top and your fingers underneath, the same as in the vacuum tube method. Remove the needle sheath.	3		
12. Grasp the patient's arm with the nondominant hand and anchor the vein with the thumb of your nondominant hand.	3		
13. With the bevel up and the needle aligned parallel to the vein, insert the needle at a 15- to 20-degree angle through the skin and into the vein with a quick but smooth motion. Observe for a flash of blood in the hub of the syringe.	5		
14. Slowly pull back the plunger of the syringe with the nondominant hand. Do not allow more than 1 mL of head space between the blood and the top of the plunger. Make sure you do not move the needle after entering the vein. Fill the barrel to the needed volume.	5		
15. Release the tourniquet when the proper volume is reached. The tourniquet must be released before the needle is removed from the arm.	5*		
16. Place sterile gauze over the puncture site at the time of needle withdrawal. Then immediately activate the needle safety device using the syringe hand and apply pressure to the site with the nondominant hand.	5*		
17. Instruct the patient to apply direct pressure on the puncture site with gauze. The patient may elevate the arm but should not bend the elbow.	3		
18. Remove the syringe safety needle and transfer the blood immediately to the required tube or tubes using a safety transfer device. Do not push on the syringe plunger during transfer.	5*		
19. Discard the entire unit in the sharps container when transfer is complete. Gently invert the tubes after the addition of blood.	5*		
20. Label the tubes with the patient's full name, date, time, and your initials or affix the preprinted tube labels and print your initials and time on the label.	3		
21. Check the venipuncture site. Make sure bleeding has stopped. Apply a new folded gauze square to the puncture site. Secure the gauze to the site with a hypoallergenic self stick wrap, tape, or a bandage.	3		
22. Disinfect the work area. Dispose of blood-contaminated materials in the biohazard waste container. Remove your eyewear and gloves.	3		

23. Wash hands or use hand sanitizer.	5*		
24. Complete the laboratory requisition form and route the specimen to the proper place. Record the procedure in the patient's health record.	3		
Total Points	100		

Affective Behavior	**Affective Behaviors Checklist** Directions: *Check behaviors observed during the role-play.*					
Critical Thinking	**Negative, Unprofessional Behaviors**	**Attempt**		**Positive, Professional Behaviors**	**Attempt**	
		1	**2**		**1**	**2**
	Coached or told of an issue or problem			Independently identified the problem or issue		
	Failed to consider alternatives; failed to ask questions that demonstrate understanding of principles/ concepts			Willing to consider other alternatives; asked appropriate questions that showed understanding of principles/ concepts		
	Failed to make an educated, logical judgment/decision; actions or lack of actions demonstrated unsafe practices			Made an educated, logical judgment/decision and actions reflected principles of safe practice		
	Other:			Other:		

Grading Rubric for the Affective Behaviors Checklist Directions: *Based on checklist results, identify the points received for the procedure checklist. Indicate how the behaviors demonstrated met the expectations.*		**Point Value**	**Attempt 1**	**Attempt 2**
Does not meet Expectation	• Response fails to show critical thinking. • Student demonstrated more than 2 negative, unprofessional behaviors during the interaction.	0		
Needs Improvement	• Response fails to show critical thinking. • Student demonstrated 1 or 2 negative, unprofessional behaviors during the interaction.	0		
Meets Expectation	• Response demonstrates critical thinking; no negative, unprofessional behaviors observed. • More practice is needed for behavior to appear natural and for student to appear comfortable and at ease.	5		
Occasionally Exceeds Expectation	• Response demonstrates critical thinking; no negative, unprofessional behaviors observed. • At times student appeared comfortable and at ease; but more practice is needed for behavior to become natural and consistent with a professional medical assistant.	5		
Always Exceeds Expectation	• Response demonstrates critical thinking; no negative, unprofessional behaviors observed. • Student's behaviors appeared natural and comfortable. Behaviors are consistent with a professional medical assistant.	5		

Documentation

Comments

CAAHEP Competencies	Step(s)
I.P.2.b. Perform the following procedures: venipuncture	Entire procedure
III.P.2. Select appropriate barrier/personal protective equipment (PPE)	1, 3
III.P.10.a. Demonstrate proper disposal of biohazardous material: sharps	19
III.P.10.b. Demonstrate proper disposal of biohazardous material: regulated wastes	23
X.P.3. Document patient care accurately in the medical record	24
A.1. Demonstrate critical thinking skills	6
ABHES Competencies	**Step(s)**
9.c. Dispose of biohazardous materials	19, 23
9.d. Collect, label, and process a specimen 1) Perform venipuncture	Entire procedure

Procedure 48.3 Perform Venipuncture: Obtain a Venous Sample with a Safety Winged Butterfly Needle Assembly

Name _____ **Date** _____ **Score** _____

Tasks: To obtain a venous sample accurately from a hand or arm vein using a butterfly needle and syringe. Document in the patient's health record.

Equipment and Supplies:
- Patient's health record
- Provider's order and/or lab requisition
- Safety winged (butterfly) needle set
- Syringe of appropriate volume for testing
- Vacuum tubes appropriate for tests ordered
- 70% isopropyl alcohol wipes
- Gauze
- Tourniquet
- Hypoallergenic self-stick wrap, tape, or bandage
- Permanent marking pen or printed labels
- Fluid-impermeable lab coat, protective eyewear, and gloves
- Biohazard waste container
- Biohazard sharps container

Standard: Complete the procedure and all critical steps in _____ minutes with a minimum score of 85% within two attempts (*or as indicated by the instructor*).

Scoring: Divide the points earned by the total possible points. Failure to perform a critical step, indicated by an asterisk (*), results in grade no higher than an 84% (*or as indicated by the instructor*).

Time: Began_____ Ended_____ Total minutes: _____

Steps:	Point Value	Attempt 1	Attempt 2
1. Check the provider's order and/or requisition form to determine the tests ordered. Gather the appropriate tubes and supplies. Put on a fluid-impermeable lab coat.	4		
2. Greet the patient. Identify yourself. Verify the patient's identity with full name, ask the patient to spell the first and last name, and give their date of birth. Explain the procedure to be performed in a manner that is understood by the patient. Answer any questions the patient may have on the procedure. Obtain permission for the venipuncture.	4*		
3. Wash hands or use hand sanitizer. Put on gloves and protective eyewear.	4*		
4. *If drawing from the antecubital region*: Ask the patient if they have a preference which arm is used for the venipuncture. Have the patient sit with their arm well supported in a slightly downward position. *If drawing from the back of the hand*: Have the patient place the venipuncture hand over the other, fisted hand with the fingers lower than the wrist.	4		

5.	*If drawing from the antecubital region*: Apply the tourniquet around the patient's arm 3-4 inches above the elbow on the patient's preferred arm. The tourniquet should never be tied so tightly that it restricts blood flow in the artery. Tourniquets should remain in place no longer than 60 seconds. *If drawing from the back of the hand*: Apply the tourniquet above the wrist just proximal to the wrist bone. Do not apply the tourniquet so tightly that blood flow in the arteries is impeded.	4		
6.	*If drawing from the antecubital region*: Select the venipuncture site by palpating the antecubital space. Use your index finger to trace the path of the vein and to judge its depth. Look at both arms and use your critical thinking skills to find the vein that will give you the greatest chance of success for the venipuncture. *If drawing from the back of the hand*: Select a vein on the back of the hand that is prominent, stable, and straight as possible. *(Refer to the Affective Behaviors Checklist – Critical Thinking and the Grading Rubric.)*	4		
7.	Remove the tourniquet and cleanse the site with a 70% alcohol wipe.	4		
8.	Assemble your equipment and supplies near your nondominant hand, next to the patient's arm for easy access during the procedure. Remove the butterfly device from the package and stretch the tubing slightly. Take care not to activate the needle-retracting safety device accidentally.	4		
9.	Attach the butterfly device firmly to the syringe. a. If using a syringe, make sure to loosen the plunger a few times after the butterfly and syringe are attached. *Note:* The Butterfly assembly can be attached to a needle holder or a syringe. Make sure the connection is firmly in place. b. If using a needle assembly, lay the first tube in the vacuum tube holder and place the unit carefully where it will not roll away.	4		
10.	Reapply the tourniquet when the alcohol is dry.	4		
11.	Hold the butterfly wings pinched in between your dominant hand thumb and index finger or hold the base of the needle. Remove the needle sheath.	4		
12.	*If drawing the antecubital region*: Grasp the patient's arm with the nondominant hand and anchor the vein by stretching the skin downward below the collection site with the thumb of the nondominant hand. *If drawing from the back of the hand*: Using your thumb, pull the patient's skin taut over the knuckles and anchor the vein.	4		
13.	With the bevel up and the needle aligned parallel to the vein, insert the needle at a 10- to 15-degree angle through the skin and into the vein with a quick but smooth motion.	4		
14.	*If drawing with a needle holder assembly*: Push the blood collecting tube into the end of the holder with your nondominant hand. *If drawing with a syringe*: Make sure the vacuum you create is slow and steady and that no more than 1 mL of head space exists between the blood and the plunger. Slowly pull back the plunger of the syringe with the nondominant hand. Fill the barrel of the syringe to the needed volume	4		
15.	Release the tourniquet when the blood appears in the tubing, or a flash of blood is seen in the hub of the syringe.	4		
16.	Always keep the tube and the holder in a downward position so that the tube fills from the bottom up.	4		

17. Place a gauze over the puncture site and gently remove the needle, engaging the safety device. Dispose of the entire unit in the sharps container.	4			
18. Apply pressure to the gauze or instruct the patient to do so. The patient may elevate the arm but should not bend the elbow.	4			
19. *If drawing with a syringe:* remove the syringe safety needle and transfer the blood immediately to the required tube or tubes using a safety transfer device. Do not push on the syringe plunger during transfer.	4			
20. Discard the entire unit in the sharps container when transfer is complete. Gently invert the tubes after the addition of blood.	4			
21. Label the tubes with the patient's full name, date, time, and your initials, or affix the preprinted tube labels and print your initials and time on the label.	4			
22. Check the venipuncture site. Make sure bleeding has stopped. Apply a new folded gauze square to the puncture site. Secure the gauze to the site with a hypoallergenic self stick wrap, tape, or a bandage.	4			
23. Disinfect the work area. Dispose of blood-contaminated materials in the biohazard waste container. Remove your eyewear and gloves.	4*			
24. Wash hands or use hand sanitizer.	4*			
25. Complete the laboratory requisition form and route the specimen to the proper place. Record the procedure in the patient's health record.	4			
Total Points	100			

Affective Behavior	Affective Behaviors Checklist Directions: *Check behaviors observed during the role-play.*					
Critical Thinking	**Negative, Unprofessional Behaviors**	**Attempt**		**Positive, Professional Behaviors**	**Attempt**	
		1	**2**		**1**	**2**
	Coached or told of an issue or problem			Independently identified the problem or issue		
	Failed to consider alternatives; failed to ask questions that demonstrate understanding of principles/concepts			Willing to consider other alternatives; asked appropriate questions that showed understanding of principles/concepts		
	Failed to make an educated, logical judgment/decision; actions or lack of actions demonstrated unsafe practices			Made an educated, logical judgment/decision and actions reflected principles of safe practice		
	Other:			Other:		

Grading Rubric for the Affective Behaviors Checklist **Directions:** *Based on checklist results, identify the points received for the procedure checklist. Indicate how the behaviors demonstrated met the expectations.*		Point Value	Attempt 1	Attempt 2
Does not meet Expectation	• Response fails to show critical thinking. • Student demonstrated more than 2 negative, unprofessional behaviors during the interaction.	0		
Needs Improvement	• Response fails to show critical thinking. • Student demonstrated 1 or 2 negative, unprofessional behaviors during the interaction.	0		
Meets Expectation	• Response demonstrates critical thinking; no negative, unprofessional behaviors observed. • More practice is needed for behavior to appear natural and for student to appear comfortable and at ease.	4		
Occasionally Exceeds Expectation	• Response demonstrates critical thinking; no negative, unprofessional behaviors observed. • At times student appeared comfortable and at ease; but more practice is needed for behavior to become natural and consistent with a professional medical assistant.	4		
Always Exceeds Expectation	• Response demonstrates critical thinking; no negative, unprofessional behaviors observed. • Student's behaviors appeared natural and comfortable. Behaviors are consistent with a professional medical assistant.	4		

Documentation

Comments

CAAHEP Competencies	Step(s)
I.P.2.b. Perform the following procedures: venipuncture	Entire procedure
III.P.2. Select appropriate barrier/personal protective equipment (PPE)	1, 3
III.P.10.a. Demonstrate proper disposal of biohazardous material: sharps	20
III.P.10.b. Demonstrate proper disposal of biohazardous material: regulated wastes	23
X.P.3. Document patient care accurately in the medical record	24
A.1. Demonstrate critical thinking skills	6
ABHES Competencies	**Step(s)**
9.c. Dispose of biohazardous materials	20, 23
9.d. Collect, label, and process a specimen 1) Perform venipuncture	Entire procedure

Procedure 48.4 Perform a Capillary Puncture: Obtain a Blood Sample by Capillary Puncture

Name _____ Date _____ Score _____

Tasks: To collect a blood specimen suitable for testing using the capillary puncture technique. Document in the patient's health record.

Equipment and Supplies:
- Patient's health record
- Provider's order and/or lab requisition
- Sterile, disposable safety lancet
- 70% alcohol wipes
- Gauze
- Hypoallergenic self-stick wrap, tape, or bandage
- Fluid-impermeable lab coat, protective eyewear, and gloves
- Appropriate collection containers (e.g., capillary tubes, Microtainer tubes)
- Permanent marking pen or printed labels
- Biohazard sharps container
- Biohazard waste container

Standard: Complete the procedure and all critical steps in _____ minutes with a minimum score of 85% within two attempts (*or as indicated by the instructor*).

Scoring: Divide the points earned by the total possible points. Failure to perform a critical step, indicated by an asterisk (*), results in grade no higher than an 84% (*or as indicated by the instructor*).

Time: Began_____ Ended_____ Total minutes: _____

Steps:	Point Value	Attempt 1	Attempt 2
1. Check the provider's order and/or requisition form to determine the tests ordered. Gather the appropriate tubes and supplies. Put on a fluid-impermeable lab coat.	5		
2. Greet the patient. Identify yourself. Verify the patient's identity with full name, ask the patient to spell the last name, and give their date of birth. Explain the procedure to be performed in a manner that is understood by the patient. Answer any questions the patient may have on the procedure. Obtain permission for the venipuncture.	5		
3. Wash hands or use hand sanitizer. Put on gloves and protective eyewear.	10*		
4. Select a puncture site, depending on the patient's age and the sample to be obtained (e.g., palmar side of middle or ring finger of nondominant hand for an adult or child; medial or lateral curved surface of the plantar surface of heel for an infant).	5		
5. Gently rub the finger or have your patient wiggle fingers and open and close hand.	5		
6. Once the finger is warm, clean the site with a 70% alcohol pad and allow it to air dry.	5		

7.	Hold onto the patient's finger above the puncture site with your nondominant hand. Select a site on the distal fingertip of the middle or ring finger. The puncture should be made across the fingerprint, not parallel to it.	5		
8.	Hold the safety lancet firmly against the patient's finger and press down on the safety trigger that activates the needle or blade to penetrate the skin. The sharp will then automatically retract into the plastic housing of the lancet.	5		
9.	Dispose of the lancet in the sharps container. Wipe away the first drop of blood with gauze	5*		
10.	Apply gentle, intermittent pressure to cause the blood to flow freely.	5		
11.	Collect the blood samples. Gently squeeze and release the finger two or three times to get a large drop of blood. Touch the capillary tube to the drop of blood. Do not scoop blood from the finger's surface. Fill the capillary to approximately 3/4 full or to the indicated line. Then tip the tube with the presealed end down. When the blood flows down and touches the sealant, hold it for 30 seconds to allow it to seal automatically.	5		
12.	Wipe the patient's finger with gauze. Express another large drop of blood in the same way and fill a Microtainer. Do not touch the container to the finger. If more blood is needed, gently squeeze, and release the finger to get another drop. Cap the Microtainer tube when the collection is complete.	10		
13.	When collection is complete, apply pressure to the site with gauze. The patient may be able to assist with this step.	5		
14.	Select an appropriate means of labeling the containers. Sealed capillary tubes can be placed in a red-topped tube, which is then labeled. Microtainers can be placed in zipper-lock biohazard bags that are subsequently labeled. Follow your institutions procedures for labeling.	5		
15.	Check the patient for bleeding and clean the site if traces of blood are visible. Apply a folded gauze square to the puncture site and secure with hypoallergenic self-stick wrap, tape, or bandage.	5		
16.	Disinfect the work area. Dispose of blood-contaminated materials in the biohazard waste container. Remove your protective eyewear.	5		
17.	Wash hands or use hand sanitizer.	5		
18.	Complete the laboratory requisition form and route the specimen to the proper location. Record the procedure in the patient's health record.	5		
	Total Points	**100**		

Documentation

Comments

CAAHEP Competencies	Step(s)
I.P.2.c. Perform: capillary puncture	Entire procedure
III.P.2. Select appropriate barrier/personal protective equipment (PPE)	1, 3
III.P.10.a. Demonstrate proper disposal of biohazardous material: sharps	9
III.P.10.b. Demonstrate proper disposal of biohazardous material: regulated wastes	16
X.P.3. Document patient care accurately in the medical record	18
ABHES Competencies	**Step(s)**
9.c. Dispose of biohazardous materials	9, 16
9.d. Collect, label, and process a specimen	Entire procedure

Procedure 48.5 Demonstrate Empathy for a Patient's Concern Related to a Procedure

Name _____ Date _____ Score _____

Task: Demonstrate empathy for the patient's concern related to a venipuncture.

Scenario: You are a medical assistant working with Dr. Walden, who ordered bloodwork for Sam Brown. Your role includes performing venipuncture when bloodwork is ordered. You obtain the order, greet Sam, identify yourself, verify Sam's identity, and explain what you need to do. You notice that Sam appears to be uncomfortable and restless. Sam states she/he didn't really want the bloodwork done.

Directions: Role-play this scenario with a peer. The peer will play Sam and you are the medical assistant.

Standard: Complete the role-play in _____ minutes with a minimum score of 100% within two attempts (*or as indicated by the instructor*).

Scoring: Divide the points earned by the total possible points. Met competency: 100% (10 points). Not met competency: 0% (0 points).

Time: Began_____ Ended_____ Total minutes: _____

Steps:	Point Value	Attempt 1	Attempt 2
1. Encourage the patient to talk about their concerns. Demonstrate active listening skills. *(Refer to the Affective Behaviors Checklist – Active Listening and the Grading Rubric)*	40*		
2. Address the patient's concerns. Demonstrate respect and empathy while addressing the concerns. *(Refer to the Affective Behaviors Checklist – Respect and Empathy and the Grading Rubric)*	40*		
3. Answer any questions the patient has.	20		
Total Points	100		

Affective Behavior	**Affective Behaviors Checklist** **Directions:** *Check behaviors observed during the role-play.*				
	Negative, Unprofessional Behaviors	**Attempt 1**	**Attempt 2**	**Positive, Professional Behaviors**	**Attempt 1**	**Attempt 2**
Active Listening	Interrupted			Refrained from interrupting		
	Did not allow for silence or pauses			Allowed for periods of silence		
	Negative nonverbal behaviors (rolled eyes, yawned, frowned, avoided eye contact)			Positive nonverbal behaviors (smiled, nodded head, appropriate eye contact)		
	Distracted (looked at watch, phone)			Focused on patient, avoided distractions		
	Biased, offensive			Remained neutral		
	Other:			Other:		
Respect	Rude, unkind, disrespectful, impolite			Courteous, polite		
	Unwelcoming, brief, abrupt			Welcoming, took time with the patient		
	Unconcerned with person's dignity			Maintained person's dignity		
	Poor eye contact with patient			Proper eye contact with patient		
	Negative nonverbal behaviors			Positive nonverbal behaviors		
	Other:			Other:		
Empathy	Didn't listen to the patient, interrupted patient; unsupportive, uninterested, or uncaring			Listened to the patient; supportive and caring		
	Did not acknowledge or respond appropriately to the patient's emotional responses; cold, aloof, insensitive, indifferent, or unfeeling			Acknowledged and responded appropriately to the patient's emotional responses; showed sensitivity		
	Failed to reassure patient; did not respond to the patient's concerns			Reassured patient by repeating and responding to the patient's concerns		
	Used language that is hard to understand (e.g., slang, generational terms, medical terminology, too scientific)			Used language that the patient can understand		
	Failed to address the patient's questions; or answers to patient's questions are inappropriate			Answered the patient's questions appropriately		
	Other:			Other:		

Grading Rubric for the Affective Behaviors Checklist **Directions:** *Based on checklist results, identify the points received for the procedure checklist. Indicate how the behaviors demonstrated met the expectations.*		Point Value	Attempt 1	Attempt 2
Does not meet Expectation	• Response lacked active listening, respect, and/or empathy. • Student demonstrated more than 2 negative, unprofessional behaviors during the interaction.	0		
Needs Improvement	• Response lacked active listening, respect, and/or empathy. • Student demonstrated 1 or 2 negative, unprofessional behaviors during the interaction.	0		
Meets Expectation	• Response demonstrates active listening, respect, and empathy; no negative, unprofessional behaviors observed. • More practice is needed for behavior to appear natural and for student to appear comfortable and at ease.	40		
Occasionally Exceeds Expectation	• Response demonstrates active listening, respect, and empathy; no negative, unprofessional behaviors observed. • At times student appeared comfortable and at ease; but more practice is needed for behavior to become natural and consistent with a professional medical assistant.	40		
Always Exceeds Expectation	• Response demonstrates active listening, respect, and empathy; no negative, unprofessional behaviors observed. • Student's behaviors appeared natural and comfortable. Behaviors are consistent with a professional medical assistant.	40		

Comments

CAAHEP Competencies	Step(s)
A.3. Demonstrate empathy for patients' concerns	2
A.4. Demonstrate active listening	1

Analysis of Blood

CAAHEP Competencies	Assessments
I.P.2.c. Perform the following procedures: capillary puncture	Procedures 49.5, 49.6, 49.7
I.P.10. Perform a quality control measure	Procedures 49.5, 49.6, 49.7
I.P.11.a. Collect specimens and perform: CLIA-waived hematology test	Procedures 49.1, 49.2, 49.4, 49.5
I.P.11.b. Collect specimens and perform: CLIA-waived chemistry test	Procedures 49.6, 49.7
II.P.2. Record laboratory test results into the patient's record	Procedures 49.1, 49.2, 49.4, 49.5, 49.6, 49.7
III.P.2. Select appropriate barrier/personal protective equipment (PPE)	Procedures 49.1, 49.2, 49.4, 49.5, 49.6, 49.7
III.P.10.a. Demonstrate proper disposal of biohazardous material: sharps	Procedures 49.1, 49.2, 49.4, 49.5, 49.6, 49.7
III.P.10.b. Demonstrate proper disposal of biohazardous material: regulated wastes	Procedures 49.1, 49.2, 49.4, 49.5, 49.6, 49.7
X.P.3. Document patient care accurately in the medical record	Procedures 49.1, 49.2, 49.4, 49.5, 49.6, 49.7
XII.P.1. Comply with safety practices.	Procedures 49.1, 49.2, 49.4, 49.5, 49.6, 49.7
ABHES Competencies	Assessments
4. Medical Law and Ethics a. Follow documentation guidelines	Procedures 49.1, 49.2, 49.4, 49.5, 49.6, 49.7
9. Medical Laboratory Procedures a. Practice Quality Control	Procedures 49.5, 49.6, 49.7
9.b. Perform selected CLIA-waived test that assist with diagnosis and treatment 2) hematology testing	Procedures 49.1, 49.2, 49.4, 49.5
9.b. Perform selected CLIA-waived test that assist with diagnosis and treatment 3) chemistry testing	Procedures 49.6, 49.7
9.c. Dispose of biohazardous materials	Procedures 49.1, 49.2, 49.4, 49.5, 49.6, 49.7
9.d. Collect, label, and process a specimen 2) Perform capillary puncture	Procedures 49.5, 49.6, 49.7

VOCABULARY REVIEW

Using the word pool, find the correct word to match the definition. Write the word on the line after the definition.

Group A

1. An old or aging cell that can no longer divide and reproduce _____

2. A cell with uncontrolled growth that spreads rapidly, with the potential for serious harm _____

3. A small plastic or glass tube designed to hold samples for laboratory tests that detect light or color changes _____

4. A substance used in a chemical reaction _____

5. An immune response against a person's own tissues, cells, or cell parts _____

6. The study of the form, shape, and structure of an organism or cell _____

7. A person trained in the nature, function, and diseases of the blood and blood-forming organs _____

8. Control center of the cell; contains chromosomes that are made up of deoxyribonucleic acid (DNA), which carries genetic information _____

9. Jelly-like substance that surrounds the nucleus and fills the cells _____

10. A substance, structure, or event that does not naturally occur in a situation _____

Word Pool

- artifact
- autoimmune
- cytoplasm
- hematologist
- malignant
- microcuvettes
- morphology
- nucleus
- reagent
- senescent cell

Group B

1. Another term for blood clot _____

2. A thick, sticky deposit that can clog arteries _____

3. Fat in the blood related to caloric intake _____

4. A fat-like substance present in cell membranes; needed to form bile acids, steroid hormones, the coverings of nerves, and some brain tissue _____

5. A condition seen during pregnancy in which the effect of insulin is partially blocked by hormones produced by the placenta _____

6. Relating to or resulting from metabolism _____

7. A laboratory or clinical technique that uses the specific binding between an antigen and antibody to identify and quantify a substance in a sample _____

Word Pool

- cholesterol
- gestational diabetes
- lateral flow immunoassay
- metabolic
- plaque
- thrombus
- triglycerides

ABBREVIATIONS

Write out what each of the following abbreviations stands for.

1. POCT _____

2. ESR _____

3. CBC _____

4. ALT _____

5. AST _____

6. PT _____

7. RBC _____

8. WBC _____

9. EDTA _____

10. Hct _____

11. Hgb _____

12. LED _____

13. INR _____

14. WHO _____

15. MCV _____

16. MCH _____

17. MCHC _____

18. FBG _____

19. GTT _____

20. LDL _____

21. HDL _____

22. T_3 _____

23. T_4 _____

24. TSH _____

25. TRH _____

Skills and Concepts
Answer the following questions.

A. Blood
Select the correct answer or fill in the blank.

1. What is the role of blood?
   a. Supplies the body's cells with nutrients and oxygen
   b. Distributes enzymes, hormones, and other chemicals needed for regulation of body activities
   c. Functions to maintain body temperature
   d. Keeps body fluids in balance and maintains pH
   e. All of the above

2. The liquid portion of whole blood is called _____.

Match the description with the correct term.

3. _____ Most abundant plasma protein in human blood and it is important in regulating the water balance of blood

4. _____ A special protein that speeds up the chemical reaction in the body

5. _____ A group of related proteins that function as antibodies and are found in plasma and other body fluids

6. _____ The liquid that remains after blood has clotted

7. _____ A chemical substance produced in an endocrine gland and transported in the blood to a specific tissue where it applies a specific effect

   a. enzymes
   b. hormones
   c. albumin
   d. immunoglobulins
   e. serum

B. Hematology in the Physician Office Laboratory
Select the correct answer or fill in the blank.

1. The _____ is a laboratory test that measures the rate at which red blood cells gradually separate from plasma and settle to the bottom of a specially calibrated tube in 1 hour.

2. Which is incorrect regarding the ESR?
   a. The ESR is not specific for any disease in particular but is used as a general indicator of inflammation.
   b. The ESR measures the time it takes to clot the blood.
   c. Normal value for males younger than age 64 are 0 to 15 mm/hr.
   d. Normal value for males older than 64 and females are 0 to 20 mm/hr.
   e. There are CLIA-waived ESR tests available.

3. Reducing the concentration of a mixture or solution by adding a known volume of liquid is called

   _____.

4. A(n) _____ is a slender tube attached to or including a bulb for transferring or measuring small amounts of a liquid; often used in a laboratory.

5. The _____ is a laboratory test that measures the time it takes for the plasma of the blood to clot.

6. Which statement is *incorrect*?
   a. PT test results are reported as the number of seconds blood takes to clot when mixed with the thromboplastin reagent.
   b. There are CLIA-waived PT tests available.
   c. The normal range for a PT result is 15-18.5 seconds.
   d. A number lower than the normal range means the blood clots more quickly than normal and a higher number means it takes longer for the blood to clot.

Match the product or condition with its action on the blood clotting process. Answers can be used more than once.

7. _____ Anticoagulant medication

8. _____ Liver disease

9. _____ Foods and supplements containing vitamin K

10. _____ Vitamin K deficiency

11. _____ Estrogen-containing medication

12. _____ Clotting factor deficiencies

a. delays the blood clotting process
b. speeds up the blood clotting process

Select the correct answer or fill in the blank.

13. The _____ is a conversion unit that considers the different sensitivities of reagents and it is widely accepted as the standard unit for reporting PT results, rather than the actual clotting time.

14. Drinking large amounts of alcohol or taking aspirin, heparin, antihistamines, antibiotics, and vitamin B can change the results of the PT/INR result. When taking warfarin, garlic and gingko biloba can increase the risk for bleeding, while St. John's wort and ginseng decrease the effects of warfarin.
    a. Both statements are correct.
    b. Both statements are incorrect.
    c. The first statement is correct, and the last statement is incorrect.
    d. The first statement is incorrect, and the last statement is correct.

C. Hematology in the Physician Office Laboratory: Complete Blood Count
Fill in the blank.

1. For a complete blood count, venous blood is collected in a(n) _____ tube containing ethylenediaminetetraacetic acid.

Match the description with the blood test.

2. _____ A measurement of the percentage of packed RBCs in a volume of blood

3. _____ Approximates the number of circulating RBCs in a person's blood

4. _____ Calculated to give the volume of the average RBC in a blood sample

5. _____ Is another way to measure the oxygen-carrying capacity of blood; can be part of the CBC or an individual test

6. _____ Measures the number of immature RBCs in the blood

7. _____ Indicates the average weight of hemoglobin compared with the cell size

8. _____ Calculated to give the average weight of hemoglobin in the RBC

9. _____ Gives an estimate of the total number of leukocytes in circulating blood

10. _____ Analyzes and counts the number of each type of WBC found in a sample of blood

a. RBC count
b. reticulocyte count
c. hematocrit
d. hemoglobin
e. mean corpuscular volume
f. mean corpuscular hemoglobin
g. mean corpuscular hemoglobin concentration
h. differential
i. WBC count

Match the description with the term.

11. _____ Consistent with the normal function of the body

12. _____ Abnormally large RBCs and a higher-than-normal MCV

13. _____ A disorder characterized by an abnormal increase in the number of RBCs in the blood

14. _____ A white layer of WBCs and platelets that form between the plasma and the RBCs when anticoagulated blood is centrifuged

15. _____ Small RBCs and have a lower-than-normal MCV

16. _____ A deficiency of hemoglobin in the blood

17. _____ Caused by or involving disease

18. _____ A machine that rotates at high speed and separates substances of different densities by centrifugal force

19. _____ Pale and lacking color

a. centrifuge
b. anemia
c. polycythemia
d. physiologic
e. pathologic
f. buffy coat
g. macrocytic
h. microcytic
i. hypochromic

Match the description with the term.

20. _____ Young neutrophils
21. _____ Smallest WBC, but most numbers in the blood
22. _____ A decrease in the WBC count; seen with viral infections, exposure to radiation and chemotherapy, and with certain drugs
23. _____ The most abundant WBC in the blood
24. _____ Has granules that contain histamine, which is involved in the inflammatory response
25. _____ Increased numbers seen with allergies, asthma, cancer, and certain parasitic infections
26. _____ An increase in the number of normal WBCs; seen with pregnancy, stress, anesthesia, and exercise
27. _____ Largest WBC which destroys foreign substances; increased numbers are seen with viral and some bacterial infections
28. _____ A higher-than-normal platelet count
29. _____ A lower-than-normal platelet count

a. leukopenia
b. leukocytosis
c. thrombocytosis
d. neutrophils
e. bands
f. eosinophil
g. basophil
h. monocytes
i. lymphocytes
j. thrombocytopenia

D. Hematology in the Reference Laboratory
Fill in the blank.

1. A(n) _____ test measures the time it takes for a blood clot to form and is used to check the function of specific coagulation factors.

2. A(n) _____ enables the examiner to microscopically view the preserved cellular structures of blood.

3. A good wedge smear should cover _____ to _____ of the slide and it should show a gradual transition from a thick to a thin end with a feathered edge.

4. Stains commonly used to make blood smears are described as _____, since they contain dyes that stain cell components different colors.

Match the description with the correct term.

5. _____ RBCs smaller than normal
6. _____ A significant variation in the shape of RBCs
7. _____ Normal-sized RBCs
8. _____ Pale-staining RBCs that have less hemoglobin than normal
9. _____ The condition in which different sizes of RBCs are present
10. _____ RBCs are larger than normal
11. _____ An RBC with a normal amount of hemoglobin

a. normocytic
b. macrocytic
c. microcytic
d. poikilocytosis
e. hypochromic
f. normochromic
g. anisocytosis

E. Immunohematology
Fill in the blank.

1. _____, also called *cross-matching*, is performed to prevent transfusion reactions in patients receiving blood from a donor.

2. A substance that stimulates the production of an antibody when introduced into the body is called a(n) _____.

3. Patients with type _____ blood are considered universal recipients.

4. Patients with type _____ blood are considered universal donors.

5. The _____ was passed in 1991 to ensure that all donor blood is tested for human immunodeficiency virus (HIV) and other blood-borne pathogens.

6. A transfusion with a person's own blood is called a(n) _____ transfusion.

F. Blood Chemistry in the Physician Office Laboratory
Select the correct answer or fill in the blank.

1. For the initial screening of a patient for diabetes type 2, a fasting blood sample is usually taken in the morning, after a fast of _____ to _____12 hours.

2. The patient's fasting blood glucose (FBG) level should be less than _____ mg/dL.

3. When coaching a patient on using the glucose monitor, the medical assistant should discuss
   a. equipment and supplies required.
   b. how to calibrate the monitor when using new container of test strips.
   c. how to perform a capillary puncture and apply the blood to the test strip.
   d. how to run the test.
   e. all of the above.

4. _____, also called *A1c*, is the result of glucose irreversibly binding to the hemoglobin molecules in the RBCs.

5. A normal A1c level for a person without diabetes ranges from _____% to _____%.

6. Cholesterol travels in the blood as distinct particles called _____.

7. The optimal LDL cholesterol level in the blood is _____.

8. A high blood level of _____ cholesterol reflects an increased risk of heart disease.

9. High levels of _____ cholesterol seem to protect against heart attack.

10. Adults should have their cholesterol levels checked every_____.

11. A(n) _____ is a series of tests that measures the total cholesterol, HDL and LDL cholesterol levels, and triglyceride levels.

12. CLIA-waived blood glucose, A1c, cholesterol, and thyroid-stimulating hormone tests are available. Patients can do home monitoring with glucose monitors and also with A1c monitors.
   a. Both statements are correct.
   b. Both statements are incorrect.
   c. The first statement is correct, and the last statement is incorrect.
   d. The first statement is incorrect, and the last statement is correct.

CERTIFICATION PREPARATION

Circle the correct answer.

1. The liquid that remains after blood has clotted is called
   a. serum.
   b. plasma.
   c. anticoagulant.
   d. none of the above.

2. The formed elements in whole blood are RBCs, WBCs, and
   a. platelets.
   b. senescent cells.
   c. thrombocytes.
   d. both a and c.

3. What is the most abundant protein in human blood?
   a. Immunoglobulins
   b. Fibrinogen
   c. Albumin
   d. Prothrombin

4. The most common anticoagulant used to collect hematology specimens is
   a. EDTA.
   b. heparin.
   c. sodium citrate.
   d. no anticoagulant is needed.

5. The layer of centrifuged blood that contains the WBCs and platelets is
   a. serum.
   b. plasma.
   c. buffy coat.
   d. both a and b.

6. An ESR is used to test for what condition?
   a. A possible heart attack
   b. Uncontrolled asthma
   c. General inflammation
   d. Diabetes mellitus

7. What test is used to monitor patients taking an anticoagulant drug?
   a. PT
   b. INR
   c. ESR
   d. Both a and b

8. What condition is defined as RBCs with different or varied sizes?
   a. Poikilocytosis
   b. Hypochromic
   c. Anisocytosis
   d. Thrombocytosis

9. The term *glycosylated hemoglobin* is described as
   a. low blood sugar.
   b. low iron hemoglobin.
   c. high blood sugar.
   d. sugar-coated hemoglobin.

10. Which two liver enzymes are used to monitor liver function?
    a. ESR and INR
    b. AST and ALT
    c. HDL and LDL
    d. Hct and Hgb

WORKPLACE APPLICATIONS

1. Bella is a 22-year-old female patient who is in to see Dr. Perez today for a routine checkup. One of the tests they performed in the lab was a capillary puncture hemoglobin test. Bella's results were a bit low; her hemoglobin was 10.8 g/dL.

   a. What is the normal hemoglobin range for an adult female?_____

   b. What factors can affect a person's hemoglobin level? _____

   _____

   c. What other test is often run with a hemoglobin level to confirm test results?_____

   _____

2. Anita is reviewing blood typing for a continuing education course she is taking. For the following, indicate the specimen's ABO blood type.

   a. Specimen has only anti-B plasma antibodies _____

   b. Specimen has no plasma antibodies _____

   c. Specimen has a B antigen on the RBCs_____

   d. Specimen has no antigens on the RBCs _____

3. Sophie is looking over her lab results for cholesterol testing. Indicate if each result is normal or abnormal.

Cholesterol component	Sophie's result	Normal	Abnormal
Total cholesterol	202 mg/dL		
LDL	104 mg/dL		
HDL	56 mg/dL		

INTERNET ACTIVITIES

1. Using online resources, research the rise in diabetes mellitus type 2 in the United States over the last 50 years. Summarize your findings in a poster or infographic.

2. Using online resources, research hemolytic disease of the newborn (HDN). Create a poster presentation, a PowerPoint presentation, or a written paper summarizing your research. Include the following points in your project:
   a. Describe how a woman becomes sensitized to the Rh antigen.
   b. Describe how HDN is treated.
   c. Describe how RhoGAM works in the body of the Rh-negative mother.

3. Using online resources, research hemoglobin A1c testing for diabetics. Create a poster presentation, infographic, or PowerPoint presentation summarizing your research. Include the following points in your project:
   a. Describe the principle of hemoglobin A1c testing.
   b. What are normal and abnormal results, and how do they relate to blood sugar?
   c. List and briefly describe two CLIA-waived hemoglobin A1c tests.

Procedure 49.1 Perform CLIA-Waived Hematology Testing: Determine the Erythrocyte Sedimentation Rate Using a Modified Westergren Method

Name _____ Date _____ Score _____

Tasks: Fill a Westergren tube properly and observe an erythrocyte sedimentation rate (ESR) obtained by using a modified Westergren method. Document the result on the lab flow sheet and patient health record.

Equipment and Supplies:
- Patient's health record
- Provider's order and/or lab requisition
- Erythrocyte sedimentation rate (ESR) laboratory log
- Ethylenediaminetetraacetic acid (EDTA)–anticoagulated blood specimen
- Safety tube decapper (if tubes do not have a Hemogard plastic top)
- Disposable transfer pipet
- Sediplast ESR system (pre-filled Sediplast vial)
- Sediplast rack
- Timer
- Fluid-impermeable lab coat, eye protection, and gloves
- Biohazard waste container
- Biohazard sharps container

Standard: Complete the procedure and all critical steps in _____ minutes with a minimum score of 85% within two attempts (*or as indicated by the instructor*).

Scoring: Divide the points earned by the total possible points. Failure to perform a critical step, indicated by an asterisk (*), results in grade no higher than an 84% (*or as indicated by the instructor*).

Time: Began _____ Ended _____ Total minutes: _____

Steps:	Point Value	Attempt 1	Attempt 2
1. Wash hands or use hand sanitizer. Put on a fluid-impermeable lab coat, eye protection, and gloves. Comply with safety practices.	10*		
2. Assemble the materials needed.	5		
3. Check the leveling bubble of the Sediplast rack.	5		
4. Bring the blood sample to room temperature if it has been refrigerated and mix the sample well by gently inverting the tube 6 to 8 times, making sure the tube has no bubbles.	5		
5. Remove the plastic Hemogard stopper on the blood sample by twisting and slowly pushing up on the stopper with your thumbs (or by using a tube decapper on rubber-stoppered blood tubes). Label with the patient's name and then remove the stopper on the prefilled Sediplast vial.	10		
6. Fill the Sediplast vial with blood to the indicated line using a disposable transfer pipet. Replace the stopper on the prefilled vial and invert it several times to mix. Recap the blood collection tube with its stopper.	10		
7. Insert a Sediplast pipet through the pierceable stopper on the prefilled vial and push down until the pipet touches the bottom of the vial. The pipet automatically draws the blood up and over the zero mark.	10		

8. Insert the filled Sediplast pipet and its vial into the Sediplast rack, making sure the vial is vertical.	10			
9. Note the start time on the ESR log sheet and allow the vial to stand undisturbed for 60 minutes.	5			
10. After 60 minutes, measure the distance the erythrocytes have fallen at the top of the tube. The scale reads in millimeters – each line is 1 mm.	10			
11. Properly dispose of all biohazard materials. Dispose of the plastic Sediplast pipet and its vial into a biohazard sharps container. Disinfect the work area. Remove your gloves, protective eyewear, and lab coat. Wash hands or use hand sanitizer.	10			
12. Record the findings in the lab's ESR log and the patient's health record. Remember: the Westergren ESR is reported in millimeters per hour (mm/hr). Using the normal range, identify if test result is normal or abnormal.	10			
Total Points	100			

ESR – Sediplast Patient Log					
Hematocrit expected values: Adult male under age 64: 0-15 mm/hr			**Adult male over age 64:** 0-20 mm/hr **Adult females:** 0-20 mm/hr		
Date	**Tech**	**Patient ID**	**Slot #**	**Results**	**Charted**
10/07/20XX	AJ	@12345	2	15 mm/hr	✓

Documentation

Comments

CAAHEP Competencies	Step(s)
I.P.11.a. Collect specimens and perform: CLIA-waived hematology test	Entire procedure
II.P.2. Record laboratory test results into the patient's record	12
III.P.2. Select appropriate barrier/personal protective equipment (PPE)	1
III.P.10.a. Demonstrate proper disposal of biohazardous material: sharps	11
III.P.10.b. Demonstrate proper disposal of biohazardous material: regulated wastes	11
X.P.3. Document patient care accurately in the medical record	12
XII.P.1. Comply with safety practices.	1
ABHES Competencies	**Step(s)**
4. Medical Law and Ethics a. Follow documentation guidelines	12
9. Medical Laboratory Procedures b. Perform selected CLIA-waived test that assist with diagnosis and treatment 2) hematology testing	Entire procedure
9.c. Dispose of biohazardous materials	11

Procedure 49.2   Perform a CLIA-Waived Protime/INR Test

Name _____ Date _____ Score _____

Tasks: Perform a capillary puncture and perform a coagulation test to determine PT/INR using the CoaguChek XS instrument with built-in quality control. Document the result on the lab flow sheet and patient health record.

Equipment and Supplies:
- Patient's health record or flow chart
- Provider's order and/or lab requisition
- PT/INR lab log
- Gauze, alcohol wipes, bandage
- CoaguChek XS PT test monitor
- CoaguChek lancet
- CoaguChek test strip container and code chip
- Package insert or flow chart with directions
- Fluid-impermeable lab coat, protective eyewear, and gloves
- Biohazard waste container
- Biohazard sharps containers

Order: Perform a protime/INR test STAT.

Standard: Complete the procedure and all critical steps in _____ minutes with a minimum score of 85% within two attempts (*or as indicated by the instructor*).

Scoring: Divide the points earned by the total possible points. Failure to perform a critical step, indicated by an asterisk (*), results in grade no higher than an 84% (*or as indicated by the instructor*).

Time: Began _____ Ended _____ Total minutes: _____

Steps:	Point Value	Attempt 1	Attempt 2
1. Wash hands or use hand sanitizer. Put on fluid-impermeable lab coat, protective eyewear, and gloves. Comply with safety practices.	10*		
2. Check the provider's order and collect the necessary equipment and supplies.	5		
3. If you are using test strips from a new, unopened container, you must change the test strip code chip. The three-number code on the test strip container must match the three-number code on the code strip. To install the code strip, follow the instructions in the Code Chip section of the user's manual.	5		
4. Place the meter on a flat surface so that it will not vibrate or move during testing.	5		
5. Greet the patient. Identify yourself. Verify the patient's identity with full name; ask the patient to spell the first and last name and to give their date of birth.	10*		
6. Explain the procedure to be performed in a manner that is understood by the patient. Answer any questions the patient may have on the procedure. Obtain permission for the capillary puncture.	5*		

7.	Examine the patient's fingers and choose the site to obtain the blood sample.	**5**		
8.	Prepare the site by: (1) Warm the hand by placing it under the arm, using a hand warmer, and/or washing the hand in warm water. (2) Have the patient hold their arm down to the side so that the hand is below the waist. (3) Massage the palm of the hand toward the base of the finger and toward the tip until the fingertip has increased color. (4) If necessary, immediately after lancing, gently squeeze the finger from its base to encourage blood flow.	**5**		
9.	When you are ready to test, remove a test strip from the container and immediately close the container. Make sure it seals tightly. Do not open the container or touch the test strips with wet hands or wet gloves.	**5**		
10.	Insert the test strip as far as you can into the meter. This powers the meter ON	**5**		
11.	Disinfect the finger with an alcohol wipe and allow the finger to air dry. Perform the fingerstick. If necessary, immediately after lancing, gently squeeze the finger to encourage blood flow. Do NOT wipe away the first drop of blood.	**5***		
12.	Hold the finger with a blood drop very close to the target (the clear area of the test strip). Apply 1 drop of blood to the top or side of the target area and wait until you hear the beep. You must apply a hanging drop of blood to the test strip within 15 seconds of the fingerstick. Do not add more blood. Do not touch or remove the test strip while the test is in progress. The flashing blood drop symbol changes to an hourglass symbol when the meter detects a sufficient sample	**10**		
13.	Read the results. *Note:* The result appears in approximately 1 minute. It may be displayed in three ways: as the international normalized ratio (INR); as the protime (PT) in seconds; or as %Quick (a unit used mainly in Europe). Laboratory reports and manufacturers must supply their own reference ranges for PT results along with each patient's results. This is because different methodologies may create different reference ranges and different units of measurement.	**5**		
14.	Dispose of the sharps into the biohazard sharps container. Dispose of regulated medical waste into the biohazard waste container. Disinfect the test area and remove your PPE.	**5**		
15.	Wash hands or use hand sanitizer.	**5**		
16.	Record the result in the lab's PT/INR log and in the patient's warfarin therapy flow sheet and/or patient health record. Using the normal range, identify if test result is normal or abnormal. For the paper log and paper patient health record, circle any results that do not fall into the Desirable Ranges. Identify critical values and take appropriate steps to notify the provider. Document the steps taken.	**10***		
	Total Points	**100**		

Protime Patient Log					
Protime expected values for both normal and therapeutic whole blood:					

			INR	PT seconds (ISI=1.0)	
Normal			0.8–1.1	11-13.5 sec	
Low anticoagulation therapy			1.5–2	19.6-26.1 sec	
Moderate anticoagulation therapy			2–3	26.1-39.2 sec	
High anticoagulation therapy			3–4	39.2-52.2 sec	

Date	Tech	Patient ID	INR	PT Seconds	Charted
10/07/20XX	AJ	@12345	1.5	19.6	✓

Documentation

Comments

CAAHEP Competencies	Step(s)
I.P.11.a. Collect specimens and perform: CLIA-waived hematology test	Entire procedure
II.P.2. Record laboratory test results into the patient's record	16
III.P.2. Select appropriate barrier/personal protective equipment (PPE)	1
III.P.10.a. Demonstrate proper disposal of biohazardous material: sharps	14
III.P.10.b. Demonstrate proper disposal of biohazardous material: regulated wastes	14
X.P.3. Document patient care accurately in the medical record	16
XII.P.1. Comply with safety practices.	1
ABHES Competencies	**Step(s)**
4. Medical Law and Ethics a. Follow documentation guidelines	16
9. Medical Laboratory Procedures b. Perform selected CLIA-waived test that assist with diagnosis and treatment 2) hematology testing	Entire procedure
9.c. Dispose of biohazardous materials	14

Procedure 49.3 Perform Preventive Maintenance for the Microhematocrit Centrifuge

Name _____ Date _____ Score _____

Tasks: Perform daily, monthly, semiannual, and annual maintenance on a microhematocrit centrifuge. Document the preventive maintenance in the laboratory logbook.

Equipment and Supplies:
- Microhematocrit centrifuge
- Maintenance logbook
- Utility gloves
- Fluid-impermeable lab coat, eye protection, and gloves
- Disinfectant
- Biohazard waste container

Standard: Complete the procedure and all critical steps in _____ minutes with a minimum score of 85% within two attempts (*or as indicated by the instructor*).

Scoring: Divide the points earned by the total possible points. Failure to perform a critical step, indicated by an asterisk (*), results in grade no higher than an 84% (*or as indicated by the instructor*).

Time: Began_____ Ended_____ Total minutes: _____

Steps:	Point Value	Attempt 1	Attempt 2
1. Wash hands or use hand sanitizer. Put on fluid-impermeable lab coat, eye protection, and gloves. In all maintenance procedures, gloves are worn under the utility gloves. *Note:* These are general recommendations. Always check the manufacturer's guidelines for specific instructions. Always unplug the power cord before cleaning or servicing the centrifuge.	10*		
Daily Maintenance 2. Clean the inside of the centrifuge and the gasket with a disinfectant recommended by the manufacturer. Plastic and nonmetal parts may be cleaned with a fresh solution of 5% sodium hypochlorite (bleach) mixed to a 1:10 dilution with water (1 part bleach plus 9 parts water).	10		
Monthly Maintenance 3. Check the reading device. Misuse and zeroing of reading devices can result in considerable error. Always use a second, simple reading device as a cross-check. Use a ruler or a flat plastic card specially made for this purpose. To use these cards, lay the spun hematocrit tube on the card and align the red cells with a line on the card to obtain the reading.	15		
4. Check the rotor for cracks or corrosion and check the interior for signs of white powder.	10		
Semiannual Maintenance 5. Check the gasket for cuts and breaks.	10		
6. Check the timer with a stopwatch to verify timer accuracy.	10		

7. Perform a maximum cell pack to verify the time required for complete packing by reading a sample after centrifugation and then recentrifuging for 1 minute. The results should be the same. If they are not, perform preventive maintenance and/or call the service technician.	**15**			
Annual Maintenance (or Maintenance Performed as Needed) 8. The centrifuge functions and maintenance verification should be performed by qualified personnel. This includes checking the centrifuge mechanism, rotors, timer, speed, and electrical leads.	**10**			
9. Record all professional service calls in the laboratory logbook.	**10**			
Total Points	**100**			

Microhematocrit Centrifuge Maintenance Log		
DATE	**SERVICE**	**INITIALS**
10/7/20XX	Performed routine daily, monthly, and annual preventive maintenance	AJ

Documentation

Comments

Procedure 49.4   CLIA-Waived Hematology Testing: Perform a Microhematocrit Test

Name _____ Date _____ Score _____

Tasks: Perform a microhematocrit test accurately. Document the result on the lab flow sheet and patient health record.

Equipment and Supplies:
- Patient's health record
- Provider's order and/or lab requisition
- Microhematocrit lab log
- Fresh sample of blood collected in a tube containing ethylenediaminetetraacetic acid (EDTA) anticoagulant (or equipment for fingerstick specimen: lancet, alcohol wipe, gauze, bandage)
- Plastic-coated self-sealing capillary tubes, or plain capillary tubes (blue-tipped)
- Sealing clay (if capillary tubes are not self-sealing)
- Gauze
- Microhematocrit centrifuge
- Fluid-impermeable lab coat, protective eyewear, and gloves
- Biohazard waste container
- Biohazard sharps containers

Standard: Complete the procedure and all critical steps in _____ minutes with a minimum score of 85% within two attempts (*or as indicated by the instructor*).

Scoring: Divide the points earned by the total possible points. Failure to perform a critical step, indicated by an asterisk (*), results in grade no higher than an 84% (*or as indicated by the instructor*).

Time: Began_____ Ended_____ Total minutes: _____

Steps:	Point Value	Attempt 1	Attempt 2
1. Wash hands or use hand sanitizer. Put on fluid-impermeable lab coat, protective eyewear, and gloves. Comply with safety practices.	10*		
2. Assemble the materials needed. 　a. If the capillary tubes are self-sealing: Fill two tubes by inserting the end opposite the sealed end into the well-mixed EDTA blood sample. *Note:* If the capillary tube and the EDTA tube are held almost parallel to the table, the capillary tubes fill easily by capillary action. When the self-sealing capillary tubes are two-thirds to three-fourths filled, tilt them upright, causing the blood sample to flow down the tube and meet the sealant. Continue to hold the tube vertical when the blood contacts the sealant for an additional 15 seconds. 　b. *Alternative:* Fill two plain (blue-tipped) capillary tubes two-thirds to three-fourths full of a well-mixed EDTA blood sample. Tip the blood tube slightly, touching the capillary tube into the blood using the side that is opposite the blue band. When enough blood has filled the capillary tube, tip the blue end of the tube down, causing the blood to flow toward the blue tip. Then readjust the tube horizontally while inserting the blue tip of the capillary tube into the clay sealant. Insert the tube as many times as needed to achieve a plug up to the blue band.	5		

3.	Wipe the outside of the tubes with clean gauze without touching the wet open end of the tube.	**5**		
4.	Place the tubes opposite each other in the centrifuge with the sealed ends securely against the gasket.	**10***		
5.	Note the numbers on the centrifuge slots and record the numbers on the log sheet, along with the patient's name.	**10***		
6.	Secure the locking top, fasten the lid down, and lock it.	**5**		
7.	Set the timer to 3 to 5 minutes and adjust the speed to 11,000 to 12,000 rpm, or as indicated by the manufacturer's instructions. Note: Check the manufacturer's instructions for time and speed, since models vary.	**5**		
8.	Allow the centrifuge to come to a complete stop. Unlock the outer locking top and then remove the inner lid.	**5**		
9.	Remove the tubes immediately and read the results. If this is not possible, store the tubes in an upright position.	**10**		

10.	Determine the microhematocrit values using one of the following methods:
	 a. Centrifuge with built-in reader using calibrated capillary tubes.
	    1. Position the tubes as directed by the manufacturer's instructions.
	    2. Read both tubes.
	    3. The average of the two results is reported.
	    4. The two values should not vary by more than 2%.
	 b. Centrifuge without a built-in reader.
	    1. Carefully remove the tubes from the centrifuge.
	    2. Place a tube on the microhematocrit reader.
	    3. Align the clay-RBC junction with the zero line on the reader. Align the plasma meniscus with the 100% line. The value is read at the junction of the red cell layer and the buffy coat. The buffy coat is not included in the reading.
	    4. Read both tubes.
	    5. The average of the two results is reported.
	    6. The two values should not vary by more than 2%.
		10*		

11.	Dispose of the capillary tubes in a biohazard sharps container.	**5***		
12.	Disinfect the work area and properly dispose of all biohazard materials. Remove your gloves, eyewear, and lab coat.	**10***		
13.	Wash hands or use hand sanitizer.	**5**		
14.	Record the results in the Hematocrit Patient Log and document the results in the patient's medical record. Using the normal range, identify if test results is normal or abnormal.	**5**		
	Total Points	**100**		

Hematocrit Patient Log					
Hematocrit expected values: Adult male: 39%-49% Adult female: 36%-45%			Newborn – 1 month: 31-57% Age: 1 month – 23 months: 27-38% Age 2-17 years: 31-50%		
Date	**Tech**	**Patient ID**	**Slot #**	**Results**	**Charted**
10/07/20XX	AJ	@12345	1 & 4	44% and 44%	✓

Documentation

Comments

CAAHEP Competencies	Step(s)
I.P.11.a. Collect specimens and perform: CLIA-waived hematology test	Entire procedure
II.P.2. Record laboratory test results into the patient's record	14
III.P.2. Select appropriate barrier/personal protective equipment (PPE)	1
III.P.10.a. Demonstrate proper disposal of biohazardous material: sharps	12
III.P.10.b. Demonstrate proper disposal of biohazardous material: regulated wastes	12
X.P.3. Document patient care accurately in the medical record	14
XII.P.1. Comply with safety practices.	1
ABHES Competencies	**Step(s)**
4. Medical Law and Ethics a. Follow documentation guidelines	14
9. Medical Laboratory Procedures b. Perform selected CLIA-waived test that assist with diagnosis and treatment 2) hematology testing	Entire procedure
9.c. Dispose of biohazardous materials	12

Procedure 49.5   Perform CLIA-Waived Hematology Testing: Perform a Hemoglobin Test

Name _____ Date _____ Score _____

Tasks: determine the level of hemoglobin present in a blood sample using the HemoCue B-Hemoglobin System. Document the result on the lab flow sheet and patient health record.

Equipment and Supplies:
- Patient's health record
- Provider's order and/or lab requisition
- Hemoglobin laboratory log
- HemoCue monitor
- HemoCue microcuvette
- Safety blood lancet
- Alcohol wipes
- Gauze
- Fluid-impermeable lab coat, protective eyewear, and gloves
- Biohazard waste container
- Biohazard sharps containers

Standard: Complete the procedure and all critical steps in _____ minutes with a minimum score of 85% within two attempts (*or as indicated by the instructor*).

Scoring: Divide the points earned by the total possible points. Failure to perform a critical step, indicated by an asterisk (*), results in grade no higher than an 84% (*or as indicated by the instructor*).

Time: Began_____ Ended_____ Total minutes: _____

Steps:	Point Value	Attempt 1	Attempt 2
1. Perform an instrument quality control check by inserting the control cuvette into the instrument. Make sure the reading is within acceptable limits before proceeding.	10*		
2. Wash your hands or use hand sanitizer. Put on fluid-impermeable lab coat, protective eyewear, and gloves. Comply with safety practices.	5*		
3. Check the provider's order and collect the necessary equipment and supplies.	5		
4. Greet the patient. Identify yourself. Verify the patient's identity with the full name; ask the patient to spell the first and last name and to give their date of birth.	5*		
5. Explain the procedure to be performed in a manner that is understood by the patient. Answer any questions the patient may have on the procedure. Obtain permission for the capillary puncture.	5*		
6. Examine the patient's fingers and choose the site to be used to obtain the blood sample.	5		
7. Clean the site with an alcohol wipe or another recommended antiseptic preparation.	10		
8. Perform a capillary puncture and wipe away the first drop of blood.	5		
9. Obtain a large drop of blood on the surface of the finger.	5		

10. Touch the microcuvette to the drop of blood. Do not touch the finger. The correct volume is drawn into the cuvette by capillary action. Wipe off any excess blood from the sides of the cuvette.	**10**		
11. Place the cuvette in the cuvette holder of the HemoCue sample door and close the door of the instrument.	**5**		
12. Read the result.	**5**		
13. Dispose of biohazard waste in the biohazard waste container and the sharps in the biohazard sharps container. Turn off the instrument. Properly disinfect the work area.	**5***		
14. Remove your gloves and dispose of them in the biohazard waste container. Remove the lab coat and protective eyewear.	**5**		
15. Wash hands or use hand sanitizer.	**5***		
16. Record the result in the lab's hemoglobin log and the patient's health record. Using the normal range, identify if test result is normal or abnormal.	**10**		
Total Points	**100**		

Hemocue B Hemoglobin System Patient Log

Test:_____ Kit Log #:_____

Hemoglobin expected values: Adult male: 13.2-16.6 g/dL Adult female: 11.6-15 g/dL	Newborn – 1 month: 10-20 g/dL Age: 1 month – 23 months: 8.9–12.7 g/dL Age 2-17 years: 10.2-16.9 g/dL

Date	Tech	Patient ID	Result	Charted
10/07/20XX	AJ	@12345	15.5 g/dL	✓

Documentation

Comments

CAAHEP Competencies	Step(s)
I.P.2.c. Perform the following procedures: capillary puncture	5-8
I.P.10. Perform a quality control measure	1
I.P.11.a. Collect specimens and perform: CLIA-waived hematology test	Entire procedure
II.P.2. Record laboratory test results into the patient's record	16
III.P.2. Select appropriate barrier/personal protective equipment (PPE)	2
III.P.10.a. Demonstrate proper disposal of biohazardous material: sharps	13
III.P.10.b. Demonstrate proper disposal of biohazardous material: regulated wastes	13
X.P.3. Document patient care accurately in the medical record	16
XII.P.1. Comply with safety practices.	2
ABHES Competencies	**Step(s)**
4. Medical Law and Ethics a. Follow documentation guidelines	16
9. Medical Laboratory Procedures a. Practice Quality Control	1
9. b. Perform selected CLIA-waived test that assist with diagnosis and treatment 2) hematology testing	Entire procedure
9.c. Dispose of biohazardous materials	13
9.d. Collect, label, and process a specimen 2) Perform capillary puncture	5-8

Procedure 49.6   Perform a Blood Glucose Test

Name _____ Date _____ Score _____

Tasks: Perform a blood test for blood glucose accurately. Document the result in the patient's health record.

Equipment and Supplies:
- Patient's health record
- Provider's order and/or lab requisition
- Glucometer glucose monitoring device
- Blood glucose test strips
- Lancet and autoloading finger-puncturing device
- Alcohol wipes
- Gauze
- Fluid-impermeable lab coat, protective eyewear, and gloves
- Biohazard waste container
- Biohazard sharps containers

Standard: Complete the procedure and all critical steps in _____ minutes with a minimum score of 85% within two attempts (*or as indicated by the instructor*).

Scoring: Divide the points earned by the total possible points. Failure to perform a critical step, indicated by an asterisk (*), results in grade no higher than an 84% (*or as indicated by the instructor*).

Time: Began_____ Ended_____ Total minutes: _____

Steps:	Point Value	Attempt 1	Attempt 2
1. Check the provider's order and collect the necessary equipment and supplies. Perform quality control measures according to the manufacturer's guidelines and office policy. *Note:* A variety of blood glucose monitors are available for testing blood glucose. Follow the specific instructions given by each individual manufacturer in the monitor/kit package insert.	5		
2. Wash hands or use hand sanitizer. Put on fluid-impermeable lab coat, protective eyewear, and gloves. Comply with safety practices.	5*		
3. Greet the patient. Identify yourself. Verify the patient's identity with full name; ask the patient to spell the first and last name and to give their date of birth.	5*		
4. Explain the procedure to be performed in a manner that is understood by the patient. Answer any questions the patient may have on the procedure. Obtain permission for the capillary puncture.	10*		
5. Ask the patient to wash their hands in warm, soapy water, then rinse them in warm water, and finally dry them completely.	5		
6. Check the patient's middle and ring fingers and select the site for puncture (both forearm and fingertip testing can be done).	5		
7. Turn on the glucometer by pressing the ON button. Coding may or may not be necessary, depending on the monitor; follow the package insert directions for the specific glucose monitor you are using.	5		
8. Check the expiration date on the test strip container. Take out a test strip and insert it into the glucometer.	5		

9. Cleanse the selected site on the patient's fingertip with an alcohol wipe and allow the finger to air dry.	5*		
10. Perform the capillary puncture and wipe away the first drop of blood.	10		
11. Apply a small blood sample to the end of the test strip.	5		
12. Give the patient gauze to hold securely over the puncture site; apply a hypoallergenic bandage or wrap if needed.	5		
13. Read the test results before the glucometer turns off. *Note:* The glucometer automatically begins the measurement process, and results are obtained as soon as 4 seconds. The test result is shown in the display window in milligrams per deciliter (mg/dL) for most glucometers. Read manufacturer's instruction on how the result is displayed. The glucometer will likely turn off automatically.	5		
14. Discard all biohazard waste in biohazard waste containers and the sharps in the biohazard sharps container.	5		
15. Clean the glucometer according to the manufacturer's guidelines. Disinfect the work area.	5		
16. Remove your gloves and dispose of them properly. Remove protective eyewear.	5		
17. Wash hands or use hand sanitizer.	5*		
18. Record the test results in the patient's health record.	5		
Total Points	**100**		

Documentation

Comments

CAAHEP Competencies	Step(s)
I.P.2.c. Perform the following procedures: capillary puncture	4-6, 9-10
I.P.10. Perform a quality control measure	1
I.P.11.b. Collect specimens and perform: CLIA-waived chemistry test	Entire procedure
II.P.2. Record laboratory test results into the patient's record	18
III.P.2. Select appropriate barrier/personal protective equipment (PPE)	2
III.P.10.a. Demonstrate proper disposal of biohazardous material: sharps	14
III.P.10.b. Demonstrate proper disposal of biohazardous material: regulated wastes	14
X.P.3. Document patient care accurately in the medical record	18
XII.P.1. Comply with safety practices.	2
ABHES Competencies	Step(s)
4. Medical Law and Ethics a. Follow documentation guidelines	18
9. Medical Laboratory Procedures a. Practice Quality Control	1
9.b. Perform selected CLIA-waived test that assist with diagnosis and treatment 3) chemistry testing	Entire procedure
9.c. Dispose of biohazardous materials	14
9.d. Collect, label, and process a specimen 2) Perform capillary puncture	4-6, 9-10

Procedure 49.7   Perform a CLIA-Waived Chemistry Test: Determine the Cholesterol Level or Lipid Profile Using a Cholestech Analyzer

Name _____ Date _____ Score _____

Tasks: Perform a Cholestech test for total cholesterol level or a lipid panel, and accurately report the results. Document the result on the lab flow sheet and patient health record.

Equipment and Supplies:
- Patient's health record
- Provider's order and/or lab requisition
- Cholestech analyzer
- Package insert or flow chart with directions
- Optics check cassette
- Test cassettes (provided by Cholestech)
- Level 1 and 2 liquid controls
- Capillary tubes and plungers for fingerstick sample (provided by Cholestech)
- Mini-Pet pipet and pipet tips for venipuncture sample (provided by Cholestech)
- Lancet, gauze, alcohol wipes, bandage for capillary blood, or lithium heparin (green-topped) tube for venous blood
- Safety tube decapper (if tubes do not have a Hemogard plastic top)
- Fluid-impermeable lab coat, protective eyewear, and gloves
- Biohazard waste container
- Biohazard sharps containers

Directions: Perform a total blood cholesterol level or lipid panel STAT.

Standard: Complete the procedure and all critical steps in _____ minutes with a minimum score of 85% within two attempts (*or as indicated by the instructor*).

Scoring: Divide the points earned by the total possible points. Failure to perform a critical step, indicated by an asterisk (*), results in grade no higher than an 84% (*or as indicated by the instructor*).

Time: Began_____ Ended_____ Total minutes: _____

Steps:	Point Value	Attempt 1	Attempt 2
1. Check the provider's order and collect the necessary equipment and supplies. Allow refrigerated testing cassettes to come to room temperature (at least 10 minutes before opening).	5*		
2. Wash hands or use hand sanitizer. Put on a fluid-impermeable lab coat, protective eyewear, and gloves. Comply with safety practices. Assemble the materials needed.	5*		
3. Perform quantitative quality control by performing a calibration check with the optics check cassette. Then test level 1 and level 2 liquid controls if using a new set of cassettes.	5*		
4. Greet the patient. Identify yourself. Verify the patient's identity with full name, ask the patient to spell the first and last name, and give date of birth.	5		

5. Explain the procedure to be performed in a manner that the patient understands. Answer any questions the patient may have on the procedure. Obtain permission for a capillary puncture.	5*			
6. Remove cassette from its pouch and place on flat surface without touching the black bar or magnetic strip.	10*			
7. Press RUN on the analyzer, allowing it to do a self-test; this will be followed by OK on the screen, then the test drawer will open. The drawer will stay open for 4 minutes while the specimen is prepared.	10			
8. Perform a fingerstick and collect the capillary blood to the black line of the Cholestech capillary tube with its plunger inserted into the red end of the tube. Or collect the fresh venous whole blood with the Cholestech Mini-Pet pipet.	10			
9. Place the whole blood sample into the well of the cassette. *Note:* The capillary specimen must be in the cassette within 5 minutes of collection.	10			
10. Immediately put the cassette into the drawer of the analyzer and press RUN. (Note: If the drawer has closed, press RUN again to open the drawer; load the specimen into the drawer and then press to close the drawer.) When the test is complete, the analyzer beeps. The screen displays and then prints out the results.	10			
11. Dispose of all sharps in the biohazard sharps container (i.e., lancet and capillary pipet with plunger). Place all regulated medical waste into the biohazard waste container (i.e., gauze, alcohol wipes, and cassettes).	5			
12. Disinfect test area, remove PPE, and dispose of gloves in biohazard waste container.	5			
13. Wash hands or use hand sanitizer.	5*			
14. Record the findings in the laboratory log and in the patient's health record. Using the normal range, identify if test result is normal or abnormal. If using paper health records, circle the results that do not fall within the Desirable Ranges column of the following table. Identify critical values and take appropriate steps to notify the provider. Document steps taken.	10			
Total Points	**100**			

TEST	DESIRABLE RANGES
Total cholesterol (TC)	<200 mg/dL
HDL cholesterol	>40 mg/dL (males); >50 mg/dL (females)
LDL cholesterol	<130 mg/dL
Triglycerides	30-190 mg/dL
TC/HDL ratio	≤4.5
Other	
Glucose	Fasting: 70-99 mg/dL
	Nonfasting: <125 mg/dL

CHOLESTECH LDX PATIENT/CONTROL LOG									
Cassette Lot #: _____ Expiration date: _____ LDX Serial #: _____									
DATE	TECH	PT ID	TC	HDL	LDL	TRG	TC/HDL	GLU	Charted
10/09/20XX	AJ	#12345	190	50	120	135	4.3	80	✓

Documentation

Comments

CAAHEP Competencies	Step(s)
I.P.2.c. Perform the following procedures: capillary puncture	5, 8
I.P.10. Perform a quality control measure	3
I.P.11.b. Collect specimens and perform: CLIA-waived chemistry test	Entire procedure
II.P.2. Record laboratory test results into the patient's record	14
III.P.2. Select appropriate barrier/personal protective equipment (PPE)	2
III.P.10.a. Demonstrate proper disposal of biohazardous material: sharps	11
III.P.10.b. Demonstrate proper disposal of biohazardous material: regulated wastes	11
X.P.3. Document patient care accurately in the medical record	14
XII.P.1. Comply with safety practices.	2
ABHES Competencies	**Step(s)**
4. Medical Law and Ethics a. Follow documentation guidelines	14
9. Medical Laboratory Procedures a. Practice Quality Control	3
9.b. Perform selected CLIA-waived test that assist with diagnosis and treatment 3) chemistry testing	Entire procedure
9.c. Dispose of biohazardous materials	11
9.d. Collect, label, and process a specimen 2) Perform capillary puncture	5, 8

Microbiology and Immunology

chapter

50

CAAHEP Competencies	Assessments
I.P.2.c. Perform: capillary puncture	Procedure 50.5
I.P.10. Perform a quality control measure	Procedures 50.4, 50.5, 50.7
I.P.11.d. Collect specimens and perform: CLIA-waived immunology test	Procedures 50.5
I.P.11.e. Collect specimens and perform: CLIA-waived microbiology test	Procedures 50.2 and 50.3 (collection only), 50.4
II.P.2. Record laboratory test results into the patient's record	Procedures 50.4, 50.5, 50.7
III.P.2. Select appropriate barrier/personal protective equipment (PPE)	Procedures 50.2, 50.3, 50.4, 50.5, 50.7
III.P.10.a. Demonstrate proper disposal of biohazardous material: sharps	Procedure 50.5
III.P.10.b. Demonstrate proper disposal of biohazardous material: regulated wastes	Procedures 50.2, 50.3, 50.4, 50.5, 50.7
V.P.3.b. Coach patients regarding: medical encounters	Procedures 50.1, 50.6, 50.8
X.P.3. Document patient care accurately in the medical record	Procedures 50.1, 50.2, 50.3, 50.6, 50.8
XII.P.1. Comply with safety practices	Procedures 50.2, 50.3, 50.4, 50.5
ABHES Competencies	Assessments
4. Medical Law and Ethics a. Follow documentation guidelines	Procedures 50.1 50.2, 50.3, 50.4, 50.5, 50.6, 50.7, 50.8
8. Clinical Procedures e. Perform specialty procedures, including but not limited to minor surgery, cardiac, respiratory, OB-GYN, neurological, and gastroenterology	Procedures 50.6, 50.7
9. Medical Laboratory Procedures a. Practice Quality Control	Procedures 50.4, 50.5, 50.7
9.b. Perform selected CLIA-waived test that assist with diagnosis and treatment 4) immunology testing	Procedure 50.5

ABHES Competencies	Assessments
9.b. Perform selected CLIA-waived test that assist with diagnosis and treatment 5) microbiology testing	Procedures 50.2 and 50.3 (collection only), 50.4
9.b. Perform selected CLIA-waived test that assist with diagnosis and treatment 6) kit testing	Procedures 50.4, 50.5
9.c. Dispose of biohazardous materials	Procedures 50.2, 50.3, 50.4, 50.5, 50.7
9.d. Collect, label, and process a specimen 2) Perform capillary puncture	Procedure 50.5
d. Collect, label, and process specimens 4) Obtain throat specimens for microbiologic testing	Procedures 50.3, 50.4
9.e. Instruct patients in the collection of 2) fecal specimen	Procedures 50.1, 50.6, 50.8

VOCABULARY REVIEW

Using the word pool, find the correct word to match the definition. Write the word on the line after the definition.

Group A

1. Any single-celled or multicellular organism that has genetic material contained in a distinct membrane-bound nucleus

   _____

2. Any animal that lacks a spine _____

3. Structures inside a cell that perform specific functions

   _____

4. Molecules needed for metabolism: carbohydrates, lipids, proteins, amino acids, and nucleic acids _____

5. Substances that inhibit the growth of microorganisms on living tissue _____

6. Thick mucus often referred to as *phlegm*

   _____

7. Growth of tiny fungi forming on a substance

   _____

8. Arthropod that carries disease and transmits to another organism through a blood meal _____

9. A glass slide that holds a specimen suspended in a drop of liquid for microscopic examination _____

10. The technique or process of keeping tissue alive and growing in a culture medium _____

Word Pool
- antiseptic
- arthropod
- eukaryote
- macromolecules
- mold
- organelles
- sputum
- tissue culture
- vector
- wet mount

Group B

1. Phase when the host recovers gradually and returns to baseline or normal health _____

2. To cultivate an organism (a bacteria) again on a new nutrient surface _____

3. Latin term meaning *in glass*; commonly known as "in the laboratory" _____

4. A liquid substance that dilutes or lessens the strength of a solution or mixture _____

5. Inflammation of the lungs with congestion of the alveoli _____

6. Phase of rapid multiplication of the pathogen; symptoms are very distinct _____

7. A medium used to keep an organism alive during transport to the laboratory _____

8. A syringe is used to gently squirt a small amount of sterile saline into the nose, and the resulting fluid is collected into a cup _____

9. A process by which a specific substance is separated from a group or solution _____

10. Occurs when the small airways of the lungs become inflamed because of a viral infection _____

Word Pool
- acute stage
- bronchiolitis
- convalescent stage
- diluent
- extraction
- in vitro
- nasal wash
- pneumonia
- subcultured
- transport medium

ABBREVIATIONS

Write out what each of the following abbreviations stands for.

1. QA _____

2. EM _____

3. CNS _____

4. ARV _____

5. AIDS _____

6. OSHA _____

7. GPC _____

8. GNB _____

9. MAC _____

10. AFB _____

11. cfu _____

12. C&S _____

13. BAP _____

14. KOH _____

15. PG _____

16. O&P _____

17. nm _____

18. GAS _____

19. RSV _____

20. HIV _____

21. EBV _____

22. UTI _____

23. Mono _____

24. DNA _____

25. RNA _____

SKILLS AND CONCEPTS

Answer the following questions. Write your answer on the line or in the space provided.

A. Introduction

Match the description with the correct term.

1. _____ A substance or medication that can destroy or inhibit the growth of bacteria

2. _____ A microorganism that lives on or in the body

3. _____ A protein substance produced in the blood or tissues in response to a specific antigen

4. _____ Any living organism of microscopic size

5. _____ Living and nonliving pathogens that can cause disease

6. _____ Infections that patients acquire while receiving treatment for other conditions within a healthcare setting

7. _____ Any various single-celled fungi, which reproduce by budding and are able to ferment sugars

8. _____ The study of the immune system, which is closely tied to microbiology

9. _____ Microorganisms that are single-celled, lack a nucleus, reproduce asexually, or can form spores

a. microorganisms
b. infectious agent
c. healthcare associated infections
d. antibiotic
e. normal flora
f. yeast
g. immunology
h. antibody
i. immunology
j. bacteria

B. Classification of Microorganisms

Match the description with the correct term.

1. _____ A system of names or terms used in science and art to categorize items

2. _____ Single-celled organisms, including molds and yeast

3. _____ A name consisting of a generic and a specific term

4. _____ Pertaining to a parasite

5. _____ Single-celled organisms that are the most primitive form of animal life, including amoebas and ciliates

a. fungi
b. protozoa
c. parasitic
d. binomial
e. nomenclature

Fill in the blank.

6. The _____ system assigns two names, which are both either italicized or underlined.

7. The first name in the binomial system is called the _____ and it begins with a capital letter.

8. After the organism's full genus and species names are given once in a report, subsequent references can just use a(n) _____ to represent the genus.

9. The second name in the binomial system is called the _____ and it begins with a lowercase letter.

C. Characteristics of Bacteria

Match the description with the correct term.

1. _____ Reagents or dyes used to prepare specimens for microscopic examination

2. _____ A long, whip-like outgrowth from a cell that helps the cell move

3. _____ The simplest unit of a chemical compound that can exist, consisting of two or more atoms held together with chemical bonds

4. _____ An inactive form of certain bacteria that can withstand poor environmental conditions

5. _____ Describes reproduction that does not involve the fusion of male and female sex cells

6. _____ Any organism that is made up of at least one cell and has genetic material that is not enclosed in a nucleus

7. _____ Able to live and grow

8. _____ Asexual reproduction in single-celled organisms during which one cell divides into two daughter cells

a. prokaryote
b. asexual
c. binary fission
d. stains
e. molecule
f. flagella
g. endospore
h. viable

Match the following description with the correct term.

9. _____ Round bacteria

10. _____ Do not stain well with a Gram stain, but they stain pink with the acid-fast stain

11. _____ Tightly coiled spirilla

12. _____ Looks deep blue/violet when stained with Gram stain

13. _____ Rod-shaped bacteria

14. _____ Looks pinkish red when stained with Gram stain

15. _____ Spiral-shaped bacteria

a. gram-positive cells
b. gram-negative cells
c. acid-fast cells
d. cocci
e. bacilli
f. spirilla
g. spirochetes

Match the following description with the correct term or prefix.

16. _____ Bacteria that require oxygen to live

17. _____ Used when bacteria are found in pairs

18. _____ Used when bacteria are in a grapelike cluster

19. _____ Used when bacteria are in a chain formation

20. _____ Bacteria that can survive in the presence of oxygen but prefer to live without oxygen

21. _____ Cocci in packets of 4

22. _____ Cocci in packets of 8 or 16

23. _____ Bacteria that die in the presence of oxygen

a. strepto-
b. diplo-
c. staphylo-
d. tetrads
e. sarcinae
f. aerobes
g. anaerobes
h. facultative anaerobes

D. Pathogens

Fill in the blank or select the correct answer.

1. _____ require host cells for growth.

2. _____ are transmitted by blood-sucking insects and cannot multiply outside a living host cell.

3. _____ do not contain peptidoglycan in their cell wall.

4. _____ is the study of fungi and the diseases they cause.

5. What is correct regarding fungi?
   a. Include yeasts and molds
   b. Present in the soil, air, and water
   c. Transmitted by direct contact with infected persons and inhalation of contaminated dust or soil
   d. Transmitted by prolonged exposure to a moist environment
   e. All of the above

6. Before microscopic observation, skin scraping samples are treated with _____ to dissolve nonfungal material, making the fungal elements easier to observe.

7. _____ are single-celled parasitic organisms that contain a nucleus and are transmitted through contaminated feces, food, and drink.

8. _____ includes the study of all parasitic organisms that live on or in the human body.

9. What is correct regarding parasites?
   a. Transmitted by ingestion and direct penetration of the skin
   b. Transmitted through injection by a vector
   c. Frequently identified in feces, blood, urine, sputum, tissue fluid, or tissue biopsy samples
   d. All of the above

10. _____ are parasitic worms that live on or in another living organism.

11. Viruses consist of a genetic core covered by a protein coat called a(n) _____.

12. A substance that stimulates the production of an antibody when introduced into the body is called a(n) _____.

13. Viruses must be cultured in fertilized eggs or in a(n) _____.

14. A blood sample is tested for a specific _____ related to the possible viral infection.

E. Specimen Collection and Transport in the Physician Office Laboratory
Fill in the blank or select the correct answer.

1. Specimens for microbiology testing must be collected carefully so that contaminating _____ are not introduced into the _____.

2. What should be done to prevent contaminating the specimen?
   a. Wash hands before collecting the sample.
   b. Cleanse the area involved with an antiseptic, if appropriate.
   c. Open sterile containers only when necessary and avoid touching the inside surfaces.
   d. Never touch a sterile swab or collection device to a nonsterile surface.
   e. All of the above.

3. To protect from pathogen exposure, the medical assistant should wear the appropriate _____ when collecting, handling, and processing specimens.

4. After the specimen has been collected on the swab, it is placed in the plastic tube with the _____.

5. Transport system swabs should be labeled with the
   a. patient's full name.
   b. date and time of collection.
   c. collector's initials.
   d. source of the specimen.
   e. all of the above.

6. Most pathogenic organisms prefer body temperatures, approximately _____°F.

7. Most pathogenic organisms will remain viable for up to _____ hours if held at room temperature or refrigerator temperature (39.2° F).

8. Stool specimens are placed into two vials, each with a preservative, and from these preparations, a(n) _____ slide is made to observe moving organisms.

9. In children, specimens to check for _____ are best collected late at night or early in the morning.

10. For a(n) _____ specimen, the swab is inserted no more than 0.5 of an inch into the nostril.

11. For a(n) _____ specimen, the swab is usually inserted no more than 1 inch.

12. For a(n) _____ specimen, the swab needs to be inserted the same distance as the nostril to the outer opening of the ear.

13. A nasal or nasopharyngeal swab should be gently rolled and then left in place for _____ to allow it to absorb secretions.

14. Which test requires a sputum specimen?
    a. Strep test
    b. Legionella test
    c. Acid-fast bacillus test
    d. All of the above
    e. Only b and c

15. When collecting a sputum specimen, patients should:

    a. Avoid food for _____ to _____ hours before collecting the sputum specimen.

    b. Rinse your mouth well to remove _____.

    c. Open the container and avoid _____ the inside of the container and cover.

    d. Inhale _____ to _____ times, breathing out hard each time, then cough deeply.

16. When obtaining a wound swab specimen, moisten the swab with _____ if the wound is dry.

17. To collect a wound swab specimen, the medical assistant should gently roll the swab stick from margin to margin using a(n) _____, using enough _____ to accumulate fluid on the swab.

F. CLIA-Waived Microbiology Testing
Fill in the blank.

1. With rapid strep testing, the test swab is placed in a(n) _____, and the extract is tested for antigens found on the surface of *S. pyogenes*.

2. With a CLIA-waived rapid strep test kit, there will be a(n) _____ with the group A strep antibodies in the testing area that occurs if the strep A pathogen is present.

3. When a rapid strep test shows a negative test result, the results should be confirmed with a(n) _____ performed in the microbiology laboratory

4. CLIA-waived rapid lateral flow immunoassays detect both influenza A and influenza B antigens from _____ or _____ swabs.

5. The CLIA-waived rapid direct immunoassay for RSV uses a(n) _____ specimen or _____ to detect the virus.

G. CLIA-Waived Immunologic Testing
Fill in the blank or select the correct answer.

1. Testing done in the immunology laboratory is designed to demonstrate the reaction between a(n) _____ and its specific _____.

2. In the acute stage of a disease, the _____ level is high.

3. During the convalescent stage, the antibody level _____.

4. Infectious mononucleosis is caused by the _____.

5. Which tests are done when mononucleosis is suspected?
   a. Herpes test
   b. CBC
   c. CLIA-waived mononucleosis test
   d. All of the above
   e. Both b and c

6. When testing for *Helicobacter pylori*, the CLIA-waived rapid immunoassay tests uses _____, which is applied to a well in a test cartridge.

7. When using CLIA-waived rapid immunoassay tests, the presence of a line in the test area of the cartridge indicates the presence of _____ to the pathogen *H. pylori*.

8. The spirochete bacterium *Borrelia burgdorferi* is the causative agent in _____.

9. Lyme disease can be detected with CLIA-waived tests and these immunoassay tests for antibodies in _____.

10. Oral HIV self-test kits require a testing device to be rubbed once over the upper and lower _____.

H. Microbiology Reference Laboratory: Identification of Pathogens
Fill in the blank.

1. The _____ stain differentiates bacteria into two categories based on the presence or absence of a waxy lipid in the cell wall.

2. Bacteria react best in the Gram stain when they are less than _____ hours old.

3. Acid-fast positive microbes stain _____.

4. Acid-fast negative microbes stain _____.

5. Bacilli that are acid-fast positive often are referred to as _____.

6. Suspicious colonies are _____ onto the appropriate medium to isolate them in pure culture.

7. For a throat culture:

   a. A throat swab is collected from the patient's throat and then the swab is streaked for isolation on a(n) _____.

   b. An antibiotic disk is placed on the _____ quadrant of the streaked plate and incubated overnight at 98.6° F.

   c. The antibiotic disk contains _____, which prevents the growth of *S. pyogenes*.

8. For urine cultures, less than 10,000 cfu/mL of urine is considered _____.

9. For urine cultures, more than 100,000 cfu/mL of urine is considered _____.

10. _____ refers to growing the organisms.

11. _____ refers to the organism's susceptibility to antibiotics.

12. With sensitivity testing, *S* means that the pathogen is _____.

13. With sensitivity testing, *R* means that the pathogen is _____.

14. With sensitivity testing, *I* means _____ or that additional testing must be performed to determine the dosage of antibiotic necessary for successful treatment.

I. Stool-Based Tests
Fill in the blank.

1. A(n) _____ detects blood in the stool specimen.

2. A(n) _____ detects genetic material from polyps and cancerous tumors in the stool specimen.

3. When developing a Hemoccult test cards, open the back of the slide and apply _____ drops of the Hemoccult developer to the guaiac paper over each smear.

4. The medical assistant should read the results within _____ seconds for the smears.

5. Any trace of _____ on the specimen smear or near the edge is considered a positive test result for occult blood.

6. The medical assistant must also apply _____ drop(s) of the developer between the positive and negative Performance Monitors areas, for quality control.

7. The quality control results for the Hemoccult test card must be read within _____ seconds.

8. The Hemoccult card and the developer are functioning if a(n) _____ color appears in the positive Performance Monitor area and does not appear in the negative Performance Monitor area.

9. The fecal immunochemical test (FIT) only detects human hemoglobin from the

   _____.

10. The _____ detects abnormal DNA, along with the presence of occult hemoglobin in the stool.

CERTIFICATION PREPARATION
Circle the correct answer.

1. Beneficial microorganisms that are responsible for breaking down organic matter are called
   a. virus.
   b. saprophyte.
   c. acid-fast bacilli.
   d. mycoplasma.

2. What color is a gram-positive bacteria?
   a. Baby blue
   b. Pink
   c. Red
   d. Purple

3. A disease-causing organism or agent is the definition of which term?
   a. Normal flora
   b. Opportunistic organism
   c. Pathogen
   d. Microorganism

4. What is a substance that inhibits the growth of microorganisms on living tissue?
   a. Antiseptic
   b. Disinfectant
   c. Antimicrobial
   d. Antifungal

5. If a bacterium is rod-shaped, it is described as
   a. cocci.
   b. spirilla.
   c. bacilli.
   d. spirochete.

6. If an organism is able to live and thrive in the presence of oxygen, it is
   a. an anaerobe.
   b. a facultative anaerobe.
   c. an aerobe.
   d. none of the above.

7. Tiny pathogenic bacteria that are transmitted by blood-sucking insects are called
   a. chlamydia.
   b. virus.
   c. mycoplasma.
   d. rickettsia.

8. Scarlet fever, rheumatic fever, and glomerulo-nephritis are all possible complications of an infection with what bacteria?
   a. *Escherichia coli*
   b. *Staphylococcus aureus*
   c. *Streptococcus pyogenes*
   d. *Clostridium difficile*

9. The causative agent for Lyme disease is
   a. *Streptococcus pyogenes*.
   b. Epstein-Barr virus (EBV).
   c. *Helicobacter pylori*.
   d. *Borrelia burgdorferi*.

10. HIV is a
    a. viral infection.
    b. blood-borne pathogen.
    c. condition that is treated with ARV medications.
    d. all of the above.

WORKPLACE APPLICATIONS

1. Laura just collected a throat swab from a 10-year-old boy. He had a fever, sore throat, and white patches on his tonsils. Laura runs a rapid strep test and it is negative. Is there any additional testing that Laura should do? Explain your answer.

_____

_____

_____

_____

_____

2. Susie Cvanshara has an appointment at WMFM clinic today because she is very tired and has swollen lymph nodes in her neck and armpits, a sore throat, and no appetite. She has had these symptoms for 5 days and they are not improving. Jean Burke, NP orders a CBC with differential and CLIA-waived Mono test. The Mono test result from the laboratory is positive.

   a. What condition does Susie have? _____

   b. What abnormalities may be seen in Susie's CBC and differential testing?_____

   _____

   _____

3. Laura is reviewing patient microbiology results received from the reference laboratory. She sees a urine culture result for Mrs. Bingley of 54,000 cfu/mL. The provider has now requested sensitivity testing be completed on this culture. Explain what this report means. Why will sensitivity testing be helpful to the provider?

_____

_____

_____

_____

INTERNET ACTIVITIES

1. Using online resources, research Lyme disease. Summarize your findings in a poster or infographic. Include the following information in your project.
   a. Description of the disease
   b. The causative agent of the disease
   c. Signs and symptoms
   d. Diagnostic procedures including CLIA-waived testing
   e. Treatment

2. Using online resources, research a CLIA-waived HIV test kit. Create a poster presentation, a PowerPoint presentation, or a written paper summarizing your research. Include the following points in your project:
   a. Description of the test
   b. Any contraindications for the test
   c. Patient preparation for the test
   d. Principle of the test

3. Using online resources, create a poster or infographic about two types of pathogenic microorganisms. Choose from bacteria, viruses, fungi, protozoa, or parasites. Include the following information in your project:
   a. Size of the microorganism
   b. Common routes of transmission
   c. 5-10 examples of infectious agents for each type of organism
   d. 5-10 examples of disease states for each type of organism

Procedure 50.1 Coach a Patient on the Collection of Fecal Specimens to Be Tested for Ova and Parasites

Name _____ Date _____ Score _____

Task: Coach a patient in the proper collection of stool for an ova and parasite microscopic examination.

Equipment and Supplies:
- Patient's health record
- Provider's order and/or lab requisition
- Clean, dry container for stool collection
- Two parasitology collection vials*
- Plastic biohazard zipper-lock bag

Note: Several types of preservatives are available. Check with the referral laboratory to make sure the patient is given the proper vials for collection. Preservatives include low-viscosity polyvinyl alcohol (LV-PVA), zinc sulfite polyvinyl alcohol (ZN-PVA), sodium acetate acetic acid formalin (SAF), and 10% neutral buffered formalin.

Standard: Complete the procedure and all critical steps in _____ minutes with a minimum score of 85% within two attempts (*or as indicated by the instructor*).

Scoring: Divide the points earned by the total possible points. Failure to perform a critical step, indicated by an asterisk (*), results in grade no higher than an 84% (*or as indicated by the instructor*).

Time: Began_____ Ended_____ Total minutes: _____

Steps:	Point Value	Attempt 1	Attempt 2
1. Greet the patient. Identify yourself. Verify the patient's identity with full name, ask the patient to spell the first and last name, and give their date of birth.	5*		
2. Explain the procedure to be performed in a manner that is understood by the patient. Answer any general questions the patient may have about the collection procedures before you give detailed instructions.	10*		
3. Instruct the patient not to take any antacids, laxatives, or stool softeners before collecting the specimen. Instruct the patient that the liquid in the vials is extremely dangerous and to keep out of the reach of children.	10		
4. Instruct the patient to urinate before collecting the specimen.	10		
5. The patient then collects the specimen. • Adults: Instruct the patient to defecate into the container. Stool cannot be retrieved from the toilet bowl. • Children: Loosely drape the toilet rim with plastic wrap and lower the seat. The child should have a bowel movement into the toilet, onto the wrap. Remove the stool using a disposable plastic spoon. • Infants: Fasten a "diaper" made of plastic wrap over the child, using tape. Remove the plastic wrap immediately after a bowel movement and remove the stool using a plastic spoon. Never leave the child unattended with the plastic wrap in place because of the risk of suffocation.	15		

6. Instruct the patient or parent/guardian to add stool to the collection containers.
   • If the stool is formed, use the scoop on the lid of the container to add a large, jellybean–sized piece of stool to the liquid in the containers
   • If the stool is liquid, pour it into the container.
   • In both of the previous cases, keep adding the specimen until the liquid preservative in the vial reaches the indicated level on the containers.
	10		

7. Instruct the patient or parent/guardian to tighten the caps completely and wipe the outside of the vials with rubbing alcohol or to wash carefully with soap and water.	15		
8. Instruct the patient or parent/guardian that the vials should be labeled, placed in a biohazard bag with a zippered closure, and transported to the laboratory immediately, if possible. The vials should not be refrigerated.	10		
9. Instruct the patient or parent/guardian to wash their hands after the specimen collection procedure.	5*		
10. Document the coaching in the patient's health record. Include the provider's name, what was taught, how the patient responded, and indicate the supplies and written directions sent home with the patient.	10		
Total Points	100		

Documentation

Comments

CAAHEP Competencies	Step(s)
V.P.3.b. Coach patients regarding: medical encounters	Entire procedure
X.P.3. Document patient care accurately in the medical record	10
ABHES Competencies	**Step(s)**
4. Medical Law and Ethics a. Follow documentation guidelines	10
9.e. Instruct patients in the collection of 2) fecal specimen	Entire procedure

Procedure 50.2   Collect a Nasal or Nasopharyngeal Specimen Using a Swab

Name _____ Date _____ Score _____

Tasks: Collect an anterior nasal specimen, a mid-turbinate nasal specimen, or a nasopharyngeal specimen using a swab. Document the procedure in the patient's health record.

Equipment and Supplies:
- Patient's health record
- Provider's order and/or laboratory requisition
- Fluid-impermeable lab coat, mask, face shield or protective eyewear, and gloves (or as indicated by healthcare facility)
- Collection kit or appropriate swab for test (e.g., sterile flocked or spun polyester tipped swab with a flexible shaft) and transport media tube
- Biohazard waste container

Standard: Complete the procedure and all critical steps in _____ minutes with a minimum score of 85% within two attempts (*or as indicated by the instructor*).

Scoring: Divide the points earned by the total possible points. Failure to perform a critical step, indicated by an asterisk (*), results in grade no higher than an 84% (*or as indicated by the instructor*).

Time: Began_____ Ended_____ Total minutes: _____

Steps:	Point Value	Attempt 1	Attempt 2
1. Wash hands or use hand sanitizer. Put on a fluid-impermeable lab coat, mask, and face shield. Comply with safety practices.	5*		
2. Review the order and gather the supplies needed.	5		
3. Greet the patient. Identify yourself. Verify the patient's identity with full name, then ask the patient to spell the first and last names and to state their date of birth.	10*		
4. Explain the procedure in a manner that the patient understands. Answer any general questions the patient may have about the collection procedures before you give detailed instructions.	5		
5. Obtain permission to perform the swab on the patient. Ask the patient if he or she has any nasal obstructions or a deviated septum. Have the patient blow his or her nose, if indicated.	5		
6. Put on gloves.	5		
7. Remove the sterile swab from the sterile wrap with your dominant hand.	5		

8.   Collect the specimen:
a.   *For an anterior nasal swab:*
   – Using the appropriate swab, insert the tip of the swab into the nostril, no more than 0. 75 inch (1.9 cm).
   – Slowly rotate the swab, gently pressing against the nasal wall. Rotate 4 times for a total of 15 seconds. Remove the swab and insert it into the other nostril. Repeat the process.
	30		

b. *For a mid-turbinate nasal specimen:*
  – Have patients tilt their head back 70 degrees.
  – Using a tapered swab, rotate the swab while inserting it. Insert it less than 1 inch (2.5 cm) into the nostril along the nasal floor until resistance is met at the nasal turbinates. Rotate the swab for about 10 to 15 seconds. Hold in place for 5 seconds. Remove swab. Repeat process on the other nostril.
c. *For a nasopharyngeal specimen:*
  – Have patients tilt their head back 70 degrees.
  – Using the unobstructed nostril, insert the swab parallel to the palate until resistance is encountered. A swab should be inserted about 3.1 to 3.9 inches (8 to 10 cm) in an adult and 2.4 to 2.8 inches (6 to 7 cm) in a child.
  – Roll the swab gently and then leave the swab in place for several sections. Rotate the swab as it is slowly removed. If the swab is not saturated with secretions, repeat the process using the other nostril if indicated by the testing procedure. The same swab can be used.				

9. Place the swab in the transport medium. Snap or cut of the applicator stick if needed. Label the tube and send it to the laboratory.	**10**			
10. Dispose of contaminated supplies in the biohazard waste container. Disinfect the work area.	**5**			
11. Remove your gloves and discard them in the biohazard waste container. Remove face shield.	**5**			
12. Wash hands or use hand sanitizer.	**5**			
13. Document the procedure in the patient's health record.	**5**			
Total Points	**100**			

Documentation

Comments

CAAHEP Competencies	Step(s)
I.P.11.e. Collect specimens and perform: CLIA-waived microbiology test	Entire procedure (collection only)
III.P.2. Select appropriate barrier/personal protective equipment (PPE)	1, 6
III.P.10.b. Demonstrate proper disposal of biohazardous material: regulated wastes	10, 11
X.P.3. Document patient care accurately in the medical record	13
XII.P.1. Comply with safety practices	1
ABHES Competencies	**Step(s)**
4. Medical Law and Ethics a. Follow documentation guidelines	13
9. Medical Laboratory Procedures b. Perform selected CLIA-waived test that assist with diagnosis and treatment 5) microbiology testing	Entire procedure (collection only)
9.c. Dispose of biohazardous materials	10, 11

Procedure 50.3   Collect a Specimen for a Throat Culture

Name _____ Date _____ Score _____

Tasks: Collect a throat culture using sterile technique for immediate testing or for transportation to the laboratory. Document the procedure in the patient's health record.

Equipment and Supplies:
- Patient's health record
- Provider's order and/or laboratory requisition
- Fluid-impermeable lab coat, mask, face shield or protective eyewear, and gloves (or as indicated by healthcare facility)
- Sterile swab if transporting to a reference laboratory, or sterile swab from the rapid strep test kit if testing patient in POL
- Sterile tongue depressor
- Transport medium
- Biohazard waste container

Standard: Complete the procedure and all critical steps in _____ minutes with a minimum score of 85% within two attempts (*or as indicated by the instructor*).

Scoring: Divide the points earned by the total possible points. Failure to perform a critical step, indicated by an asterisk (*), results in grade no higher than an 84% (*or as indicated by the instructor*).

Time: Began_____ Ended_____ Total minutes: _____

Steps:	Point Value	Attempt 1	Attempt 2
1. Wash hands or use hand sanitizer. Put on fluid-impermeable lab coat and face shield. Put on a mask if required by the facility. Comply with safety practices.	5*		
2. Review the order and gather the supplies needed.	5		
3. Greet the patient. Identify yourself. Verify the patient's identity with full name, ask the patient to spell the first and last name, and give their date of birth.	5*		
4. Explain the procedure to be performed in a manner that is understood by the patient. Answer any questions the patient may have on the procedure.	10		
5. Obtain permission to perform the throat culture on the patient.	5		
6. Put on gloves. Position the patient so that the light shines into the mouth.	5		
7. Remove the sterile swab from the sterile wrap with your dominant hand and grasp the sterile tongue depressor with your nondominant hand.	5		
8. Instruct the patient to open the mouth and say, "Ah." Depress the tongue with the depressor.	10		
9. Swab the back of the throat between the tonsillar pillars in a figure-8 pattern, especially any reddened, patchy areas of the throat, white pus pockets, purulent areas, and the tonsils; take care not to touch any other areas in the mouth.	10		
10. Place the swab in the transport medium, label it, and follow appropriate procedures to send it to the referral laboratory. If rapid strep testing is requested, it may be done in the POL or sent to a reference laboratory.	10		

11. Dispose of contaminated supplies in the biohazard waste container. Disinfect the work area.	**10**			
12. Remove your gloves and discard them in the biohazard waste container. Remove the face shield.	**5**			
13. Wash hands or use hand sanitizer.	**10**			
14. Document the procedure in the patient's health record.	**5**			
Total Points	**100**			

Documentation

Comments

CAAHEP Competencies	**Step(s)**
I.P.11.e. Collect specimens and perform: CLIA-waived microbiology test	Entire procedure (collection only)
III.P.2. Select appropriate barrier/personal protective equipment (PPE)	1, 6
III.P.10.b. Demonstrate proper disposal of biohazardous material: regulated wastes	11, 12
X.P.3. Document patient care accurately in the medical record	14
XII.P.1. Comply with safety practices	1
ABHES Competencies	**Step(s)**
4. Medical Law and Ethics a. Follow documentation guidelines	14
9. Medical Laboratory Procedures b. Perform selected CLIA-waived test that assist with diagnosis and treatment 5) microbiology testing	Entire procedure (collection only)
9.c. Dispose of biohazardous materials	11, 12
9.d. Collect, label, and process specimens 4) obtain throat specimens for microbiologic testing	Entire procedure

Procedure 50.4 Perform a CLIA-Waived Microbiology Test: Perform a Rapid Strep Test

Name _____ Date _____ Score _____

Tasks: To perform a rapid strep screening test to assist in the diagnosis of strep throat. Document the results in the patient's health record.

Equipment and Supplies:
- Patient's health record
- Provider's order and/or lab requisition
- QuickVue In-Line Strep A test kit contents, CLIA-waived kit
  - Extraction solution bottle
  - Individually packaged test cassette
  - Individually wrapped sterile rayon swab provided in kit
  - Positive (+) control swab provided in kit
  - Visual flow chart outlining the steps of the test
- Rapid Strep Test Log Sheet (Work Product 50.1)
- Stopwatch or laboratory timer
- Fluid-impermeable lab coat, mask, face shield or protective eyewear, and gloves (or as indicated by healthcare facility)
- Biohazard waste container

Standard: Complete the procedure and all critical steps in _____ minutes with a minimum score of 85% within two attempts (*or as indicated by the instructor*).

Scoring: Divide the points earned by the total possible points. Failure to perform a critical step, indicated by an asterisk (*), results in grade no higher than an 84% (*or as indicated by the instructor*).

Time: Began_____ Ended_____ Total minutes: _____

Steps:	Point Value	Attempt 1	Attempt 2
1. Wash hands or use hand sanitizer. Put on fluid-impermeable lab coat and face shield or protective eyewear. Put on a mask if required by the facility. Comply with safety practices.	5*		
2. Collect all necessary supplies and equipment. Bring all reagents to room temperature. Check the expiration date on the test kit package. *Note:* Before running the first patient test from a new test kit, positive and negative controls must be run using the control swabs provided in the kit. Confirm that both controls reacted correctly and record the control results on the log sheet.	5		
3. Greet the patient. Identify yourself. Verify the patient's identity with full name, ask the patient to spell the first and last name, and give their date of birth.	5*		
4. Explain the procedure in a manner that the patient understands. Answer any general questions the patient may have about the collection procedures before you give detailed instructions. Obtain permission to collect a throat culture.	10*		
5. Put on gloves. Collect a throat specimen using the rayon swab provided in the test kit.	10		

6.	Remove the test cassette from the foil pouch and place it on a clean, dry, level surface. Using the notch at the back of the chamber as a guide, insert the patient's swab completely into the swab chamber.	**10**		
7.	Place the extraction bottle between your thumb and forefinger and squeeze once to break the glass ampule inside the extraction solution bottle. Vigorously shake the bottle five times to mix the solutions. The solution should turn green.	**10**		
8.	Immediately remove the cap on the extraction solution bottle, hold the bottle vertically over the chamber, and quickly fill the chamber to the rim (approximately 8 drops).	**5**		
9.	Remove your face shield. Wait 5 minutes to read the results and record them in the lab log. • Positive result: A pink line shows in the T area, indicating the presence of *Streptococcus pyogenes* antigen; a blue line appears in the C area, indicating that the fluid activated the internal control. • Negative result: No pink line appears in the T test area; a blue line appears in the C control area, indicating that the internal control worked. • Invalid result: The blue control line does not appear next to the letter C at 5 minutes. The test result cannot be reported.	**10**		
10.	Discard all the test materials in the appropriate biohazard waste container. Disinfect the work area.	**5**		
11.	Remove your gloves. Wash hands or use hand sanitizer.	**10***		
12.	Record the test results in the patient's health record.	**10**		
13.	If the test results are negative, a second throat swab should be obtained and sent to the reference laboratory for a throat culture. Often two swabs are used simultaneously when the sample is initially collected from the throat to prevent the need to recollect a specimen.	**5**		
	Total Points	**100**		

Documentation

Comments

CAAHEP Competencies	Step(s)
I.P.10. Perform a quality control measure	2
I.P.11.e. Collect specimens and perform: CLIA-waived microbiology test	Entire procedure
II.P.2. Record laboratory test results into the patient's record	12
III.P.2. Select appropriate barrier/personal protective equipment (PPE)	1, 5
III.P.10.b. Demonstrate proper disposal of biohazardous material: regulated wastes	10
XII.P.1. Comply with safety practices	1
ABHES Competencies	**Step(s)**
4. Medical Law and Ethics a. Follow documentation guidelines	12
9. Medical Laboratory Procedures a. Practice Quality Control	2
9. b. Perform selected CLIA-waived test that assist with diagnosis and treatment 5) microbiology testing	Entire procedure
9.b. Perform selected CLIA-waived test that assist with diagnosis and treatment 6) kit testing	Entire procedure
9.c. Dispose of biohazardous materials	10
9.d. Collect, label, and process specimens 4) obtain throat specimens for microbiologic testing	4-5

Work Product 50.1   Rapid Strep Test Log Sheet

To be used with Procedure 50.4.

Name _____   Date _____   Score _____

Directions: Complete the documentation

QUALITATIVE CONTROL/PATIENT LOG SHEET

TEST: <u>Strep A test</u>

KIT NAME AND MANUFACTURER: QuickVue In-Line Strep A Test – Quidel

LOT # <u>12345</u>   EXPIRATION DATE: <u>11/22/20XX</u>

STORAGE REQUIREMENTS: <u>Room Temp</u> TEST FLOW CHART <u>yes</u>

DATE	SPECIMEN I.D. (CONTROL/PATIENT)	RESULT (+ OR –)	INTERNAL CONTROL PASSED (Y or N)	CHARTED IN PATIENT RECORD	TECH INITIALS
7/11/20XX	POSITIVE CONTROL	+	Y		LP
7/11/20XX	NEGATIVE CONTROL	–	Y		LP
7/11/20XX	PT ID: 5432	+	Y	✓	LP

Procedure 50.5   Perform a CLIA-Waived Immunology Test: Perform the QuickVue+ Infectious Mononucleosis Test

Name _____ Date _____ Score _____

Tasks: Perform a capillary puncture. To perform and interpret a rapid CLIA-waived test for infectious mononucleosis. Document the results in the patient's health record.

Equipment and Supplies:
- Patient's health record
- Provider's order and/or lab requisition
- CLIA-waived QuickVue+ test kit for infectious mononucleosis and blood collecting supplies
  - Package with test kit supplies
  - Color-coded bottles of positive and negative controls and the developer
  - Test cassette in its foil-wrapped protective pouch
  - Pipets supplied in kit with black line indicating amount of capillary blood to collect
- Alcohol wipes, gauze, and bandage
- Lancet
- Laboratory timer, stopwatch, or wristwatch with sweep second hand
- Fluid-impermeable lab coat, protective eyewear, gloves
- Biohazard waste container
- Qualitative Control/Patient Log Sheet (Work Product 50.2)

Standard: Complete the procedure and all critical steps in _____ minutes with a minimum score of 85% within two attempts (*or as indicated by the instructor*).

Scoring: Divide the points earned by the total possible points. Failure to perform a critical step, indicated by an asterisk (*), results in grade no higher than an 84% (*or as indicated by the instructor*).

Time: Began_____ Ended_____ Total minutes: _____

Steps:	Point Value	Attempt 1	Attempt 2
1. Wash hands or use hand sanitizer. Put on the fluid-impermeable lab coat. Comply with safety practices.	5*		
2. Remove the test kit from the refrigerator and allow the reagents to warm to room temperature. Check the expiration date of the kit.	5		
3. Before running the first patient test from a new test kit, run the positive and negative liquid controls provided in the kit to see whether they react correctly. Record your control results on the log sheet.	10*		
4. Greet the patient. Identify yourself. Verify the patient's identity with full name, ask the patient to spell their first and last name, and give their date of birth.	5*		
5. Explain the procedure in a manner that the patient understands. Answer any general questions the patient may have about the collection procedures before you give detailed instructions. Obtain permission for the capillary puncture.	10*		
6. Put on gloves and protective eyewear.	5		
7. Remove the test device from its protective pouch, and label it with the patient's identification.	5		

8.	Disinfect the patient's finger with an alcohol wipe. Allow it to air dry and then perform a capillary puncture.	**10***		
9.	Wipe away the first drop of blood and then fill the disposable pipet provided in the kit to the calibration mark with capillary blood.	**10**		
10.	Dispense all the blood from the capillary tube into the "Add" well of the testing device. (Or, if you are using venous blood, transfer a large drop from the venous whole blood specimen using the longer capillary pipet provided in the kit.)	**5**		
11.	Hold the developer bottle vertically above the "Add" well and allow 5 drops to fall freely.	**5**		
12.	Read the results at 5 minutes. Note: The "Test Complete" box must be visibly colored by 10 minutes. • *Positive result*: A vertical line in any shade of blue forms a plus sign in the "Read Result" window, along with a blue "Test Complete" line. Even a faint blue plus sign should be reported as a positive. • *Negative result*: No vertical blue line appears, leaving a minus sign in the "Read Result" window, along with a blue "Test Complete" line. • *Invalid result*: After 10 minutes, no line is seen in the "Test Complete" window, or a blue color fills the "Read Result" window. If either of these is noted, the test must be repeated with a new testing device. If the problem continues, request technical support.	**10**		
13.	Dispose of biohazard waste in the biohazard waste container. Disinfect the work area.	**5**		
14.	Remove your gloves and protective eyewear. Wash hands or use hand sanitizer.	**5**		
15.	Document control results in the appropriate laboratory log. Document patient results in the appropriate laboratory log and in the patient's health record.	**5***		
	Total Points	**100**		

Documentation

Comments

CAAHEP Competencies	Step(s)
I.P.2.c. Perform: capillary puncture	5, 8
I.P.10. Perform a quality control measure	3
I.P.11.d. Collect specimens and perform: CLIA-waived immunology test	Entire procedure (collection only)
II.P.2. Record laboratory test results into the patient's record	15
III.P.2. Select appropriate barrier/personal protective equipment (PPE)	1, 6
III.P.10.a. Demonstrate proper disposal of biohazardous material: sharps	13
III.P.10.b. Demonstrate proper disposal of biohazardous material: regulated wastes	13
XII.P.1. Comply with safety practices	1
ABHES Competencies	**Step(s)**
4. Medical Law and Ethics a. Follow documentation guidelines	15
9. Medical Laboratory Procedures a. Practice Quality Control	3
9.b. Perform selected CLIA-waived test that assist with diagnosis and treatment 4) immunology testing	Entire procedure
9.b. Perform selected CLIA-waived test that assist with diagnosis and treatment 6) kit testing	Entire procedure
9.c. Dispose of biohazardous materials	13
9.d. Collect, label, and process a specimen 2) Perform capillary puncture	5, 8

Work Product 50.2 Qualitative Control/Patient Log Sheet

To be used with Procedure 50.5.

Name _____ Date _____ Score _____

Directions: Document the patient's result and the control sample results on the log.

QUALITATIVE CONTROL/PATIENT LOG SHEET

TEST: <u>Mononucleosis Rapid Test</u>

KIT NAME & MANUFACTURER: QUICK VUE+ Infectious Mononucleosis Test -QUIDEL

LOT # <u>12345</u>   EXPIRATION DATE: <u>11/22/20XX</u>

STORAGE REQUIREMENTS: <u>Refrigerator</u> TEST FLOW CHART <u>yes</u>

DATE	SPECIMEN I.D. (CONTROL/PATIENT)	RESULT (+ OR −)	INTERNAL CONTROL PASSED (Y or N)	CHARTED IN PATIENT RECORD	TECH INITIALS
7/11/20XX	POSITIVE CONTROL	+	Y		LP
7/11/20XX	NEGATIVE CONTROL	−	Y		LP
7/11/20XX	PT ID: 5432	−	Y	✓	LP

Procedure 50.6 Coach a Patient on the Guaiac Fecal Occult Blood Test

Name _____ Date _____ Score _____

Tasks: Coach a patient on the guaiac fecal occult blood test (gFOBT), while considering the patient's developmental life stage. Document the coaching in the health record.

Background: When coaching patients, it is important to consider their developmental life stage. When working with older adults, it is important to communicate with dignity and respect. Use simpler language. Speak clearly and allow time for the patient to respond. It is important to find out what they know about the topic and respectfully correct any inaccuracies. Make sure to listen to their concerns and provide resources as needed.

Scenario: You work at WMFM Clinic. You are working with Dr. David Kahn, who asked you to coach Charles Johnson (date of birth [DOB] 03/03/19XX) on the gFOBT. He is to receive three Hemoccult cards for stool smears.

Directions: Role-play the scenario with a peer, who is the patient. Your instructor is the provider. Use the following as the patient instructions:

Patient Instructions for Guaiac Fecal Occult Blood Test

To prepare for the test, avoid the following for 3 days prior to the test and while collecting the sample(s):
- Aspirin and nonsteroidal antiinflammatory drugs (NSAIDs) (e.g., ibuprofen and naproxen)
- More than 250 mg of vitamin C daily from supplements and foods (e.g., fruit and fruit juices)
- Red meats (e.g., pork, beef, and lamb)
- Horseradish, cantaloupe, raw turnips, broccoli, cauliflower, red radishes, and parsnips
- Antacids
- Antidiarrheal medications
- Iron supplements

To store cards and collect the specimens:
- Keep the Hemoccult test cards in their envelopes (if given that way). Keep the cards at room temperature, away from heat, light, chemicals, children, and pets.
- Prepare the card by writing your name, age, and address on the front of the card, if they are not prelabeled by the provider.
- Before collecting the sample, write the date on the front of the card.
- Prepare to collect the stool, using one of these three ways:
  - Either use a clean disposable container.
  - If given a flushable collection tissue with the Hemoccult card, unfold the tissue paper. Float it on the surface of the toilet water. The edges will stick to the side of the bowl and your stool will fall on the tissue. Sometimes water will collect on the tissue and this is fine.
  - Apply plastic wrap to the bowl.
- Remove the Hemoccult test card from the envelope and place it with the applicator stick in a dry location in the bathroom. Do not get them wet.
- Open the large flap on the front of the card. Sometimes there is a blue discoloration on the squares marked A and B, but this will not affect the test results.
- After collecting the stool, use the applicator stick and place a thin smear of stool in the square marked A.
- Do the same thing for the square marked B but take a sample from another part of the stool. Wrap the applicator stick in toilet paper and discard in the wastebasket. Empty the stool in the toilet and flush.
- Close the flap on the Hemoccult test card and insert the front flap under the tab. Store the card in the envelope until you have completed collecting all the samples. Keep the card in a cool dark place. Do not place it in a plastic bag or in the refrigerator.

- Wash your hands well with soap and water.
- Repeat these directions on days 2 and 3.
- Return the Hemoccult cards to the provider or the laboratory. If you are to mail the cards back, allow the last Hemoccult card to dry overnight. Then place the cards in the special mailing pouch you received and seal. Return the cards immediately.

Equipment and Supplies:
- Hemoccult test kit (Hemoccult cards, applicator sticks, and if available flushable collection tissue)
- Patient instructions
- Patient's health record
- Pen

Standard: Complete the procedure and all critical steps in _____ minutes with a minimum score of 85% within two attempts (*or as indicated by the instructor*).

Scoring: Divide the points earned by the total possible points. Failure to perform a critical step, indicated by an asterisk (*), results in grade no higher than an 84% (*or as indicated by the instructor*).

Time: Began_____ Ended_____ Total minutes: _____

Steps:	Point Value	Attempt 1	Attempt 2
1. Wash hands or use hand sanitizer.	10		
2. Greet the patient. Identify yourself. Verify the patient's identity with full name and date of birth. Explain what you will be doing.	10		
3. Use simpler language when talking. Speak clearly. Communicate with dignity and respect. Allow time for the patient to respond. Listen to the patient's concerns.	15*		
4. Ask the patient if he has ever taken a guaiac fecal occult blood test. If so, ask him what he remembers about it.	10		
5. Discuss the purpose of the test and the supplies needed (e.g., Hemoccult cards, applicator kits, and if available, flushable collection tissue). Show the supplies to the patient.	10		
6. Discuss how the patient needs to prepare for the tests and refer to the written instructions.	15		
7. Discuss how the patient should collect and return the Hemoccult cards. Use the written directions when coaching the patient. Write the patient's name, date of birth, and address on the Hemoccult cards if required by the agency.	10		
8. Ask the patient to teach back the preparation and the collection to you. Clarify any misconceptions or inaccuracies. Answer any questions the patient may have.	10		
9. Document the coaching in the patient's health record. Include the provider's name, what was taught, how the patient responded, and indicate the supplies and written directions sent home with the patient.	10		
Total Points	100		

Documentation

Comments

CAAHEP Competencies	Step(s)
V.P.3.b. Coach patients regarding: medical encounters	Entire procedure
X.P.3. Document patient care accurately in the medical record	9
ABHES Competencies	**Step(s)**
4. Medical Law and Ethics a. Follow documentation guidelines	9
9.e. Instruct patients in the collection of 2) fecal specimen	Entire procedure

Procedure 50.7 Developing a Hemoccult Card and Performing Quality Control

Name _____ Date _____ Score _____

Tasks: Develop a stool specimen using a Hemoccult card and perform a quality control test. Document the test results in the patient's health record.

Scenario: Charles Johnson (DOB 03/03/19XX) returns his Hemoccult card(s). Dr. David Kahn is his provider. You need to develop (test) the sample.

Equipment and Supplies:
- Hemoccult card with stool smear applied
- Hemoccult developer
- Gloves
- Biohazard waste container
- Waste container
- Patient's health record
- Timer

Standard: Complete the procedure and all critical steps in _____ minutes with a minimum score of 85% within two attempts (*or as indicated by the instructor*).

Scoring: Divide the points earned by the total possible points. Failure to perform a critical step, indicated by an asterisk (*), results in grade no higher than an 84% (*or as indicated by the instructor*).

Time: Began_____ Ended_____ Total minutes: _____

Steps:	Point Value	Attempt 1	Attempt 2
1. Wash hands or use hand sanitizer. Put on gloves.	10		
2. Identify when the specimen was applied and if testing can be done.	10		
3. Open the back of the card and apply two drops of the Hemoccult developer to the guaiac paper directly over each smear.	15		
4. Within 60 seconds, read the result accurately.	10		
5. Perform quality control on the card by applying one drop of the Hemoccult developer between the positive and negative Performance Monitors area.	10*		
6. Within 10 seconds, accurately read the results.	10*		
7. Discard the Hemoccult card in the biohazard bag. Clean up the area. Remove gloves and discard in the waste container.	10		
8. Wash hands or use hand sanitizer.	10		
9. Document the test result and the provider notified in the patient's health record.	15		
Total Points	**100**		

Documentation

Comments

CAAHEP Competencies	Step(s)
I.P.10. Perform a quality control measure	5, 6
II.P.2. Record laboratory test results into the patient's record	9
III.P.2. Select appropriate barrier/personal protective equipment (PPE)	1
III.P.10.b. Demonstrate proper disposal of biohazardous material: regulated wastes	7
ABHES Competencies	**Step(s)**
4. Medical Law and Ethics a. Follow documentation guidelines	9
8. Clinical Procedures e. Perform specialty procedures, including but not limited to minor surgery, cardiac, respiratory, OB-GYN, neurological, and gastroenterology	Entire procedure
9. Medical Laboratory Procedures a. Practice Quality Control	5, 6
9.c. Dispose of biohazardous materials	7

Procedure 50.8   Coach a Patient on Collecting a Stool Specimen for the Cologuard Test

Name _____ **Date** _____ **Score** _____

Tasks: Coach a patient on collecting a stool specimen for a Cologuard test, while considering their developmental level. Document the coaching in the health record.

Background: When coaching patients, it is important to consider their developmental life stage. When working with older adults, it is important to communicate with dignity and respect. Use simpler language. Speak clearly and allow time for the patient to respond. It is important to find out what they know about the topic and respectfully correct any inaccuracies. Make sure to listen to their concerns and provide resources as needed.

Scenario: You work at WMFM Clinic. You are working with Dr. David Kahn, who asked you to coach Charles Johnson (DOB 03/03/19XX) on the Cologuard test.

Directions: Role play the scenario with a peer, who is the patient. Your instructor is the provider.

Equipment and Supplies:
- Cologuard test kit (box with plastic bag, sample container, bottle of preservative, bracket, tube, sample labels, and directions)
- Patient instructions (optional)
- Patient's health record
- Pen

Patient Instructions for a Cologuard Test

- Purpose of the Cologuard test: to identify altered DNA and blood in the stool
- Do not collect a stool sample if they have diarrhea, bleeding hemorrhoids, rectal bleeding, menstrual period, or cuts or wounds on their hands.
- Make sure the sample can be returned within a day of collecting it. The laboratory must have the sample within 72 hours, so consider mailing delays such as holidays and weekends.
- When collecting the sample:
  - The box, zippered plastic bag, and the tray will be used to return the sample.
  - Remove the bracket from the box and unfold the sides. Please the bracket under the toilet seat near the back of the toilet. Lower the toilet seat.
  - Remove the sample container from the box. Remove the lid of the container and set the lid aside. Place the sample container in the hole in the center of the bracket.
  - Empty your bladder first. Avoid getting urine, toilet paper, or other material in the sample container.
  - Have a bowel movement. The stool sample should be no larger than the bottle of preservative, which is found in the box. Make sure the toilet paper is not placed in the container.
- After completing the bowel movement:
  - Remove the sample (specimen) container from the bracket and place a counter or other stable surface.
  - Remove the bracket from the toilet and discard.
  - Remove the tube from the box and unscrew the cap. Pull the probe from the tube. Use the probe to scrap the surface of the stool in the container until the probe has stool on it. Make sure the grooves on the probe are filled with stool, but do not fill the tube with stool. Place the probe back into the tube and tighten the cap. Set the tube aside.
  - Remove the bottle of preservative out of the box and remove the cap. Pour all of the preservative into the sample container. The preservative bottle and cap can be discarded.

- Place the lid on the sample container and tighten the lid. Remove the Sample Label Card from the box and complete both labels. Write your first and last name, date of birth (MM/DD/YY), the date you collected the sample (MM/DD/YY) and the time you collected the sample. Circle AM or PM. Remove one of the labels from the paper and wrap the label around the tube. Remove the other label and place it on the sample container.
- Place the tube and the sample container into the tray, which sits in the plastic bag in the box. Close the bag, removing the air. Close the box, peel the paper backing off the tape on the box lid, and secure the top of the box. Return the box within a day.

Standard: Complete the procedure and all critical steps in _____ minutes with a minimum score of 85% within two attempts (*or as indicated by the instructor*)

Scoring: Divide the points earned by the total possible points. Failure to perform a critical step, indicated by an asterisk (*), results in grade no higher than an 84% (*or as indicated by the instructor*).

Time: Began_____ Ended_____ Total minutes: _____

Steps:	Point Value	Attempt 1	Attempt 2
1. Wash hands or use hand sanitizer.	10		
2. Greet the patient. Identify yourself. Verify the patient's identity with full name and date of birth. Explain what you will be doing.	10		
3. Use simpler language when talking. Speak clearly. Communicate with dignity and respect. Allow time for the patient to respond. Listen to the patient's concerns.	15		
4. Ask the patient if he has ever collected a specimen for a Cologuard test. If so, ask him what he remembers about it.	10		
5. Discuss the purpose of the test, time to take the sample, and the supplies in the box.	10*		
6. Discuss how the patient should prepare to collect the sample.	10*		
7. Discuss the activities the patient needs to do after the collection, including the use of the probe, adding the preservative to the sample, and packing the box.	10		
8. Ask the patient to teach back the preparation and the collection to you. Clarify any misconceptions or inaccuracies. Answer any questions the patient may have.	10		
9. Document the coaching in the patient's health record. Include the provider's name, what was taught, how the patient responded, and indicate the supplies and written directions sent home with the patient.	15		
Total Points	100		

Documentation

Comments

CAAHEP Competencies	Step(s)
V.P.3.b. Coach patients regarding: medical encounters	Entire procedure
X.P.3. Document patient care accurately in the medical record	9
ABHES Competencies	**Step(s)**
4. Medical Law and Ethics a. Follow documentation guidelines	9
9.e. Instruct patients in the collection of 2) fecal specimen	Entire procedure

Intravenous Therapy

CAAHEP Competencies	Assessment
I.P.4.a. Verify the rules of medication administration: right patient	Procedures 51.2, 51.3
I.P.4.b. Verify the rules of medication administration: right medication	Procedures 51.1, 51.3
I.P.4.c. Verify the rules of medication administration: right dose	Procedures 51.1, 51.3
I.P.4.d. Verify the rules of medication administration: right route	Procedures 51.1, 51.3
I.P.4.e. Verify the rules of medication administration: right time	Procedure 51.3
I.P.4.f. Verify the rules of medication administration: right documentation	Procedures 51.2, 51.3
III.P.2. Select appropriate barrier/personal protective equipment (PPE)	Procedures 51.2, 51.4
III.P.10.a. Demonstrate proper disposal of biohazardous material: sharps	Procedures 51.2, 51.4
X.P.3. Document patient care accurately in the medical record	Procedures 51.2, 51.4

ABHES Competencies	Assessment
4. Medical Law and Ethics a. Follow documentation guidelines	Procedures 51.2, 51.4
8. Clinical Procedures a. Practice standard precautions and perform disinfection/ sterilization techniques	Procedures 51.1, 51.2, 51.3, 51.4
8. f. Prepare and administer oral and parenteral medications and monitor intravenous (IV) infusions	Procedures 51.1, 51.2, 51.3, 51.4

VOCABULARY REVIEW

Using the word pool on the right, find the correct word to match the definition. Write the word on the line after the definition.

Group A

1. Administered into a vein _____
2. Administration and monitoring of fluid and medication by intravenous infusion _____
3. Another name for the medication port on an IV solution bag

    _____
4. Located next to the medication port on an IV solution bag

    _____
5. Created when solutes are dissolved in a solvent

    _____
6. A glucose solution administered intravenously

    _____
7. A substance that is dissolved in a liquid to form a solution

    _____
8. A liquid that is able to dissolve other substances

    _____
9. Liquid found between the cells of the body

    _____
10. A medical term for low sodium _____

Word Pool
- crystalloid solution
- dextrose
- hyponatremia
- injection port
- interstitial fluid
- intravenous
- intravenous therapy
- IV tubing port
- solute
- solvent

Group B

1. Another name for an infusion set _____
2. The number of drops per milliliter of fluid

    _____
3. The number of drops in 1 minute required to infuse the ordered solution _____
4. Open condition of a body cavity or canal

    _____
5. Inflammation of a vein _____
6. The volume of fluid infused per hour _____
7. To run IV fluid through the tubing to remove all of the air

    _____
8. Occurs when the IV solution leaks or is administered into the surrounding tissues _____
9. Occurs when medication leaks into and damages the surrounding tissues _____
10. A medication that can damage tissue and produce blisters

    _____
11. An immune response that causes the body to react with an exaggerated response to a foreign agent or antigen

    _____
12. Circulatory or fluid overload _____

Word Pool
- drop factor
- extravasation
- flow rate
- hypersensitivity
- infiltration
- infusion rate
- patency
- phlebitis
- primary infusion set
- priming
- pulmonary edema
- vesicant medication

ABBREVIATIONS

Write out what each of the following abbreviations stands for.

1. IV _____

2. CT _____

3. 0.9% NaCl _____

4. D$_5$W _____

5. D$_5$LR _____

6. gtt _____

7. mL _____

8. DOB _____

SKILLS AND CONCEPTS

Answer the following questions. Write your answer on the line or in the space provided.

A. Introduction

1. Which of the following is a reason for IV therapy in ambulatory care?
    a. To replace fluids and electrolytes
    b. For treatment of infections and cancer
    c. For diagnostic tests
    d. All of the above

B. IV Solutions

1. What must be checked on the IV solution bag?
    a. IV solution type
    b. Amount of fluid in the bag
    c. Expiration date
    d. All of the above

2. What is a reason to discard an IV solution bag?
    a. Contains precipitate or looks cloudy
    b. Has expired or become contaminated
    c. Is no longer needed for the patient
    d. All of the above

3. _____ and plasma have a similar dissolved particle concentration.

4. What occurs when an isotonic solution is administered in the bloodstream?
    a. The fluid is distributed between the bloodstream, the interstitial fluid, and cells.
    b. It causes the fluid from the cells to move into the bloodstream, increasing the blood volume.
    c. The fluid moves out of the blood vessels and into the interstitial fluid and cells.
    d. None of the above.

5. Which is *not* an isotonic IV solution?
    a. 0.45% sodium chloride
    b. Dextrose 5% in lactated Ringer's
    c. 0.33% sodium chloride
    d. 2.5% dextrose in water

6. Which is a potential complication of administering isotonic IV solutions?
    a. Hypervolemia and hypertension
    b. Pulmonary crackles, dyspnea, and shortness of breath
    c. Peripheral edema
    d. All of the above

7. _____ have a lower concentration of dissolved particles than plasma.

8. What occurs when a hypotonic solution is administered in the bloodstream?
    a. The fluid is distributed between the bloodstream, the interstitial fluid, and cells.
    b. It causes the fluid from the cells to move into the bloodstream, increasing the blood volume.
    c. The fluid moves out of the blood vessels and into the interstitial fluid and cells.
    d. None of the above.

9. Which is a hypotonic IV solution?
    a. 0.45% sodium chloride
    b. 0.33% sodium chloride
    c. 2.5% dextrose in water
    d. All of the above

10. Which is a potential complication of administering hypotonic IV solutions?
    a. Hypervolemia and peripheral edema
    b. Pulmonary crackles, dyspnea, and shortness of breath
    c. Hypotension, dizziness, and confusion
    d. All of the above

11. _____ have a higher concentration of dissolved particles than plasma.

12. What occurs when a hypertonic solution is administered in the bloodstream?
    a. The fluid is distributed between the bloodstream, the interstitial fluid, and cells.
    b. It causes the fluid from the cells to move into the bloodstream, increasing the blood volume.
    c. The fluid moves out of the blood vessels and into the interstitial fluid and cells.
    d. None of the above.

13. Which is *not* a hypertonic IV solution?
    a. 3% sodium chloride
    b. Dextrose 5% in 0.45% sodium chloride
    c. 0.45% sodium chloride
    d. Dextrose 5% in lactated Ringer's

14. Which is a potential complication of administering hypertonic IV solutions?
    a. Hypervolemia and peripheral edema
    b. Pulmonary crackles, dyspnea, and shortness of breath
    c. Hypotension, dizziness, and confusion
    d. Both a and b

C. IV Infusion Sets

1. Which is a characteristic of macrodrip infusion sets?
   a. Create larger drops
   b. Create small drops
   c. Come in a variety of sizes
   d. Both a and c

2. When is a macrodrip infusion set used?
   a. For routine IV therapy in adults
   b. For routine IV therapy in children
   c. For delivering larger volume of fluid in an hour
   d. All of the above
   e. Both a and c

3. Which is a characteristic of minidrip infusion sets?
   a. Create larger drops
   b. Create small drops
   c. Come in a variety of sizes
   d. Both a and c

4. When is a minidrip infusion set used?
   a. When an adult needs a smaller volume of fluid
   b. For routine IV therapy in children
   c. For delivering larger volume of fluid in an hour
   d. All of the above
   e. Both a and b

5. A sterile _____ is inserted into an IV bag using the IV tubing port.

6. The _____ is used to count the drip rate of the IV if an IV pump is not used.

7. The _____ is used to control the rate at which the IV flows with a gravity infusion.

8. A(n) _____ is a cylinder holding a device that limits the amount of IV solutions given.

9. Why is a secondary infusion set used? _____

    _____

10. Which statement is correct regarding a secondary infusion set and IV bag?
    a. The secondary infusion set and IV bag hang higher than the primary infusion set.
    b. The secondary IV bag will infuse first.
    c. After the secondary IV bag is empty, the primary IV bag infuses.
    d. All of the above.

D. Additional Supplies and Equipment for IV Therapy

1. Which is the size range for IV catheters for adult infusions?
   a. 16- to 18-gauge
   b. 20- to 24-gauge
   c. 22- to 26-gauge
   d. 24- to 28-gauge

2. Catheters with a larger gauge than 20 can increase the risk of _____.

3. A(n) _____ is used to help engorge the vein during the insertion procedure.

4. Which of the following is an antiseptic that can be used to clean the IV insertion site?
   a. Chlorhexidine
   b. Betadine
   c. Alcohol
   d. All of the above

E. Pump and Gravity Infusions

Find the infusion rate. Round the answer to the nearest whole number and label the answer.

1. Order: 0.9% NS IV 250 mL over 5 hours. Infusion rate: _____

2. Order: 0.9% NS IV 250 mL over 2 hours. Infusion rate: _____

3. Order: 0.9% NS IV 250 mL over 3 hours. Infusion rate: _____

4. Order: 0.9% NS IV 500 mL over 10 hours. Infusion rate: _____

5. Order: 0.9% NS IV 1000 mL over 8 hours. Infusion rate: _____

6. Order: 0.9% NS IV 250 mL over 6 hours. Infusion rate: _____

7. Order: 0.9% NS IV 100 mL over 1 hour. Infusion rate: _____

8. Order: 0.9% NS IV 500 mL over 5 hours. Infusion rate: _____

9. Order: 0.9% NS IV 1000 mL over 6 hours. Infusion rate: _____

10. Order: 0.9% NS IV 1000 mL over 5 hours. Infusion rate: _____

11. Order: 0.9% NS IV 500 mL over 6 hours. Infusion rate: _____

12. Order: 0.9% NS IV 500 mL over 8 hours. Infusion rate: _____

13. Order: 0.9% NS IV 1000 mL over 7 hours. Infusion rate: _____

14. Order: 0.9% NS IV 1000 mL over 12 hours. Infusion rate: _____

15. Order: 0.9% NS IV 100 mL over 2 hours. Infusion rate: _____

16. Order: 0.9% NS IV 50 mL over 40 minutes. Infusion rate: _____

17. Order: 0.9% NS IV 100 mL over 40 minutes. Infusion rate: _____

18. Order: 0.9% NS IV 100 mL over 45 minutes. Infusion rate: _____

19. Order: 0.9% NS IV 50 mL over 50 minutes. Infusion rate: _____

20. Order: 0.9% NS IV 100 mL over 30 minutes. Infusion rate: _____

Find the flow rate. Round the answer to the nearest whole number and label the answer.

21. Order: 0.9% NS IV 50 mL over 60 min; Infusion set: Drop factor of 20 gtt/ml. Flow rate:

   _____

22. Order: 0.9% NS IV 75 mL over 50 min; Infusion set: Drop factor of 10 gtt/ml. Flow rate:

   _____

23. Order: 0.9% NS IV 50 mL over 30 min; Infusion set: Drop factor of 15 gtt/ml. Flow rate:

_____

24. Order: 0.9% NS IV 100 mL over 60 min; Infusion set: Drop factor of 20 gtt/ml. Flow rate:

_____

25. Order: 0.9% NS IV 50 mL over 60 min; Infusion set: Drop factor of 60 gtt/ml. Flow rate:

_____

26. Order: 0.9% NS IV 50 mL over 45 min; Infusion set: Drop factor of 60 gtt/ml. Flow rate:

_____

27. Order: 0.9% NS IV 50 mL over 45 min; Infusion set: Drop factor of 20 gtt/ml. Flow rate:

_____

28. Order: 0.9% NS IV 50 mL over 40 min; Infusion set: Drop factor of 20 gtt/ml. Flow rate:

_____

29. Order: 0.9% NS IV 100 mL over 80 min; Infusion set: Drop factor of 15 gtt/ml. Flow rate:

_____

30. Order: 0.9% NS IV 100 mL over 80 min; Infusion set: Drop factor of 10 gtt/ml. Flow rate:

_____

Find the infusion rate and then the flow rate. Round the answer to the nearest whole number and label the answer.

31. Order: 0.9% NS IV 250 mL over 4 hours; Infusion set: Drop factor of 20 gtt/ml.

Infusion rate: _____ Flow rate: _____

32. Order: 0.9% NS IV 100 mL over 2 hours; Infusion set: Drop factor of 10 gtt/ml.

Infusion rate: _____ Flow rate: _____

33. Order: 0.9% NS IV 250 mL over 3 hours; Infusion set: Drop factor of 15 gtt/ml.

Infusion rate: _____ Flow rate: _____

34. Order: 0.9% NS IV 1000 mL over 8 hours; Infusion set: Drop factor of 20 gtt/ml.

Infusion rate: _____ Flow rate: _____

35. Order: 0.9% NS IV 100 mL over 4 hours; Infusion set: Drop factor of 60 gtt/ml.

Infusion rate: _____ Flow rate: _____

36. Order: 0.9% NS IV 250 mL over 4 hours; Infusion set: Drop factor of 60 gtt/ml.

Infusion rate: _____ Flow rate: _____

37. Order: 0.9% NS IV 500 mL over 6 hours; Infusion set: Drop factor of 20 gtt/ml.

Infusion rate: _____ Flow rate: _____

38. Order: 0.9% NS IV 500 mL over 5 hours; Infusion set: Drop factor of 20 gtt/ml.

Infusion rate: _____ Flow rate: _____

39. Order: 0.9% NS IV 250 mL over 4 hours; Infusion set: Drop factor of 15 gtt/ml.

    Infusion rate: _____ Flow rate: _____

40. Order: 0.9% NS IV 250 mL over 3 hours; Infusion set: Drop factor of 10 gtt/ml.

    Infusion rate: _____ Flow rate: _____

F. Initiating IV Infusions

1. Which of the following items must an IV order include?
   a. Patient's name and date of birth (DOB)
   b. Type of IV solution
   c. Amount of fluid to infuse over a specific time period or the rate of the infusion for a specific time period
   d. All of the above

2. The IV tubing is _____, which prevents air from entering the patient's circulatory system.

3. If an IV attempt is unsuccessful, all future sites must be _____ to that site.

4. What must be considered if the IV is to remain in over a longer period of time, such as a few days?
   a. Use the nondominant hand/arm.
   b. Avoid inserting the catheter in the hand if the patient is using an assistive device.
   c. Avoid inserting the catheter near the wrist or elbow.
   d. All of the above.

5. What strategy can be used to help engorge a vein for an IV insertion?
   a. Using a tourniquet
   b. Stroking the vessel
   c. Applying a warm pack to the site for a few minutes
   d. Have the patient open and close his or her hand, making a fist
   e. All of the above

6. When using _____, scrub back and forth and up and down for 30 seconds. Allow the product to dry on the skin for at least _____ seconds.

7. If using _____ or _____, place the applicator at the intended site of insertion and work outward in a circular pattern, making larger circles as the area is cleaned.

8. With the bevel _____, insert the needle/catheter unit using a(n) _____-degree angle.

9. When is a blood flashback seen in the clear flashback chamber initially? _____

    _____

    _____

10. Jan, the patient, is having tingling and numbness while you are inserting the IV. What should you do?

    _____

    _____

G. Monitoring IV Therapy

1. When an IV is infusing, the patient must be checked every _____ minutes.

2. What must the medical assistant check when monitoring the IV infusion?
    a. The provider's order
    b. The name and amount of fluid
    c. The IV insertion site and flow rate (if it is a gravity infusion)
    d. All of the above

3. The IV tubing and insertion site must be changed every _____ hours.

4. The IV solution bag must be changed every _____ hours.

H. Complications of IV Therapy

1. The medical assistant should notify the _____ or _____ if they suspect a complication during IV therapy.

2. _____ occurs when the IV solution leaks or is administered into the surrounding tissues.

3. Which of the following causes infiltration?
    a. Improper placement of the IV catheter
    b. The catheter slips out of the blood vessel
    c. The catheter punctures through the blood vessel
    d. All of the above

4. Which of the following are *not* signs or symptoms of infiltration?
    a. Swelling, discomfort, or pain at the site
    b. Coolness, blanching, and tightness of the skin at the site
    c. Dyspnea and labored breathing
    d. Slowed or stopped IV flow rate

5. What step(s) should the medical assistant take if infiltration occurs?
    a. Stop the infusion.
    b. Remove the IV catheter.
    c. Elevate the extremity and apply a warm compress to the site.
    d. All of the above.

6. What can a medical assistant do to prevent infiltration?
    a. Insert the IV at a joint.
    b. Properly secure the catheter.
    c. Use the appropriate flow rate.
    d. All of the above.

7. _____ is the inflammation of a vein.

8. Which of the following does *not* cause phlebitis?
    a. The IV catheter rubbing on the walls of the vein
    b. Prolonged use of the site
    c. Air in the IV tubing
    d. Trauma during the insertion process
    e. Acidic, alkaline, or hypertonic IV solutions or medications

9. Which of the following are *not* signs or symptoms of phlebitis?
   a. Redness and tenderness at the insertion site
   b. Coolness, blanching, and tightness of the skin at the insertion site
   c. Heat or swelling at the insertion site
   d. Pain at the insertion site

10. _____ occurs when medication leaks into and damages the surrounding tissues.

11. How can a medical assistant prevent a local or systemic infection related to IV therapy?
    a. Wash their hands or use hand sanitizer before putting on gloves to start an IV.
    b. Use sterile technique when priming IV tubing and attaching the tubing to the catheter.
    c. Use aseptic technique during IV insertion.
    d. All of the above.

12. Which of the following are *not* signs or symptoms of pulmonary edema?
    a. Shortness of breath and dyspnea
    b. Productive cough and wheezing
    c. Peripheral edema
    d. Rapid pulse and a decreased blood pressure

13. List two ways a medical assistant can prevent an air embolism during IV therapy. _____

_____

_____

CERTIFICATION PREPARATION

Circle the correct answer.

1. Which is a reason for IV therapy in ambulatory healthcare facilities?
   a. To replace fluids and electrolytes
   b. To administer IV antibiotics for an infection
   c. To administer chemotherapy as a cancer treatment
   d. All of the above

2. Which is used to insert the infusion set into the IV solution bag?
   a. IV tubing port
   b. Drip chamber
   c. Roller clamp
   d. Slide clamp

3. Which of the following solutions is an isotonic solution?
   a. 10% dextrose in water
   b. 0.45% sodium chloride
   c. 0.9% sodium chloride
   d. 2.5% dextrose in water

4. Which statement is *not* correct regarding hypotonic solutions?
   a. Hypotonic solutions have a lower concentration of dissolved particles than plasma.
   b. Hypotonic solutions move out of the blood vessels and into the interstitial fluid and cells.
   c. Hypotonic solutions are typically ordered for patients with diabetic ketoacidosis.
   d. Hypotonic solutions can cause hypervolemia.

5. Which is *not* a sign of hypervolemia?
   a. Hypotension
   b. Pulmonary crackles
   c. Dyspnea
   d. Shortness of breath

6. Which device prevents fluids or medication from traveling up the IV tubing and into the IV solution bag?
   a. Luer connector
   b. Backcheck valve
   c. Injection port
   d. Drip chamber

7. What is the infusion rate for this order? Order: 0.9% NS IV 300 mL over 4 hours. Infusion set: Drop factor of 20 gtt/mL
   a. 20 gtt/min
   b. 25 gtt/min
   c. 25 mL/hr
   d. 75 mL/hr

8. Which is the flow rate for this order? Order: 0.9% NS IV 50 mL over 40 minutes. Infusion set: Drop factor of 20 gtt/mL
   a. 30 gtt/min
   b. 25 gtt/min
   c. 75 mL/hr
   d. 25 mL/hr

9. Which is the flow rate for this order? Order: 0.9% NS IV 400 mL over 6 hours. Infusion set: Drop factor of 60 gtt/mL
   a. 67 gtt/min
   b. 400 gtt/min
   c. 15 mL/hr
   d. 67 mL/hr

10. The insertion site of an IV is in a joint area. This increases the risk for _____ to occur.
    a. extravasation
    b. phlebitis
    c. infiltration
    d. hypersensitivity

WORKPLACE APPLICATIONS

1. Dr. Martin orders IV therapy for Mr. Sam Jones. Gabe initiates the IV therapy. After 40 minutes, the patient has swelling and pain at the insertion site. The insertion site is cool to touch and the skin is tight.

   a. What might be occurring? _____

   _____

   _____

   b. What should Gabe do? _____

   _____

   _____

   c. What can be done to reduce the swelling at the insertion site? _____

   _____

2. Gabe is helping the registered nurse monitor an IV infusion. The patient starts to have burning and pain at the insertion site and blistering occurs.

   a. What might be happening? _____

   _____

   b. What should Gabe do? _____

   _____

3. When Gabe is helping the RN monitor an antibiotic IV infusion, the patient has a hypersensitivity reaction. What medications might the provider order to help treat the hypersensitivity reaction?

   _____

   _____

INTERNET ACTIVITIES

1. Using online resources, research the equipment and supplies used for IV therapy in ambulatory care. Create a poster presentation, a PowerPoint presentation, or write a paper summarizing your research. Include a description of the product and how it is used for IV therapy.

2. Using online resources, research one of the complications of IV therapy. Create a poster presentation, a PowerPoint presentation, or write a paper summarizing your research.

Procedure 51.1   Prime an IV Infusion Set

Name _____   **Date** _____   **Score** _____

Task: Prime an IV infusion set with IV solution.

Scenario: Dr. Martin ordered LR 500 mL over 5 hours for Celia Tapia (DOB 05/18/19XX). You need to administer the IV infusion.

Equipment and Supplies:
- Provider's order
- Patient's health record
- Primary IV infusion set
- IV fluid (LR 500 mL)
- Time label and marker or pen
- Waste container
- Sink or basin

Standard: Complete the procedure and all critical steps in _____ minutes with a minimum score of 85% within two attempts (*or as indicated by the instructor*).

Scoring: Divide the points earned by the total possible points. Failure to perform a critical step, indicated by an asterisk (*), results in grade no higher than an 84% (*or as indicated by the instructor*).

Time: Began_____ Ended_____ Total minutes: _____

Steps	Point Value	Attempt 1	Attempt 2
1. Wash your hands or use hand sanitizer. Review the order. Clarify any questions you have with the provider.	5		
2. Select the IV solution bag from the storage area. Check the IV solution label against the order. Check for the right name, form, and route. Check the expiration date to make sure the IV solution is not expired. Verify the right dose and the right time.	10*		
3. Assemble the supplies required for the procedure. Remove the IV solution from the outer plastic packaging if present.	5		
4. Check the IV bag for leaks. Check the IV fluid for unusual color, precipitate, or cloudiness.	10*		
5. Remove the primary IV tubing from the packaging. Position the roller clamp about 1 inch below the drip chamber. Close the roller clamp. Keep the spike and luer connector sterile.	10*		
6. Perform the second medication check. Check the IV solution label against the order. Check for the right name, form, and route.	5*		
7. Remove the covers from the IV solution port and the IV tubing spike. Maintain the sterility of both during the removal process.	10*		
8. Insert the IV tubing spike into the IV solution port, using a twisting motion. Hang the IV solution bag on the IV pole or hook. Hold the luer connector end of the IV tubing.	5		
9. Gently squeeze the drip chamber so it fills about half full.	5		

10. Slowly open the roller clamp to prime the tubing. Invert the ports and any valves as the fluid passes. Tap the air out of the ports and valve. Remove the cover on the luer connector and keep end sterile. Hold the luer connector end over a sink or basin and allow a small amount of fluid to drain out of the tubing.	10		
11. Close the roller clamp. Check the tubing for air. If air is found, reposition the tubing as needed to help move the air either to the drip chamber or out through the luer connector. Slowly open the roller clamp and allow a small amount of fluid to drain to remove the air. When the tubing is free of air, cover the luer connector end with the sterile cover.	10*		
12. Place the tubing on the IV hook or pole. Perform the third medication check. Check the IV solution label against the order. Check for the right name, form, and route.	5		
13. Following the healthcare facility's policy, complete the IV bag label with a pen or marker and place label on the solution.	5		
14. Clean up the work area. Packaging and other waste should be discarded in the waste container.	5		
Total Points	100		

Comments

CAAHEP Competencies	Step(s)
I.P.4.b. Verify the rules of medication administration: right medication	2, 6, 12
I.P.4.c. Verify the rules of medication administration: right dose	2, 6, 12
I.P.4.d. Verify the rules of medication administration: right route	2, 6, 12
ABHES Competencies	**Step(s)**
8. Clinical Procedures a. Practice standard precautions and perform disinfection/ sterilization techniques	1
8. f. Prepare and administer oral and parenteral medications and monitor intravenous (IV) infusions	Entire procedure

Procedure 51.2   Administer IV Fluids

Name _____ **Date** _____ **Score** _____

Tasks: Insert an IV catheter, attach the primed IV tubing with the IV solution, and document in the patient's health record.

Scenario: Dr. Martin ordered LR 500 mL over 5 hours for Celia Tapia (DOB 05/18/19XX). You need to administer the IV infusion.

Equipment and Supplies:
- Provider's order
- Patient's health record
- Primed IV infusion set attached to the IV solution bag with an IV stand or hook
- Infusion pump (optional)
- Short extension tubing with syringe containing 1 to 3 mL of 0.9% sodium chloride (optional)
- IV safety catheter
- IV start kit
- Gloves
- Biohazard sharps container
- Waste container

Standard: Complete the procedure and all critical steps in _____ minutes with a minimum score of 85% within two attempts (*or as indicated by the instructor*).

Scoring: Divide the points earned by the total possible points. Failure to perform a critical step, indicated by an asterisk (*), results in grade no higher than an 84% (*or as indicated by the instructor*).

Time: Began_____ Ended_____ Total minutes: _____

Steps:	Point Value	Attempt 1	Attempt 2
1. Wash your hands or use hand sanitizer. Review the order. Clarify any questions you have with the provider.	3		
2. Calculate the infusion rate. Calculate the flow rate if needed.	5*		
3. Gather the supplies and equipment needed, included the primed IV tubing with the IV solution and the IV pole or hook. If using short extension tubing, remove any protective covers, prime with the 0.9% sodium chloride, and replace protective cover to maintain the sterility of the tubing.	2		
4. Prior to entering the exam room, knock on the door and wait a moment. Greet the patient. Identify yourself. Verify the patient's identity with full name and date of birth. Make sure the patient's information matches the order and the record. Explain what you are going to do.	5*		
5. Provide the right education to the patient. Explain the medication ordered, the desired effect, and common side effects; also identify the provider who ordered it. Answer any questions the parent/patient may have. Use language the parent/patient can understand. Ask if the patient has any allergies. If the parent/patient refuses the medication, notify the provider.	5*		
6. Use hand sanitizer and put on gloves.	5		

7.	Ask the patient which arm they prefer. Apply the tourniquet about 4 to 6 inches above the intended site. Do not apply the tourniquet too tight to injury the tissue. Check for a radial pulse. If the radial pulse is absent, loosen the tourniquet.	5*		
8.	Palpate the vein with your index finger. Select a straight well-dilated vein that is large enough for the IV catheter. Stroke the vessel or have the patient open and close his or her hand, making a fist.	5		
9.	Release a tourniquet.	5*		
10.	Clean the intended site with the antiseptic swab or applicator as indicated by the facility's policies. If chlorhexidine is used, do a 30-second friction scrub back and forth and up and down at the site. Let the site dry. If using Betadine or alcohol, clean in a circular pattern working outwardly. Allow the Betadine to dry.	5*		
11.	Using the dominant hand, firmly grip the catheter on each side of the hub. Use the nondominant hand to hold the skin tautly. Apply distal traction and anchor the vein with the thumb.	5		
12.	With the bevel up, position the needle unit parallel and directly above the vein. Inform the patient of the insertion.	5		
13.	Insert the needle in the skin using a 10- to 30-degree angle. Aim toward the vein and slowly advance until blood flashback is seen in the clear flashback chamber. Loosen the tourniquet.	5		
14.	Lower the angle of the needle unit. Advance the cannula over the needle until the hub sits on the skin.	5		
15.	Stabilize the catheter. With the dominant hand, withdraw the needle and activate the safety device if needed. Depending on the type of device used, apply pressure over the vein above the catheter if needed.	5*		
16.	Secure the luer connector on the tubing to the catheter hub without contaminating the hub. If the extension tubing is used, occlude the tubing with the slide clamp, remove the syringe, and connect the extension tubing to the primary infusion set.	5		
17.	Tape the catheter hub to the skin. Per the facility's policy, place the transparent dressing over the insertion site or place a 2x2-inch gauze dressing over the insertion site and the hub.	5		
18.	Create a loop with the IV tubing and secure the tubing to the skin with tape.	5		
19.	Set the infusion rate if using a pump and ensure the clamps are opened. If using gravity infusion, count the drops and adjust the roller clamp to get the correct flow rate.	5*		
20.	Observe the site for swelling during the infusion of the fluid.	3*		
21.	Discard the needle in the biohazard sharps container. Clean up the area. Discard the supplies per the facility's policy. Remove gloves and wash or sanitize hands.	2		
22.	Document the procedure, including the ordering provider's name, IV order, the type and size of the catheter inserted, number of attempts, IV solution, and the infusion rate.	5*		
	Total Points	100		

Documentation

Comments

CAAHEP Competencies	Step(s)
I.P.4.a. Verify the rules of medication administration: right patient	4
I.P.4.f. Verify the rules of medication administration: right documentation	22
III.P.2. Select appropriate barrier/personal protective equipment (PPE).	6
III.P.10.a. Demonstrate proper disposal of biohazardous material: sharps	21
X.P.3. Document patient care accurately in the medical record	22
ABHES Competencies	**Step(s)**
4. Medical Law and Ethics a. Follow documentation guidelines	22
8. Clinical Procedures a. Practice standard precautions and perform disinfection/ sterilization techniques	1, 6
8. f. Prepare and administer oral and parenteral medications and monitor intravenous (IV) infusions	20

Procedure 51.3 Changing an IV Bag

Name _____ Date _____ Score _____

Task: Change an IV bag

Scenario: Dr. Martin ordered LR 500 mL over 5 hours for Celia Tapia (DOB 05/18/19XX). The first bag you hung was 250 mL and now you need to switch bags to give the last 250 mL.

Equipment and Supplies:
- Provider's order
- IV bag

Standard: Complete the procedure and all critical steps in _____ minutes with a minimum score of 85% within two attempts *(or as indicated by the instructor).*

Scoring: Divide the points earned by the total possible points. Failure to perform a critical step, indicated by an asterisk (*), results in grade no higher than an 84% *(or as indicated by the instructor).*

Time: Began_____ Ended_____ Total minutes: _____

Steps:	Point Value	Attempt 1	Attempt 2
1. Wash your hands or use hand sanitizer. Review the order. Clarify any questions you have with the provider.	10		
2. Select the IV solution bag from the storage area. Check the IV solution label against the order. Check for the right name, form, and route. Check the expiration date to make sure the IV solution is not expired. Verify the right dose and the right time.	10*		
3. Remove the IV solution from the outer plastic packaging if present. Check the IV bag for leaks. Check the IV fluid for unusual color, precipitate, or cloudiness.	10*		
4. Perform the second medication check. Check the IV solution label against the order. Check for the right name, form, and route.	10*		
5. Prior to entering the exam room, knock on the door and wait a moment. Greet the patient. Identify yourself. Verify the patient's identity with full name and date of birth. Make sure the patient's information matches the order and the record. Explain what you are going to do.	10*		
6. Perform the third medication check. Hang the new IV solution bag on the IV pole.	10*		
7. Pause the IV infusion pump or close the roller clamp if giving the IV by gravity.	10		
8. Remove the protective plastic cover over the tubing port. Remove the old IV bag from the pole and turn the bag upside down. Using a twisting motion remove the IV tubing spike from the IV bag. Using a twisting motion, insert the spike in the new IV bag at using the tubing port. Keep the spike sterile during this procedure.	10*		

9. If the drip chamber is less than 1/3 to 1/2 filled, squeeze the drip chamber to fill it to this level. Check for air in the tubing before restarting the infusion pump or opening and regulating the roller clamp.	10		
10. Label the bag per the healthcare facility's policy. If the facility requires documentation when administering a new bag of fluid, document at this time.	10		
Total Points	100		

Documentation

Comments

CAAHEP Competencies	Step(s)
I.P.4.a. Verify the rules of medication administration: right patient	5
I.P.4.b. Verify the rules of medication administration: right medication	2, 4, 6
I.P.4.c. Verify the rules of medication administration: right dose	2, 4, 6
I.P.4.d. Verify the rules of medication administration: right route	2, 4, 6
I.P.4.e. Verify the rules of medication administration: right time	2, 4, 6
I.P.4.f. Verify the rules of medication administration: right documentation	10
ABHES Competencies	**Step(s)**
8. Clinical Procedures a. Practice standard precautions and perform disinfection/ sterilization techniques	1
8. f. Prepare and administer oral and parenteral medications and monitor intravenous (IV) infusions	Entire procedure

Procedure 51.4   Remove an IV Catheter

Name _____   Date _____   Score _____

Tasks: Remove an IV catheter and document the patient care.

Scenario: Dr. Martin ordered LR 500 mL over 5 hours for Celia Tapia (DOB 05/18/19XX). The fluid has been infused and the IV needs to be discontinued or removed.

Equipment and Supplies:
- Provider's order
- Sterile gauze (e.g., 2x2s)
- Gloves
- Hypoallergenic self-stick wrap, tape, or bandage
- Patient's health record

Standard: Complete the procedure and all critical steps in _____ minutes with a minimum score of 85% within two attempts (*or as indicated by the instructor*).

Scoring: Divide the points earned by the total possible points. Failure to perform a critical step, indicated by an asterisk (*), results in grade no higher than an 84% (*or as indicated by the instructor*).

Time: Began_____ Ended_____ Total minutes: _____

Steps:	Point Value	Attempt 1	Attempt 2
1. Wash your hands or use hand sanitizer. Review the order. Clarify any questions you have with the provider.	10		
2. Gather the supplies needed.	10		
3. Prior to entering the exam room, knock on the door and wait a moment. Greet the patient. Identify yourself. Verify the patient's identity with full name and date of birth. Make sure the patient's information matches the order and the record. Explain what you are going to do.	10*		
4. Apply gloves. Open the supplies. If an IV is infusing, stop the flow.	10		
5. Remove tape that secured the tubing to the skin. Hold the IV catheter with one hand. With the other hand, start to remove the transparent dressing, by loosening one side and stretching the dressing. Then loosen and stretch the dressing on the opposite side. Completely remove the transparent dressing.	10		
6. Hold the sterile gauze above the insertion site. Pull the IV catheter back and straight out.	10		
7. Once the catheter is removed, place the sterile gauze over the site and hold pressure until the bleeding has stopped, which may be 2 to 3 minutes.	10		
8. Inspect the catheter tip for any breakage. Discard the catheter in the biohazard sharps container.	10*		
9. Once the bleeding has stopped, replace the gauze with a new piece of sterile gauze. Secure the gauze with a hypoallergenic self-stick wrap, tape, or bandage. Ensure the patient has adequate blood flow below the site.	5		
10. Clean up the area. Discard the supplies per the facility's policy. Remove gloves and wash or sanitize hands.	5		
11. Document the IV catheter removal. Include ordering provider's name, the order, the amount of fluid infused and the appearance of the catheter tip.	10		
Total Points	**100**		

Documentation

| |
| |
| |
| |
| |
| |
| |
| |
| |
| |

Comments

CAAHEP Competencies	Step(s)
III.P.2. Select appropriate barrier/personal protective equipment (PPE).	4
III.P.10.a. Demonstrate proper disposal of biohazardous material: sharps	8
X.P.3. Document patient care accurately in the medical record	11
ABHES Competencies	**Step(s)**
4. Medical Law and Ethics a. Follow documentation guidelines	11
8. Clinical Procedures a. Practice standard precautions and perform disinfection/sterilization techniques	1, 4
8. f. Prepare and administer oral and parenteral medications and monitor intravenous (IV) infusions	Entire procedure

Radiology Basics

CAAHEP Competencies	Assessment
None	

ABHES Competencies	Assessment
None	

VOCABULARY REVIEW

Using the word pool on the right, find the correct word to match the definition. Write the word on the line after the definition.

Group A

1. The organization that publishes the curriculum for the limited x-ray machine operator is the _____.

2. A device that contains a moving grid is the _____.

3. _____ is a cassette-based digital imaging system where the image of the body part is obtained using storage phosphor plate.

4. The source of the x-rays is the _____.

5. The organization that writes the certification examination for limited x-ray machine operators is the _____.

6. _____ is generated from the patient.

7. The radiation that leaves the tube is _____.

8. The squared area of the x-ray beam that strikes the patient and x-ray table is the _____.

9. _____ is a cassetteless imaging system where the phosphor is bonded to a flat panel detector or the system converts x-ray energy directly to an electronic signal.

10. The device that receives the energy of the x-ray beam and forms the image of the body part is the _____.

Word Pool
- American Registry of Radiologic Technologists (ARRT)
- American Society of Radiologic Technologists (ASRT)
- Bucky
- computed radiography
- digital radiography
- image receptor
- primary radiation
- radiation field
- scatter radiation
- x-ray tube

Group B

1. Radiation that is created when an electron enters the tungsten anode of the x-ray tube, misses the tungsten electrons, and gets very near the nucleus is _____.
2. The relationship between the actual focal spot on the anode surface and the effective focal spot size is the _____.
3. The unit of measure for the voltage _____.
4. _____ is the process of removing the long-wavelength photons from the x-ray beam.
5. _____ is the ability to do work.
6. Radiation created when an electron enters the tungsten anode of the x-ray tube and knocks out a K-shell electron is _____.
7. _____ is anything that occupies space and has a shape or form.
8. The rate of current flow across the x-ray tube each second is known as _____.
9. _____ refers to the lower field intensity toward the anode in comparison to the cathode due to lower x-ray emissions from the target material at angles perpendicular to the electron beam.
10. When the filament is heated and electrons begin to "boil off" is known as _____.

Word Pool
- anode heel effect
- Bremsstrahlung radiation
- characteristic radiation
- energy
- filtration
- kilovolts peak (kVp)
- line focus principle
- matter
- milliampere seconds (mAs)
- thermionic emission

Group C

1. _____ terminates the exposure time when a certain quantity of radiation has been detected at the image receptor.
2. _____ is the process of changing alternating current to direct current so it flows in one direction only.
3. The _____ supplies a low current to heat the x-ray tube filament for thermionic emission of electrons.
4. The distance between the tube target and the image receptor is called the _____.
5. _____ is the difference between the actual subject and its radiographic image.
6. The distance between the subject and the image receptor is the _____.
7. _____ delivers the electrical power to the x-ray tube and permits the selection of x-ray energy, x-ray quantity, and exposure time.
8. The _____ supplies the x-ray tube with voltage high enough to create x-rays.
9. _____ is the result of unequal magnification of the actual shape of the structure.
10. The _____ expresses the relationship between SID and intensity.

Word Pool
- high-voltage circuit
- source-image receptor distance (SID)
- distortion
- filament circuit
- inverse square law
- shape distortion
- object-image receptor distance
- generator
- automatic exposure control (AEC)
- rectification

ABBREVIATIONS
Write out what each of the following abbreviations stands for.

1. kVp _____

2. mAs _____

3. AEC _____

4. OID _____

5. FPD _____

6. ASRT _____

7. DR _____

8. ARRT _____

9. CR _____

10. SID _____

11. APR _____

12. EI _____

13. IR _____

14. PSP _____

SKILLS AND CONCEPTS
Answer the following questions.

A. Limited X-Ray Machine Operator

1. Describe the limited x-ray machine operator in your own words. _____

   _____

2. Describe the curriculum for limited x-ray machine operators. _____

   _____

   _____

3. Is state licensure required to practice as a limited x-ray machine operator? Explain your answer.

   _____

   _____

B. Primary X-Ray Beam and Scatter Radiation
Fill in the blank.

1. _____ radiation comes from the x-ray tube.

2. _____ radiation comes from the patient in the form of scatter radiation.

3. Absorption of the x-ray beam is known as _____.

Match the tissue density with the correct appearance description.

4. _____ Blood and muscles absorb fewer x-rays than bones and appear darker on the image than bones

5. _____ Appears darker than fluid and soft tissues

6. _____ Absorbs fewer x-rays and thus appears the darkest on images; air is most visible in the lungs on chest x-rays

7. _____ Are dense and thus absorb more x-rays; bones appear white on the image

a. fat
b. fluid and soft tissue
c. air
d. bones

C. Introduction to Radiographic Equipment
Match the equipment with the correct description.

1. _____ Produces x-rays

2. _____ Contains the Bucky and provides support for the patient

3. _____ Utilized for upright imaging procedures

4. _____ Where the LXMO selects the technical factors for the examination

5. _____ Provides electricity to the x-ray tube

a. upright image receptor
b. control console
c. radiographic table
d. x-ray tube
e. transformer cabinet

D. Basic Radiation Safety

1. _____ are the measures taken to safeguard patients, personnel, and the public from unnecessary exposure to ionizing radiation.

Match the description with the characteristics of a cell that determined cell radiosensitivity (as stated by Bergonie and Tribondeau).

2. _____ Younger patient cells are more sensitive than older ones.

3. _____ Simple cells are more sensitive than highly complex ones.

4. _____ Cells that use energy rapidly are more sensitive than those that have a slower metabolism.

5. _____ Cells that divide and multiply rapidly are more sensitive than those that replicate slowly.

a. mitotic rate
b. differentiation
c. age
d. metabolic rate

Fill in the blank using the terms.

6. _____ is the use of lead walls for the control booth and lead aprons, gloves, and thyroid shields.

7. The amount of exposure is directly proportional to the _____ spent in the radiation field, so the occupational dose is decreased when this time is minimized.

8. Increasing the _____ between yourself and a radiation source decreases your exposure in proportion to the square of the _____.

    a. time
    b. distance
    c. shielding

Fill in the blank

9. The _____ states that all radiation exposure should be limited to levels that are "as low as reasonably achievable."

E. Basic Physics for Radiography
Select the correct answer or fill in the blank.

1. _____ is any process by which electrically neutral atoms or molecules are converted to electrically charged atoms or molecules (ions).

2. _____ is the spectrum of energies that includes radio waves, microwaves, visible light, ultraviolet light, x-rays, gamma rays, and cosmic rays.

3. What is a characteristic of x-rays?
    a. They have no mass.
    b. Are highly penetrating and invisible.
    c. Electrically neutral.
    d. Produce a wide range of energies and wavelengths.
    e. All of the above.

4. What is *not* a characteristic of x-rays?
    a. Travel in a curved line at the speed of light
    b. Can ionize matter
    c. Produce biological changes in tissue
    d. Produce secondary and scatter radiation

Match the term with the correct description.

5. _____ Hinders the flow of current.

6. _____ The quantity of electrons flowing in a circuit. The ampere (A) is the unit of measure for current.

7. _____ Is the force or speed of the electron flow in the current. The volt (V) is the unit for potential difference. In radiology, we use milliamperes (mA) and kilovolt peak (kVp).

8. _____ Occurs when a conductor is placed in a magnetic field and electric current creates a magnetic field.

    a. potential difference
    b. current
    c. resistance
    d. electromagnetic induction

Fill in the blanks.

9. A(n) _____ consists of primary and secondary coils, usually surrounding an iron core.

10. _____ always flows from the primary to the secondary coils.

11. When there are more turns, or "windings," in the secondary coil than in the primary coil, the voltage on the secondary side is greater, and the transformer is called a(n) _____ transformer.

12. If the secondary side has fewer turns, the secondary voltage and the transformer will be a(n) _____ transformer.

F. X-Ray Production
Fill in the blank or select the correct answer.

1. When Roentgen discovered x-rays, he was experimenting with a(n) _____ tube.

2. What is an essential requirement for the production of x-rays?
   a. Vacuum
   b. Source of electrons
   c. Target
   d. High potential difference (voltage) between the electron source and the target
   e. All of the above

3. A(n) _____ forms the basic structure of the x-ray tube.

4. Radiation that is created when an electron enters the tungsten anode of the x-ray tube, misses the tungsten electrons, and gets very near the nucleus is _____.

5. Radiation that is created when an electron enters the tungsten anode of the x-ray tube and knocks out a K-shell electron is _____ _____.

6. The _____ is the negative side of the x-ray tube.

7. The _____ is the positive side of the x-ray tube.

8. The term _____ refers to the area on the target surface struck by the electron stream.

9. The _____ refers to the vertical projection of the actual focal spot onto the patient and image receptor.

10. Due to the anode heel effect, the _____ portion of the body part should be placed toward the anode end of the tube.

11. _____ is the process of removing the long-wavelength photons from the x-ray beam.

G. X-Ray Circuit
Fill in the blank.

1. The x-ray circuit is divided into three sections: _____, _____, and _____.

2. The primary function of the _____ is to vary the voltage to the primary side of the step-up transformer.

3. The primary purpose of the _____ is to supply a low current to heat the x-ray tube filament for thermionic emission.

4. What type of transformer is located in the high-voltage circuit? _____

H. Rectification

1. _____ is changing alternating current into direct current, so it flows in one direction only.

2. In _____, the negative phase of the electric cycle is completely removed, and a gap remains.

3. During _____, the current is redirected during the negative half of the electric cycle so that the current will flow in the same direction during the positive and negative halves of the cycle.

I. Generators

1. List the three types of generators. _____

   _____

   _____

2. Which type of generator is powered by a single source of alternating current?_____

   _____

3. Which type of generator is the most efficient? _____

J. X-Ray Control Panel

1. Which is a component of the control panel?
   a. Some means for selecting kVp, mA, exposure time, and focal spot size
   b. Switches to control power to the console and the Bucky
   c. Rotor and exposure switches
   d. All of the above

2. What device controls the power to the control panel? _____

3. The _____ control adjusts the mA.

4. The _____ control adjusts the kVp.

5. What are the options for the Bucky control? _____

6. _____ allows the operator to select the body part to be imaged and the technical factors are predetermined.

K. Principles of Exposure and Image Quality
Select the correct answer or fill in the blank.

1. Which is a prime factor of radiographic exposure?
   a. mAs
   b. kVp
   c. SID
   d. All of the above

2. Which is a principal factor that affects x-ray quantity?
   a. mAs
   b. kVp
   c. SID
   d. Filtration
   e. All of the above

3. Which is *not* a principal factor that affects x-ray quality?
   a. mAs
   b. kVp
   c. Filtration

4. What is the relationship between milliamperage and the rate of exposure?_____

_____

5. What is the relationship between kilovoltage and the penetrating power of the x-ray beam? _____

_____

6. The distance between the target and the image receptor is known as _____.

7. The _____ expresses the relationship between SID and intensity, which states that the intensity is inversely proportional to the square of the distance.

8. What are the two primary factors that affect the appearance of the x-ray image? _____

_____

9. _____ is when a body part appears shorter than it actually is.

10. Which is a factor that controls distortion?
    a. OID
    b. SID
    c. CR angle
    d. Part position and IR position
    e. All of the above

11. _____ is the actual anatomic area, body part, or structure shown in the radiographic image.

12. The _____ describes the "unsharp edges" of the umbra or body part.

13. Motion causes a(n) _____ of the image.

14. _____ is a term used to describe the situation in which a grainy or mottled (spotty) image is created.

15. What causes quantum mottle to occur?
    a. Either the mAs or the kVp is set too high.
    b. Either the mAs or the kVp is set too low.

L. Digital Imaging

1. The imaging plate that contains a photostimulable phosphor (PSP) that stores the _____ image of the body part until it is processed.

2. The _____ consist of either a scintillation screen or a photoconductor that converts the x-ray photons directly into electrical signals.

3. _____ and _____ are digital terms used to describe the viewing monitor and the image.

4. _____ is the ability to distinguish anatomical structures of similar subject contrast.

5. The _____ is a graph of the minimum and maximum signals in the image.

6. The window _____ controls the brightness in the image.

7. The window _____ controls the contrast in the image.

8. Which of the following is a postprocessing option?
   a. Electronic cropping and image stitching
   b. Annotation and edge enhancement
   c. Smoothing and rescaling
   d. All of the above

9. The _____ is a numerical value indicating the quantity of ionizing radiation received by a digital radiographic image receptor; also called an *exposure index*.

10. What does PACS stand for? _____

Match the definition with the correct type of artifact.

11. _____ Caused by inadequate exposure techniques. Either low mAs or low kVp can cause this.

12. _____ Occurs when the grid lines are not aligned with the laser scanning frequency of the CR reader.

13. _____ Caused by dust on the IP.

14. _____ Appear along the length of travel on the image due to dust on the light guide.

15. _____ May be caused by any of the following: improper collimation, importer technique, beam alignment error, scatter, and extreme subject density differences.

16. _____ Phantom or ghost images may appear as a result of incomplete IP erasure. This artifact requires troubleshooting of both the CR plate and display systems. Extreme overexposure may require two erasure cycles to remove the image completely.

17. _____ Scratches or tears are permanent artifacts caused by damage to CR plates. Replacement of CR plates is costly but is the only solution to repair these artifacts.

18. _____ Extraneous line patterns are linear artifacts caused by noise in the image reader electronics. They can run lengthwise or crosswise.

19. _____ Fogging from background or scatter radiation can sometimes be seen on the CR plates.

a. fogging
b. histogram analysis errors
c. white line artifacts
d. moiré pattern
e. quantum mottle
f. extraneous line patterns
g. scratches or tears
h. phantom or ghost images
i. light spots

CERTIFICATION PREPARATION

Circle the correct answer.

1. When were x-rays discovered?
   a. November 8, 1985
   b. November 8, 1895
   c. November 8, 1875
   d. November 8, 1905

2. Exposure, dose, and dose equivalent are _____.
   a. radiologic quantities
   b. fundamental quantities
   c. derived quantities
   d. all of the above

3. The positive electrode of the x-ray tube is the _____.
   a. cathode
   b. diode
   c. canode
   d. anode

4. The device that restricts the x-ray beam to the area of interest is the _____.
   a. tube housing
   b. mirror
   c. collimator
   d. crosshair

5. The three main parts of the x-ray imaging system are the x-ray tube, _____, and _____.
   a. operating console, high-voltage generator
   b. protective barrier, tabletop
   c. crane assembly, tabletop
   d. rectification circuit, operating console

6. The automatic exposure control (AEC) terminates the exposure when _____.
   a. sufficient radiation reaches the image receptor
   b. set radiation leaves the x-ray tube
   c. the set time is reached
   d. the correct mAs is reached

7. Thermionic emission at the filament determines the _____ across the x-ray tube during an exposure.
   a. resistance
   b. milliamperage
   c. kilovoltage
   d. magnetism

8. Because of the line focus principal, the effective focal spot size decreases with decreasing _____.
   a. rotor speed
   b. window thickness
   c. target angle
   d. thermionic emission

9. The inverse square lay has the same effect on x-ray _____ and x-ray _____.
   a. intensity, quantity
   b. intensity, exposure
   c. quantity, exposure
   d. intensity, energy

10. The principal source of noise in computed radiography is _____.
    a. computer noise
    b. background radiation
    c. phosphor scatter
    d. scatter radiation

WORKPLACE APPLICATIONS

1. Working in family medicine, Kayla performs multiple x-ray examinations per day. Kayla just completed an abdomen image that displays quantum mottle. Describe the adjustments that can be made to the factors to decrease quantum mottle.

   a. kVp_____

   _____

   b. mAs _____

   _____

    c. x-ray tube, part, and image receptor_____

_____

2.   Kayla has just completed an imaging examination of a hip on an older patient. Upon evaluation of the image, Kayla notices artifacts in the image. What is the cause of these artifacts?

    a. Moiré pattern _____

_____

    b. Light spots _____

_____

    c. Phantom image _____

_____

3.   Kayla just completed a scoliosis x-ray examination that consisted of three exposures. List and define the postprocessing feature that Kayla will need to use on the images before she completes the examination and sends the images to PACS.

_____

_____

_____

INTERNET ACTIVITIES

1.   Using appropriate online resources, research the typical duties of a limited x-ray machine operator. Create a poster, PowerPoint, or paper summarizing your research. Focus on these areas:
    a. What procedures are LXMO trained to perform?
    b. What are the licensure and educational requirements for LXMOs?

2.   Using your skills and knowledge, how do you respond to a patient when asked about radiation exposure? Write a brief paper and address these points:
    a. Radiation is part of our natural environment.
    b. Compare the radiation dose of a chest x-ray to background radiation.
    c. Discuss methods to reduce the patient's radiation dose.

Positioning for Radiology	chapter 53

CAAHEP Competencies	Assessment
None	

ABHES Competencies	Assessment
None	

VOCABULARY REVIEW

Using the word pool on the right, find the correct word to match the definition. Write the word on the line after the definition.

1. To the outside; at or near the surface of the body or body part
_____

2. Referring to the sole of the foot _____

3. Pertaining to organs _____

4. Away from the central mass of an organ, toward its outer limits; the opposite of central _____

5. Referring to the walls of a cavity _____

6. Deep, near the center of the body or a body part; opposite of external _____

7. Pertaining to the middle area or main part of an organ or body part _____

8. Away from the head _____

9. The method of restricting and confiding the x-ray beam to a given area _____

10. Contains a moveable grid device that absorbs scatter radiation and also contains the image receptor _____

11. The width is greater than its height _____

12. The height is greater than its width _____

13. The distance between the subject and the image receptor
_____

14. The distance between the tube target and the image receptor
_____

Word Pool
- Bucky
- caudal
- central
- collimation
- external
- internal
- landscape orientation
- object-to-image receptor distance
- parietal
- peripheral
- plantar
- portrait orientation
- source-to-image-receptor distance
- visceral

ABBREVIATIONS

Write out what each of the following abbreviations stands for.

1. RAO _____

2. mAs _____

3. HIPAA _____

4. OID _____

5. LPO _____

6. CR _____

7. LAO _____

8. kVp _____

9. SID _____

10. RPO _____

11. IR _____

12. MCP _____

13. ASIS _____

SKILLS AND CONCEPTS

Answer the following questions.

A. Introduction to Radiographic Positioning

Match the term with the correct definition.

1. _____ Forward or front portion of the body or body part

2. _____ Backward or back portion of the body or body part; opposite of anterior

3. _____ Away from the source or point of origin

4. _____ Toward the source or point of origin

    a. distal
    b. anterior
    c. proximal
    d. posterior

Fill in the blank.

5. For a(n) _____ position, the patient is recumbent with the central (CR) horizontal or parallel to the floor.

6. A(n) _____ position is achieved by placement of the body or body part with the sagittal plane parallel to the IR.

7. A(n) _____ position results in angulation of the coronal plane of the chest with the IR.

8. A(n) _____ position is achieved when the body part or entire body is placed so that the coronal plane is not parallel with the radiographic table or IR.

Match the projection with the correct description.

9. _____ Produced by directing the CR to "skim" the profile of the subject

10. _____ The image is taken with a longitudinal angulation of the CR of 10 degrees or more

11. _____ The CR enters the anterior surface and exits the posterior surface of the body or anatomic structure

12. _____ The body is rotated so that the CR travels through the body on an oblique plane rather than following an anatomic plane

13. _____ The sagittal plane of the body or body part is parallel to the IR

14. _____ The CR enters the posterior surface and exits the anterior surface of the body or anatomic structure

a. anteroposterior (AP) projection
b. posteroanterior (PA) projection
c. lateral projection
d. oblique projection
e. axial projection
f. tangential projection

B. Radiographic Procedures

1. Which action is done to prepare for the radiographic procedure?
   a. Select the patient and projection from the computer worklist
   b. Choose IR
   c. Call the patient from the waiting area
   d. Explain procedure to the patient
   e. All of the above

2. When instructing the patient just prior to a radiographic procedure, what topic would *not* be discussed?
   a. Clothing that needs to be removed
   b. Artifact items that need to be removed
   c. Medications needing to be stopped
   d. Both a and b

C. Upper Limb and Shoulder Girdle Images

1. Label the image using these terms: capitate, hamate, lunate, pisiform, radius, scaphoid, trapezium, trapezoid, triquetrum, and ulna.

    a. _____

    b. _____

    c. _____

    d. _____

    e. _____

    f. _____

    g. _____

    h. _____

    i. _____

    j. _____

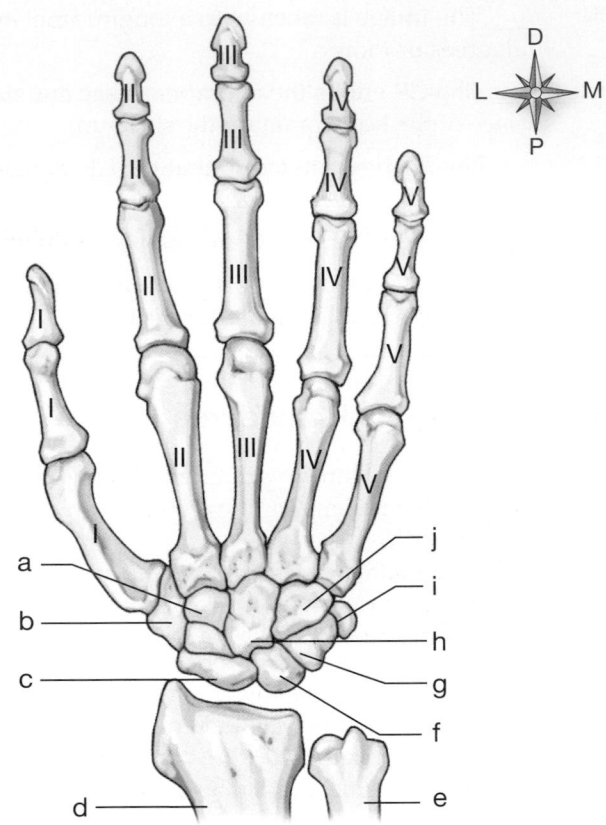

(Figure from Patton KT, Thibodeau GA: *The Human Body in Health and Disease*, ed 7, St. Louis, 2018, Elsevier.)

Match the direction of the central ray with the correct projection description.

2. _____ For the lateral projection of the elbow

3. _____ For the oblique projection of the wrist

4. _____ For the PA projection of the hand

5. _____ For the lateral projection of the scapula

6. _____ For the AP projection of the humerus

7. _____ For the AP projection of the forearm

8. _____ For the AP projection of the shoulder

a. perpendicular to the 3rd MCP joint
b. perpendicular to the midcarpal area
c. perpendicular to the midpoint of the forearm
d. lateral epicondyle
e. perpendicular to midhumerus
f. perpendicular to a point 1 inch inferior to the coracoid process
g. midpoint of the medial border of the scapular body

9. Which of the following is a traumatic condition of the upper extremity?
    a. Bursitis
    b. Tendonitis
    c. Scaphoid fracture
    d. Osteoarthritis
    e. Osteomyelitis

10. Which of the following is a nontraumatic condition of the upper extremity?
    a. Boxer's fracture of the 5th metacarpal
    b. Arthritis
    c. Colles fracture of distal radius
    d. Monteggia fracture of ulna with dislocation of radial head
    e. Radial head fracture

D. Lower Limb and Pelvis Images

1. Label the image using these terms: calcaneus bone, cuboid bone, cuneiform bones, distal phalanx, metatarsals, middle phalanx, navicular bone, phalanges, proximal phalanx, talus, and tarsals.

    a. _____

    b. _____

    c. _____

    d. _____

    e. _____

    f. _____

    g. _____

    h. _____

    i. _____

    j. _____

    k. _____

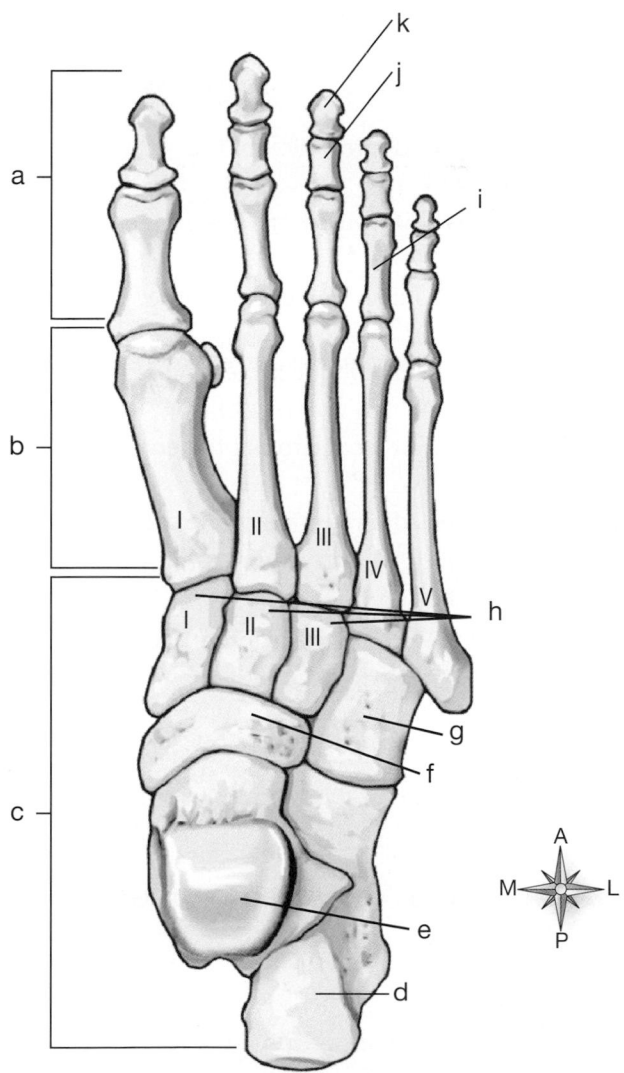

(Figure from Patton KT, Thibodeau GA: *The Human Body in Health and Disease*, ed 7, St. Louis, 2018, Elsevier.)

Match the direction of the central ray with the correct projection description.

2. _____ For the AP projection of the lower leg
3. _____ For the oblique projection of the ankle
4. _____ For the AP projection of the pelvis
5. _____ For the AP projection of the toes
6. _____ For the AP projection of the knee on a patient with an ASIS measurement of <19 cm
7. _____ For the lateral projection of the foot

a. angled 15 degrees posteriorly (toward heel) to MTP joints
b. perpendicular to base of 3rd metatarsal
c. perpendicular to point midway between malleoli
d. perpendicular to center of IR entering midshaft of the tibia
e. entering 0.5 inch distal to apex of patella angled 3-5 degrees caudad
f. perpendicular to midpoint of IR

E. Spine

Match the direction of the central ray with the correct projection description.

1. _____ For the AP projection of the thoracic spine
2. _____ For the AP projection of the sacroiliac joints
3. _____ For the lateral projection of the coccyx
4. _____ For the AP oblique projection of the cervical spine
5. _____ For the AP projection of the entire spine
6. _____ For the AP projection of the sacrum
7. _____ For the AP oblique projection of the lumbar spine
8. _____ For the lateral projection of the lumbar spine

a. angled 15 degrees cephalad to center of IR through body of C4
b. perpendicular to center of IR at T7
c. perpendicular to center of IR through L4
d. perpendicular to center of IR through L3. CR enters at point 2 inches medial to ASIS farthest from IR and 1.5 inches superior to iliac crest
e. angled 30 degrees cephalad for males and 35 degrees cephalad for females. Directed to center of IR through lumbosacral junction, midline, 1 inch inferior to the ASIS
f. angled 15 degrees cephalad to enter body at midline, 1 inch inferior to ASIS
g. perpendicular to center of IR through center of coccyx. CR enters at point 2 inches inferior to ASIS level and 3.5 inches posterior to ASIS
h. aligned perpendicular to center of IR, entering at midline approximately at level of xiphoid process

9. What is the SID for the lateral projection of the cervical spine? _____

F. Bony Thorax, Chest, and Abdomen

1. Which body habitus is considered average and about 50% of the population has this body type?

_____

2. Which projection is performed to demonstrate the posterior right ribs? _____

Match the direction of the central ray with the correct projection description.

3. _____ For the PA oblique projection of the ribs

4. _____ For the PA projection of the chest

5. _____ For the AP lateral decubitus projection of the chest

6. _____ For the AP projection of the abdomen

7. _____ For the AP axial projection of the chest

a. perpendicular to center of IR. Center point should be at the level of T7, which corresponds to the level of the inferior angle of the scapulae

b. horizontal and perpendicular to center of IR. Center point should be midsagittal and at the level of T7

c. perpendicular to center of IR. Center point should be at the level of the midsternum

d. perpendicular to center of IR. CR enters at point on posterior surface midway between spine and midaxillary line of affected side at approximate level of axillary fold

e. perpendicular to center of IR through a point in midline at level of iliac crest

G. Skull, Facial Bones, and Paranasal Sinuses

Match the direction of the central ray with the correct projection description.

1. _____ For the lateral projection of the skull

2. _____ For the PA projection of the mandible

3. _____ For the PA axial projection of the skull

4. _____ For the lateral projection of the facial bones

5. _____ For the axiolateral projection of the mandible

6. _____ For the PA axial projection of the sinuses

7. _____ For the AP axial projection of the skull

a. angled 15 degrees caudad to center of IR through nasion

b. angled 30 degrees caudad to center of IR through the foramen magnum at the level of the EAM. CR enters skull in midsagittal plane, approximately 2.5 inches superior to the glabella

c. perpendicular to center of IR through a point approximately 2 inches superior to the EAM

d. perpendicular to center of IR to exit through acanthion

e. angled 10 degrees cephalad through the mandible

f. perpendicular to center of the IR through a point approximately halfway between the outer canthus and the EAM

g. directed horizontal to exit the nasion

H. Image Evaluation

1. What is the recommended light setting for reviewing images? _____

2. The _____ is described as the patient is standing erect, with the face directed forward, arms extended by the sides, with the palms facing forward, and the toes pointing anteriorly.

3. When reviewing images, the acronym I AM ExpERT is helpful. What does the acronym stand for?

_____

_____

4. The correct right or left _____ should be clearly visible on each image.

5. Which is an image quality factor to consider as part of the image evaluation?
   a. Image brightness
   b. Radiographic contrast
   c. Spatial resolution
   d. Distortion
   e. All of the above

6. _____ refers to the visual appeal of the image.

7. Which two radiation safety factors can be visually evaluated on the image? _____

   _____

8. Define troubleshooting as part of image review. _____

   _____

I. Closing Comments

1. When imaging patients, it is imperative that the _____, _____, and
   _____ are properly aligned.

2. What does ALARA stand for? _____

   _____

3. What organization publishes the Standards of Ethics? _____

   _____

4. Who is the primary liaison among patients, licensed practitioners, and other support team members?

   _____

5. What organization publishes the practice standards for the profession? _____

   _____

CERTIFICATION PREPARATION

Circle the correct answer.

1. The radial tuberosity is located at the
   a. distal end on the posterior surface.
   b. proximal end, distal to the head of the radius.
   c. proximal end, proximal to the head of the radius.
   d. distal end on the anterior surface.

2. Which of the following describes the proper position of the forearm when taking a lateral projection of the forearm?
   a. Elbow extended, coronal plane through wrist and elbow parallel to the IR, hand supinated
   b. Elbow extended, coronal plane through wrist and elbow perpendicular to the IR, hand pronated
   c. Elbow flexed at 90 degrees, coronal plane through wrist and elbow perpendicular to IR, medial surface of the forearm in contact with the IR
   d. Elbow flexed at 90 degrees, coronal plane through wrist and elbow parallel to IR, anterior surface of the forearm in contact with the IR with hand pronated

3. The rounded, superior part of the ileum that is used as a palpable landmark is called the
   a. wing.
   b. ala.
   c. anterior superior iliac spine.
   c. iliac crest.

4. How much is the plantar surface of the foot rotated medially from the IR for the AP oblique projection of the foot?
   a. 10 degrees
   b. 25 degrees
   c. 30 degrees
   d. 45 degrees

5. On which projection of the spine is the "Scottie dog" configuration demonstrated?
   a. Lateral projection of the cervical spine
   b. AP axial projection of the sacrum
   c. Oblique projection of the lumbar spine
   d. Oblique projection of the thoracic spine

6. When the patient is upright, the midsagittal planes of body and head are parallel to IR with infraorbital line parallel to floor, the CR is directed to C4, the resulting image is a(n) _____.
   a. lateral projection of the cervical spine
   b. AP projection of the upper cervical spine (open-mouth technique)
   c. PA oblique projection of the cervical spine
   d. AP projection of the lower cervical spine

7. The inferior lateral "corners" of the lungs, visible on a PA chest image, are called the _____.
   a. hila
   b. costophrenic angles
   c. apices
   d. cardiophrenic angles

8. How many ribs should be visible above the diaphragm on a PA projection of the chest, as a demonstration of proper inspiration?
   a. 4
   b. 8
   c. 6
   d. 10

9. Which radiographic baseline is used to position the PA axial projection (Caldwell method) of the skull?
   a. OML
   b. IOML
   c. mentomeatal
   d. either the OML or the IOML

10. Which projection of the skull demonstrates the petrous ridges within the orbits?
    a. AP axial (Towne method)
    b. Lateral
    c. PA axial (Caldwell method)
    d. PA

WORKPLACE APPLICATIONS

1. Working in family medicine, Alexis performs multiple x-ray examinations per day. Alexis just completed a lateral knee image, and the condyles are not superimposed. Answer the following questions related to this image.

   a. Should the image be repeated? _____

   b. What (if any) positioning adjustment should be made? _____

   _____

   c. Should adjustments be made to the technical factors? _____

2. Alexis has just completed an imaging examination of a hip series on an older patient. Upon evaluation of the first image, the AP, Kayla notices the patient has had a hip replacement with a long rod extending to the knee. Answer the following questions related to this imaging series.

   a. Should the image be repeated? _____

   _____

    b.   What (if any) positioning adjustment should be made? _____

_____

    c.   Should adjustments be made to the technical factors? _____

3.   Alexis just completed a chest x-ray examination. Upon evaluation of the first image, the PA, Kayla notices the image demonstrates six sets of ribs.

    a.   Should the image be repeated? _____

    b.   What (if any) positioning adjustment should be made? _____

_____

    c.   Should adjustments be made to the technical factors? _____

INTERNET ACTIVITIES

1.   Using appropriate online resources, research the components of image evaluation. Create a poster, PowerPoint, or paper summarizing your research. Focus on these areas:
    a.   I AM ExpERT
    b.   Anatomy and positioning errors

2.   Using your skills and knowledge, how do you respond to a patient when asked about shielding? Write a brief paper and address these points:
    a.   Radiation is part of our natural environment
    b.   Recent research related to radiation exposure
    c.   Recent research related to shielding guidelines

Procedure 53.1 Perform a 2-View Chest X-Ray Examination

Name _____ Date _____ Score _____

Task: Perform the 2-view chest x-ray examination.

Equipment and Supplies:
- Patient's x-ray requisition
- Image receptor

Scenario: You are working with Jean Burke, NP. She just finished seeing Ken Thomas (date of birth [DOB] 10/25/19XX) and orders a 2-view chest x-ray examination.

Directions: Role play the scenario with a peer. You are the limited x-ray machine operator, and the peer is the patient.

Standard: Complete the procedure and all critical steps in _____ minutes with a minimum score of 85% within two attempts (*or as indicated by the instructor*).

Scoring: Divide the points earned by the total possible points. Failure to perform a critical step, indicated by an asterisk (*), results in grade no higher than an 84% (*or as indicated by the instructor*).

Time: Began_____ Ended_____ Total minutes: _____

Steps:	Point Value	Attempt 1	Attempt 2
1. Read the provider's order. Assemble supplies needed for the provider's order. Ensure that the patient can read and understand the directions. Verify the order if you have any questions.	5		
2. Greet the patient. Identify yourself. Verify the patient's identity with the full name and date of birth. Explain the order from the provider. Obtain a patient history. Answer any questions the patient may have.	10		
3. Accurately instruct the patient on the procedure. Use words that the patient can understand. Refrain from jargon and medical terminology. Use professional verbal and nonverbal communication.	10		
Scenario Update: After explaining the procedure, Mr. Thomas states he is not sure he will be able to extend his arm for the examination. 4. Using therapeutic communication techniques (e.g., reflection, restatement, and summarizing), show the patient you are aware of his concerns.	10		
5. Based on the patient's concerns, provide positioning alternatives that would meet the requirements for the examination.	10		
6. Evaluate the patient's understanding of the teaching by asking the patient to summarize the positioning plan. Answer any questions the patient may have.	10		
7. Position the patient for the first projection for the examination.	10		
8. Step up to the control console and set the technical factors for the exposure and take the exposure.	5		
9. Position the patient for the second projection for the examination.	10		
10. Step up to the control console and set the technical factors for the exposure and take the exposure.	5		

11. Evaluate the images and make adjustments as needed. Send the images to PACS.	**10**		
12. Dismiss the patient and provide follow-up instructions (if needed).	**5**		
Total Points	**100**		

Comments

Skills and Strategies

CAAHEP Competencies	Assessment
X.C.9. Identify legal and illegal applicant interview questions	Skills and Concepts – K. 3-5; Certification Preparation – 7

ABHES Competencies	Assessment
10. Career Development a. Perform the essential requirements for employment, such as resume writing, effective interviewing, dressing professionally, time management, and following up appropriately	Procedures 54.1 through 54.6
b. Demonstrate professional behavior	Procedure 54.5
c. Explain what continuing education is and how it is acquired	Certification Preparation – 10; Internet Activities – 3

VOCABULARY REVIEW

Using the word pool on the right, find the correct word to match the definition. Write the word on the line after the definition.

1. Allowing the listener to recap and review what was said

   _____

2. Rewording a statement to check the meaning and interpretation; also shows you are listening and understanding the speaker

   _____

3. The ability to communicate and interact with others; sometimes referred to as *soft skills* _____

4. Websites where employers post jobs _____

5. Putting words to the patient's emotional reaction, which acknowledges the person's feelings _____

6. The act of working with another person or multiple individuals

   _____

7. Allows the listener to get additional information by explaining a specific statement or topic _____

8. Exchange of information among others in your field

   _____

Word Pool
- clarification
- collaboration
- compassion
- counteroffer
- dignity
- interpersonal skills
- job boards
- mock
- networking
- paraphrasing
- proofread
- reflecting
- reverse chronologic order
- skill set
- summarizing

9. The inherent worth or state of being worthy of respect
   _____

10. To have a deep awareness of another's suffering and the desire to lessen it _____

11. The most recent item is listed first, and the oldest item is last
    _____

12. To read and mark corrections _____

13. Simulated; intended for imitation or practice
    _____

14. A person's abilities, skills, or expertise in an area
    _____

15. Return offer made by one who has rejected an offer or a job
    _____

ABBREVIATIONS

Write out what each of the following abbreviations stands for.

1. CPR _____

2. CMA _____

3. BLS _____

4. AAMA _____

5. RMA _____

6. AMT _____

7. CCMA _____

8. NHA _____

9. NCMA _____

10. NCCT _____

11. HIPAA _____

12. CMAC _____

13. AMCA _____

SKILLS AND CONCEPTS
Answer the following questions. Write your answer on the line or in the space provided.

A. Understanding Personality Traits Important to Employers
Fill in the blank or select the correct answer.

1. Which traits help new employees blend with the existing staff?
   a. Collaboration and interpersonal skills
   b. Professionalism and compassion
   c. Genuine interest in the job
   d. All of the above

2. Which interpersonal skill(s) should a new employee have?
   a. Flexible and dependable
   b. Supportive of peers
   c. Remain calm under pressure
   d. All of the above

3. Effective _____ communication involves using clear, thoughtful, and easily understood language.

4. _____ communication relays more information to others than any words you could use and includes eye contact, posture, voice, and gestures.

5. Which is *not* a trait of effective nonverbal communication?
   a. Being focused, calm, and polite
   b. Being distracted and rushed
   c. Showing interest in the other person

6. For communication to be effective, _____ must occur and this can be shown by asking appropriate questions that can draw others into the conversation.

7. A person can demonstrate professionalism by
   a. being flexible, punctual, and honest.
   b. paying attention to details.
   c. using time-management skills.
   d. demonstrating the ability to follow directions and prioritize.
   e. all of the above.

B. Assessing Your Strengths and Skills
Fill in the blank, select the correct answer, or answer the question.

1. Describe four personality traits you have and list the "evidence" to support your claim. _____

   _____

   _____

   _____

2. Which are *not* technical skills of a medical assistant?
   a. Phlebotomy and injections
   b. Electrocardiograms and obtaining vital signs
   c. Compassion and flexibility
   d. Software proficiency and reception duties

3. List at least four technical skills you possess and indicate where you developed each skill. _____

_____

_____

_____

_____

4. _____ job skills are developed in one job or experience that can be transferred to another job.

5. List at least two transferable skills that you have and indicate where you developed each skill.

_____

_____

C. Identifying Career Objectives and Personal Needs

Answer the question.

1. Identify career objectives for yourself.

   a. What area and skills did you enjoy in class and/or in practicum? _____

   _____

   b. Where do you want to be in 5 years? _____

   _____

   c. Where do you want to be in 10 years? _____

   _____

   d. What additional skills do you need to get where you want to go? _____

   _____

   e. Based on these answers, describe at least two goals you have for yourself. _____

   _____

   _____

2. Identify your personal needs by answering the following questions.

   a. Do you need a specific wage and/or benefits? If so, describe your needs. _____

   _____

   b. Do you need specific hours? If so, describe the hours. _____

   _____

   c. How far are you willing to travel? _____

   _____

d. Do you have a reliable mode of transportation?_____

_____

_____

D. Finding Job Openings
Match the credentialing examinations with the correct agency.

1. _____ National Certified Medical Assistant
2. _____ Certified Clinical Medical Assistant
3. _____ Certified Medical Assistant
4. _____ Clinical Medical Assistant Certification
5. _____ Registered Medical Assistant

a. American Association of Medical Assistants
b. American Medical Technologists
c. National Healthcareer Association
d. National Center for Competency Testing
e. American Medical Certification Association

Fill in the blank, select the correct answer, or answer the question.

6. _____ is the exchange of information among others in your field.

7. Larger healthcare facilities post job openings on their websites, and these are considered _____ job boards.

8. _____ job boards contain jobs from a variety of employers.

9. List four possible job search methods you can use in your area. These can include job boards, newspapers, and so on.

_____

_____

_____

_____

E. Developing a Resume
Fill in the blank or select the correct answer.

1. A(n) _____ summarizes your qualifications, education, and experience and its purpose is to "market" yourself.

2. A(n) _____ resume is the most popular format and focuses on the person's employment history.

3. A(n) _____ resume; also called a *hybrid resume*, lists a person's abilities and skill sets, along with listing the employment history.

4. A(n) _____ resume is customized to a unique job posting

5. What information is found in the education section on a resume?
   a. Schooling after high school
   b. Coursework completed
   c. Diplomas obtained and academic recognition
   d. Practicum information
   e. All of the above

6. What is *not* included in the work experience information on a resume?
   a. The reason you left
   b. The name of the facility and the city and state
   c. Dates in that position
   d. Title of the position held

7. For those in the workforce for a decade or more, employers want to see _____ years of employment information.

8. What information should be included for certifications?
   a. Title of the certification or license
   b. Awarding agency
   c. Expiration date
   d. All of the above

9. How should a person create a visually appealing resume?
   a. Bold only important information.
   b. Use simple bullets to help organize information.
   c. Change font size in certain areas to emphasize more important elements.
   d. Pay attention to the spacing and avoid too much "white space."
   e. All of the above.

F. Developing a Cover Letter
Fill in the blank or select the correct answer.

1. The goal of the _____ is to create enough interest that the reader wants to look at the resume.

2. Which strategy can be used to create a professional cover letter?
   a. Match the appearance of the cover letter and resume.
   b. Address the inside address and the salutation to a specific person.
   c. Be professional and sell yourself to the reader.
   d. Reaffirm that you are an excellent match for the job.
   e. All of the above

3. The cover letter should include the _____ and posting number.

G. Completing Online Profiles and Job Applications
Fill in the blank or select the correct answer.

1. What is the advantage of online profiles?
   a. An applicant completes the profile once and updates the information as needed.
   b. The employer can track the activities of applicants.
   c. The employer can easily read a person's information.
   d. The employer can advertise new postings to potential applicants whose profiles meet certain requirements.
   e. All of the above.

2. If you need to complete an application before an interview, come prepared with your information and arrive at least _____ minutes before the interview so you can complete the application.

3. What information is needed when completing an application or profile?
   a. Educational institution's name and address with dates and titles of coursework or diploma
   b. Past and present job information
   c. Certifications and credentials
   d. References
   e. All of the above

4. What information is *not* required for references?
   a. Person's name and title
   b. Email address
   c. Social media sites
   d. Contact information

5. Before using a person as a reference, they must be _____ and agree to be a reference.

H. Career Portfolios
Fill in the blank or select the correct answer.

1. The _____ is a tool that can show a potential employer that a person has the skills required for the job.

2. Which education-related documents could be included in a career portfolio?
   a. Copies of letters of recommendation
   b. Copies of transcripts, awards, and honors
   c. A list of the courses successfully completed with a short description of each course
   d. Copies of student clinical experience evaluation forms and skill document form
   e. All of the above

3. What information could be included in a career portfolio?
   a. Prior employment documents, such as letters of recommendation and employment evaluations
   b. References
   c. Certifications
   d. All of the above

I. Preparing for the Interview
Select the correct answer.

1. What should a job seeker do to prepare for an interview?
   a. Research the facility.
   b. Practice answering potential questions.
   c. Select interview attire.
   d. Prepare for the day of the interview.
   e. All of the above.

2. What should the job seeker research about the healthcare facility?
   a. Mission and value statements
   b. Size of the organization
   c. Size of the department with the open position
   d. Names and types of providers in the department
   e. All of the above

3. What should *not* be worn to an interview?
    a.   A business suit
    b.   Ripped jeans and flipflops
    c.   Clean, wrinkle-free, and well-fitting dress pants and shirt/blouse

4. What should be brought to an interview?
    a.   An interview portfolio
    b.   A copy of your cover letter and resume for each interviewer
    c.   A notepad and pen to take notes
    d.   A list of references on resume paper and a list of questions for the interviewer
    e.   All of the above

J. Types of Interviews
Fill in the blank or select the correct answer.

1. During a face-to-face interview, do not fidget and maintain good _____ contact.

2. Why might phone interviews be done?
    a.   To screen applicants and narrow the candidate pool
    b.   To provide additional information and verify that the applicant wants an interview
    c.   To replace a face-to-face interview
    d.   All of the above

3. When finishing a phone interview, the job seeker should _____ the interviewer at the end of the call.

4. The benefit of a virtual interview over a phone interview is that the interviewer can actually see the interviewee and allow the interviewer to assess the _____ and the _____ being presented.

5. When participating in a virtual interview, the camera is positioned to show your _____ and _____.

K. Professionalism During and After the Interview
Select the correct answer.

1. How should a job seeker answer a question such as "Tell me about yourself"?
    a.   Inform if you are married or single
    b.   Describe your hobbies and social activities
    c.   Describe your career to date
    d.   Detail your personal life
    e.   All of the above

2. What should the job seeker do during the interview?
    a.   Pause before simple, straightforward questions.
    b.   Fill in silence with filler words such as "um."
    c.   Be honest, and do not exaggerate experiences or length of employment.
    d.   Share negative experiences about past employers.

3. Which question is considered legal during an interview?
    a. When did you move to this country?
    b. Who will look after your infant when you are at work?
    c. What medications are you taking?
    d. Can you work the weekend?
    e. All of the above.

4. Which question is considered illegal during an interview?
    a. Have you ever been arrested?
    b. Have you ever been convicted of a crime?
    c. Are you 18 or older?
    d. Are you eligible to work in this state?

5. Which question is considered legal during an interview?
    a. How old are you?
    b. Where do you attend church services?
    c. Can you perform the essential job functions with or without reasonable accommodation?
    d. Have you ever been convicted of a crime?
    e. Both c and d.

L. Improving Your Opportunities
Fill in the blank or select the correct answer.

1. When a person is not having success with the job search, what should be reevaluated?
    a. Am I being too selective?
    b. Am I looking for the correct job title?
    c. Can the geographic search area be enlarged?
    d. All of the above.

2. When a person is not getting calls for interviews, what should be reevaluated?
    a. Is the cover letter, resume, online profile, or application negatively affecting the job search?
    b. Are there spelling and grammar errors in the information?
    c. Do the cover letter and resume need to be reformatted or revised?
    d. Are the cover letter and resume customized to the job posting?
    e. All of the above

3. _____ interviews can help you refine your interview skills and behavior.

M. Starting and Keeping Your Job
Match the description to the correct form.

1. _____ Used to check the person's past for criminal activity and listing in sex offender database

2. _____ Required to be completed so funds can be transferred into the employee's bank account instead of the employee receiving a paper paycheck

3. _____ Completion of paperwork is required as part of the insurance enrollment activities

4. _____ Newly hired employee must sign forms related to the Health Insurance Portability and Accountability Act and computer security

5. _____ Used to verify a person's identity and employment authorization

6. _____ New hires must provide their tax status and how many withholding allowances they are claiming, which is used to withhold money from their paycheck

a. Form I-9
b. Form W-4
c. insurance benefit form
d. background check form
e. direct deposit form
f. agreement forms

Fill in the blank.

7. The purpose of the _____ period is to see if the new employee is the right fit for the job.

8. With _____-degree style performance appraisals, supervisors evaluate their employees based on their observations of job performance over a given time period.

9. With _____-degree style performance appraisals, supervisors gather input from your coworkers and others with whom you interact on a regular basis.

10. Always offer at least _____ weeks notice when resigning from a job, since you would want this length of notice from your employer if your job was terminated.

CERTIFICATION PREPARATION
Circle the correct answer.

1. _____ means to have a deep awareness of another's suffering and a desire to lessen it.
   a. Interpersonal skills
   b. Reflecting
   c. Compassion
   d. Dignity

2. "Communicates well" is a _____.
   a. technical skill
   b. personality trait
   c. transferable job skill
   d. both a and b

3. What is the best and most effective way to find employment?
   a. Checking job boards and newspaper ads
   b. Using the school career placement office
   c. Networking and checking job boards
   d. Using employment agencies

4. Which is the most popular type of resume that is used when people are seeking employment in the same field as their education or experience?
   a. Reverse chronologic
   b. Chronologic
   c. Combination
   d. Targeted

5. What is true regarding the header in the resume and cover letter?
    a. The information should appear on all pages of the cover letter and resume.
    b. Contains the person's name and mailing address.
    c. Contains a phone number and a professional email address.
    d. All of the above are true.

6. Which item is typically presented in a reverse chronologic order on a resume?
    a. Education information
    b. Work experience
    c. Skills
    d. Both a and b

7. What is an illegal interview question?
    a. "Are you eligible to work in this state?"
    b. "Who looks after your children when you work?"
    c. "Are you able to work 8 AM to 3 PM on the weekends?"
    d. "Have you ever been convicted of a federal offense?"

8. Form _____ is the Employee's Withholding Allowance Certificate.
    a. W-3
    b. W-2
    c. I-9
    d. W-4

9. Form _____ is the Employment Eligibility Verification Form.
    a. W-3
    b. W-2
    c. I-9
    d. W-4

10. What is the importance of continuing education for a medical assistant?
    a. Helps keep the person updated and current
    b. Needed to maintain a certification or registration
    c. Important for professional development
    d. All of the above

WORKPLACE APPLICATIONS

1. Select six interview questions from Figure 54.7 and write a response for each question. Your answer should be at least five sentences in length.

    _____

    _____

    _____

    _____

    _____

    _____

    _____

    _____

2. During an interview, Michelle was asked her age. Michelle knew this was not a legal interview question. If you were in this situation, how would you respond?

    _____

    _____

    _____

INTERNET ACTIVITIES

1. Using appropriate online resources, research one of the five national certification exams:
   - Certified Medical Assistant (CMA) through the American Association of Medical Assistants (AAMA)
   - Registered Medical Assistant (RMA) through the American Medical Technologists (AMT)
   - Medical Assistant Certification (CCMA) through the National Healthcareer Association
   - Medical Assistant (NCMA) through the National Center for Competency Testing (NCCT)
   - Clinical Medical Assistant Certification (CMAC) through the American Medical Certification Association (AMCA)

   In a PowerPoint presentation, poster, or paper, address the following points:
   a. List the credential and the sponsoring agency
   b. Describe the exam (e.g., number of questions, coverage of topics, time limit)
   c. Describe the registration process
   d. Describe the requirements for maintaining the credential (e.g., continuing education, fees, retaking the exam)

2. Using online resources, identify four potential job openings that interest you. Describe each position in a brief paper and provide the websites for the openings.

3. Using online resources, identify two resources for continuing education for medical assistants. Briefly describe the resources and list the websites.

4. Using online resources, identify 8-10 potential job postings that interest you.

Procedure 54.1   Prepare a Chronologic Resume

Name _____   Date _____   Score _____

Task: Write an effective resume for use as a tool in obtaining employment.

Equipment and Supplies:
- Computer with word processing software and a printer
- Current job posting
- Resume paper
- Paper and pen

Standard: Complete the procedure and all critical steps in _____ minutes with a minimum score of 85% within two attempts (*or as indicated by the instructor*).

Scoring: Divide the points earned by the total possible points. Failure to perform a critical step, indicated by an asterisk (*), results in grade no higher than an 84% (*or as indicated by the instructor*).

Time: Began_____   Ended_____   Total minutes: _____

Steps:	Point Value	Attempt 1	Attempt 2
1. Apply critical thinking skills as you create a list of the personality traits (wanted by employers), technical skills, and transfer job skills that you possess. Also write down your career goal(s).	5		
2. Using the current job posting, identify the required and recommended qualifications and credentials needed for the position.	10		
3. Using the computer with word processing software, create a professional-looking header for your document. Include your name, address, telephone number(s), and email address. Select an appropriate font style for your name and a smaller font size for your contact information.	10		
4. Create a section header for "Education." For the learning institution(s) you attended, list the school's name, city and state, degree obtained or coursework successfully completed, and the year. Include any additional educational information, such as awards and the student clinical experience information.	10		
5. Create a section header for "Healthcare Experience" and/or "Work Experience." Provide details about your work experience, including the facility's name, city and state, title of your position, start and end date (month and year), and job duties. The job duties must start with an active verb using the appropriate tense (e.g., a past job would have past tense verbs and a current job would include present tense verbs).	10		
6. Create a section header for "Special Skills," and list your special language skills, computer proficiencies, and other unique skills you possess that relate to the position.	10		
7. Create a section header for "Certifications and Credentials," and list the active credentials and certifications you have. Include the title of the certification, awarding agency, and the expiration date. *Note:* You may want to consider adding the date you are taking a credentialing examination. Employers like to know the status of your credentialing examination.	10		

8.	All information on the resume needs to appear in reverse chronologic order (i.e., newest information is listed first). Work experiences should include both the start and end month and year.	10		
9.	The resume needs to look professional and interesting. Use font styles (e.g., bold, underline, italic) to emphasize important words and phrases. Use professional-looking bullets to list job duties and other information. Use the key words from the posting throughout the resume.	15*		
10.	Proofread the resume. Correct any spelling, grammar, punctuation, or sentence structure errors you find. If time allows, have another person review your resume, and use the feedback to revise it.	5		
11.	Print the resume on resume paper, and proofread it one final time. Any errors should be corrected and the document should be reprinted or emailed to the instructor.	5		
	Total Points	100		

Comments

ABHES Competencies	Step(s)
10. Career Development a. Perform the essential requirements for employment, such as resume writing, effective interviewing, dressing professionally, time management, and following up appropriately	Entire procedure

Procedure 54.2   Create a Cover Letter

Name _____ Date _____ Score _____

Task: Write an effective cover letter that will accompany the resume.

Equipment and Supplies:
- Computer with word processing software and a printer
- Current job posting
- Resume paper
- Pen

Standard: Complete the procedure and all critical steps in _____ minutes with a minimum score of 85% within two attempts (*or as indicated by the instructor*).

Scoring: Divide the points earned by the total possible points. Failure to perform a critical step, indicated by an asterisk (*), results in grade no higher than an 84% (*or as indicated by the instructor*).

Time: Began_____ Ended_____ Total minutes: _____

Steps:	Point Value	Attempt 1	Attempt 2
1. Using the job posting, read through the job description. With a pen, circle the position requirements and the key phrases.	5		
2. Using the computer with word processing software, create a professional-looking header in the document's header that matches your resume header. Include your name, address, telephone number(s), and email address.	10		
3. Type the date in the correct location using the correct format. Have one blank line between the date line and the last line of the letterhead.	10		
4. Type the inside address using the correct spelling, punctuation, and location for the information. Leave 1 to 9 blank lines between the date and the inside address, depending on the location of the body of the letter.	10		
5. Starting on the second line below the inside address, type the salutation using the correct format. Use a colon after the person's name.	10		
6. Type the message in the body of the letter using the proper location and format. There should be a blank line after the salutation and between each paragraph. The message should be clear, concise, and professional. Use proper grammar, punctuation, capitalization, and sentence structure.	10		
7. The first paragraph should contain the title and number of the job posting. The middle paragraph(s) should summarize your strengths and include key phrases from the posting. The final paragraph should discuss your availability for an interview. The body should end with an expression of gratitude to the reader.	10		
8. Type a proper closing, leaving one blank line between the last line of the body and the closing. Use the correct format and location.	10		
9. Type the signature block using the correct format and location. There should be four blank lines between the closing and the signature block.	10*		
10. Spell-check and proofread the document. Check for proper tone, grammar, punctuation, capitalization, and sentence structure. Check for proper spacing between the parts of the letter.	10		

11. Make any final corrections. Print the document on resume paper and sign the letter or email the document to your instructor or potential employer.	5		
Total Points	**100**		

Comments

ABHES Competencies	**Step(s)**
10. Career Development a. Perform the essential requirements for employment, such as resume writing, effective interviewing, dressing professionally, time management, and following up appropriately	Entire procedure

Procedure 54.3 Complete a Job Application

Name _____ Date _____ Score _____

Task: Complete an accurate, detailed job application legibly to secure a job offer.

Equipment and Supplies:
- Pen
- Application form
- Information regarding your past education, job experiences, and the skill sets you have developed (e.g., computer skills, keyboarding speed)
- Contact information for former supervisors and references
- Current resume

Standard: Complete the procedure and all critical steps in _____ minutes with a minimum score of 85% within two attempts (*or as indicated by the instructor*).

Scoring: Divide the points earned by the total possible points. Failure to perform a critical step, indicated by an asterisk (*), results in grade no higher than an 84% (*or as indicated by the instructor*).

Time: Began_____ Ended_____ Total minutes: _____

Steps:	Point Value	Attempt 1	Attempt 2
1. Read the entire job application before completing any part of the document.	5		
2. Refer to your information on past jobs, education experiences, and skill sets you have developed as you complete the application. Answers to the questions need to be accurate and honest.	45		
3. Use proper grammar, sentence structure, punctuation, spelling, and capitalization. Handwriting should be legible to the reader.	15		
4. Do not leave any space blank. Answer each question on the document. If the question does not apply, write "not applicable."	10		
5. Do not write "See resume" anywhere on the document.	5		
6. Include information on the application that exhibits dependability, punctuality, teamwork, attention to detail, a positive work ethic and initiative, the ability to adapt to change, a responsible attitude, and use of technology.	10		
7. Sign the document and date it.	5		
8. Proofread the document and make sure none of the information conflicts with the resume.	5		
Total Points	100		

Comments

ABHES Competencies	Step(s)
10. Career Development a. Perform the essential requirements for employment, such as resume writing, effective interviewing, dressing professionally, time management, and following up appropriately	Entire procedure

Work Product 54.1   Job Application

To be used with Procedure 54.3.

Name _____   Date _____   Score _____

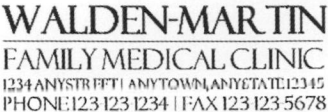

APPLICATION FOR EMPLOYMENT

Walden-Martin Family Medical Clinic is an equal opportunity employer and upholds the principles of equal opportunity employment. It is the policy of Walden-Martin Family Medical Clinic to provide employment, compensation and other benefits related to employment based on qualifications and performance, without regard to race, color, religion, national origin, age, sex, veteran status or disability, or any other basis prohibited by federal or state law. As an equal opportunity employer, Walden-Martin Family Medical Clinic intends to comply fully with all federal and state laws, and the information requested on this application will not be used for any purpose prohibited by law. Disabled applicants may request any needed accommodation. Please complete this application using ink, answer all questions completely, and sign the application.

Date: _____

Name: (First, Middle Initial, Last) _____

Social Security No.:_____   Phone: _____

Address:_____

City, State, Zip: _____

Have you been previously employed by Walden-Martin Family Medical Clinic?
☐ Yes ☐ No
If "Yes", when and job title?

How did you learn of the position for which you are applying?
☐ Newspaper/Print Advertisement ☐ Friend/Relative ☐ Employment Agency
☐ Job Service
☐ Radio/TV Advertisement ☐ Clinic Staff Person Name:

EMPLOYMENT DESIRED

Position(s) applied for: _____

☐ Full-time ☐ Part-time (If "Part time", number of shifts/hours desired _____)

Date available to start: _____ Salary requested: _____

PERSONAL HISTORY

Are you a United States citizen or do you have an entry permit which allows you to lawfully work in the U.S.? ☐ Yes ☐ No
    If applicable, Visa Type: _____ Immigration No.: _____

Are you at least 18 years old? ☐ Yes ☐ No

Are you ineligible to be employed with an AnyState licensed health care entity as a result of being found guilty by a court of law for abusing, neglecting, or mistreating individuals in a health care related setting? ☐ Yes ☐ No

    If "Yes," please explain: _____

Are you able to perform all of the duties required by the position for which you are applying, without endangering yourself or compromising the safety, health, or welfare of the patients or other staff member? ☐ Yes ☐ No

    If "No," please explain: _____

EDUCATION

	Name, City, State	Graduation Date	Course of Study/ Degree Obtained
High School:			
College:			
Other:			

LICENSURE/CERTIFICATION/REGISTRATION

Type of Certification, License or Registration	Agency/State	Registration Name

List any special skills or qualifications which you possess and feel are relevant to health care and the position for which you are applying.

_____

_____

_____

_____

_____

MILITARY SERVICE

From: _____   To: _____

Branch: _____

Duties: _____

Did you receive any specialized training? ☐ Yes ☐ No
If "Yes", describe: _____

EMPLOYMENT HISTORY

Please give accurate and complete information. Start with present or most recent employer.
May we contact and communicate with your present employer? ☐ Yes ☐ No

Employer:		Phone:	
Address:		**Supervisor:**	
Employed	Start: Month/Year: _____ Ended: Month/Year: _____	**Hourly Pay:**	Start: _____ Ended: _____
Position title and responsibilities:			
Reason for leaving:			

Employer:		Phone:	
Address:		**Supervisor:**	
Employed	Start: Month/Year: _____ Ended: Month/Year: _____	**Hourly Pay:**	Start: _____ Ended: _____
Position title and responsibilities:			
Reason for leaving:			

Employer:		Phone:	
Address:		Supervisor:	
Employed	Start: Month/Year: _____ Ended: Month/Year: _____	Hourly Pay:	Start: _____ Ended: _____
Position title and responsibilities:			
Reason for leaving:			

Employer:		Phone:	
Address:		Supervisor:	
Employed	Start: Month/Year: _____ Ended: Month/Year: _____	Hourly Pay:	Start: _____ Ended: _____
Position title and responsibilities:			
Reason for leaving:			

REFERENCES

Names of co-workers (no relatives) you have worked with and whom we may contact for a reference.

Name:	
Address:	
Phone:	
Job Title:	

Name:	
Address:	
Phone:	
Job Title:	

Name:	
Address:	
Phone:	
Job Title:	

Please read the following statements completely and carefully before you sign your name.

The Applicant HEREBY CERTIFIES that the answers given on this Application For Employment, including any statements or answers provided by the Applicant during interview, are true and correct. The Applicant fully authorizes Walden-Martin Family Medical Clinic to contact any references, past and present employers, persons, schools, law enforcement agencies and any other sources of information which may be relevant to the Applicant and this Application For Employment. It is understood and agreed that any misrepresentation, false statement, or omission by the Applicant will be sufficient reason for rejection of the Application For Employment or for dismissal from employment at any time, without recourse or liability to Walden-Martin Family Medical Clinic.

I have read, understand and agree to the above statement.

Sign: _____

Date: _____

Procedure 54.4 Create a Career Portfolio

Name _____ Date _____ Score _____

Task: Create a custom portfolio that provides potential employers evidence of your skills and knowledge as a medical assistant.

Equipment and Supplies:
- Three-ring binder or folder
- Plastic sleeves for the three-ring binder
- Dividers with tabs for the three-ring binder
- Current resume and cover letter
- Documents providing evidence of your skills and knowledge (e.g., transcripts, job evaluations, student clinical experience evaluation forms and skill checklist, projects completed in school, letters of recommendation, and copies of certifications [e.g., CPR card])

Standard: Complete the procedure and all critical steps in _____ minutes with a minimum score of 85% within two attempts (*or as indicated by the instructor*).

Scoring: Divide the points earned by the total possible points. Failure to perform a critical step, indicated by an asterisk (*), results in grade no higher than an 84% (*or as indicated by the instructor*).

Time: Began_____ Ended_____ Total minutes: _____

Steps:	Point Value	Attempt 1	Attempt 2
1. Group documents in a logical manner, putting similar documents together. Identify the arrangement for the portfolio. An arrangement could include cover letter and resume, education section (e.g., transcript, evaluation form and skills checklist, awards), prior job-related documents (e.g., evaluations), reference letters, and work products (e.g., projects you created in your medical assistant program).	25		
2. Insert one document per plastic pocket. Place all documents in plastic pockets.	15		
3. Neatly write the topic area on the tab of the dividers. Insert the tabbed dividers in the binder or folder.	15		
4. Place all documents in the binder or folder behind the correct divider. Place your cover letter and resume in the front of all the other documents.	15		
5. Create a table of contents to identify the tabbed areas.	15		
6. After the portfolio is assembled, review the entire portfolio to ensure it looks professional and the documents provide positive support of your skill set and knowledge.	15		
Total Points	100		

Comments

ABHES Competencies	Step(s)
10. Career Development a. Perform the essential requirements for employment, such as resume writing, effective interviewing, dressing professionally, time management, and following up appropriately	Entire procedure

Procedure 54.5 Practice Interview Skills During a Mock Interview

Name _____ Date _____ Score _____

Tasks: Project a professional appearance during a job interview and be able to express the reasons the medical assistant is the best candidate for the position.

Equipment and Supplies:
- Current job posting
- Resume
- Cover letter
- Interview portfolio (optional)
- Application (optional)
- Interviewer
- Mock interview questions

Standard: Complete the procedure and all critical steps in _____ minutes with a minimum score of 85% within two attempts (*or as indicated by the instructor*).

Scoring: Divide the points earned by the total possible points. Failure to perform a critical step, indicated by an asterisk (*), results in grade no higher than an 84% (*or as indicated by the instructor*).

Time: Began_____ Ended_____ Total minutes: _____

Steps:	Point Value	Attempt 1	Attempt 2
1. Wear interview-appropriate attire and be groomed professionally.	15		
2. Portray a professional image by shaking hands firmly prior to the start of the interview. Ensure that each interviewer has a copy of your resume and cover letter. Refrain from nervous behaviors (e.g., saying "um," tapping a pen or your foot) during the interview.	10		
3. Answer introductory questions by providing only professional information. This may include information about your education, experience, and career goals.	10		
4. Answer interview questions with open, honest, and positive responses. Completely answer questions, provide information or examples, and do not answer in single sentences or with limited responses.	25		
5. Use key words from the job posting when answering the interview questions.	10		
6. Ask the interviewer two to three appropriate questions about the facility or the position.	20		
7. Express interest in the job, and politely complete the interview by shaking hands and thanking the interviewer for the opportunity for the interview.	10		
Total Points	**100**		

Comments

ABHES Competencies	Step(s)
10. Career Development a. Perform the essential requirements for employment, such as resume writing, effective interviewing, dressing professionally, time management, and following up appropriately	Entire procedure
10. b. Demonstrate professional behavior	Entire procedure

Procedure 54.6 Create a Thank-You Note for an Interview

Name _____ Date _____ Score _____

Task: Create a meaningful, thank-you note to be sent after the interview process.

Equipment and Supplies:
- Computer with word processing software and a printer
- Job description
- Contact name from interview

Standard: Complete the procedure and all critical steps in _____ minutes with a minimum score of 85% within two attempts (*or as indicated by the instructor*).

Scoring: Divide the points earned by the total possible points. Failure to perform a critical step, indicated by an asterisk (*), results in grade no higher than an 84% (*or as indicated by the instructor*).

Time: Began_____ Ended_____ Total minutes: _____

Steps:	Point Value	Attempt 1	Attempt 2
1. Using word processing software, compose a professional letter using the business letter format. Include all of the required elements in the letter. Use correct spacing between the elements.	30		
2. Emphasize the particulars of the interview in the body of the letter.	20		
3. Include positive information you wish you had covered in the interview.	20		
4. Create a message that is concise and to the point.	20		
5. Proofread the letter and make any revisions as needed. Sign and send the thank-you note.	10		
Total Points	**100**		

Comments

ABHES Competencies	Step(s)
10. Career Development a. Perform the essential requirements for employment, such as resume writing, effective interviewing, dressing professionally, time management, and following up appropriately	Entire procedure